# Pathology of Genetically Engineered

# MICE

# Pathology of Genetically Engineered Engineered

# MICE

Jerrold M. Ward  ∘  Joel F. Mahler  ∘  Robert R. Maronpot  ∘  John P. Sundberg

Richard M. Frederickson,  Imaging and Graphics Editor

Iowa State University Press / Ames

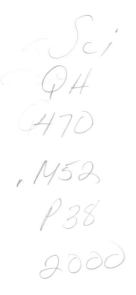

**Jerrold M. Ward,** DVM, PhD, Chief, Veterinary and Tumor Pathology Section, Office of Laboratory Animal Resources, National Cancer Institute, Frederick, MD

**Joel F. Mahler,** DVM, Staff Pathologist, Laboratory of Experimental Pathology, National Institute of Environmental Health Sciences, National Institutes of Health, Research Triangle Park, NC

**Robert R. Maronpot,** DVM, Chief, Laboratory of Experimental Pathology, National Institute of Environmental Health Sciences, National Institutes of Health, Research Triangle Park, NC

**John P. Sundberg,** DVM, PhD, Senior Staff Scientist and Head, Pathology Program, The Jackson Laboratory, Bar Harbor, ME

**Richard M. Frederickson,** AA, Scientific Graphics Specialist, Publications Department, National Cancer Institute–Frederick Cancer Research and Development Center, SAIC Frederick, Frederick, MD

Iowa State University Press
2121 South State Avenue, Ames, Iowa 50014

Orders: 1-800-862-6657
Office: 1-515-292-0140
Fax: 1-515-292-3348
Web site: www.isupress.edu

Authorization to photocopy items for internal or personal use, or the internal or personal use of specific clients, is granted by Iowa State University Press, provided that the base fee of $.10 per copy is paid directly to the Copyright Clearance Center, 222 Rosewood Drive, Danvers, MA 01923. For those organizations that have been granted a photocopy license by CCC, a separate system of payments has been arranged. The fee code for users of the Transactional Reporting Service is 0-8138-2521-0/2000 $.10.

♾ Printed on acid-free paper in the United States of America

First edition, 2000

**Library of Congress Cataloging-in-Publication Data**

Pathology of genetically engineered mice / Jerrold M. Ward — [et al.].
     p. cm.
  Includes bibliographical references and index.
  ISBN 0-8138-2521-0
  1. Transgenic mice—Diseases. I. Ward, Jerrold Michael.

  QH470.M52 P38 2000
  619'.93—dc21                                    00-038477

The last digit is the print number:   9   8   7   6   5   4   3   2   1

# Contents

# Editors and Contributors

## EDITORS

**Jerrold M. Ward, DVM, PhD**
Veterinary and Tumor Pathology Section
Office of Laboratory Animal Resources
National Cancer Institute, NCI-FCRDC
National Institutes of Health
Frederick, MD 21702-1201
Ward@mail.ncifcrf.gov
http://www.ncifcrf.gov/vetpath

**Joel F. Mahler, DVM**
Laboratory of Experimental Pathology
National Institute of Environmental Health Sciences
National Institutes of Health
PO Box 12233
Research Triangle Park, NC 27709
Mahler@niehs.nih.gov

**Robert R. Maronpot, DVM**
Laboratory of Experimental Pathology
National Institute of Environmental Health Sciences
National Institutes of Health
PO Box 12233
Research Triangle Park, NC 27709
Maronpot@niehs.nih.gov
http://dir.niehs.nih.gov/dirlep/home.htm

**John P. Sundberg, DVM, PhD**
The Jackson Laboratory
600 Main Street
Bar Harbor, ME 04609-1500

## IMAGING AND GRAPHICS EDITOR

**Richard M. Frederickson**
Publications Department
National Cancer Institute
Frederick Cancer Research and Development Center
SAIC Frederick
Frederick, MD 21702-1201
fredericksonr@mail.ncifcrf.gov

## CONTRIBUTORS

**Louise C. Abbott, PhD, DVM**
Department of Veterinary Anatomy and Public Health
College of Veterinary Medicine
Texas A&M University
College Station, TX 77843-4458

**Miriam R. Anver, DVM, PhD**
Pathology/Histotechnology Laboratory
NCI-FCRDC, SAIC-Frederick
PO Box B
Frederick, MD 21702-1201
M_anver@mail.ncifcrf.gov

**Hendrick G. Bedigian, PhD**
Laboratory Animal Sciences Program
NCI-FCRDC, SAIC Frederick
PO Box B, Frederick, MD 21702-1201
bedigianh@mail.nciferf.gov

**Roderick T. Bronson, DVM**
USDA Human Nutrition Research Center on Aging
    at Tufts University
711 Washington Street
Boston, MA 02111
bronson_pa@hnrc.tufts.edu

**Michele Cottler-Fox, MD**
Cell Therapy and Graft Engineering
University of Maryland Cancer Center
Baltimore, MD 21201

**Jacqueline N. Crawley, PhD**
Section on Behavioral Neuropharmacology
Experimental Therapeutics Branch
National Institute of Mental Health, NIH
Building 10, Room 4D11
Bethesda, MD 20892
jncrawle@codon.nih.gov

Maria L.Z. Dagli, DVM, PhD
Department of Pathology
Faculty of Veterinary Medicine and Zootechny
University of Sao Paulo
Av.Prof.Dr. Orlando Marques de Paiva
87 CEP 05508-900
Sao Paulo—SP
Brazil
and International Agency for Research on Cancer
150, cours Albert Thomas
69008 Lyon
France

Charles A. Dangler, DVM, PhD
Division of Comparative Medicine
Massachusetts Institute of Technology
Cambridge, MA 02139
Cdangler@mit.edu

Deborah E. Devor-Henneman, BS, LATG
Veterinary and Tumor Pathology Section
National Cancer Institute, NCI-FCRDC
Frederick, MD 21702-1201
Ddh@mail.ncifcrf.gov

Michael A. Eckhaus, VMD
Chief, Pathology Section
Veterinary Resources Program
Office of Research Services, NIH
Bethesda, MD 20892

Akiko Enomoto, DVM
Institute of Environmental Toxicology
4321 Uchimoriya-cho
Mitsukaido-shi
Ibaraki 303-0043
Japan

Norris D. Flagler, BS
Laboratory of Experimental Pathology
NIEHS, NIH
PO Box 12233
Research Triangle Park, NC 27709

Julie F. Foley, BS
Laboratory of Experimental Pathology
NIEHS, NIH
PO Box 12233
Research Triangle Park, NC 27709

Cecil H. Fox, PhD
Molecular Histology, Inc.
18536 Office Park Drive
Montgomery Village, MD 20879
jwgibbs@us.net, www.us.net/mol.hist

James G. Fox, DVM
Division of Comparative Medicine
Massachusetts Institute of Technology
Cambridge, MA 02139
Jgfox@mit.edu

Richard M. Frederickson
Publications Department
National Cancer Institute
Frederick Cancer Research and Development Center
Frederick, MD 21702-1201
frederickson@mail.ncifcrf.gov

John W. Gillespie, MD
Laboratory of Pathology
National Cancer Institute, NIH
Bethesda, MD 20895

Thomas L. Goldsworthy, PhD
Director of Toxicology
Integrated Laboratory Systems, Inc.
PO Box 13501
Research Triangle Park, NC 27709

Shelley B. Hoover, BS, HTL (ASCP)
Molecular Histology, Inc.
18536 Office Park Drive
Montgomery Village, MD 20879

Eric A. Hudson, BS
Analytical, Cellular, and Molecular Microscopy
  Laboratory
National Cancer Institute-FCRDC
Frederick, MD 21702-1201
and The Van Andel Research Institute
201 Monroe Avenue, Suite 400
Grand Rapids, MI 49503

Sakae Ikeda, DVM
The Jackson Laboratory
Bar Harbor, Maine 04609-1500

David M. Jacobowitz, PhD
Section on Histopharmacology
Laboratory of Clinical Science
Building 10, Room 3D-48
National Institute of Mental Health, NIH
Bethesda, MD 20892
dwj@helix.nih.gov

Priscilla Jewett, BS
The Jackson Laboratory
Bar Harbor, Maine 04609-1500

**Simon W.M. John, PhD**
The Jackson Laboratory
Bar Harbor, Maine 04609-1500
and The Howard Hughes Medical Institute
Bar Harbor, Maine 04609-1500
USA
swmj@aretha.jax.org

**Abraham T. Kallarakal, PhD**
Laboratory of Clinical Science
National Institute of Mental Health, NIH
Building 10, Room 3D-48
Bethesda, MD 20892

**Matthew H. Kaufman, PhD, DSc, FRCP Edin.**
Department of Biomedical Sciences (Anatomy)
University Medical School
Teviot Place
University of Edinburgh
Edinburgh EH8 9AG
United Kingdom
M.Kaufman@ed.ac.uk
http://genex.hgu.mrc.ac.uk/

**Lloyd E. King, Jr., MD, PhD**
Skin Disease Research Center
Department of Medicine
Vanderbilt University
Nashville, TN 37232-5227
lloyd.king@mcmail.vanderbilt.edu

**Jeffrey B. Kopp, MD**
Kidney Disease Section
Metabolic Diseases Branch
NIDDK, NIH
Bethesda, MD 20892

**Francis C. Lau, PhD**
Laboratory of Clinical Science, Building 10, Rm. 3D-48
National Institute of Mental Health, NIH
Bethesda, MD 20892

**Liat Lomnitski, PhD**
Department of Neurobiochemistry
The George S. Wise Faculty of Life Sciences
Tel-Aviv University, 69978
Israel

**Joel F. Mahler, DVM**
Laboratory of Experimental Pathology
National Institute of Environmental Health Sciences
National Institutes of Health
PO Box 12233
Research Triangle Park, NC 27709
Mahler@niehs.nih.gov

**Michael Mähler, DVM**
Central Animal Facility
Medical School Hannover
30625 Hannover
Germany
maehler.michael@mh-hannover.de

**Robert R. Maronpot, DVM**
Laboratory of Experimental Pathology
National Institute of Environmental Health Sciences
National Institutes of Health
PO Box 12233
Research Triangle Park, NC 27709
Maronpot@niehs.nih.gov
http://dir.niehs.nih.gov/dirlep/home.htm

**Glenn Merlino, PhD**
Molecular Genetics Section
Laboratory of Molecular Biology
National Cancer Institute, NIH
Building 37, Room 2E24
Bethesda, MD 20892
merlinog@dc37a.nci.nih.gov

**Daniel M. Michaelson, PhD**
Department of Neurobiochemistry
The George S. Wise Faculty of Life Sciences
Tel-Aviv University, 69978
Israel

**Larry E. Mobraaten, PhD**
The Jackson Laboratory
600 Main Street
Bar Harbor, ME 04609-1500

**Herbert C. Morse III, MD**
Laboratory of Immunopathology
National Institute of Allergy and Infectious Diseases
National Institutes of Health
Bethesda, Maryland 20892
hmorse@atlas.niaid.nih.gov

**Michele S. Moss, PhD**
Vector Laboratories, Inc.
30 Ingold Road
Burlingame, CA 94010

**Patsy M. Nishina, PhD**
The Jackson Laboratory
Bar Harbor, Maine 04609-1500

Abraham Nyska, DVM
Laboratory of Experimental Pathology
NIEHS, NIH
PO Box 12233
Research Triangle Park, NC 27709
Nyska@niehs.nih.gov

Craig S. Pow, PhD
Vector Laboratories, Inc.
30 Ingold Road
Burlingame, CA 94010
Vector@vectorlabs.com
www.vectorlabs.com

James H. Resau, PhD
Analytical, Cellular and Molecular Microscopy
   Laboratory
National Cancer Institute-FCRDC
Frederick, MD 21702-1201
and The Van Andel Research Institute
201 Monroe Avenue, Suite 400
Grand Rapids, MI 49503
james.resau@vai.org

Björn Rozell, DDS, PhD, DVM
Unit for Embryology and Genetics
Clinical Research Center
Huddinge Hospital, F61
141 86 Huddinge
Sweden
bjorn.rozell@kfc.hs.sll.se

B.K. Sathyanarayana, PhD
Analytical, Cellular and Molecular Microscopy
   Laboratory
National Cancer Institute-FCRDC
Frederick, MD 21702-1201

David B. Schauer, DVM, PhD
Division of Comparative Medicine
Massachusetts Institute of Technology
Cambridge, MA 02139
Schauer@mit.edu

John J. Sharp, PhD
The Jackson Laboratory
600 Main Street
Bar Harbor, ME 04609-1500
jjs@jax.org
http://www.jax.org/resources/documents/imr/

Richard S. Smith, MD, Dr. Med. Sci.
The Jackson Laboratory
Bar Harbor, Maine 04609-1500
and the Howard Hughes Medical Institute
Bar Harbor, Maine 04660
Rss@aretha.jax.org

Colin L. Stewart, DPhil
Laboratory of Cancer and Developmental Biology
NCI-FCRDC
PO Box B
Frederick, MD 21702
stewartc@mail.ncifcrf.gov

John P. Sundberg, DVM, PhD
The Jackson Laboratory
600 Main Street
Bar Harbor, ME 04609-1500

Cynthia Sung, PhD
Bioengineering and Physical Science Program
NIH
Bethesda, MD 20892

Lekidelu Taddesse-Heath, MD
Laboratory of Immunopathology
National Institute of Allergy and Infectious Diseases
and Laboratory of Pathology, National Cancer Institute
National Institutes of Health
Bethesda, MD 20892

Chihiro Tohda, PhD
Research Center for Ethnomedicines
Institute of Natural Medicines
Toyama Medical and Pharmaceutical University
2630 Sugitani, Toyoma 930-0194
Japan

Thai-Vu T. Ton, BS
Laboratory of Experimental Pathology
NIEHS, NIH
PO Box 12233
Research Triangle Park, NC 27709

Jerrold M. Ward, DVM, PhD
Veterinary and Tumor Pathology Section
Office of Laboratory Animal Resources
National Cancer Institute, NCI-FCRDC
National Institutes of Health
Frederick, MD 21702-1201
Ward@mail.ncifcrf.gov
http://www.ncifcrf.gov/vetpath

James S. Whitehead, PhD
Vector Laboratories, Inc.
30 Ingold Road
Burlingame, CA 94010
Vector@vectorlabs.com
www.vectorlabs.com

Adriana Zabaleta, MS
The Jackson Laboratory
Bar Harbor, Maine 04609-1500

# Preface

This book contains chapters derived from presentations at the symposium called "The Pathology of Genetically-Engineered Mice" held at the National Institutes of Health (NIH) in 1999. The 1990s have been called "the decade of the mouse." In the twenty-first century, the biomedical research revolution in technology will clearly emphasize the mouse to an even greater extent. During the past 20 years, spontaneous mutations occurring in wild and captive mice have resulted in collections of mutant mice with phenotypes corresponding to a wide variety of human diseases. The advent of recombinant DNA technology and creation of transgenic (Tg), targeted mutagenesis (Tm; so-called knockout), and inducible mutagenesis mice have led to an overwhelming array of models for diseases and biochemical pathway analysis. Repositories of these genetically engineered and natural mutant mice have been created to preserve these valuable research models. The technology to induce mutant mice has become simplified. Many institutions now have core facilities whereby investigators only need to provide a DNA construct and wait for the mice to be delivered with the transgene or targeted mutation in place. Consequently, the generation of new genetically modified mouse models is expected to continue at a rapid rate.

The biological characterization of mutant mice, particularly on a systemic basis beyond a particular anatomic structure or biochemical cascade, requires pathologists and physiologists with specialized skills. Few pathologists and physiologists have been trained specifically to deal with mutant laboratory mice as a species. This book brings together the collective expertise of many of these specialists to cover approaches to organ-specific evaluations, to provide examples of many currently available mutant mice to illustrate how specific defects can be studied, and to present methods for evaluation of live mice. It is impossible to cover all organ systems and physiological processes in one book, but the detail and breadth of this book provide good starting points for the neophyte, the refinement of ideas for experts, and an overall appreciation for the value of

mice and the progress that has been made in this decade. When possible, references and web pages are given for the tissues and organs not discussed in detail in the book. Some important general references on mouse pathology are given at the end of the book.

Nomenclature guidelines for mouse strains and mutations have been well reported by organizations such as the International Committee on Standardized Genetic Nomenclature for Mice. Relevant information is available on the Internet *(http://jaxmice.jax.org/html/nomenclature/nomen_memo.shtml; http://jaxmice.jax.org/html/infosearch/searchDB_index.html; http://www.taconic.com/anmodels/animlmod.htm)*. Scientists are encouraged to use appropriate nomenclature when publishing their work. While editing this book, we continually ran into inconsistencies in mouse strain and mutant locus/gene nomenclature. Because of the large number of genetically engineered mice described or listed in this book and the variety of mixed-strain backgrounds reported by the authors, we found it impossible to trace and verify all the designations provided, nor did we attempt to change designations to conform to a standard.

All images and graphic elements were prepared electronically. Images were scanned from 35 mm color slides and adjusted for reproduction. All 35 mm slides were prepared from tissue sections stained with hematoxylin and eosin, unless otherwise noted. Illustrations, charts, and graphs were drawn with appropriate software. We are very grateful for the important graphic support of Jennifer L. Smith (The Jackson Laboratory), Beth W. Gaul (Experimental Pathology Laboratories), Norris Flagler (National Institute of Environmental Health Sciences [NIEHS]), and Maria L. Tennis and Allen R. Kane (National Cancer Institute–Frederick Cancer Research and Development Center [NCI-FCRDC]). This work was supported, in part, with federal funds from the National Cancer Institute, NIH, under contract number NO1-CO-56000, and from the NIEHS, NIH, under a contract to Experimental Pathology Laboratories, Inc.

# Pathology of Genetically Engineered

# MICE

# 1
# Mutant Mouse Resources

John J. Sharp, Larry E. Mobraaten, and Hendrick G. Bedigian

## GENETICALLY ENGINEERED MICE

Here we present the role of a repository in maintaining and distributing genetically engineered strains of mice and review the existing repositories and informatics resources that support their use. Genetically engineered mice (GEM) for the purposes of this chapter include strains or stocks carrying transgenes, targeted mutations, and chemically induced mutations, primarily ENU (N-ethyl-N-nitrosourea). Following is a review of the technology of producing transgenic, targeted mutant, and chemically induced mutants.

### Transgenic Mice

The production of the first transgenic mouse was preceded by several technological advancements, including increased knowledge of mouse reproductive physiology (Palmiter and Brinster 1986) and the ability to culture mouse embryos (Brinster 1963); the development of recombinant DNA technology (Cohen and Boyer 1992; Cohen et al. 1992); and the development of microinjection techniques (Lin 1966). The first transgenic strain was reported in 1980 when segments of herpes simplex virus and simian virus 40 viral DNA were shown to integrate into the mouse genome following pronuclear microinjection. (Gordon et al. 1980) This initial report did not mention transgene expression or germline trans-

Current support for the IMR is derived from Howard Hughes Medical Institute grant 76196-502403, from National Institutes of Health National Center for Research Resources grants 1 P40 RR09781 (with supplements from NIAID and NIAMS), 1 P40 RR11081, 1 P40 RR01262, and Cancer Center Support (CORE) Grant CA34196. The IMR is also supported by revenues generated by the distribution of mice and by TJL institutional funds. The IMR was initially supported by funds from the March of Dimes Birth Defects Foundation grant TY92-1314, American Cancer Society grant RD-366, Cystic Fibrosis Foundation grant 5901, the Howard Hughes Medical Institute grant 76193-502402, the American Heart Association, the National Multiple Sclerosis Society, and the ALS Foundation.

mission, but it was quickly followed by others that did (Wagner 1981; Harbers 1981; Brinster 1981; Costantini 1981; Gordon and Ruddle 1981). The term "transgenic" was first proposed by Gordon and Ruddle in 1981.

Following pronuclear microinjection, the transgene integrates randomly into the mouse genome, usually in concatameric arrays at a single site (Palmiter and Brinster 1986). Thus, founders carrying identical transgenes represent a unique line since there will be variation in integration site and copy number between founders. Because transgene integration can occur within an endogenous gene or regulatory region, it is necessary to verify that the observed phenotype results from transgene expression and not from insertional mutagenesis. Recovery of two or more founders with similar phenotypes is usually considered sufficient verification that the phenotype is a result of transgene expression. The level of transgene expression is, to a large extent, dependent on the number of copies that integrate with high copy number usually resulting in high expression. There are, however, poorly understood positional effects that affect expression (Palmiter and Brinster 1986), and a recent report indicates that in some cases an increased copy number may actually result in reduced expression (Garrick et al. 1998).

The utility of transgenic strains is widespread. Initially utilized to study mammalian gene expression (i.e., Brinster et al. 1984), they now provide models for human diseases such as cancer, diabetes, and atherosclerosis (for reviews see Bedell et al. 1997a, 1997b). Transgenics have also been used to generate human monoclonal antibodies and to investigate antisense-mediated gene inhibition. Cre recombinase transgenic strains are a requisite component of the Cre-lox conditional mutagenesis system (Kuhn et al. 1995; Sauer and Henderson 1988). Likewise, transgenic mice provide the key components of the tetracycline (Furth et al. 1994; Kistner et al. 1996) and FLP recombinase regulatory systems (Dymecki 1996; Logie and Stewart 1995). Transgenic strains carrying selectable markers or markers such as LacZ serve as valuable research tools by allowing selection or identification of tissue or cell types arising from these strains (e.g., Zambrowicz et al. 1997).

Transgenes, as mentioned above, may integrate within a gene or regulatory region. Given an identifiable phenotype, the disrupted gene (or DNA segment) may be mapped and cloned. This characteristic of insertional mutagenesis has recently been exploited as a gene discovery tool (Friedrich and Soriano 1993) through the use of specifically designed gene-trap vectors carrying a promoterless LacZ reporter gene. An expansion of this technology not requiring insertion into an expressed gene is now a commercial gene discovery tool (Zambrowicz et al. 1998).

## Targeted Mutant Mice

Gene-targeting technology, or homologous recombination, makes it possible to alter or remove the function of specific genes within the mouse genome. The determination that the blastocyst could be colonized by multipotent teratocarcinoma cells (Brinster 1974), the isolation and in vitro maintenance of pluripotent embryonic stem (ES) cell lines from mouse preimplantation embryos (Evans and Kaufman 1981), and the demonstration that these ES cells could recolonize blastocysts and be transmitted in the germline (Bradley et al. 1984) were among the major contributing factors leading to the development of gene targeting in the mouse (Smithies et al. 1985; Thomas and Capecchi 1987).

The initial step in targeting a gene, or any endogenous DNA sequence, is the design of a vector that will undergo homologous recombination with the endogenous target. In the case of gene targeting, this vector also contains selectable marker(s) and the sequences necessary to inactivate or alter the targeted gene. This targeting vector is introduced into ES cells, usually by electroporation, after which correctly targeted ES cells are enriched by the utilization of the selectable markers (Mansour et al. 1988). A major influence on the recovery of correctly targeted cells is the extent of homology between the targeting vector and the host genome. The use of isogenic DNA in the targeting vector versus random insertion greatly increases the frequency of homologous recombination (te Riele et al. 1992). Correctly targeted ES cells are then microinjected into host blastocysts or aggregated with morulae-stage embryos (Wood et al. 1993) and are subsequently implanted into recipient pseudopregnant females. Targeted 129-derived ES cells are most often injected or aggregated with C57BL/6 blastocysts or morulae in order to identify chimeric mice by their coat color. Chimeric offspring are then mated to determine if the mutation is transmissible in the germline (i.e., the gonads are also chimeric). If transmissible, a homozygous or heterozygous colony carrying the targeted allele is then established.

To date, the majority of targeted mutant strains that have been produced carry null mutations in the targeted gene. These strains provide valuable experimental systems for understanding mammalian gene function and regulation, even if the homozygous null mutation presents a developmentally lethal phenotype. Targeted mutant strains also provide specific models for human genetic diseases for which the mutated gene has been determined (i.e., Bedell et al. 1997a, 1997b). Experimentation that would be impossible or inappropriate in human beings may be carried out in these model systems, thus furthering our understanding of disease processes and leading to the development and testing of new therapies.

More recently, conditional targeted mutagenesis systems have been developed that allow control of both the tissue specificity and the onset (temporal control) of the mutation. The most fully developed conditional mutagenesis system is the patented (Du Pont) Cre recombinase (or Cre-lox) system (Sauer and Henderson 1988), where both tissue-specific and temporal control of the mutagenesis have been demonstrated (i.e., Gu et al. 1994; Kuhn et al. 1995). Other conditional mutagenesis systems include the tetracycline inducible system (Furth et al. 1994; Kistner et al. 1996) and the FLP recombinase system (Dymecki 1996; Logie and Stewart 1995).

## ENU Mutagenesis

Treatment of mouse gametes or ES cells with the chemical mutagen N-ethyl-N-nitrosourea (ENU) results in random point mutations within the mouse genome (McDonald et al. 1990). This random mutagenesis approach produces both dominant and recessive mutations and is a useful gene discovery tool. Following mutagenesis, mice carrying mutations in genes (or other functional DNA) are identified by their phenotype. Thus, the class of mutants recovered is dependent on the phenotypic screen(s) utilized. In order to take full advantage of the procedure, a rapid, high-throughput phenotype screening system must be available. In addition, the resources for mapping and cloning these genes must be available. Several large-scale ENU mutagenesis projects are currently underway including the Medical Research Council (MRC) Mammalian Genetics Unit, SmithKline Beecham, Imperial College consortium [*http://www.mgu.har.mrc.ac.uk/mutabase/*] and the Max Planck Institute program [*http://www.gsf.de/isg/ENU.index.html*].

## Genetic Background Affects the Phenotype

It is well-known that the genetic background of a mutation can have a dramatic effect on the observed phenotype (see Chap. 10). Individual mice from stocks carrying a mutation on a mixed genetic background are likely to show a wide variability on the observed phenotype, and it is preferable to transfer the mutation onto a stable inbred background by a series of backcrosses. Not only is the phenotype stabilized on an inbred background but the range of experimentation is increased, including the potential for mapping and cloning other genes that affect the given phenotype (quantitative trait loci).

## REPOSITORIES FOR GENETICALLY ENGINEERED MICE

The generation of genetically engineered mice has increased rapidly in the last few years and is expected to continue to grow (Fig. 1.1). This increase has created the need for repositories, or distribution centers, to make important strains and stocks available to the greater scientific community.

In 1993, the Jackson Laboratory established the Induced Mutant Resource (IMR), whose function is to

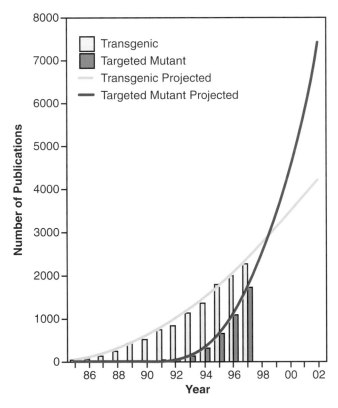

**FIGURE 1.1** The number of publications that cite either transgenic mice (*black bars*) or gene-targeted mice (*white bars*). Values for 1985–1997 were obtained using SilverPlatter to search MEDLINE. Values for 1998–2002 were projected utilizing a three-order polynomial equation generated from Microsoft Chart.

select, rederive (rid of disease), cryopreserve, develop, and distribute genetically engineered mice (see next section). The IMR has received operating funds from six voluntary health care agencies, the Howard Hughes Medical Institute, and the National Institutes of Health (NIH) (including the National Center for Research Resources [NCRR], National Institute of Allergy and Infectious Diseases [NIAID], and National Institute of Arthritis and Musculoskeletal and Skin Diseases [NIAMS]). These funds offset the costs of rederivation, cryopreservation, and strain development (transferring mutations on inbred backgrounds, i.e., generating congenic strains). Without this support only the most widely distributed strains would be available, drastically reducing the number of available strains and inhibiting the pace of research in many important human disease areas. As of February 1999, the IMR had accepted 624 strains and was distributing 397 of these. Forty-five new strains were being rederived. Ninety strains had been removed from the shelf because of low demand and were available as frozen embryos. Eight to nine new strains were being added each month. The NCRR has recently initiated a plan to create a "node" system of mouse mutant resources, with the IMR serving as the prototype. There will likely be at least two other regional repositories for genetically engineered mice underway in the United States by the time this article is published.

In addition to the IMR, three other repositories for genetically engineered mice exist. The European Mouse Mutant Archive (EMMA) has recently opened, with the IMR serving as its operating prototype. Initially EMMA plans to cryopreserve strains and to distribute frozen embryos to regional nodes where they will be recovered and distributed. The Mammalian Genetic Unit, Harwell, U.K., distributes over 200 mutant, chromosome anomaly, inbred, and chemically mutagenized lines. The NIH Animal Genetic Resource maintains rats, guinea pigs, and cotton rats in addition to mice maintained as inbred and congenic strains and as outbred and mutant stocks. The Internet locations for these repositories are listed in Table 1.1. It is anticipated that a repository for

**TABLE 1.1.  The URL for each mouse repository**

**Repository web sites**

The Induced Mutant Resource
    *http://www.jax.org/resources/documents/imr/*
European Mouse Mutant Archive
    *http://www.emma.rm.cnr.it/*
MGU Harwell
    *http://www.mgu.har.mrc.ac.uk/*
NIH Animal Genetic Resource
    *http://dirs.info.nih.gov/intramur/vrp/open/geneinfo.htm*

genetically engineered mice may soon be established in Japan. In addition several commercial distributors offer genetically engineered strains of mice.

# REPOSITORY FUNCTIONS

To function effectively, a repository must be able to (1) rederive acquired stocks to a pathogen-free health status, (2) perform both health and genetic quality control procedures, (3) breed stocks having widely varying husbandry requirements, (4) cryopreserve germ plasm, (5) distribute animals, and (6) provide information to researchers.

## Stock Rederivation

Stocks to be maintained in a repository will come from many different sources with various levels of health quality. It is now clear that the presence of certain pathogens or the health status, in general, can affect phenotype and experimental results. Therefore, mice that are to be distributed to research laboratories from a repository must have a high health status. This is especially important since an increasing number of research laboratories are now utilizing barrier-maintained animals for their research. Thus, animals from sources with lower health status must be rederived for introduction into the barrier facility.

Methods commonly used for rederivation include hysterectomy derivation (cesarean section) and embryo transfer. The long-established method of hysterectomy derivation consists of cesarean removal of fetuses and fostering them into a pathogen-free female recipient who has just delivered a litter herself. This method has been used successfully for many years at the Jackson Laboratory. The relatively more recent method of embryo transfer into pathogen-free recipients has been shown to be effective, and its use is increasing. Several reports have documented the efficacy of this method (Carthew et al. 1983, 1985; Okamoto and Matsumoto 1999; Okamoto et al. 1990; Reetz et al. 1988). Rederivation by embryo transfer can also be used to facilitate the exchange of strains between institutions where differences in health quality may exist or be suspected. Embryos can be frozen and shipped to the recipient institution where they will be transferred into pathogen-free foster mothers as the means of rederivation for introduction into a barrier facility (Mobraaten 1997).

## Quality Control

### HEALTH MONITORING
Since a repository will supply mice to a wide variety of institutions, it is important that the animals distributed be of the highest health quality to avoid spread of disease or unnecessary rederivations. Health monitoring must be carried out routinely, and documentation of health status must be made available to investigators receiving animals. In addition, the maintenance of a high level of health quality in colonies within the repository will prevent miscasting phenotypes that are affected by pathogens.

### GENETIC MONITORING
Because errors can occur during breeding, especially in large colonies, and because many genetically modified mice have no visible phenotype, genetic monitoring becomes an essential function within a repository. Most genotyping protocols are available from the developer of the strain, but personnel in a repository must be prepared to develop genotyping protocols where none have been published or where published protocols are not sufficiently robust. In addition to verifying the presence of the correct mutated gene, or transgene, monitoring the genetic background by use of molecular or enzymatic markers is also a strict requirement of genetic quality control.

## Breeding

Induced mutants, as well as spontaneous mutants, pose many challenges to the breeder since the mutation frequently negatively affects reproductive performance. It is often necessary for experienced animal technicians to determine optimal husbandry and breeding procedures for difficult strains. To produce a more genetically defined model, some stocks having a mixed genetic background will need to be backcrossed to a common inbred strain. This requires expertise and experience in genetics as well as in husbandry.

Reproductive performance and demand will determine the size of a colony for any particular strain, and strains with little or no demand present a dilemma. A decision must be made to either maintain a breeding stock or keep cryopreserved germ plasm only. For strains with few numbers of requests, frozen storage is more economical than maintaining a breeding colony. A drawback of relying on frozen storage is the time required for reestablishing a breeding colony to the level where sufficient numbers of animals can be provided for research.

## Cryopreservation

Frozen germ plasm preservation primarily provides assurance that strains will not be inadvertently lost, but it additionally permits investigators to maintain infrequently used strains with a minimum number of breeders because loss of a breeding colony can always be replaced from frozen germ plasm. Because of the large number of laboratories now developing genetically manipulated strains, more strains are being created than can be simultaneously used. Economical management of such a large number of strains, especially in the face of limited and expensive animal facilities, is best aided by the cryopreservation of germ plasm in one of several forms, embryos or sperm being the most common at present.

Embryo cryopreservation has proven reliable for most strains although the efficiency of obtaining embryos will vary depending upon the genetic background of the strain and, in some cases, on the mutant or transgene carried. Embryo cryopreservation is the method preferred for inbred strains that require diploid germ plasm for intact reconstitution or for mutant and transgenic strains in which the induced gene is best kept homozygous.

Since 1972, when mammalian embryos were first successfully frozen (Whittingham et al. 1972; Wilmut 1972), many different methods of freezing embryos have proven successful, but the methods are, for the most part, variations of two basic approaches (Mazur 1990). The first is often referred to as equilibrium freezing, in which the rate of cooling is sufficiently slow to allow embryos to dehydrate as a result of achieving equilibrium with the surrounding medium during the cooling process. Dehydration prevents the formation of intracellular ice crystals that are detrimental to the survival of the embryo during the freezing or thawing process. Conversely, no-equilibrium methods consist of ultrarapid cooling rates, often referred to as vitrification methods. Ice crystal formation does not occur in either the embryos or medium and, instead, a glass state results from the rapid cooling rate in combination with prior exposure to relatively high concentrations of cryoprotective agents.

Methodology for the cryopreservation of mouse sperm is not presently as reliable as embryo cryopreservation, but the need for it is greater because of the economy it offers. Sperm collected and frozen from a single male mouse can generally result in well over 1000 offspring if the mouse is a hybrid or has a mixed genetic background. In contrast, an average of four offspring can be derived from frozen embryos of a typical female mouse (Sharp and Mobraaten 1997). However, recovering offspring from cryopreserved sperm is generally not successful for most inbred strains of mice. New methods for the recovery of offspring from frozen sperm are now under development, and foremost among these is the method of intracytoplasmic sperm injection (ICSI). ICSI has been shown to be effective using sperm rendered nonviable from freezing as well as with freeze-dried sperm (Wakayama et al. 1998; Wakayama and Yanagimachi 1998).

## Distribution

Distribution of mice, of course, must be carried out as one of the functions of a repository, and it must be done in such a manner as to preserve high health quality as well as to provide the mice to an investigator in a timely fashion. The latter goal is perhaps difficult to achieve in a repository setting in that many strains will be maintained either in small numbers or in the preserved state. The basic dilemma for "low-demand" strains is whether to keep a colony on the shelf or to recover it from frozen germ plasm. It is difficult to financially support an active breeding colony when the demand for its mice is small and infrequent; recovering costs from proceeds of selling the mice would make the price of such animals prohibitively high. On the other hand, the cost in time of reconstituting a strain from frozen storage may also be prohibitively high for some researchers, but the alternative of not having such mice available at all would be more intolerable. The amount of available breeding capacity affects this issue.

## INFORMATION RESOURCES

TBASE (Targeted/Transgenic Mutant Database) is a database for transgenic and targeted mutant animals originally developed by Richard Woychik (Woychik et al. 1993). It has recently been transferred to the Jackson Laboratory, where it is undergoing revisions to better fit within the structure of the Mouse Genome Database maintained at the laboratory. TBASE contains information on, among other items, the correct nomenclature, biology, and literature for transgenic and targeted mutants and is intended to represent all transgenic and targeted mutant mouse strains and stocks.

The IMR maintains an online database that provides information on strains available from the IMR, including brief phenotype descriptions, creation of the mutation or transgene, available genetic backgrounds, animal husbandry, genotyping protocols, and initial references. The IMR database also links to the Mouse Genome Database (MGD) for descriptive information on genes. Information on the availability and pricing of IMR strains can be obtained from the Jax Mice database [*http://jaxmice.jax.org/index.shtml*].

The International Mouse Strain Resources (IMSR) database is intended to be a central database where one may obtain the location of any existing inbred, outbred, or mutant strain or stock. It currently lists all stocks and strains held by the Mammalian Genetics Unit (MGU) at Harwell and the Jackson Laboratory.

The BioMedNet Mouse Knockout and Mutation Database is a valuable subscription database available through BioMedNet. The URLs of these databases are listed in Table 1.2.

**TABLE 1.2.   The URL for each mouse database**

Informatics web sites

TBASE
  *http://tbase.jax.org/*
International Mouse Strain Resources
  *http://www.jax.org/pub-cgi/imsrlist*
BioMedNet Mouse Knockout and Mutation Database
  *http://www.biomednet.com/home*
Mouse Genome database
  *http://www.informatics.jax.org/*

# REPOSITORIES IN THE FUTURE

Genetically engineered strains of mice are now critical research tools for basic biomedical research and for genomic approaches to developing new therapeutic treatments for human disease. Because of today's fast-paced scientific research, investigators want immediate access to reagents and resources. For mice, this creates a particular problem since mouse production is dependent on the mouse reproductive cycle. One solution is to maintain large colonies of mice in order to meet any anticipated demand. This would be expensive and impractical, especially when one considers the large number of new mutants that are being produced (Fig. 1.1). Compromises on availability level will have to be made. One potential compromise might be to make high-demand strains available in moderate numbers and small-demand strains available only in small numbers. The investigator could breed, or contract to breed, larger numbers of mice if they were required.

Cryopreservation is another alternative to maintaining live breeding colonies of low-demand strains. The recovery of animals from the cryopreserved state takes longer than if they were maintained on the shelf, but it is possible that technological improvements could make this process more efficient than it is today. These improvements might include expanding the utilization of mouse sperm cryopreservation to inbred as well as hybrid background strains, improving and utilizing ICSI to recover strains from the frozen or freeze-dried state, and technology that would reduce the costs of embryo cryopreservation.

Genetically engineered mice will be in even greater demand in the near future than they are today as sequencing the human and mouse genomes nears completion and as the Human and Mouse Genome Projects shift to understanding of gene function and gene interaction. New central repositories like the IMR will soon be coming online, but the production of important new strains will certainly outstrip these planned resources. The challenge for the future will be to innovate and manage a vastly increasing number of strains in a demanding scientific environment.

# ADDITIONAL ACKNOWLEDGMENT

Supported by National Cancer Institute (NCI) contract NO1-CO-5600 to SAIC-Frederick.

# REFERENCES

Bedell, M.A., Jenkins, N.A., Copeland, N.G. 1997a. Mouse models of human disease. Part I: techniques and resources for genetic analysis in mice. Genes Dev. 11:1–10.

Bedell, M.A., Largaespada, D.A., Jenkins, N.A., et al. 1997b. Mouse models of human disease. Part II: recent progress and future directions. Genes Dev. 11:11–43.

Bradley, A., Evans, M., Kaufman, M.H., et al. 1984. Formation of germ-line chimaeras from embryo-derived teratocarcinoma cell lines. Nature 309:255–256.

Brinster, R.L. 1963. A method for in vitro cultivation of mouse ova from two-cell to blastocyst. Exp. Cell Res. 32:205–208.

Brinster, R.L. 1974. The effect of cells transferred into the mouse blastocyst on subsequent development. J. Exp. Med. 140:1049–1056.

Brinster, R.L., Chen, H.Y., Trumbauer, M., Senear, A.W., Warren, R., Palmiter, R.D. 1981. Somatic expression of herpes thymidine kinase in mice following injection of a fusion gene into eggs. Cell 27:223–231.

Brinster, R.L., Chen, H.Y., Messing, A., et al. 1984. Transgenic mice harboring SV40 T-antigen genes develop characteristic brain tumors. Cell 37:367–379.

Carthew, P., Wood, M.J., Kirby, C. 1983. Elimination of Sendai (parainfluenza type 1) virus infection from mice by embryo transfer. J. Reprod. Fertil. 69:253–257.

Carthew, P., Wood, M.J., Kirby, C. 1985. Pathogenicity of mouse hepatitis virus for preimplantation mouse embryos. J. Reprod. Fertil. 73:207–213.

Cohen, S.N., Boyer, H.W. 1992. Process for producing biologically functional molecular chimeras. 1979 [classical article]. Biotechnology 24:546–555.

Cohen, S.N., Chang, A.C., Boyer, H.W., et al. 1992. Construction of biologically functional bacterial plasmids in vitro. Biotechnology 24:188–192.

Costantini, F., Lacy, E. 1981. Introduction of a rabbit beta-globin gene into the mouse germ line. Nature 294:92–94.

Dymecki, S.M. 1996. Flp recombinase promotes site-specific DNA recombination in embryonic stem cells and transgenic mice. Proc. Natl. Acad. Sci. USA 93:6191–6196.

Evans, M.J., Kaufman, M.H. 1981. Establishment in culture of pluripotential cells from mouse embryos. Nature 292:154–156.

Friedrich, G., Soriano, P. 1993. Insertional mutagenesis by retroviruses and promoter traps in embryonic stem cells. Methods Enzymol. 225:681–701.

Furth, P.A., St Onge, L., Boger, H., et al. 1994. Temporal control of gene expression in transgenic mice by a tetracycline-responsive promoter. Proc. Natl. Acad. Sci. USA 91:9302–9306.

Garrick, D., Fiering, S., Martin, D.I., et al. 1998. Repeat-induced gene silencing in mammals. Nat. Genet. 18:56–59.

Gordon, J.W., Ruddle, F.H. 1981. Integration and stable germ line transmission of genes injected into mouse pronuclei. Science 214:1244–1246.

Gordon, J.W., Scangos, G.A., Plotkin, D.J., et al. 1980. Genetic transformation of mouse embryos by microinjection of purified DNA. Proc. Natl. Acad. Sci. USA 77:7380–7384.

Gu, H., Marth, J.D., Orban, P.C., Mossmann, H., et al. 1994. Deletion of a DNA polymerase beta gene segment in T cells using cell type-specific gene targeting [see comments]. Science 265:103–106.

Harbers, K., Jahner, D., Jaenisch, R. 1981. Microinjection of cloned retroviral genomes into mouse zygotes: integration and expression in the animal. Nature 293:540–542.

Kistner, A., Gossen, M., Zimmermann, F., et al. 1996. Doxycycline-mediated quantitative and tissue-specific control of gene expression in transgenic mice. Proc. Natl. Acad. Sci. USA 93:10933–10938.

Kuhn, R., Schwenk, F., Aguet, M., et al. 1995. Inducible gene targeting in mice. Science 269:1427–1429.

Lin, T.P. 1966. Microinjection of mouse eggs. Science 151:333–337.

Logie, C., Stewart, A.F. 1995. Ligand-regulated site-specific recombination. Proc. Natl. Acad. Sci. USA 92:5940–5944.

Mansour, S.L., Thomas, K.R., Capecchi, M.R. 1988. Disruption of the proto-oncogene int-2 in mouse embryo-derived stem cells: a general strategy for targeting mutations to non-selectable genes. Nature 336:348–352.

Mazur, P. 1990. Equilibrium, quasi-equilibrium, and nonequilibrium freezing of mammalian embryos. Cell Biophys. 17:53–92.

McDonald, J.D., Bode, V.C., Dove, W.F., et al. 1990. The use of N-ethyl-N-nitrosourea to produce mouse models for human phenylketonuria and hyperphenylalaninemia. Prog. Clin. Biol. Res. 340C:407–413.

Mobraaten, L.E. 1997. Cryopreservation and strain re-derivation. Lab. Anim. 26:21–25.

Okamoto, M., Matsumoto, T. 1999. Production of germfree mice by embryo transfer. Exp. Anim. 48:59–62.

Okamoto, M., Matsushita, S., Matsumoto, T. 1990. [Cleaning of Sendai virus-infected mice by embryo transfer technique]. Jikken Dobutsu 39:601–603.

Palmiter, R.D., Brinster, R.L. 1986. Germ-line transformation of mice. Annu. Rev. Genet. 20:465–499.

Reetz, I.C., Wullenweber-Schmidt, M., Kraft, V., et al. 1988. Rederivation of inbred strains of mice by means of embryo transfer. Lab. Anim. Sci. 38:696–701.

Sauer, B., Henderson, N. 1988. Site-specific DNA recombination in mammalian cells by the Cre recombinase of bacteriophage P1. Proc. Natl. Acad. Sci. USA 85:5166–5170.

Sharp, J., Mobraaten, L. 1997. To save or not to save: the role of repositories in a period of rapidly expanding development of genetically engineered strains of mice. In Transgenic Animals: Generation and Use, ed. L.M. Houdebine, pp. 525–532. Switzerland: Harwood Academic Publishers.

Smithies, O., Gregg, R.G., Boggs, S.S., et al. 1985. Insertion of DNA sequences into the human chromosomal beta-globin locus by homologous recombination. Nature 317:230–234.

te Riele, H., Maandag, E.R., Berns, A. 1992. Highly efficient gene targeting in embryonic stem cells through homologous recombination with isogenic DNA constructs. Proc. Natl. Acad. Sci. USA 89:5128–5132.

Thomas, K.R., Capecchi, M.R. 1987. Site-directed mutagenesis by gene targeting in mouse embryo-derived stem cells. Cell 51:503–512.

Wagner, T.E., Hoppe, P.C., Jollick, J.D., Scholl, D.R., Hodinka, R.L., Gault, J.B. 1981. Microinjection of a rabbit beta-globin gene into zygotes and its subsequent expression in adult mice and their offspring. Proc. Natl. Acad. Sci. USA 78:6379–6380.

Wakayama, T., Yanagimachi, R. 1998. Development of normal mice from oocytes injected with freeze-dried spermatozoa. Nat. Biotechnol. 16:639–641.

Wakayama, T., Whittingham, D.G., Yanagimachi, R. 1998. Production of normal offspring from mouse oocytes injected with spermatozoa cryopreserved with or without cryoprotection. J. Reprod. Fertil. 112:11–17.

Whittingham, D.G., Leibo, S.P., Mazur, P. 1972. Survival of mouse embryos frozen to −196 degrees and −269 degrees C. Science 178:411–414.

Wilmut, I. 1972. The effect of cooling rate, warming rate, cryoprotective agent and stage of development on survival of mouse embryos during freezing and thawing. Life Sci. II 11:1071–1079.

Wood, S.A., Allen, N.D., Rossant, J., et al. 1993. Non-injection methods for the production of embryonic stem cell-embryo chimaeras. Nature 365:87–89.

Woychik, R.P., Wassom, J.S., Kingsbury, D., Jacobson, D.A. 1993. TBASE: a computerized database for transgenic animals and targeted mutations [published erratum appears in Nature 1993 Jun 17;363(6430):656]. Nature 363:375–376.

Zambrowicz, B.P., Imamoto, A., Fiering, S., et al. 1997. Disruption of overlapping transcripts in the ROSA beta geo 26 gene trap strain leads to widespread expression of beta-galactosidase in mouse embryos and hematopoietic cells. Proc. Natl. Acad. Sci. USA 94:3789–3794.

Zambrowicz, B.P., Friedrich, G.A., Buxton, G.C., et al. 1998. Disruption and sequence identification of 2,000 genes in mouse embryonic stem cells. Nature 392:608–611.

# I
# Techniques

# 2
# In Situ Hybridization Techniques for Studying Gene Expression in the Genetically Altered Mouse

Shelley B. Hoover, Cynthia Sung, Michele Cottler-Fox, and Cecil H. Fox

When in situ hybridization with nucleic acid probes was first reported, it seemed to be an interesting but exotic technique for the study of chromosomes. At the present time it is no less exotic and interesting, but applications have extended far beyond to include gene expression, viral pathobiology, detection of bacteria in tissues, and the presence or absence of specific genes following genetic manipulations. Due to the variety of applications, we confine our remarks to those that can be used to study gene expression of the genetically altered mouse. In situ hybridization work must be carefully planned, with clear goals and objectives. While this might be said of any scientific endeavor, in situ techniques are particularly sensitive, require a great amount of time and expense, and involve many variables. The most important considerations follow.

## CONSIDERATIONS FOR IN SITU HYBRIDIZATION

### Resolution

The first decision should be the level of resolution of the target required. For example, if embryos are to be probed for expression of a gene in an organ such as the liver, entire embryo hybridizations may be acceptable using chromogenic probes. On the other hand, if only 20–100 cells express the gene and the morphology of the tissue is important, radioactive probes in formaldehyde-fixed tissue would be preferable. The two different approaches are not always interchangeable but may be supportive of each other.

## Sensitivity

Despite years of advertising about how sensitive nonradioactive probes are, these assertions are difficult to place on an objective scale. In general, radioactive probes have the advantage because they may be measured with great precision and they give a more sensitive indication of hybridization. Nonradioactive probes may be favored because of speed, optical properties, or the regulatory inconveniences of radioisotopes.

Another issue is the relative amount of mRNA that is present. If only a small amount of RNA per cell is being expressed, it may be below the limits of detection by a particular probe. Further, if the probe represents only a small portion of the target RNA, once again the sensitivity may be too low. We may state our rule of thumb for estimating successful hybridization as follows. To obtain 200 silver grains in a 400 $\mu m^2$ area over a cell by emulsion autoradiography in our standard protocol, the cell must contain 100,000 copies of mRNA with a 500 base probe sequence, or 10,000 copies with a 1000 base probe sequence, or 100 copies with a 10,000 base probe sequence.

(This "rule" is conservative but allows an estimate of the probable success of hybridization with formaldehyde-fixed paraffin-embedded 6 $\mu m$ sections and assumes that probes will be reduced in size to about 200 bases by alkaline hydrolysis.)

13

Alternatively, one may estimate the sensitivity based on Northern blots. If a Northern develops on film within 6–8 hours, the target molecule is probably abundant enough to detect by autoradiography. Unfortunately, we are unaware of similar estimates for nonradioactive probes.

## Choosing a Probe System

In this section we address only the procedure after a sequence is isolated, purified, and subcloned in an appropriate expression vector. Faced with the question of DNA or RNA probes, there no longer seem to be compelling reasons for using DNA except in special circumstances. Oligo probe cocktails, when they consist of both significant amounts of antisense sequence and corresponding sense oligos, are a cumbersome and expensive step but may remain stable for years. DNA is generally "stickier" than RNA, it gives high background, and suitable controls are difficult to employ. Greater hybrid duplex stability and enzymatic hydrolysis of single-stranded RNA are further reasons for using riboprobes. Expression vectors are increasingly convenient to use, and the presence of two promoters and multiple cloning sites make probe synthesis much easier. For the novice, cDNA is obtained by reverse transcription or by long-chain polymerase chain reaction (PCR). The strands of cDNA are inserted into an expression vector, and a single colony of bacteria is selected. The bacteria are grown into a large culture and ruptured, and the plasmid is removed and purified. The plasmid, which is circular, can then be cut with restriction enzymes at one end or the other of the insert. This "linearized" cDNA has the sequence of the plasmid, the promoter, and the insert cDNA. When an RNA polymerase is added in the presence of nucleotide triphosphates, starting at the promoter, the sequence is "read off" by the enzyme and makes a copy of RNA complementary to the insert (Fig. 2.1). At this point, the nomenclature can become confusing. An antisense probe is the probe sequence that is complementary to the mRNA of the target. A sense probe is the same size and composition (same sequence but in reverse order) but will not hybridize to the target. Consequently, the sense probe serves as a molecular control for the antisense probe.

Once cDNA is obtained and linearized (a confirmatory gel is useful to show linearization), probe synthesis can begin. For a number of years we have used T7, Sp6 promoters, but T7, T3 combinations are equally satisfactory for polymerization. Most molecular biology companies have reagents in kit form for probe synthesis. At this point, the next decision is whether to use radioactive probes or nonradioactive

ones. Either reagent can be made with kit-type reagents.

Nonradioactive probes may be made by incorporating nucleotide triphosphates with marker molecules attached to them: fluorescein, bromodeoxyuridine, biotin, or digoxygenin are common. These probes may be detected with polyclonal, monoclonal or Fab fragment antibodies using standard immunological methods. More recently, a variety of intensification methods have been used to increase the sensitivity of immune-based reagents. Most producers of antibodies have at least one type, usually based on tyramide amplification.

If radioactive probes are chosen, an isotope must be selected. Here again there is a choice. The usual isotopes for making radioactive probes are $^{35}$S, $^{33}$P, $^{3}$H, and $^{125}$I. These isotopes are used because commercial supplies of NTPs are available. Each has advantages and disadvantages. Sulfur is used as a thionyl phosphate group on nucleotide phosphates and is notorious for moving around spontaneously; that is, the radioactive atoms are shed from nucleotides and may be released into the air or transferred to other reagents. Phosphorus is about twice as expensive, is more stable, but has a rather short half-life (25.4 days), and while it has greater decay energy than sulfur, it must be used immediately for any advantage to ensue. Tritium gives the best resolution, but its low energy makes exposure times quite long (3–50 weeks). Iodine, which is attached to the nucleotide ring and is stable, produces γ emissions in addition to secondary β, thus making laboratory personnel wary of this isotope. For economic reasons, most investigators use sulfur for routine labeling of probes.

The riboprobes should be purified on a column and alcohol precipitated. Nonradioactive probes may be assayed by serial dilutions on nitrocellulose, while radioactive probes may be precipitated and counted in a scintillation counter. Nonradioactive probes are stable at −70°C for months or years, but we prefer to use radioactive probes within 2 weeks of synthesis.

## Selecting a Protocol

Using a published protocol taken from the journal literature is risky as to reproducibility and even accuracy. There are, however, standard protocols that appear in texts that are generally well thought out and proven to work (Fox and Cottler-Fox 1993; Zeller and Rogers 1996). By experience we have found that once a protocol has been determined to provide satisfactory results, any deviation is suspect, even to substituting different lot numbers of reagents and enzymes. In most protocols there are steps that seem illogical or are included in an arbitrary way. We suggest that though they may seem that way, deviation from the protocol will result in

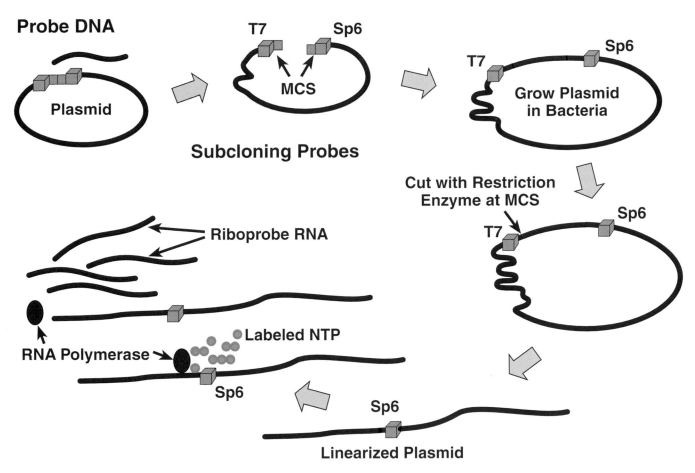

**FIGURE 2.1**   A general plan for producing probes for in situ hybridization. A fragment of DNA is ligated into a plasmid that is grown in a bacterium. The plasmid is recovered and linearized at either end of the insert with a promoter in place allowing transcription in either orientation. The probe is run off using radiolabeled nucleotides in the reaction mixture and the finished riboprobes used in hybridizations. MCS = multiple cloning site; NTP = nucleotide triphosphate.

technical failures that will invalidate results. A simplified in situ hybridization cartoon is shown in Fig. 2.2.

## Preparing Tissue

There are a number of misconceptions about how to prepare tissues for in situ hybridization. These usually arise from trying to combine protocols or from a misconception of basic histologic techniques. If whole mounts are not to be used, the preferable method is to fix tissues in aqueous formaldehyde and cut paraffin sections. Formaldehyde should be prepared by depolymerizing paraformaldehyde. Paraformaldehyde is to formaldehyde as dry ice is to carbon dioxide. It is a white powder that in a base catalyzed reaction becomes hydrated to form a solution. There is no reason to add buffers, saline, or physiological buffered saline (PBS) to freshly prepared formaldehyde solutions at the appropriate pH. Formaldehyde solution should be added to

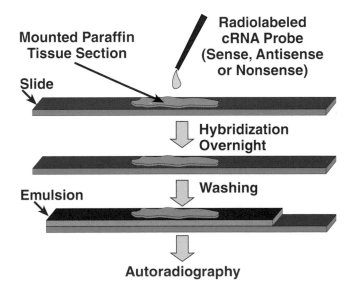

**FIGURE 2.2**   A simplified outline of in situ hybridization.

tissues in a proportion of 20 parts of 1.3M formaldehyde to each part of tissue, and the tissue should not be thicker than 0.5 cm at any point. The formaldehyde solution should be at 24°C, and the tissues should remain at 24°C for 24 hours, preferably on a reciprocating shaker. For large embryos it may be desirable to either inject formaldehyde into the abdominal cavity with a fine needle or to fix the tissues at 38°C for 24 hours. If tissues are to be stored for longer periods, they may be transferred to 70 percent ethanol. Because we have the option of manual processing, we prefer to process tissues on different time schedules, depending on size and development of the tissue. Most larger labs use machine processing for embryos. When tissues are embedded in paraffin, there is the option of section thickness. One may argue that thin (4–8 μm) sections are superior because they give the highest resolution of signal. The reverse of this, that 8–15 μm sections will give greater signals, is especially true for nonradioactive probes and may be true for some types of tissue. Until more quantitative data exists, we continue to use 6 μm sections.

## Visualizing Results

After a successful hydridization, the problem of visualizing results is critical to obtaining useful information from the tissues. If nonradioactive probes are used, signal is revealed by an immunological system. Nonradioactive probes may be used for fluorescence in situ hybridization (FISH), cosmid probes, and whole-mount in situ hybridization (ISH) (embryos, larvae, etc.) when your isotope license gets revoked, when detecting small amounts of mRNA is not important, and for qualitative experiments. An antibody to the marker on the nTPs is employed, followed by a color reaction to show deposition of the antibody. Usually an alkaline phosphatase marker is added to the antibody and a 5-bromo-4-chloro-3-indolyl phosphate (BCIP)-nitroblue tetrazolium substrate is deposited at the site of the enzyme. The solubility of the colored complex is such that slides may be mounted and are more or less permanent. A number of other dye systems including fluorescent ones are available, as are immunogold reagents.

If radioactive probes are used (Fig. 2.3), the alternatives are somewhat greater. The simplest and most immediate is to make autoradiograms of the slides. In the past, two types of autoradiography were used. In one, no longer common, emulsion was stripped from glass plates and allowed to adhere to the slides as a film. These manipulations, done in the dark, require more patience than it is reasonable to expect. Another method was to simply place a film, emulsion side down, over the slide and expose in the dark. The spatial resolution of this system is generally only about 50 μm. The

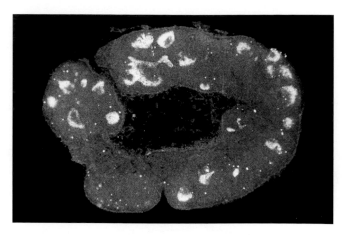

**FIGURE 2.3**  Use of the low-power dark-field condenser allows large structures to be viewed in their entirety. This image, made at 2×, shows HIV RNA distribution in a human lymph node.

majority of autoradiographic slides are now made with liquid emulsion. While methods abound for diluting emulsion prior to dipping, we use undiluted emulsion in handy resealable lightproof containers from Kodak, usually the NTB2 grade. Before use, the emulsion is heated to 45°C in a water bath; then the slides are dipped by immersing them in the melted emulsion. With practice, the entire process can be conducted in the dark (Fox and Cottler-Fox 1993).

Once the slides are developed, they are stained to define the tissues. For general use, hematoxylin and eosin provide good tissue differentiation. The emulsion on the slides retains some eosin, giving them a pink cast. Other useful stains include Giemsa and toluidine blue. We use no. 1 1/2 coverslips for slides, both for optical reasons and for consistency.

Cleaning slides of emulsion is most easily done by allowing the mounting medium to set and then washing the backs of the slides with conventional scouring powder and a piece of cellulose sponge. This is an important step for further examination of the slides.

Viewing slides in the microscope is a specialized endeavor (Fox and Dreyfuss 1992). Many investigators are not expert in microscopy and use a compound bright-field microscope at a magnification of 100× or greater to inspect slides. We use a very low power fiber optic dark-field microscope condenser (available from most dealers) at magnifications of 10–15× for initial screening of the slides (Fig. 2.4). Once the distribution of positive areas has been made, it is then possible to identify organs and cellular types at greater magnification. Methods employing image analysis and grain counting are highly idiosyncratic and cumbersome to use.

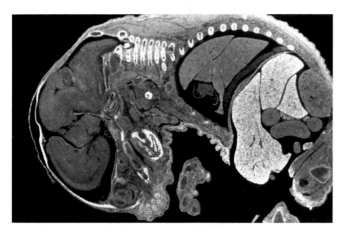

**FIGURE 2.4** A low-power image of a mouse embryo hybridized with a specific probe. 5×

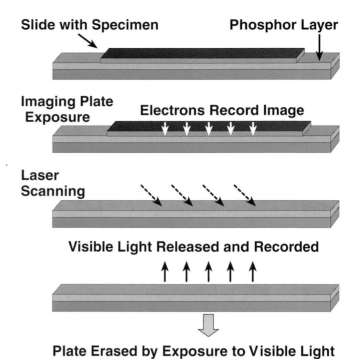

**Plate Erased by Exposure to Visible Light**

An additional method for imaging from in situ hybridization comes from the development of phosphor storage imaging for β emissions by electron capture (Fig. 2.5). We first reported this application some time ago (Fox et al. 1994), and instruments have steadily improved. Currently we use either a high-resolution Fuji instrument (Fuji BAS 5000, Fuji Medical Instruments Division, Stamford, CT) or a more compact Packard "Cyclone" (Packard Instruments, Meriden, CT). Both instruments use screens for detection manufactured by Fuji.

In practice, slides, following in situ hybridization and before dipping in emulsion, are placed on "screens" in a conventional X-ray film cassette. The slides are "exposed" for 1 to 4 days, and the screens removed. The screen is "read" by a laser-photomultiplier combination, and the light signals recorded as an image of the plate and slides (Fig. 2.5). This procedure has a number of advantages over emulsion autoradiography. The images are stored in a computer and are useful in morphological analysis of the tissue as well as in quantitation of the amounts of radiolabeled probe hybridized to the tissue. Both instruments have software that is powerful enough to allow planimetric measurements and feature extraction without a high level of computer skill. Both instruments make reference to units of radiation that are different and confusing. Fuji uses "psl" (photostimulated luminescence) for its units, while Packard refers to its as "dlu" (digital light units), both of which are simply arbitrary names for the phosphorescent signal induced by the laser beam as measured by the detector. In both instruments the values are proportional to the β radiation absorbed but are not more closely comparable without the use of standards. The digital images derived from the measuring screens may be converted to color through a variable lookup table or may be used directly in black and white. In addition,

**FIGURE 2.5** A simplified explanation of the basic principle of phosphor storage imaging as it applies to specimens on microscope slides. Beta electrons are captured by a phosphor screen as a "latent" image. The image is revealed by sweeping the plate with a laser beam and measuring the light emitted. This is converted into digital data stored in a computer. The phosphor plate can then be erased and reused.

images may be transferred to popular image analysis shareware programs such as NIH Image.

The ready availability of these instruments allows performing experiments where relative distributions of radioactivity are easily derived (Fig. 2.6). These procedures fall into two different categories. In one, a measurement is made of the amounts of radioactive probe hybridized as a function of area. The amounts of hybridization might be compared between brain and liver, for example. The sensitivity and resolution of the Fuji instrument is such that single cells may be detected so that a developing organ can be accurately located at the inception of gene expression. With knockouts, objective comparisons may be very useful.

A second use of phosphor storage imaging is in estimating actual amounts of hybridizable RNA in tissue sections. This is more difficult than it appears due to the matrix in which the target RNA is embedded (i.e., in cells and tissues). Neither fixed nor frozen sections are ideal for quantitation. However, we have constructed several artificial tissues that are satisfactory for calibration standards (Cottler-Fox and Fox 1991). The reference object

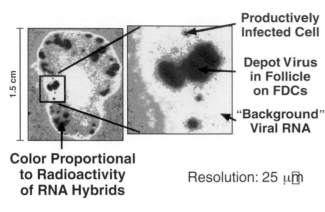

**Productively Infected Cell**

**Depot Virus in Follicle on FDCs**

**"Background" Viral RNA**

1.5 cm

**Color Proportional to Radioactivity of RNA Hybrids**

Resolution: 25 μm

**FIGURE 2.6** Applications of phosphor imaging to the analysis of an HIV-infected lymph node section. The Fuji BAS 5000 instrument resolves 25 μm pixels, allowing identification of single expressing cells.

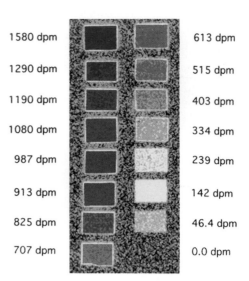

| | |
|---|---|
| 1580 dpm | 613 dpm |
| 1290 dpm | 515 dpm |
| 1190 dpm | 403 dpm |
| 1080 dpm | 334 dpm |
| 987 dpm | 239 dpm |
| 913 dpm | 142 dpm |
| 825 dpm | 46.4 dpm |
| 707 dpm | 0.0 dpm |

**FIGURE 2.8** A microscope slide with standard samples of [14]C-labeled plastic allows direct calibration of quantities of hybridization in tissues as well as a control for hardware.

## Cylinder of RNA

A. **RNA suspension**
B. **Fibrin "Glue"**
C. **Thrombin**

**Combine, fix in 1.3 M formaldehyde, process, cut 6 μm sections, mount on slides, hybridize with** [35]**S sense or antisense.**

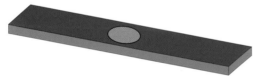

## Calculation:
## RNA per unit area X area of Section.

**FIGURE 2.7** Constructing a test object containing viral particles, synthetic DNA, or synthetic RNA is relatively simple using fibrinogen coagulated by thrombin to yield an "artificial tissue" with a known amount of target material per unit volume.

(Fig. 2.7) consists of an extremely dense block of fibrin prepared from a blood product called "fibrin glue." Fibrin glue may be obtained from transfusion medicine centers or pharmacies (sold by Baxter as "Tisseel"). A solution of RNA is prepared with a known molar amount of nucleic acid. This is suspended in the fibrin glue liquid and mixed thoroughly. The mixture is solidified by addition of bovine thrombin. The resulting clot is fixed in formaldehyde and processed for sectioning and hybridization in the same way a tissue would be.

An alternative is to take a transfected cell line, determine the amounts of RNA and the numbers of cells, and then suspend cells in a clot for sectioning. Other possibilities include homogenized fixed tissue to which is added cRNA and immobilization in a matrix such as polyacrylamide or other gel.

Reference matrices may be made with dilutions of RNA to provide concentration curves that allow calculation of amounts of hybridization per unit of area. We have found it helpful to also include radiation standards of [14]C on glass slides to verify linearity of signal to radioactivity (Fig. 2.8). To use this system, we hybridize radiolabeled probes to the reference object(s) and to the test slides. The plates are exposed to the slides for from 1 to 4 days, whereupon the slides are removed in the dark and the exposed plates are read in the imaging device. The finished image may be stored on computer memory or, as we do, on read-only CDs (Fig. 2.9). The genetically altered mouse does not offer special problems in using in situ hybridization to detect gene expression (Fig. 2.10). In our experience, the success of the technique depends on good probes, on adequate amounts of mRNA in the tissues, and in selecting the correct stage of fetal development (Fig. 2.11). In studying transgenic animals, the requirement of adequate controls is important. We prefer to make cell clots of transfected cell lines and use these as positive controls. Under any circumstances, we strongly recommend the inclusion of as many controls as possible. In our own work we like to have

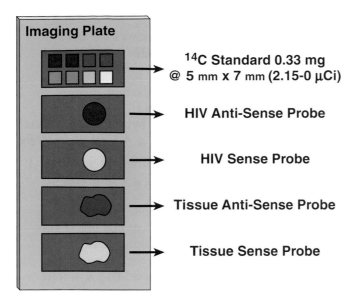

**FIGURE 2.9** A diagram of a typical experiment showing controls and test objects as they would appear on an actual phosphor image.

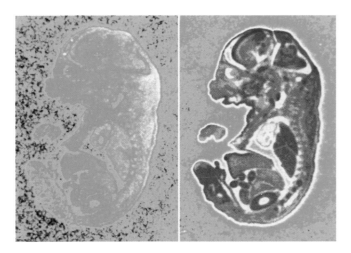

**FIGURE 2.10** Image of a 16-day mouse fetus and the sense control. An alternative to the sense control is a "nonsense" control that will account for any antisense strand transcription of the DNA.

1. A protease-digested antisense slide run in duplicate
2. An undigested antisense slide
3. A sense slide
4. A nonsense slide using an irrelevant probe. The nonsense control is especially important when there is a suspicion that translation of both the sense and antisense configuration by the target DNA may be occurring.
5. If a transfected cell culture is used as a positive control, an untransfected cell line since cell culture in

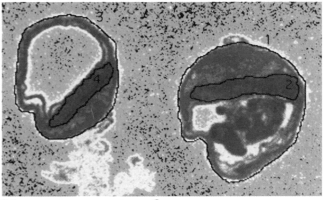

Measurements of areas:
1   18840 PSL
2   3749 PSL (20% of total signal)
3   9008 PSL
4   2712 PSL (30% of total signal)

**FIGURE 2.11** The placenta is an often ignored but important structure in mouse development. These placentas show amount of probe binding to the labyrinth.

high serum sometimes introduces nonspecific probe binding

6. If emulsion is used, a control slide dipped and developed to determine the actual amounts of background

The possible artifacts that may occur are extensive. For example, eosinophils will strongly bind probe nonspecifically. If washes are not stringent enough, false-positive signals will result. Many beginners have trouble developing slides coated with emulsion. Streaking of emulsion is a constant problem. Holes in tissues will fill with emulsion and give the impression of a positive signal. Becoming adept at in situ hybridization of tissues in our experience requires at least a year of practice and is so labor-intensive that we liken it to producing one's own tissue culture media.

Comparing knockouts with controls must involve some caution in interpreting weak signals and in ensuring that the tissues are run in parallel. The greatest problems are biological, particularly when there are lethal changes that result in intrauterine death at an early stage of development. In such instances, making a "Swiss roll" (spiral) of the uterus allows serial sectioning to detect embryos at 6–7 days of development. A nagging concern with knockouts is the necessity of proving a "null" hypothesis, that is, that something is not there.

13. **Counterstaining and Mounting.** Slides may be stained with a simple H&E stain as follows:

Mayer's hematoxylin—3 to 5 minutes
Distilled water—twice, 5 minutes each
0.3 percent ammonium hydroxide—20 dips
Distilled water—twice, 5 minutes each
95 percent ethanol—twice for 2 minutes each
Eosin/phloxine solution—1 minute
95 percent ethanol—twice for 2 minutes each
100 percent ethanol—three times for 2 minutes each
Hemo-D® or xylenes—three times for 2 minutes each

Mount slides with Permount® or DPX® mounting media, and dry flat on a warming tray for several days.

14. **Cleaning Slides.** After slides are thoroughly dried, remove excess emulsion from the back of slides with scouring powder and a cube of sponge. Wash slides in running water, rinse in distilled water, and dip in absolute ethanol. Allow the slides to air dry. The slides are now ready to be examined.

# REFERENCES

Cottler-Fox, M. and Fox, C.H. 1991. Examining cells for infectious agents: a novel approach. J. Infect. Dis. 164:1239–40.

Fox, C.H. and Cottler-Fox, M. 1993. In situ hybridization for the detection of HIV RNA in cells and tissues. In Current Protocols in Immunology (Coligan, J., Kruisbeek, A., Margulies, D., Shevach, E., Strober, W., eds.), Wiley: New York.

Fox, C.H. and Dreyfuss, R. 1992. Photography and molecular biology: in situ hybridization, autoradiography and immunogold. J. Biol. Photog. 60: 39–44.

Fox, C.H., Hoover, S., Currall, V.R., Bahre, H.J., and Cottler-Fox, M. 1994. HIV in infected lymph nodes. Nature 370:256.

Zeller, R.M. and Rogers, M. 1996. In situ hybridization and immunohistochemistry. In Current Protocols in Molecular Biology. 14.0.1 Supplement 35. Wiley: New York.

# 3
# Immunohistochemistry: Methods and Troubleshooting

Craig S. Pow, James S. Whitehead, and Michele S. Moss

Immunohistochemistry (IHC) has proven to be invaluable for investigators in biological sciences. Through IHC, the presence of a particular protein within a tissue, the extent of its distribution in that tissue, and its precise location within a single cell can be elucidated. By observation and interpretation of the specific staining patterns obtained with IHC in normal (control) tissue compared with samples from a treated case, or during proliferation and differentiation, information about a given protein's regulation and possible function can be determined.

For any IHC method to be useful, however, it is essential that it is sensitive, produces no or little background, and gives reliable and reproducible results. To help the user to achieve these goals, this chapter highlights problem areas in applying the technique, presents information on how to troubleshoot effectively, and brings to light considerations that are often overlooked. Finally, a novel approach is available to researchers hoping to use mouse monoclonal antibodies on murine transgenic, gene knockout, and xenograft models. Established IHC methodologies, terminology, and basic fundamentals have been well illustrated in existing literature, and we refer the reader to the following references for these overviews: Carson 1997; Polak and Van Noorden 1997; Larsson 1988; and Sheehan and Hrapchak 1980.

## ENZYME- AND FLUORESCENCE-BASED DETECTION

When commencing "immunodetection," the choices of what specific technique to use can be overwhelming. At the light microscope level, IHC, defined here as an enzyme-based detection, encompasses several amplification methods utilizing mostly horseradish peroxidase

(HRP) or alkaline phosphatase (AP). Immunofluorescence requires similar procedures but does not involve a chemical color reaction. While either an enzymatic or fluorescence approach may yield a result in a given application, a number of key differences should be noted (Table 3.1). IHC offers more in terms of morphological detail and sensitivity, while yielding a permanent color precipitate that can be archived for future reference or photography. One advantage that immunofluorescence has over IHC is that a greater degree of exquisite detail and resolution can be obtained. This is particularly

**TABLE 3.1. Comparison of enzyme- and fluorescence-based detection**

| Enzyme immunohistochemistry | Immunofluorescence |
| --- | --- |
| Choice of enzyme—HRP or AP | Choice of fluorochrome |
| Most sensitive method | Less sensitive than enzyme method |
| Performed on frozen or paraffin-embedded tissue sections | Best results achieved on nonaldehyde-fixed sections |
| Several substrate colors available for multiple antigen labeling in same tissue section | Recommended for colocalization of antigens on the same tissue section |
| Tissue morphology visible | Not able to distinguish cellular detail |
| Endogenous enzyme activity must be quenched | Autofluorescence may be present |
| Permanent color development | Long-term storage may be a problem |
| | Best suited for confocal/3-D reconstruction |

Note: Generalized comparisons are based on current standard detection procedures.

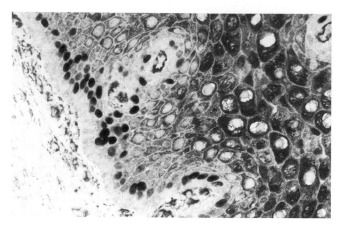

**FIGURE 3.1** Triple immunohistochemistry staining on a paraffin-embedded human epithelial tissue section. Proliferating cells detected with avidin biotin peroxidase-complex (ABC) method 3,3'-diaminobenzidine (DAB) (brown) peroxidase substrate; anti-Ki67 mouse monoclonal antibody, endothelial cells detected with anti-CD34 mouse monoclonal antibody using Vector® Blue (blue) alkaline phosphatase substrate; and epithelial cells detected with anti-multicytokeratin mouse monoclonal antibody using Vector® Red (red) alkaline phosphatase substrate. The detection systems used were Vectastain® ABC peroxidase and alkaline phosphatase kits.

helpful where different antigens are colocalized in the same cell compartment and can each be labeled separately with a fluorochrome (e.g., one fluorescein, the other rhodamine) and subsequently visualized under their respective filters. It should be noted, though, that in situations where multiple antigen labeling involves different cell types in the same tissue section or different cell compartments of the same cell (e.g., nuclear versus cytoplasmic), IHC would usually be recommended (Fig. 3.1). One of the most widely used IHC detection and amplification systems for single or multiple antigen labeling is the highly sensitive avidin biotin peroxidase-complex (ABC) method (Hsu et al. 1981a, 1981b). Given the benefits that enzyme detection provides over immunofluorescence in standard IHC applications, it is a more popular method and will be the focus of this chapter.

A key decision in IHC is which enzyme system should be used. This choice may depend on several factors, such as the advice from a previous user, the procedures given in a published reference, the desired color or quality of the final staining, the specific application, and the tissue preparation. While both HRP- and AP-based systems can essentially be used interchangeably in the same application without loss of specificity or sensitivity, there are some subtle differences between the two

that should be listed and may help in making a decision. HRP-based detection procedures are more widely referenced, and the substrates tend to produce a more dense, though very discrete, label. Ideal applications would include localization of cell surface markers and fine neuronal projections. AP substrates, on the other hand, do not produce as dense a precipitate and therefore may allow for easier examination of cell morphology. The characteristics of the test tissue, though, may determine which enzyme system would be the most appropriate. High endogenous peroxidase activity, for example, could prove difficult to quench, and hence, an AP-based system would ultimately give less background in this situation and make interpretation of the results easier. The reverse can also be stated where endogenous AP is present in the test sample (e.g., intestine).

One less subtle difference between the two systems would be of interest for researchers anticipating using IHC for neuronal tract tracing and localization of nerve axons and projections, particularly in the central nervous system. It has been the experience of many investigators that HRP provides superior results over AP in this application. For reasons as yet not fully characterized, the AP substrates do label cell bodies in this tissue; however, they do not precipitate consistently along pathways. This phenomenon seems to be related to the difference in the substantivity of the reaction products in various tissues.

## TISSUE PREPARATION

The importance of careful preparation of tissue intended for IHC use cannot be overstated. Antigen preservation and retention of tissue morphology are crucial to the success of the application. To optimize both of these variables, consideration must be given to many related topics including the fixative, the method of fixation, the size of the tissue sample, the length of time in and temperature of fixative, and whether the sample is to be frozen or processed for embedding into paraffin blocks. Unfortunately, we cannot do justice to this vast topic in this chapter. However, we refer the reader to the numerous detailed book chapters and research papers that focus on this area (Carson 1997; Larsson 1993; Brandtzaeg 1982; Sheehan and Hrapchak 1980).

A factor often overlooked at this initial stage is what primary antibodies are available (commercially or otherwise) for identification of the target antigen. If all of the primary antibodies that are available work only on frozen sections, then there is no alternative except to freeze the specimen. In some instances, an antibody developed for other techniques such as immunoprecipitation and Western blotting may have unknown suitability for IHC. For this evaluation it would be recommended to prepare both frozen and paraffin-embedded tissues.

The decision to freeze or paraffin embed the specimen should take into consideration the desired quality of the tissue morphology, which directly affects the final IHC result. Freezing the sample is certainly faster; however, the morphology can be greatly compromised. Paraffin embedding is a much more time-consuming technique, but the enhanced results through improved morphology are worth the extra effort.

There is certainly no universal fixative to use for all IHC applications. A fixative suitable for one antigen may provide very poor reactivity or no staining for another antigen. Much has been written about this subject, and here, the only point to be made is to emphasize that the method of fixation can be critical. Perhaps the most sound recommendation to be made is to use a fixative that has been published to work for the tissue specimen and target antigen intended for investigation. Beyond this, trying several different fixatives is a good approach to finding one that will provide optimal morphology and tissue staining.

# TISSUE-STAINING PROCEDURE

Once the specimen has been adequately prepared, the IHC procedure itself is relatively straightforward. A series of steps involving the blocking of various tissue components, antibody and detection reagent incubations, and buffer washes constitutes the majority of the protocol. Table 3.2 shows a typical IHC staining sequence for paraffin-embedded sections and frozen sections using a peroxidase-based avidin-biotin method.

The procedures shown in Table 3.2 list the essential features found in a standard indirect IHC amplification detection system. However, the considerable variation in antibody incubation times, incubation temperatures, and additional blocking steps that may be required in some methods is not emphasized. The prevalence of the target antigen, the tissue specimen characteristics (e.g., endogenous biotin, section thickness), and even the source of primary antibody (e.g., ascites fluid, hybridoma supernatant, serum) all contribute to procedural modifications. To achieve the best results, each investigator must optimize all the steps in the IHC assay, and inclusion of the appropriate control sections helps to monitor the effectiveness of each step.

Certain fixatives, in combination with infiltration and paraffin embedding of a tissue specimen, have been found to produce profound masking effects on some antigens. Proteolytic enzymes, such as trypsin, were first utilized to unmask these antigens so that subsequent IHC detection could be performed (Hautzer et al.

## TABLE 3.2. Typical IHC staining sequences

### Staining procedure for paraffin sections

1. Deparaffinize and hydrate tissue sections through xylene or other clearing agents and graded alcohol series.
2. Rinse for 5 min in tap water.
3. If quenching of endogenous peroxidase activity is required, incubate the sections for 30 min in 0.3% hydrogen peroxide in either methanol or water. Incubation times may be shortened by using higher concentrations of hydrogen peroxide. If endogenous peroxidase activity does not present a problem, step 3 may be omitted.
4. Wash in buffer for 5 min.
5. Incubate sections for 20 min with diluted normal blocking serum that was prepared from the species in which the secondary antibody is made. (In cases where nonspecific staining is not a problem, steps 5 and 6 may be omitted.)
6. Blot excess serum from sections.
7. Incubate sections for 30 min with primary antiserum diluted in buffer.
8. Wash slides for 5 min in buffer.
9. Incubate sections for 30 min with diluted biotinylated secondary antibody solution.
10. Wash slides for 5 min in buffer.
11. Incubate sections for 30 min with ABC peroxidase complex.
12. Wash slides for 5 min in buffer.
13. Incubate sections in peroxidase substrate solution until desired stain intensity develops.
14. Rinse sections in tap water.
15. Counterstain, clear, and mount.

### Staining procedure for frozen sections

1. Sections are air dried.
2. Immediately before staining, fix sections with acetone or the appropriate fixative for the antigen under study.
3. Transfer slides into buffer.
4. If quenching of endogenous peroxidase is required, follow the procedure in step 3 of the paraffin section protocol. In some cases, especially when using monoclonal antibodies, the antigen may be destroyed by treatment with hydrogen peroxide. In these cases, this treatment should be used only after incubation with biotinylated antibody.
5. Follow steps 4–15 of the procedure recommended for paraffin sections.

1980). More recently, various heating procedures using microwaves, pressure cookers, and other heating devices have been used with great success for enhancing the unmasking of some antigens (Figs. 3.2, 3.3; Shi et al. 1995a; Norton et al. 1994; Cattoretti et al. 1993). These high-temperature antigen-unmasking methods require the use of defined buffers to achieve maximal unmasking and hence staining intensity. Antigen unmasking may be the most difficult part of the tissue-staining

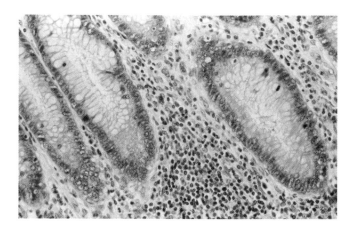

**FIGURE 3.2** Paraffin-embedded section of human colon adenocarcinoma stained using proliferating cell marker Ki67 mouse monoclonal antibody and brown DAB peroxidase substrate and counterstained with hematoxylin. No high-temperature antigen unmasking was performed.

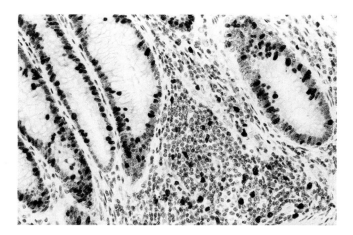

**FIGURE 3.3** Adjacent section to Figure 3.2. The high-temperature antigen-unmasking technique was used (pressure cooker).

procedure since not all heating regimes or buffer solutions work with equivalent effectiveness for all antigens (Shi et al. 1995b). For any given antigen, optimization of the unmasking step is required.

# INTERPRETATION OF RESULTS AND TROUBLESHOOTING

Assuming that staining is achieved on the test sample, the most important point to establish is whether or not it is "specific." Any study is based entirely on the validity of this factor, and the correct use of appropriate positive and negative controls in each separate IHC experiment is imperative.

A positive control tissue is required to determine that the IHC procedure and reagents are working correctly. If staining is achieved on the positive control, the colored precipitate of the substrate should be visible at the presumed site of the target antigen (e.g., cell nuclei). Positive control sections should be consulted first, since absence of staining in these sections will invalidate any staining on the test specimen. It is important that the tissue used for a positive control be processed in an identical manner to that of the test tissue and strongly expresses the target antigen. The positive control tissue need not necessarily be from the same organ or species as the test specimen, but confirmation that the primary antibody does recognize or cross react with the antigen must be demonstrated for each species. When commencing a study, it is also recommended to have a sufficient supply of the positive control tissue on hand to optimize the IHC detection system prior to working with an unknown. If no or very weak staining is seen on the positive control tissue, the problem may be due to one or several contributing factors. Table 3.3 features some of the most likely causes and solutions.

Negative controls are necessary to help confirm the specificity of the primary antibody and to identify the source of any background problems. When run correctly, an appropriate negative control with no background problems should result in no staining on a tissue section. Table 3.4 lists some of the most commonly used negative controls to establish primary antibody specificity. The most commonly used *in*appropriate negative control is substitution of the primary antibody with buffer. As indicated in Table 3.4, a negative control using a suitable substitute for the primary antibody may be used on the test specimen, or the negative control may be a tissue sample that does not contain the target antigen.

When background staining is present, it can obscure the view of the target antigen and throws into question the specificity of the primary antibody and the detection system. Background may arise from more than one part of the procedure and is best overcome by identifying the source(s) or origin of the nonspecific staining. This requires troubleshooting through a series of additional negative controls aimed at pinpointing the most likely cause of the problem. Table 3.5 was designed for this purpose, and by working through the control steps A to D, the vast majority of background staining encountered can be eliminated.

**TABLE 3.3.  Tests to perform if IHC staining is weak or absent in positive control tissues**

| A. Enzyme/substrate | B. Primary antibody |
|---|---|
| **For peroxidase substrate:** Add 1–2 drops of Vectastain ABC reagent to 1 ml substrate solution (DAB; Vector· NovaRED; Vector· VIP; Vector· SG, AEC, TMB). Color of solution should change within about 5 seconds. | Be sure primary antibody is used at an appropriate concentration and that it is active. If potency is lost over time, a higher concentration of primary antibody may be required to achieve optimal staining. Harsh treatment such as freezing/thawing, especially with monoclonal antibodies, may result in a partial or complete inactivation of the antibody. High concentrations of antibodies may also reduce staining. |
| **For any substrate:** Place 1 drop ABC reagent on a small piece of nitrocellulose, and then immediately dip the nitro-cellulose into substrate solution. A colored spot will develop where the ABC reagent was dotted. | **Testing the antibody on sections taken from another known positive block may provide information on the activity of the antibody. If the known positive block is positive, but the test section is negative, SEE NOTES.** |
| **If color develops, SEE B. If no color develops, SEE BELOW.** | |
| Deionized water can contain inhibitors of the peroxidase reaction. Even if the water has very low conductivity, the peroxidase reaction can be severely compromised. | If the pH of the diluent for the primary antibodies is incorrect, the antibody may not bind well to the antigen. |
| **Use glass distilled water for the preparation of the substrate solution.** | **Check the pH of the diluent. Generally TBS or PBS, pH 7.0–8.2, is recommended.** |
| Check the pH of the substrate buffer. Buffers of different pH values are recommended for different substrates. Use freshly diluted hydrogen peroxide to prepare substrate solution. The final hydrogen peroxide concentration should be about 0.01%. Use clean glassware to prepare substrate: traces of chlorine, cleaning solutions, etc., may inhibit the peroxidase reaction. | If the primary antibody recognizes an antigen that is present in biological fluids, it may bind to the antigen in solution rather than on the tissue section. Common diluent additives that may contain significant antigen concentrations are normal serum, fetal bovine serum, or nonfat dry milk. |
| **The substrate should be made according to instructions.** | **Take care that the diluent for the antibody does not contain the antigen.** |
| | **If negative, SEE C.** |

| C. Biotinylated secondary antibody | Notes |
|---|---|
| Inappropriately high dilutions of biotinylated secondary antibody can result in diminished staining. | **Procedure check** |
| **Generally a range of 3–10µg/ml dilution biotinylated secondary antibodies will give optimal staining.** | An equal volume of reagent A and then reagent B, from Vectastain ABC kit, should be added to a defined volume of buffer. Do not mix reagent A and reagent B and then dilute. This procedure may result in an inactive complex. |
| If the diluent contains any neutralizing antibodies, diminished staining could result. For example, biotinylated anti–mouse IgG should not be diluted in mouse serum. The immunoglobulins in mouse serum will bind the biotinylated anti–mouse IgG and prevent this secondary antibody from binding to the primary antibody. | Avoid adding potential sources of biotin to the diluent for ABC. Serum, nonfat dry milk, and culture media are common sources of biotin. Some grades of bovine serum albumin (BSA) may also interfere with the avidin/biotin interaction. **Avoid using Fraction V-grade BSA. If BSA is added, use only an immunohistochemical grade.** |
| **Remove source of neutralizing antibodies.** | **Blocking** |
| If the biotinylated antibody is incorrect, no staining will occur. The biotinylated antibody should be specific for the species in which the primary antibody is made. For example, biotinylated anti–rabbit IgG should be used with primary antibodies made in the rabbit. | Some animals from which blocking serum was obtained may have developed antibodies to the antigen in question. If present, the antibodies may bind to the antigen and prevent the primary antibody from binding. **Try other blocking proteins such as an immunohistochemical grade of BSA, gelatin, fetal bovine serum, nonfat dry milk, etc., or 0.1% detergent.** |
| **Use correct biotinylated antibody.** | **Fixation check** |
| | If a certain tissue section does not stain, but other sections stain with the same detection system, the antigen may have been destroyed by fixation or embedding. If possible, be sure that the method employed for preparing the section is appropriate to preserve antigen and provide access to all the detection system reagents. **Use an antigen-unmasking technique employing heat or protease digestion to recover antigen damaged by fixation.** |
| | **Counterstain/mounting** |
| **If negative, SEE NOTES.** | Some enzyme reaction products are soluble in alcohol, xylenes, or other solvents used for nonaqueous permanent mounting. **Be certain that the enzyme reaction product is compatible with the counterstain and mounting medium.** |

Source: Developed by Vector Laboratories, Inc., using the Vectastain® ABC detection kits.

**TABLE 3.4.  Suitable negative controls to confirm primary antibody specificity**

- Preabsorb the primary antibody with purified specific target antigen, and evaluate on test specimen.
- Use immunoglobulin matching the class of the primary antibody, and substitute for the primary antibody at the same concentration on test sample.[a]
- Use a nonbinding antibody of the same species and subclass as the primary antibody on the test tissue.[a]
- Use tissue (treated in an identical manner as the test tissue) that does not express the target antigen.
- Use preimmune serum or immunoglobulin from the same animal that the antibody was developed in.

[a]These negative controls are especially important when staining for more than one antigen in the same tissue section.

# APPLYING MOUSE PRIMARY ANTIBODIES ON MOUSE TISSUE

The use of an unconjugated primary antibody developed in the same species as the IHC test tissue is particularly problematic. Such a situation exists when using mouse monoclonal antibodies on tissues of mouse origin. The main concern is that, in order to detect the mouse primary antibody, an anti–mouse secondary antibody must be used. In the vast majority of cases, the anti–mouse secondary antibody is unable to differentiate between the primary (immunoglobulin) antibody and any endogenous tissue immunoglobulin that may be present. As a consequence of this nonspecific binding, background staining will occur and interfere directly with the specific reactivity. Given the popularity of mice as research subjects and that most monoclonal antibodies are generated in mice, this is a frequently encountered problem.

Some clarification is required for the phrase "using mouse monoclonal antibodies on tissues of mouse origin." These antibodies may or may not cross react with

**TABLE 3.5.  Controls to use on tissue sections if background staining occurs**

| A. Substrate alone | | B. • Blocking serum<br>• ABC reagent<br>• Substrate | |
|---|---|---|---|
| Staining | No staining, see B.→ | Staining | No staining, see C. |
| ↓ | | ↓ | |
| Endogenous enzyme may be developing the substrate. | | ABC reagent may be binding to tissues for three main reasons: | |
| When running this control, use the same time and conditions that would be appropriate for antibody staining. Color that develops with long exposure to substrate may not be seen within the development time used for specific staining. | | Endogenous protein-bound biotin<br>Endogenous lectins<br>Ionic interactions | |
| If staining is of a generalized nature, it may be due to endogenous enzyme smeared across the section when the section was prepared. | | Various techniques can be used depending on the specific cause: | |
| Block endogenous enzyme appropriately: | | Endogenous protein-bound biotin—Use **avidin/biotin block.** | |
| Peroxidase— Use 0.3% hydrogen peroxide in methanol for 30 minutes or 3% hydrogen peroxide in water for 5 minutes. | | Endogenous lectins—Add **0.2M alpha-methyl mannoside to the ABC diluent.** | |
| Alkaline phosphatase —Add levamisole to alkaline phosphatase substrate unless endogenous enzyme is the intestinal isoform. | | Ionic interactions—Make up ABC reagent in buffer containing **0.5M sodium chloride.** | |
| | | **An avidin/biotin blocking step after the normal serum blocking step will eliminate the binding of the ABC regardless of the cause.** | |
| | | Some protocols suggest the use of bovine serum albumin (BSA) in the blocking procedure. Certain grades of BSA may contain contaminants (bovine IgG, lipids, etc.) that can contribute to background staining. | |
| Repeat control A. | | **Use an immunohistochemical grade of BSA or omit BSA.** | |
| | | Repeat control B. | |

**TABLE 3.5. Continued**

| | |
|---|---|
| • Blocking serum<br>• Biotinylated secondary antibody<br>• ABC reagent<br>C. • Substrate | • Blocking serum<br>• Primary antibody<br>• Biotinylated secondary antibody<br>• ABC reagent<br>D. • Substrate |
| Staining        No staining, see **D.**→<br>↓ | Inappropriate staining<br>↓ |
| Cross-reactivity may occur between the biotinylated secondary antibody and endogenous immunoglobulins or other tissue proteins. | Too much primary antibody has been used. |
| This can occur when the secondary antibody recognizes identical or closely related amino acid sequences of these proteins. | The concentration of primary antibody should be the amount that produces clean specific staining without background. |
| **Add 2% or more normal serum from tissue species to the biotinylated secondary antibody diluent, and/or reduce concentration of the biotinylated secondary antibody.** | **Reduce primary antibody concentration.** |
| Biotinylated antibody may bind nonspecifically to tissue components. | The primary antibody may cross react with other tissue epitopes or bind nonspecifically. |
| **Use additional blocking agents such as 2% immunohistochemical grade BSA, nonfat dry milk, gelatin, or 0.1% detergent.** | **Add normal serum, BSA, nonfat dry milk, gelatin, or detergent to primary antibody diluent.** |
| The wrong species of blocking serum was used. | **Change source or species of primary antibody.** |
| **Use serum from the same species in which the biotinylated secondary antibody was produced.** | The diluent for the primary antibody contains little or no sodium chloride. |
| Egg white or egg white products were used for coating slides, diluting buffers, or blocking tissues. Traces of avidin may be present that bind to the tissue section. Biotinylated secondary antibodies can bind to bound avidin, resulting in unwanted staining. | **Be sure that the diluent for the primary antibody has sufficient salt to block nonspecific binding. Generally diluents should contain from 0.15M (0.9%) to 0.6M sodium chloride.** |
| **Avoid using egg white proteins.** | If the section shows small, amorphous, punctate staining, the primary antibody may have some denatured precipitated immunoglobulin. |
| Repeat control C. | **Centrifuge primary antibody; use supernatant.** |
| | **Tissue sections dried out during procedure.** |
| | Be sure tissue sections are kept moist during all steps in the procedure. |
| | Repeat control D. |

mouse antigens, and the application does not have to involve a direct study of mouse antigen expression to encounter the background problem. For example, the localization of a bacterial or viral infectious agent in a mouse tissue sample, using an unconjugated mouse primary antibody directed against the microbial insult, may generate nonspecific staining when subsequently detected using an anti–mouse secondary antibody. Quite obviously, the problem does not lie with the primary antibody, but rather with the anti–mouse secondary antibody.

Some methodologies have arisen over recent years to overcome this problem. In the past, the method of choice has been to avoid using antibodies made in mice altogether. Rabbits and other species have been used as sources of primary antibodies for IHC in mice. However, differential affinities and lack of epitope specificity of these polyclonal antibodies may present certain unrealized limitations on these studies. Conjugation of the mouse primary antibody to either biotin or an enzyme has also been attempted with some success. This direct conjugation allows detection of the primary antibody without using an anti–mouse secondary antibody, but this method has been found to compromise the sensitivity of IHC, requires purification of the antibody, and may become expensive as this must be done for each antibody of interest. Another method is to preincubate the primary antibody with the secondary antibody, and subsequently use normal mouse serum to absorb any unbound sites on this antibody complex (Hierck et al. 1994; Fung et al. 1992).

The method described herein is based on the use of a straightforward blocking methodology that is effective in producing consistent and reproducible specific staining and that does not compromise sensitivity or require tedious antibody concentration calculations. Developed and offered commercially by Vector Laboratories, Inc., it is referred to as the Vector® Mouse on Mouse

(M.O.M.™) immunodetection kit and is intended for the explicit use of mouse primary antibodies on mouse tissues. It should be noted that other kits intended for use with mouse primary antibodies on mouse tissues are available through different vendors and no direct performance comparisons have been made between those kits and the Vector® M.O.M.™ reagents.

The kit itself contains four components: a protein-blocking solution, a specific mouse IgG blocking reagent, a biotinylated anti–mouse IgG reagent, and the Vectastain® Elite ABC reagent. It is a peroxidase-based system and can be used with any appropriate peroxidase substrate. Background-free, specific staining has been achieved on a variety of mouse tissues, both frozen and paraffin-embedded, including adult liver, kidney, intestine, brain (Figs. 3.4–3.6), and embryonic mouse tissues (Figs. 3.7, 3.8). Double labeling of two different antigens on the same mouse tissue section has also been successfully performed using the Vector® M.O.M.™ kit (Figs. 3.9, 3.10).

One prime consideration when commencing this application is whether the mouse primary antibody, which may have been produced by immunizing mice with an antigen not of mouse origin, will specifically cross react with the mouse target antigen. Some monoclonal antibodies raised against a highly conserved antigen (or part thereof) exhibit a very broad species cross-reactivity, and these could probably be applied

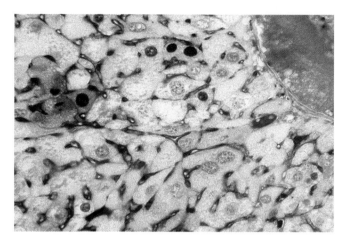

FIGURE 3.4   Adult mouse liver (paraffin section) staining for proliferating cell nuclear antigen (PCNA) using the PC10 mouse monoclonal antibody, a standard biotinylated anti–mouse secondary antibody, and an ABC peroxidase detection system with brown DAB substrate. Significant intercellular staining of endogenous immunoglobulin is present. Hematoxylin counterstain.

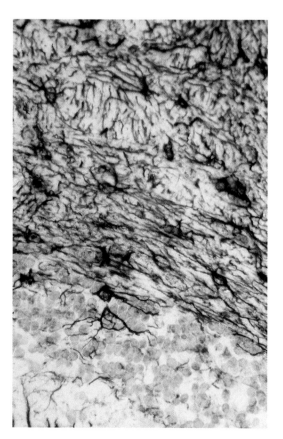

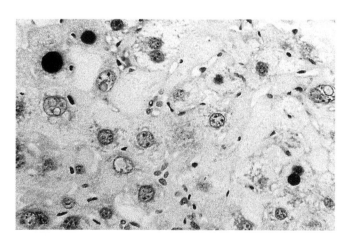

FIGURE 3.5   Mouse liver section similar to Figure 3.4 and utilizing the same PCNA mouse monoclonal antibody but using the Vector® (M.O.M.)™ immunodetection kit. Note specific nuclear reactivity for PCNA without the background. Hematoxylin counterstain.

FIGURE 3.6   Adult mouse brain stained for glial fibrillary acidic protein (GFAP) using mouse primary antibody (clone GA5), Vector® M.O.M.™ immunodetection kit, and Vector® VIP (purple) peroxidase substrate. Methyl green counterstain.

successfully onto mouse tissue. Studies involving normal embryonic and adult mouse tissues or gene knockout models may benefit from using these mouse monoclonal antibodies. Special attention should be drawn to gene knockout studies as these require the demonstration of *no* IHC staining for the gene product. This example emphasizes the need for positive controls and a detection system that will not cause background staining.

It is quite clear, however, that not every mouse monoclonal antibody is suitable for the detection of mouse antigens. Given the high degree of specificity of monoclonal antibodies, and the fact that not all regions of a given antigen may be conserved, many mouse monoclonal antibodies are quite limited in their use in mice. For

example, mouse monoclonal antibodies generated against human antigens are very common, but many of these may not recognize the equivalent mouse antigen because of absence of the epitope, which is present in the human antigen.

In some applications, though, such as human to mouse xenografts, it may be more useful or even desirable for the mouse primary antibody *not* to bind the mouse antigens, but rather to be specific for the human antigen in the graft tissue. This would enable the positive identification of cells of just human origin in

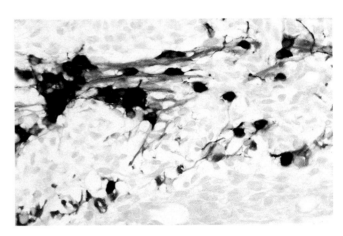

FIGURE 3.9   Mouse embryo (day 10) double labeled for (1) tyrosine hydroxylase (mouse primary antibody clone 1B5) using DAB/NiCl (gray/black) peroxidase substrate and (2) synapsin 1 (mouse primary antibody clone A10C) using Vector® NovaRED (red) peroxidase substrate (brown) and the Vector® M.O.M.™ immunodetection kit for both antibodies.

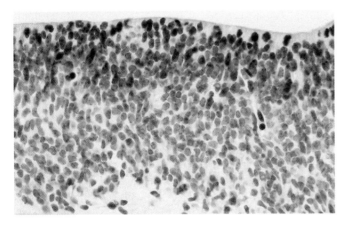

FIGURE 3.7   Mouse embryo (day 10) neuroepithelium stained for Ki67 using mouse primary antibody (clone MM1), Vector® M.O.M.™ immunodetection kit, and DAB (brown) peroxidase substrate. Hematoxylin counterstain.

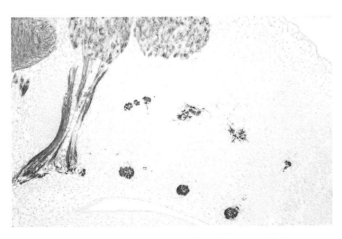

FIGURE 3.8   Mouse embryo (day 10) stained for synapsin 1 using mouse primary antibody (clone A10C), Vector® M.O.M.™ immunodetection kit, and (DAB, brown) peroxidase substrate.

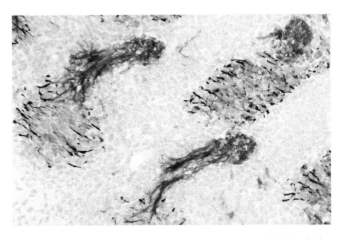

FIGURE 3.10   Mouse embryo (day 10) double labeled for (1) desmin (mouse primary antibody clone DE-R-11) using Vector® VIP peroxidase substrate and (2) synapsin 1 (mouse primary antibody clone A10C) using DAB (brown) peroxidase substrate and the Vector® M.O.M.™ immunodetection kit for both antibodies.

instances of angiogenesis, cell migration, proliferation, and differentiation in the mouse xenograft recipient. To avoid background staining of the mouse host tissue in this situation, specific blocking methodologies must still be employed.

In certain circumstances, endogenous immunoglobulin may not be present in the tissue and hence allows unhindered specific staining to be achieved using a standard anti–mouse secondary antibody. Cell culture preparations, early embryos, and even some perfuse fixed adult tissues may be relatively free of endogenous mouse immunoglobulin. Care must be exercised, though, as the amount of immunoglobulin in a given tissue may vary depending on a number of factors including the disease state. In any preparation therefore, the use of both positive and negative controls will help determine what effective blocking methods need to be utilized.

# REFERENCES

Brandtzaeg, P. 1982. Tissue preparation methods for immunohistochemistry. Pp. 1–75. In: Bullock, G.R. and Perusz, P., eds. Techniques in Immunocytochemistry. Vol. 1. London: Academic Press.

Carson, F.L. 1997. Histotechnology. A self-instructional text. 2nd Ed. Chicago: ASCP Press.

Cattoretti, G., Pileri, S., Parravicini, C., et al. 1993. Antigen unmasking on formalin-fixed, paraffin-embedded tissue sections. J. Pathol. 171:83–98.

Fung, K.-M., Messing, A., Lee, V.M.-Y., et al. 1992. A novel modification of the avidin-biotin complex method for immunohistochemical studies of transgenic mice with murine monoclonal antibodies. J. Histochem. Cytochem. 40:1319–1328.

Hautzer, N.W., Wittkuhn, J.F., and McCaughey, W.T.E. 1980. Trypsin digestion in immunoperoxidase staining. J. Histochem. Cytochem. 28:52–53.

Hierck, B.P., Iperen, L.V., Gittenberger-De Groot, A.C., et al. 1994. Modified indirect immunodetection allows study of murine tissue with mouse monoclonal antibodies. J. Histochem. Cytochem. 42:1499–1502.

Hsu, S.-M., Raine, L., and Fanger, H. 1981a. A comparative study of the peroxidase-antiperoxidase method and an avidin-biotin complex method for studying polypeptide hormones with radioimmunoassay antibodies. Am. J. Clin. Pathol. 75:734–738.

Hsu, S.-M., Raine, L., and Fanger, H. 1981b. Use of avidin-biotin-peroxidase complex (ABC) in immunoperoxidase techniques: a comparison between ABC and unlabeled antibody (PAP) procedures. J. Histochem. Cytochem. 29:577–580

Larsson, L.-I. 1988. Immunocytochemistry: theory and practice. Boca Raton, FL: CRC Press.

Larsson, L.-I. 1993. Tissue preparation methods for light microscopic immunohistochemistry. Appl. Immunohistochem. 1:2–16.

Norton, A.J., Jordan, S., and Yeomans, P. 1994. Brief, high temperature heat denaturation (pressure cooking): a simple and effective method of antigen retrieval for routinely processed tissues. J. Pathol. 173:371–379.

Polak, J.M. and Van Noorden, S. 1997. Introduction to immunocytochemistry. 2nd Ed. New York: Springer-Verlag, by arrangement with BIOS Scientific Publishers Ltd., Oxford, UK.

Sheehan, D.C. and Hrapchak, B.B. 1980. Theory and practice of histotechnology. 2nd Ed. St. Louis, MO: C.V. Mosby Co.

Shi, S.-R., Gu, J., Kalra, K.L., Chen, T., Cote, R.J., and Taylor, C.R. 1995a. Antigen retrieval technique: a novel approach to immunohistochemistry on routinely processed tissue sections. Cell Vision 2:6–22.

Shi, S.-R., Iman, S.A., Young, L., et al. 1995b. Antigen retrieval immunohistochemistry under the influence of pH using monoclonal antibodies. J. Histochem. Cytochem. 43:193–201.

# 4

# Use of Confocal Microscopy Techniques in the Study of Transgenic and Knockout Mouse Genetics

James H. Resau, Eric A. Hudson, and B.K. Sathyanarayana

Genetically engineered mice have produced a revolution in the study of pathology and development. Their use and applications have expanded exponentially in recent years. Several informative reviews document the use of genetically engineered mice (Hanahan 1988; Jaenisch 1988; Adams and Cory 1991; Merlino 1994). In general, a known gene or DNA sequence is inserted into a mouse gamete, and the resulting animal will ordinarily either have the gene knocked out or amplified. The resultant animal may then express a different phenotype. The phenotype may be lethal, occult, or not expressed at all. Methods that identify, quantify, and characterize the phenotype are vital in the understanding of how certain genes affect development, anatomy, histology, pathology, and physiology.

Microscopy of these animals is one of the most obvious and useful methods to characterize phenotype. The use of digital and confocal microscopy is increasing all the time. The techniques are new, but they build on the established principles and techniques of fixation, staining, and image analysis. There are numerous types of microscopy that can be employed in the characterizations of genetically engineered mice. Reviews of the newer confocal laser scanning microscope (CLSM) type microscopic techniques are readily available. A partial but by no means all-inclusive list would include Cavanagh et al.

1993; Matsumoto 1993; Tekola et al. 1994; Pawley 1995; Kimura et al. 1997; and Hasegawa 1998.

Confocal microscopy, which now includes two-photon instruments, produces focused images of a defined volume that are free of out-of-focus fluorescence. These images can be collected rapidly and stored to optical disk or the hard drive. They utilize lasers rather than mercury lamps to produce monochromatic light of defined wavelength. They require high-numerical aperture lenses, pinhole apertures, and computers to produce images in the $x$, $y$, and $z$ directions. These images can be superimposed on each other, rotated, paired for stereo effects, quantified using image analysis, and pseudo-colored for maximum interpretation. Their resolution is still dependent on the laws and formulas of all light microscopy, so they will never match the resolution of electron microscopes, but they have produced a level of excitement in microscopy that has been missing since the days of Keith Porter and the unraveling of the cellular organelles.

In general, one uses CLSM for light microscopic imagery. Fluorescent antibodies or probes are used rather than histochemical dyes since there is a proportional and specific emission for a defined excitation wavelength that can be controlled and quantified by dilutions of antibodies. One chooses specimens, antibodies (primary and secondary), dyes, and so on in accordance with standard experimental guidelines. The wavelength, numerical aperture, specimen thickness, and dye characteristics will determine the resolution. Resolution is still dependent primarily on wavelength (Pawley 1995). The theoretical limit of light microscopy

The authors wish to thank Ave Cline for excellent administrative and clerical support. Research was sponsored by the National Cancer Institute, DHHS, under contract with ABL.

is at the wavelength of UV light. Most CLSM systems have three standard options or modes. The first is transmitted light. This will ordinarily be phase, bright-field, Hoffman-Modulation, or Nomarski/differential interference contrast (DIC) imagery. Visible light microscopy enables one to define the area of interest and narrow the field of view. The principles of Kohler illumination still apply, and one should make sure that the microscope system is optimally aligned. Nomarski/DIC requires a glass substrate (e.g., slide, dish), while phase, bright-field, dark-field, and Hoffman can be applied to either glass or plastic substrates (e.g., dishes, chamber slides). Bright-field is also quite flexible but is dependent on staining of the cells. The stains may be a problem, and they are usually omitted in fluorescent work as many are auto-fluorescent.

Once the area of interest or region of interest is chosen, then one ordinarily switches with a click of a mouse from transmitted to either reflected or fluorescent mode. Usually CLSM microscopes are able to use two or three additional laser lines for fluorescence to complement the transmitted light in channel one. Depending on the sophistication of the instrument, one will either select or rotate lens/condenser, laser line, and mode to produce the fluorescent image. Usually the laser line selection is coordinated to the mode. Typically one will have an HeNe, Argon, or Krypton/Argon/Neon combination for the lasers. Other lasers/lines are available for the UV and higher-red excitations. The images are collected and then stored to memory. The images are either viewed sequentially or simultaneously depending on filter sets or selection of diachronic beam-splitting systems.

The images are then easily printed or manipulated using software systems available from many sources (Salisbury 1994; Hamilton and Allen 1995; Furness 1997; Lehr et al. 1997). We have used combinations of Nomarski images with fluorescein isothiocyanate (FITC) –labeled images to analyze and rank a series of breast cancer cases (Tsarfaty et al., 1999; Klineberg et al. 1996). We hypothesized that the ranking of cases would be improved if we would compare the expression of the oncogene *met* in human breast tumor to the expression of the same protein in adjacent histologic-appearing "normal" tissue. We would then rank cases not on absolute amounts but on the ratio of their normal to tumor. The details of how we identified the regions of interest and measured and quantified the cases are detailed in Klinberg et al. 1996 and Alstock et al. (in preparation, 1999). In general, we drew a mask using the Nomarski image based on the histology of normal and tumor, then overlaid that image with the corresponding FITC image for *met*. *Met* expression was then quantified by pixel intensity and depicted using a spreadsheet computer program.

Similar analytical measurements have been done for the determination of estrogen and progesterone receptors in primary breast carcinomas (Allred et al. 1998). Originally ER/PR quantification was based on a biochemical analysis of a portion of the tumor, selected at resection and sent to the lab frozen, where a radioimmunoassay (RIA) procedure determined receptor expression. The deficiency of that technique was that one never knew for sure if one was measuring all tumor, all normal, or some mixture. Later, it was determined that using immunocytochemistry would enable the pathologist to accurately determine whether the receptor expression was in the normal, in the tumor, or, most often, in mixed areas. We then ranked the breast cancer cases on the basis of their ratios and not whether the level of *met* was high in tumor or low in normal tissue. This form of ranking will control the different fixatives used since the absolute amount will change but the relative ratio will not be affected. Using alcoholic formalin versus a neutral buffered formalin (NBF) will change fluorescent expression, but the relative amount will remain constant, and one can mix different centers' material and develop coherent data (Tsarfaty et al., 1999). In general, this outline could be applied to any tissue, organ, or cell line from a knockout, transgenic, or wild-type mouse to determine and quantify the changes induced by the specific genetic manipulation. This type of analysis requires the application of identical parameters of the instrument. The advantage of the CLSM system is that one can save parameter files and later recall them to apply to new/same samples. No longer does one have to remember the type of alignment or selection of filters. Everything is now in a stored image/parameter file.

So far this chapter has not been specifically about genetically engineered mice, but the information is a good introduction to the use of CLSM in the study of genetically engineered animals. The current expansion of research into the genetics of development and pathology has contributed to a substantial increase in histological-based analysis. Once founder animals have produced a developing embryo or a term pregnancy, researchers immediately are calling upon anatomists, histologists, and pathologists to explain, analyze, and diagnose the mouse or embryo phenotype. It has similarly spiked the role and significance of graduate students' education (Askew and Heffelfinger 1998). Currently we have replaced many of the anatomy- and cell biology–based graduate programs with molecular biology–based programs. This has been an appropriate transition since we need molecular skills to answer those questions only blots, gels, and in situ hybridization can answer. The expanded role of genetically engineered animals, though, is once again rapidly changing the direction of research, just as the electron microscope did a half century ago. Many mutant mice may not show any easily observed pathologic or developmentally distorted phenotypes. One may need to stress or challenge these mice in order to produce the changes that can be diagnosed by microscopy. The histology section stained with hematoxylin and eosin and certain basic immunohistochemical stains is the first line in characterizing these mice, but many animals require additional and sophisticated types of analyses.

We also have need for an increase in the number of individuals knowledgeable about comparative anatomy and histology. Pathologists should be familiar with more than one species. Nucleated red cells are pathologic in man but normal in birds. The human stomach is all glandular epithelium, while many rodents have a large epidermoid component. Numerous other examples abound in the human/veterinary anatomy textbooks. One has to know the normal histology of the wild-type mouse in order to understand knockout/transgenic mouse histopathology. Askew and Heffelfinger (1998) report that in their observations incoming graduate students can not distinguish anatomic detail and that they are unaware of the research applications of histology.

There are other techniques that will increase the specificity of molecular techniques and lead to the quantification of images. The new technology of microdissection developed in the Liotta laboratory of the National Cancer Institute (NCI) (Dean-Clower et al. 1997) similarly uses knowledge of microanatomy. In order to accurately "draw" the outline of the area or region of interest to remove for analysis, one must understand the histology. If one takes a mixture of normal and tumor in both the "normal" and "tumor" samples, then there will probably be no difference in the molecular characterizations, regardless of the specificity or sensitivity of the probe, polymerase chain reaction (PCR) primer, or reagent purity. The microscopist is, therefore, a significant collaborator in most research projects.

In the following, we present several examples of how CLSM can be applied to the study of genetically engineered mice and explain the general rules for the application of microscopy to these mice and the cell lines that evolve from them. CLSM depends on one's knowledge of the microscopes, the sensitivity and specificity of the reagents, and the quality of one's instrumentation. Most important is the knowledge and analytical capabilities of the microscopist.

One starts with representative sections taken by a trained investigator. The sections should be harvested from a representative area of the animal in a manner that will not induce any artifacts. One must be knowledgeable of gross anatomy to select from areas that are "viable" and not injured, ischemic, or infected foci. The criteria that distinguish between normal injury (sub-

lethal) and lethal injury (necrosis apoptosis) have been well characterized (Majno and Joris 1995). Ischemic/necrotic injury ordinarily is caused by disruption of the cytosolic mitochondrial energy production capacity of the cell. Damage to the membrane of the cell ordinarily spares nuclear morphology until late in the sequence. The membranes of injured cells show swelling and blebs. The mitochondria are damaged and swollen. In programmed or developmental cell death, the nucleus is the first to be changed, and the classic enzymatic breakdown of the nucleus precedes the cytoplasmic morphologic change. One must be able to distinguish between injured, damaged, and undeveloped tissues or the molecular characterizations will be uninformative.

Once a representative sample is secured, it must be fixed before sections can be prepared. The choice of fixative is quite important. Ordinarily one would use neutral buffered formalin, and that is still acceptable, but care must be given to compounds that are fluorescent or produce fluorescence. Paraformaldehyde is superior to NBF in many fluorescent staining procedures, but knowledge of what was used should be made known to the microscopist and the individuals who do the immunostaining. Alcoholic fixatives like Bouin's or Omnifix are coagulative or precipitating fixatives and will denature the specimen. This will create the equivalent of a "permeabilized" sample as opposed to aldehyde or additive fixatives that cross-link tissues and reduce swelling. Aldehyde fixation may inhibit penetration of the immunoreagents, while alcohol-based fixatives will increase the staining intensity. Certain aldehydes also will fluoresce, so care must be taken to understand the nature of specimen preparation.

NBF-fixed tissues may require "permeabilization" procedures like the use of Tween or enzymes. Standard immunotechniques then follow with the only general change that one may use slightly more concentrate secondary reagents because of the nature of the images produced. This is explained in detail later. Excellent references for histologic techniques include Kok and Boon 1992; Prophet et al. 1992; Hyatt 1993; Javois 1994; and Kerr and Thorpe 1994.

## CLSM METHODS

In general, one uses the most dilute concentration of the primary antibody to decrease the likelihood of nonspecific staining. Typical concentrations are in the order of a magnitude of 1:100, 1:250, or 1:500. The secondary antibody that is bound to the fluorophore is usually slightly more concentrated in the order of 1:100 or 1:50. Increased concentrations of the secondary are required since images are of a defined single slice of the sample and there must be adequate intensity in that

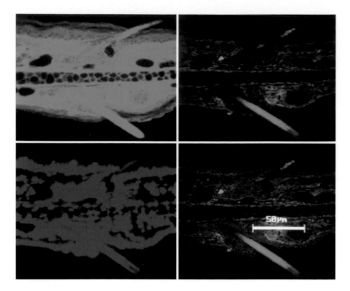

**FIGURE 4.1** Nonconfocal images of mouse skin (two images on left side). The tissue is stained with DAPI, which is a histochemical stain that binds to the groove of DNA and is routinely used as a DNA stain. The keratinocytes are stained with a primary antibody against a pan-cytokeratin protein and then amplified using a FITC-stained secondary against the primary antibody (IgG) species. FITC is green, and DAPI is blue. Confocal images (two images on right side) of the same mouse skin. The images are sharper and cleaner now that out-of-focus fluorescence staining has been eliminated by the pinhole aperture.

smaller slice, while standard epifluorescence is of the whole-cell thickness. Reduced concentrations, shorter incubation periods, and lowered temperatures will reduce nonspecific staining, but there is a trade-off where too little stain will result when one examines small incremental $z$ levels of the specimen. What actually happens in CLSM is that the focal plane for excitation is equivalently focused (e.g., confocal) with the excitation level/point. Therefore, all image planes above and below the focused point are eliminated from the image. The elimination is achieved by the use of a pinhole aperture placed in the beam. Brightness and contrast are determined electronically by settings within the parameter files. Nonconfocal images of a mouse embryo are shown in Figure 4.1—both figures on the left side. The corresponding images using the pinhole aperture are shown in Figure 4.1—both figures on the right side. All of these are of the same section and same $x, y, z$ coordinates. The areas that are intensely bright in the nonconfocal image are clear, focused, and sharp using the CLSM system because all out-of-focus planes have been eliminated. The CLSM image is a uniform thickness (volume).

Depending on the system one uses, multiple fluorphores can be imaged serially or simultaneously. The key determinants are the wavelength, the filter sets, the type of diachronic/mirror beam splitter, the excitation wavelength, and the characteristics of the microscope system. If the CLSM is designed for four-channel operation, like the Zeiss 310 and 410 systems, that allows one to have a red, green, and blue file/image and to put another image (e.g., DIC) into a fourth, which is then simultaneously depicted with the other three channels (Fig. 4.2). Combinations of the three primary colors, red, green, and blue (RGB), produce our perceived colored images. Within an RGB image there are actually three different files, be they tif, jpg, or some other format. They are then simultaneously displayed. Should both green and red occupy the same $x, y$ coordinate, then that pixel would be perceived as yellow. Each coordinate will have an amount of stain that is excited by the proper wavelength. The intensity of that emission is graded according to a photometer. Ordinarily the intensity is expressed as a shade of gray ranging from black (0) to intense white (255). The intensity is measured, and an actual gray scale or intensity level is known for each coordinate/pixel of the image.

The image is scanned using a rasterlike pattern and galvanometer motor–driven lenses that focus within a defined $z$ plane all the $x, y$ coordinates for that image. Since the dilutions are known and the volume is defined by the pinhole and all the parameter settings of the microscope are controlled, then one can objectively measure or quantify the image produced. This is one of the most significant advantages of digital, CLSM imagery.

One can use immunostaining (Fig. 4.1), histochemical stains (Figs. 4.2A, 4.3, 4.6), reflected light (Fig. 4.4), in situ hybridization (Fig. 4.4), and/or transmitted light of unstained material by either phase or Nomarski/DIC (Fig. 4.5). The images can subsequently be combined and simultaneously displayed (Fig. 4.2D) to facilitate the visualization of where exactly in the tissue or organ the protein is located. Multiple immunostaining is usually done with grouped stains such as FITC, rhodamine, and DAPI. These excite with three distinct different wavelength lights at 488, 543, and 364, respectively. Fluorescence is always of a longer wavelength than the incident beam and filter sets, and diachronic mirrors can compensate for these and allow simultaneous imagery. A composite set of images is shown in Figure 4.7. *The Handbook of Biological Confocal Microscopy,* second edition, by Pawley (1995) explains these techniques and cites both review and primary references for all aspects of CLSM. The width and the length of the focused beam are known as a raster size. The raster, or "box" that defines the area or region of interest (ROI), is of a defined pixel size (e.g., 512 × 512 or 1024 × 1024). The larger the raster size, the greater the potential resolution. However, the length of the excitation wavelength and the numerical aperture (NA) of the lens determine

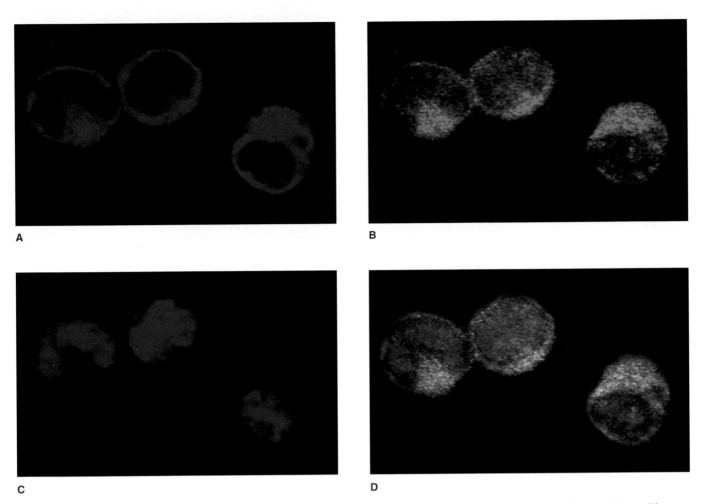

**FIGURE 4.2** Composite image that is made up of red, green, and blue images. The histochemical stain Evans Blue fluoresces red when imaged using a green laser line (**A**) and produces a rhodaminelike image that is confocal. The green image is produced using FITC labeled secondary (**B**), while the histochemical stain DAPI is used to label the DNA in blue (**C**). Shown are individual red, green, and blue images and then an overlay of all three (**D**).

the ultimate resolution. One inherent disadvantage of CLSM is that high-energy, focused excitation wavelengths are focused onto this ROI. This will at least "photo-bleach" this region (Fig. 4.6), but it does outline the raster as well. At worst, in living cells or tissue systems, visible light will induce damage through heat and secondarily by inducing membrane damage to cells. If the excitation wavelength is in the ultraviolet range, the damage can be even more severe as UV damage to DNA, cell membranes, and cellular organelles can induce oxidative damage, free radical generation, and DNA mutations.

The newer two-photon or multiphoton systems will greatly reduce this potential problem. The underlying principle of the multiphoton systems is based on wavelength and energy. In a single-photon system, one unit of energy of an appropriate wavelength will excite on a fluorescent molecule of the appropriate receptor substance. In the case of FITC, the maximum absorbency

or excitation is 488 or 490 nm. One photon of 490 nm will cause the FITC molecule to excite, and its emission is the longer wavelength of about 525. Fluorescence is always a longer wavelength than excitation, since emission is of a "weaker" energy level. In general the shorter the wavelength, the "stronger" the energy of the wave. This is proportional such that wavelengths of 980 will be approximately half the energy of a similar light wave of 490 nm in length. This principle has been applied to the newer two-photon microscope systems. In these instruments, instead of sending a continuous wavelength laser, the excitation is pulsed. The laser emits bursts of photons of light at wavelengths of 1100 nm, for example. The theory is that if two photons of half-maximum intensity strike the target fluorescent molecule "simultaneously" then two wavelengths of half intensity will equal one photon of appropriate intensity. This hypothesis has now been proven correct, and two-photon microscope systems are commercially

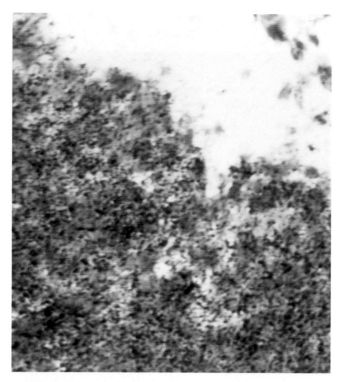

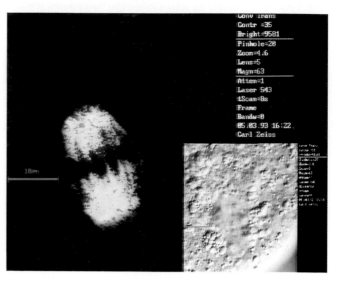

**FIGURE 4.5** Nomarski or differential interference contrast image of a mouse oocyte is shown in black-and-white (inset), while the corresponding confocal image of the DAPI-stained nuclei and FITC-stained tubulin protein structures is shown in blue and green respectively, and colocalized pixels are in yellow.

**FIGURE 4.3** Reflected light image that is confocal of light that reflects back off the dye-stained cells. There is a pinhole aperture in the path but no emission filter. This tissue section is stained with the methylene blue histochemical stain and used in an isotopic autoradiographic image.

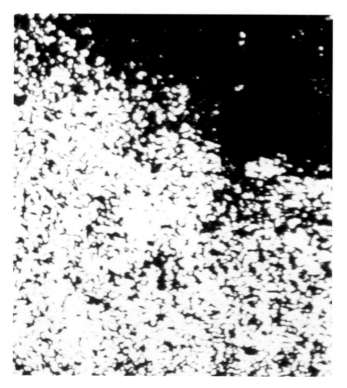

**FIGURE 4.4** The image in Figure 4.3 is now shown using reflected light that comes back off the silver grains. There is a pinhole aperture but no emission filter in this pathway.

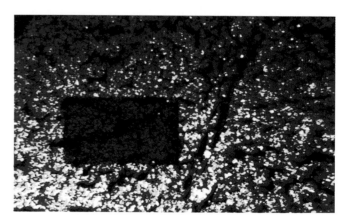

**FIGURE 4.6** This is an FITC-stained tissue section that has been colored using the Zeiss look-up table color profile that artificially colors pixels in a pattern of black through red, orange, yellow, and white according to intensity. The black is lowest, and the white is highest. The confocal image is a raster image of a defined rectangle. As the raster moves across the field, it can photo-bleach the tissue, as is demonstrated in this image. The "looked at" area is darker than the surrounding area. The original confocal image was made at a higher power, and this is a lower-power image that examines a larger area.

available from several vendors. The original work that led to the development of the two-photon system was carried out at Cornell University (Denk et al. 1990). A ti:sapphire laser usually creates the pulse laser system. Detailed information on two-photon systems is available in Pawley's book (1995). An exciting potential application of two-photon microscopy is that the long wavelength laser lines are in the infrared range and are capable of deep penetration into tissues. The intensity of these wavelengths is of considerably less potential energy than those of the visible or ultraviolet spectrum so that damage to cells and tissues is much less severe and these cells and tissues should be viable and injury free for a longer period of time. The other exciting application of two-photon microscopy is that the only excitation occurs at the focus point since that is the only spot within the $z$ dimension (volume) that two simultaneous wavelengths coincide. As a consequence, photo-bleaching, as well as injury, are greatly reduced in cells and tissues. The third advantage is that a number of fluorophores can be imaged simultaneously. Using proper filter sets will enable one to excite with a wavelength of 1100 (ti:sapphire laser) the DNA dye DAPI (345 ex/425 em), the green dye FITC (490 ex/525 em), and the red dye rhodamine (543–560 ex/580 em) with one laser. This will greatly improve our understanding of dynamic cellular processes, the colocalization of proteins, and the three-dimensional structure of cells and tissues.

Using the techniques mentioned above, we have imaged a series of embryos, tissues, and cells to demonstrate the application of CLSM to transgenic/ knockout technology. The following are examples of the application.

The mouse microphthalmia (*mi*) gene affects the development of the eye among other organs. It has been linked to the Waardenburg syndrome and an inherited hearing loss disorder as well as aberrant skin coloration. The defect involves a transcription factor. We evaluated mouse embryos (embryo day [E] 13.5). The image shown in Figure 4.7A is of a mutant mouse carrying the microphthalmia eyeless white (mi ew) mutation. A wild-type embryo is shown in Figure 4.8. The mi gene product is shown by the green FITC staining, nuclear DNA is shown by the blue DAPI staining, and the β-tubulin protein in rhodamine red. In the wt mouse the mi protein goes only to the nucleus (Fig. 4.7B, right side) of the retinal pigmented epithelium (RPE) cells where a transcription factor would be expected. In the mutant mouse the mi protein goes to both the nucleus and the cytoplasm of the RPE cells (Fig. 4.7B, left side). Where both green and red colocalize, the color produced is yellow. This can be easily visualized in most images, but if quantification of the colocalization observation is needed, then additional image analysis can be

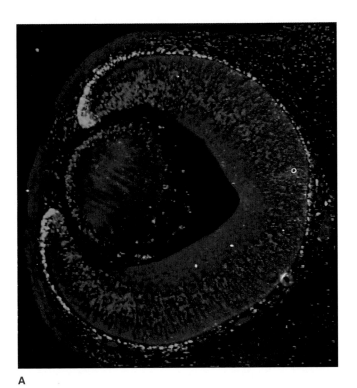

A

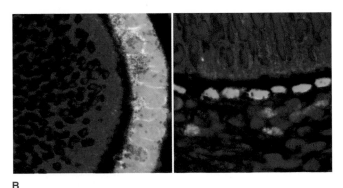

B

**FIGURE 4.7** (A) This is an image of a mutant mouse embryo taken at low power using confocal optics. The nuclei are in blue (DAPI), the microphthalmia (mi) protein is in green (FITC), and the tubulin protein is in red (rhodamine). The mi protein is in both the nucleus and the cytoplasm of the mutant mouse. Wherever red and green colocalize, the color produced is yellow. There is a higher magnification of mi protein in **B** (left side). On right side is higher power of wt.

done. The Zeiss CLSM system has a colocalization program. The red image is loaded into one channel ($x$ axis), and the green image into the other channel ($y$ axis; Figs. 4.9–4.12). The pixels ($x$ and $y$ coordinates) that contain both are displayed in blue (Fig. 4.10). These are the same pixels that are yellow in traditional colocalized images. One can then use the mouse cursor to draw an area that is composed of the colocalized pixels of given values. Those that are highest for both red and green will be in the upper right corner of the graph, while

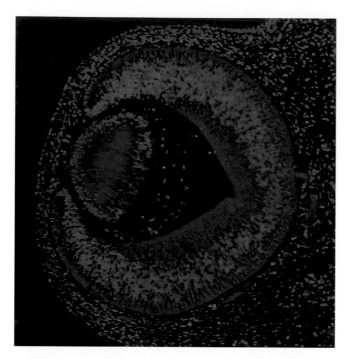

**FIGURE 4.8** The wild-type mouse that corresponds to the mutant in Figure 4.7 is shown in an identical staining pattern here. There is little if any mi protein in the red tubulin areas of the eye (cytoplasm)(Fig. 4.7B, right side).

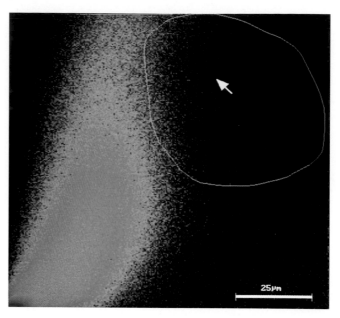

**FIGURE 4.10** Colocalization of Figure 4.9 imagery. FITC pixels on *y* axis, rhodamine in *x* axis, and colocalized pixels are shown in a scatterlike diagram. Highest for both are in upper right; lowest for both in lower left. A degree or amount of intensity is selected and circled in green.

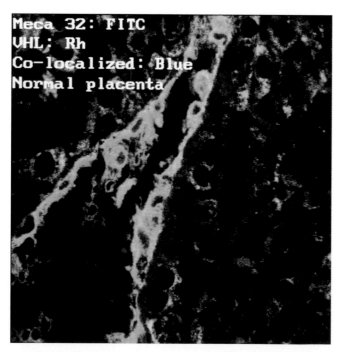

**FIGURE 4.9** Placental tissue is a highly vascularized tissue. Shown here is a red, green, and blue (RGB) image of the labyrinth of the mouse placenta. The red is loaded into channel 1, the green in channel 2, and the blue in channel 3. Using the Zeiss colocalization program, one can ask (Figs. 4.10, 4.11, 4.12) where the area of intense overlap is.

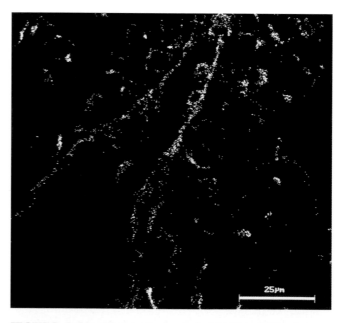

**FIGURE 4.11** Those pixels circled in Fig. 4.10 are shown as blue in an RGB image (Fig. 4.12). They can also be shown as a separate mask of white dots on a black background as shown here.

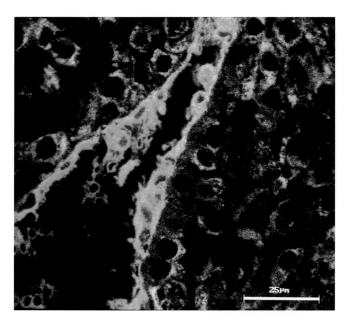

**FIGURE 4.12** The RGB image is loaded now, and those white dots (Fig. 4.11) are now blue in the RGB image.

those high for green and lower for red will be in the upper left quadrant (Fig. 4.10). A mask of these is shown in black-and-white in Figure 4.11. These are then selected and highlighted in blue (Fig. 4.12). The actual number of *x, y* coordinates and their area are also available in the image file. Factors, constructs, and agents that increase or decrease colocalization can be identified and quantified using this digital technology and instrumentation. One can not only colocalize red-green images but also whatever pair of fluorophores is in question; the pair can be placed into the appropriate channels and analyzed as described. This can be done using the Zeiss programs, but most other image analysis programs can do this or be written to do this using their "macro" program capabilities.

CLSM was helpful in understanding the phenotype of transgenic mice that carried an androgen-sensitive flanking region to the SV40 large T antigen (Shibata et al. 1998). When the SV40 T antigen expression was targeted to the genitourinary systems in a series of transgenic mice, adenocarcinoma developed in these tissues (urethral and bulbourethral glands) after 7 months. These sites in humans ordinarily do not develop adenocarcinomas. Since *met* has been implicated in certain tumors and is known to be involved in the transformation of mesenchyme to epithelium (Tsarfaty et al. 1994), we evaluated the expression of *met* in these transgenic animals. *Met* was weakly evident in the normal glands and overexpressed in certain areas of the tumors.

Identification and localization of pigments within brain tissue has also been accomplished using CLSM. In a series of investigations, we evaluated brain sections

from mice. The pathology of these animals is associated with a unique localization to the brain of vacuolated lesions. These vacuoles were hypothesized to be the result of an accumulation of a pigmented product. The pigment was evaluated to see if it could be visualized by CLSM. Using unstained, deparaffinized sections, we examined the tissues using the reflection mode of CLSM. This is similar to immunohistochemistry (see Chap. 13) in its visual effect but does not involve any immuno-staining. Certain pigments, proteins, and structures will reflect light better than other similar compounds, tissues, or structures. Obviously, silver mirrors are excellent reflection compounds, as are metallic silver granules. The reflected light will appear in the CLSM image as a signal that can be focused and defined to a definite volume, just like an immunosignal. The reflection is either yes or no, and the reflection depends on the ability of the material to reflect and the angle and focus of the incident and reflection beams. In the brains of these animals, we recorded definite reflection signals in the locations of certain nuclei that corresponded to the sites of the known lesions within these mice. We then did immunostaining to confirm the locations and to identify the materials within these lesions. Representative images of the mouse brain regions are shown in Figure 4.13. The reflected light (RF) from the green (543) laser are shown in red, while the RF of the blue laser (490) are shown in green. Colocalized spots are shown in yellow. Within mouse placenta and embryo sections, we studied the expression of *VHL* and MECA-32. *VHL* was expressed in placental trophoblasts and yolk sac endoderm (Fig. 4.12).

In addition to examining embryos and newborn animals of transgenic/knockout mice, one can also establish primary cultures or cell lines from both embryos and newborns. In the case of lethal constructs, often the cell lines are the only possible method to obtain cell biologic characterizations of the induced changes. The isolated cells are established using standard tissue culture techniques (Freshney 1994). CLSM or two-photon analysis of living cells is best done using specialized culture substrates. The working distance of many lenses used in CLSM is less than that of ordinary lenses. It is, therefore, best if the substrate is thin so that valuable focusing/working distance is available for the depth into cells and tissues rather than penetrating the glass or plastic culture vessel substrate. The optimal lenses currently used in biological microscopy are the water immersion, long working distance lenses. One should use water-based lenses that have a refractive index near to that of water ($n = 1.33$). Zeiss uses a C-Apochromat as its water immersion lens. The working distance for its lens is 220 μm as opposed to 75–100 μm for ordinary lenses. Using such lenses requires one to use cover glass of matching thickness. One should use number

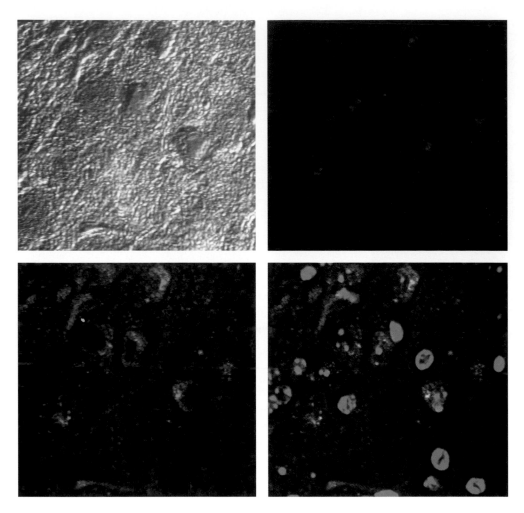

**FIGURE 4.13** These are images from a transgenic mouse. Using reflected light that will identify pigments within the tissue, we imaged using both green and blue laser lines. The blue laser will induce a green emission (lower left), while the green line will induce a red emission (upper right). These R and G images have been overlaid onto a DAPI-stained image (lower right) to produce this RGB image of the mouse transgenic brain. The Nomarski/DIC image is in the upper left.

1 (0.17 mm) cover glasses. If one uses the standard flask-ette, chamber slide, or any similar product with an inverted microscope CLSM, the actual thickness of the glass or plastic substrate will reduce the working distance and distort the resolution of one's lens. If one uses an upright type of microscope, then one should place onto the slide or substrate an appropriate cover glass after staining.

The clarity of the cell structure is noted by using the Nomarski/DIC optics. This transmitted light image provides optimal structure orientation for the subsequent fluorescent imagery. FITC images can be overlaid onto the Nomarski image for improved understanding of the light-fluorescent relationship. In a recent paper by Huang et al. (1999) isolated dendritic cells from a transgenic/knockout animal were imaged using CLSM. The hypothesis was that pigments were transported along cytoskeletal filaments. To prove this hypothesis by microscopy, the compound was colabeled using a marker for the intermediate filaments as well as the actin fibers. The colocalization of the two probes is evident in the yellow-stained areas. Huang et al. (1999) used CLSM to supplement the molecular data to show how cells can use their microtubule networks for long-range transport of cellular components and their actin microfilaments for short-range transport. The coordination for these parallel and supplementary transports are coordinated by motor proteins although the actual mechanisms are poorly understood.

We have also utilized green fluorescent protein (GFP) and all its variants to identify the expression of proteins within cells and organs. GFP has many varieties. There are mitoses that express in the visible range as well as the UV range. In a recent publication by Stauber et al. (1998), the full range of GFP mutants have been explained in detail. The multiple phenotypes of GFP

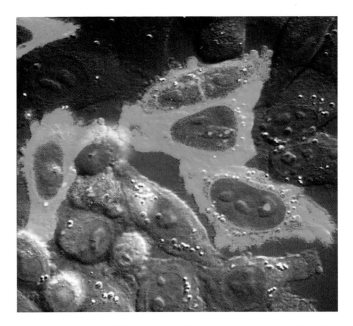

**FIGURE 4.14** GFP is green fluorescent protein that is a jellyfish protein. The gene that codes for this protein has been obtained from the aquatic animal and transfected into cells or tissue. The protein (GFP) is an indicator protein that marks where the transgene or transfected gene has inserted and produced protein in the target tissue. Wherever there is green, there is also the protein of choice. These cells produce an intracytoplasmic HIV-associated protein. Cells are imaged using Nomarksi optics.

enable researchers to use them in dual-color tagging in living cells. Isolated cells can be analyzed by CLSM, and the observations correlated with Western and Northern analysis to scc if the cells are making the protein of interest. A representative image of a GFP-expressing cell is shown in Figure 4.14. Although not a transgenic or knockout experiment as such, we examined the change in phenotype that resulted when *met* was expressed in a fibrosarcoma cell line. In a series of experiments (Rong et al. 1993, 1994), coexpression of met and hepatocyte growth factor (HGF) in fibroblasts led to the development of a rapidly invasive, autocrine loop–mediated fibrosarcoma. We also noted that certain areas within the tumor expressed an epithelial phenotype. In a series of experiments (Tsarfaty et al. 1992, 1994), we observed how the expression of Met proteins induced an epithelial phenotype. If such a hypothesis was proposed for similar signaling proteins, then the measurement of the protein could be done in a similar manner to the analysis that we did in Tsarfaty et al. 1992 and 1994. We showed coexpression, quantitated the fluorescent expression, and correlated light, CLSM, and electron microscopy to precisely and quantitatively determine the role of Met in changing cellular phenotypes.

## REFERENCES

Adams, J.M., and Cory, S. 1991. Transgenic models of tumor development. Science 254: 1161–1167.

Allred, D.C., Harvey, J.M., Berardo, M., et al. 1998. Prognostic and predictive factors in breast cancer by immunohistochemical analysis. Mod. Pathol. 11: 155–168.

Askew, D.S., and Heffelfinger, S. 1998. Graduate education in microscopic anatomy. Anat. Rec. 253: 143–146.

Cavanagh, H.D., Petroll, W.M., and Jester, J.V. 1993. The application of confocal microscopy to the study of living systems. Neurosci. Biobehav. Rev. 17: 483–498.

Dean-Clower, E., Vortmeyer, A.O., Bonner, R.E., et al. 1997. Micro-dissection based genetic discovery and analysis applied to cancer progression. Cancer Sci. Am. J. 3: 259–265.

Denk, W., Strickler, J.H., and Webb, W.W. 1990. Two-photon laser scanning fluorescence microscopy. Science 248: 73–76.

Freshney, R.I., 1994. Culture of Animal Cells: A Manual of Basic Technique. New York: Wiley-Liss.

Furness, P.N. 1997. The use of digital images in pathology. J. Pathol. 183: 253–263.

Hamilton, P.W., and Allen, D.C. 1995. Morphometry in histopathology. J. Pathol. 175: 369–379.

Hanahan, D. 1988. Dissecting multistep tumorigenesis in transgenic mice. Annu. Rev. Genet. 22: 479–519.

Hasegawa, S. 1998. Multi-photon fluorescence microscopy. Acat. Hist. Cyto. 31: 293–296.

Huang, J.D., Brady, S.T., Richards, B.W., et al. 1999. Direct interaction of microtubule- and actin-based transport motors. Nature 397: 267–270.

Hyatt, M. 1993. Stains and Cytochemical Methods. New York: Plenum Press.

Jaenisch, R. 1988. Transgenic animals. Science 240: 1468–1474.

Javois, L. 1994. Methods in Molecular Biology, in Immunocytochemical Methods and Protocols. Totowa, NJ: Humana Press.

Kerr, M., and Thorpe, R. 1994. Immunochemistry Lab Fax Bios. Oxford, UK: Academic Press.

Kimura, K., Sasano, H., Shimosegawa, T., et al. 1997. Ultrastructural and confocal laser scanning microscopic examination of TUNEL-positive cells. J. Pathol. 181: 235–242.

Klineberg, E., Tsarfaty, I., Alvord, W.G., et al. 1996. Correction and Quantification of Normal Differentiation in Human Epithelium: Application for Optimas 4.0 Image Analysis Program. Cell Vision 3: 402–406.

Kok, L., and Boon, M. 1992. Microwave cookbook for microscopists. Leyden, Netherlands: Coulomb Press.

Lehr, H.A., Mankoff, D.A., Corwin, D., et al. 1997. Application of Photoshop-based image analysis to quantification of hormone receptor expression in breast cancer. J. Histochem. Cytochem. 45: 1559–1565.

Majno, G., and Joris, I. 1995. Apoptosis, oncosis and necrosis: an overview of cell death. Am. J. Pathol. 146: 3–15.

Matsumoto, B. 1993. Methods in cell biology, in Cell Biological Applications of Confocal Microscopy. San Diego: Academic Press.

Merlino, G. 1994. Transgenic mice as models for tumorigenesis. Cancer Invest. 12: 203–213.

Pawley, J. 1995, Handbook of Biological Confocal Microscopy, 2nd ed. New York: Plenum Press.

Prophet, E., Mills, B., Arrington, J., et al. 1992. Laboratory Methods in Histotechnology. Washington, DC: AFIP.

Rong, S., Oskarsson, M., Faletto, D., et al. 1993. Tumorigenesis induced by co-expression of human hepatocyte growth factor and the human *met* protooncogene leads to high levels of expression of the ligand and receptor. Cell Growth Differ. 4: 563–569.

Rong, S., Segal, S., Anver, M., et al. 1994. Invasiveness and metastasis of NIH 3T3 cells induced by Met-hepatocyte growth factor/scatter factor autocrine stimulation. Proc. Natl. Acad. Sci. USA 91: 4731–4735.

Salisbury, J. 1994. Three-dimensional reconstruction in microscopial morphology. Histol. Histopathol. 9: 773–780.

Shibata, M.A., Jorcyk, C.L., Devor, D.E., et al. 1998. Altered expression of transforming growth factor betas during urethral and bulbourethral gland tumor progression in transgenic mice carrying the androgen-responsive C3(1)5′ flanking region fused to SV40 large T antigen. Carcinogenesis 19: 195–205.

Stauber, R.H., Horie, K., Carney, P., et al. 1998. Development and applications of enhanced green fluorescent protein mutants. Biotechniques 24: 462–466, 468–471.

Tekola, P., Zhu, Q., and Baak, J.P. 1994. Confocal laser microscopy and image processing for three-dimensional microscopy: technical principles and an application to breast cancer. Hum. Pathol. 25: 12–21.

Tsarfaty, I., Resau, J.H., Rulong, S., et al. 1992. The met proto-oncogene receptor and lumen formation. Science 257: 1258–1261.

Tsarfaty, I., Rong, S., Resau, J.H., et al. 1994. The Met proto-oncogene mesenchymal to epithelial cell conversion. Science 263: 98–101.

Tsarfaty, I., Alvord, W.G., Resau, J.H., et al. 1999. Alteration of Met protooncogene product expression and prognosis in breast carcinomas. Anal. Quant. Cytol. Histol. 21(5): 397–408.

## Web Sites

[*http://www.cs.ubc.ca/spider/ladic/confocal.html*]
This home page indicates what one can do with the 3-D techniques. Information is provided in six areas: introduction to 3-D, specimen preparation, data acquisition, image processing, volume visualization, and references.

*http://listserv.acsu.buffalo.edu/archives/confocal.html*]
This page is devoted to a series of questions and answers about CLSM.

[*http://pharmacy.arizona.edu/centers/toxcenter/swehsc/exp_path/conf_www.html*]
This is a complete list of CLSM resources on the World Wide Web.

[*http://www.isc.tamu.edu/BIO/cellvolumes*]
This is a site that is devoted to three-dimensional reconstruction applications of CLSM.

# 5
# Measurement of Cell Replication and Apoptosis in Mice

Robert R. Maronpot, Norris D. Flagler, Thai-Vu T. Ton, Julie F. Foley, and Thomas L. Goldsworthy

This chapter focuses primarily on practical methods for assessing cell proliferation and apoptosis in tissue sections from mice. Alternative methods (e.g., biochemical, flow cytometric, molecular) that may also be used to assess cell cycle and apoptotic activity have been covered in the literature (Baserga and Wiebel 1969; Zietz and Nicolini 1978; Hall and Levison 1990; Alison et al. 1994; Amati and Land 1994; Baserga et al. 1994; Gong et al. 1994; Loyer et al. 1994; Piwnica-Worms 1994; Levine and Broach 1995) and will not be presented in this chapter. Information on apoptosis can be found in recent books (Bowen and Bowen 1990; Tomei and Cope 1991; Lavin and Watters 1993; Slyuser 1996). The emphasis in this chapter is on the authors' experience. The approaches and techniques described apply equally to genetically engineered and conventional mice. It is assumed that the ultimate goal of studies on cell growth is assessment of organ or tissue status as influenced by the balance between cell birth and cell death. Thus, in most instances, obtaining measurements of both cell proliferation and cell death parameters is warranted.

## CELL PROLIFERATION

Since passage through S-phase is an obligatory step in cell proliferation, this measurement has been frequently used to measure cell proliferation. Passage through S-phase, however, is not absolute proof that the cell will ultimately undergo cell division since cells that have undergone replicative DNA synthesis may arrest prior to undergoing mitosis (Wilke et al. 1988) and subse-quently may be removed from the proliferating pool by undergoing apoptosis. For some rodent tissues, such as liver and salivary glands, replicative DNA synthesis may result in increased ploidy without cell division (Carriere 1967; Brodsky and Uryvaeva 1977; Stein and Kudryav-tsev 1992; Lin and Allison 1993). This is a frequent occurrence in mouse liver, where the proportion of tetraploid and octaploid cells increases as the animal ages (Fig. 5.1). Despite these potential limitations, calculation of the S-phase labeling index remains a primary means of quantitating the cell proliferative state; thus, S-phase is indicative of cell replication. The ability to

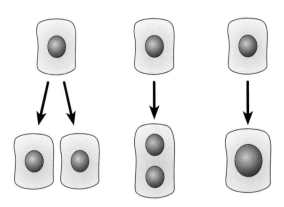

**FIGURE 5.1** Replicative DNA synthesis of diploid hepatocytes in the mouse may result in production of two diploid daughter cells, a binucleated original cell that is tetraploid by virtue of having two diploid nuclei, or the original cell with a single tetraploid nucleus. As the mouse ages, the proportion of tetraploid and octaploid hepatocytes increases.

detect S-phase cells in tissue sections allows for corre-lating the proliferative state in specific target cells with histopathological changes (Goldsworthy et al. 1991).

The identification of S-phase cells involves (1) use of exogenously introduced labeling agents that can ulti-mately be visualized in tissue sections, (2) staining of intrinsic tissue proteins reflective of cycling cells, or (3) a combination of both approaches. Even if one relies primarily on a single methodological approach, it is reassuring to generate at least a limited amount of data by an alternative method as a means of confirming the primary selected approach or, alternatively, linking to other measurements of the cell cycle such as mitosis.

## Exogenous Labeling Agents

Tritiated thymidine ($^3$H-TdR) and bromodeoxyuridine (BrdU) are two frequently used labeling agents for iden-tifying cells undergoing replicative DNA synthesis. When present in the nucleotide pool, these thymidine analogues are incorporated into newly synthesized DNA by substituting for thymidine. The extent of incor-poration is dependent upon the amount of labeling agent present as well as the duration of labeling. The amount of labeling agent (the dose) should be sufficient to allow enough incorporation into newly synthesized DNA to permit the ultimate visualization of cells that are in S-phase of the cell cycle but should be below the level of toxicity. High doses of these potentially toxic agents can induce cellular damage resulting in either unscheduled DNA synthesis or overt cytotoxicity with subsequent compensatory enhanced cell proliferation. Either situation could obviously compromise interpre-tation of a study. The extent of labeling is directly dependent upon the amount of exogenous labeling agent incorporated and the length of S-phase. These two factors will directly affect the intensity of the stain. For example, if labeling agent is present and available throughout a 10-hour period of S-phase, a relatively large amount of the agent will be incorporated into the newly synthesized DNA, providing the cells are in S-phase for a large portion of the 10-hour period. Cells leaving the S-phase compartment just as labeling agent becomes available and cells just entering the S-phase compartment at the end of the 10-hour period will incorporate small amounts of labeling agent and, thus, will be more difficult to score as positive. On the other hand, if the labeling agent is present for only 30 min-utes during a 10-hour S-phase, small amounts of label-ing agent will be incorporated into newly synthesized DNA, subsequent visualization will be less dramatic, and the number of cells scored as positive will be less. The approximate durations of various phases of the cell cycle for epithelial cells are given in Table 5.1. These times are intended as a relative comparison and do not

**TABLE 5.1. Duration of phases of the cell cycle for rapidly proliferating mouse epithelial cells**

| Cell cycle phase | Average duration (h) | Range (h) |
|---|---|---|
| $G_0$ | 24 | 12–50 |
| $G_1$ | 11 | 3–38 |
| S | 10 | 5–25 |
| $G_2$ | 3 | 1–15 |
| M | 1 | 0.4–1.4 |

Source: From data in Bisconte 1979 and Wright and Alison 1984.

take into account the observation that cells may remain in $G_0$ for days or weeks, and cells in the proliferating pool may arrest in $G_1$ or $G_2$ (Pederson and Gelfant 1970; Gelfant 1981).

Tritiated thymidine ($^3$H-TdR) has been used as a labeling agent for decades. Once incorporated into newly synthesized DNA, it can be visualized by cover-ing the tissue section with a photographic emulsion and allowing a sufficient time for the energy emitted by the radioactive thymidine to expose the silver grains in the overlying photographic emulsion. Application and sub-sequent exposure of the photographic emulsion is car-ried out in the dark and typically requires days to months to sufficiently expose the emulsion. The emulsion-coated slides are developed, much as photo-graphic film is developed, and then the tissue is stained with a histologic dye, "coverslipped," and visualized microscopically. Positive cells are identified by discrete silver grains that overlie the nucleus of any cell that incorporated the $^3$H-TdR. Cells are scored as positive when the number of silver grains exceeds whatever background silver grains are present on the section. As an indicator of proper systemic exposure to the $^3$H-TdR as well as a positive control for the histoautoradio-graphic technique, it is recommended that a section of small intestine be included on each slide that is to be evaluated. Technical factors and pitfalls in use of $^3$H-TdR and autoradiography have been reviewed (Bisconte 1979; Maurer 1981; Simpson-Herren 1987). Some advantages and disadvantages of labeling S-phase cells with $^3$H-TdR are listed in Table 5.2.

Bromodeoxyuridine (BrdU) has been used in recent years in lieu of $^3$H-TdR and has been reported to yield quantitatively similar results (Lanier et al. 1989; Eldridge et al. 1990). Once incorporated into newly synthesized DNA, the label can be visualized immuno-histochemically using commercially available anti-BrdU antibody. The antibody binds to single-stranded DNA. Positive cells are identified by chromogen-staining of the nuclei. There should be virtually no background staining with this procedure. Setting the threshold for

**TABLE 5.2.  Advantages and disadvantages of exogenously adminstered labeling agents**

Tritiated thymidine ($^3$H-TdR)
Advantages
   Well-established procedure
   Sensitive
   Lower-end cutoff is clear
   Automated morphometric grain count possible
Disadvantages
   Long emulsion exposure times
   Radioactive containment issues
   Potential toxicity
   Difficult to assess tissue morphology

Bromodeoxyuridine (BrdU)
Advantages
   Well-established procedure
   Rapid procedure
   As sensitive as $^3$H-TdR
   No radioactive disposal costs
Disadvantages
   Poorly defined lower-end cutoff for positive cells
   Potential toxicity

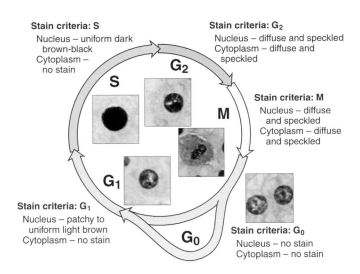

**FIGURE 5.2**  Characteristic features of PCNA-stained hepatocytes in different phases of the cell cycle.

when to score weakly stained nuclei as positive represents a shortcoming of this immunohistochemical approach. It is recommended that a piece of small intestine from each animal be included on each slide to serve as a control to indicate appropriate delivery of the BrdU and to simultaneously show the sensitivity of the immunohistochemical technique. Small intestine has a high intrinsic rate of cell proliferation and should always be positive even with short exposure to BrdU. The current BrdU staining method used at the National Institute of Environmental Health Sciences can be found on the Internet [*http://dir.niehs.nih.gov/dirlep/immuno.html*]. The advantages and disadvantages of labeling S-phase cells with BrdU are listed in Table 5.2.

# Intrinsic Measures of Cell Proliferation

Counting mitotic figures in tissue sections has long been used as a measure of cellular proliferative activity. This is generally done on hematoxylin and eosin stained histopathological sections, and the results reflect the percentage of cells undergoing morphologically recognizable mitosis at the moment the tissue is harvested. Since the duration of mitosis represents a relatively transient portion of a cell's proliferative cycle (see Table 5.1), only a few cells may be in the mitotic phase at a particular moment in time. Thus, measurement of the mitotic index is relatively insensitive. One way to increase the sensitivity of mitotic index measurements is to administer a stathmokinetic agent such as colcemid or vinblastin an hour or two before collecting tissue (Tannock 1965; Wright and Appleton 1980; Alabi and Alison

1984). Colcemid, a mitotic spindle poison, maintains any cells undergoing mitosis in metaphase, allowing accumulation of recognizable mitotic cells and, thereby, increasing the sensitivity of this measure of cell proliferative activity. Arrested metaphase cells begin to undergo visible degenerative changes 60 to 90 minutes following administration of colcemid (Wright and Appleton 1980). Thus, care should be taken to harvest tissues between 1 and 2 hours after administration of this compound.

Proliferating cell nuclear antigen (PCNA) is a 36,000–molecular weight auxiliary protein of DNA polymerase delta, an enzyme vital for DNA replication (Kurki et al. 1986; Bravo et al. 1987). PCNA is differentially expressed during different phases of the cell cycle. Synthesis begins in late $G_1$ of the cell cycle and peaks during S-phase. It is a relatively stable protein found in all tissues. Commercially available antibodies allow for immunohistochemical staining of PCNA. For many tissues, intensity and cellular localization of staining allows for classifying cells into $G_1$, S, $G_2$, and M fractions (phases) of the cell cycle (Figs. 5.2, 5.3). The PCNA labeling index is a measure of cell cycle activity at the time the tissue was harvested, taking into account the ~18-hour half-life of PCNA in tissue. The PCNA S-phase index is similar to a 30-minute pulse dose BrdU or $^3$H-TdR S-phase index (Eldridge et al. 1993; Foley et al. 1993). Immunohistochemical procedures for PCNA staining have been described (Greenwell et al. 1991, 1993; Foley et al. 1993). The current procedure used at the National Institute of Environmental Health Sciences can be found on the Internet [*http://dir.niehs.nih.gov/dirlep/immuno.html*]. The advantages and disadvantages of PCNA as a measure of cell cycle activity are presented in Table 5.3.

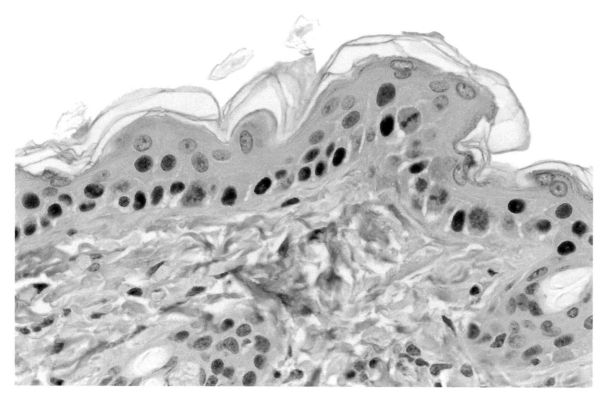

**FIGURE 5.3** Section of mouse skin stained for PCNA. Darker brown basal cells are considered to be in S-phase, while faintly staining nuclei are in $G_1$. Diffuse, speckled cytoplasmic staining is present in mitotic epidermal cells.

**TABLE 5.3. Advantages and disadvantages of PCNA immunohistochemistry as a method for assessing cell proliferation**

Advantages
  Does not require administration of an exogenous labeling
    agent
  Works on archival fixed samples
  Provides rapid results for evaluation
  Allows for identification of cells in various phases of the
    cell cycle
Disadvantages
  May not be useful in tissues with slow cell turnover
  May not be reliable in transformed cells (potentially
    influenced by perturbations in growth factors,
    oncogenes, DNA repair, etc.)
  May miss early or late proliferation spikes (e.g., snapshot
    view only)

**TABLE 5.4. Examples of intrinsic tissue capacity for cell replication**

High
  Skin
  Esophagus
  Intestine
  Bone marrow
Medium
  Liver
  Salivary glands
  Bone and cartilage
  Kidney
Low
  Neurons
  Cardiac muscle
  Skeletal muscle

Another intrinsic cell proliferation marker, Ki-67 (MIB-5), has recently been shown to yield acceptable immunohistochemical staining in rodent tissues (Gerlach et al. 1997; Ito et al. 1998; Reed et al. 1998). Ki-67 provides a proliferative index by labeling all cells in $G_1$, S, $G_2$, and M fractions. While we have no hands-on experience with this intrinsic marker of cell prolifer-

ation, interested investigators are encouraged to consult these relevant references.

## Considerations in Selecting Methods for Identifying Proliferating Cells

Different tissues have different inherent rates of cell proliferation (Table 5.4). Normal small intestinal epithelium, for example, is completely replaced by newly pro-

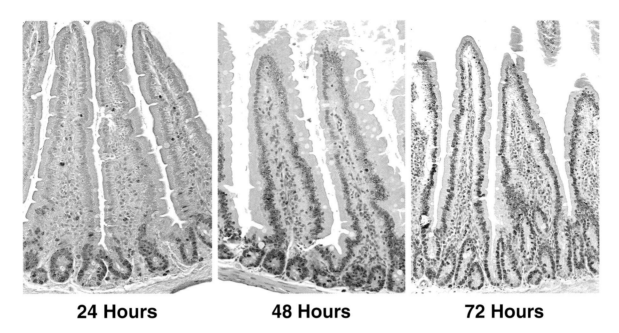

24 Hours        48 Hours        72 Hours

**FIGURE 5.4** Immunohistochemical staining of incorporated BrdU in the small intestine of the mouse following 24, 48, or 72 hours of administration by osmotic minipump. While predominantly crypt epithelium is labeled during 24 hours of BrdU administration, progressively more of the villous epithelium becomes labeled with longer periods of continuous administration.

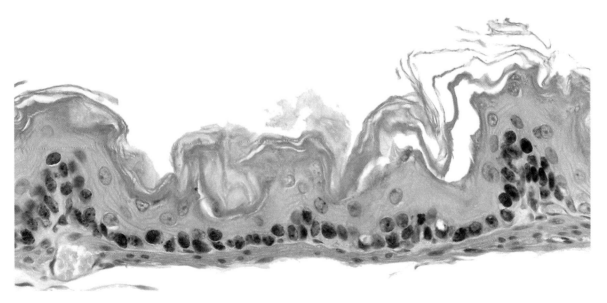

**FIGURE 5.5** The entire basal layer of the forestomach mucosal epithelium is labeled following 24 hours of continuous BrdU administration.

liferating cells in approximately 72 hours (Fig. 5.4). Lymphoid and myeloid tissue may, likewise, maintain an inherently high rate of proliferation. The entire population of basal cells in the rodent forestomach is labeled following a 24-hour dosing with BrdU (Fig. 5.5). Other tissues in a normal state, such as liver and kidney, have a slow rate of normal cell proliferation, on the order of weeks or months. Neural tissue or skeletal

muscle has yet a slower rate of cell proliferation. Because of different inherent rates of cell proliferation between tissues, a given labeling technique is unlikely to be ideal for all tissues. While a pulse dose of BrdU would identify a quantifiable number of S-phase cells in the small intestinal crypts, only a few hepatocytes or renal tubule cells would be labeled by the same pulse dose, making it difficult to generate a sensitive S-phase count for these latter tissues. For obtaining cell proliferation rates from tissues with an inherently slower rate of proliferation than intestine, multiple injections of an exogenous labeling agent or continuous administration of an exogenous labeling agent for several days may be necessary to generate a measurable S-phase labeling index (LI). Some tissues, such as liver, are conditionally highly proliferative. Comparison of LIs in control animals, where cell proliferation is low, to those in animals exposed to a hepatocytotoxic agent or a hepatomitogenic agent, where cell proliferation would be conditionally high, requires selection of a labeling interval that will capture data from both groups of animals. In this example with liver, a pulse dose of exogenous labeling agent might be adequate for the treated group but would be insufficient for a reliable measure of cell proliferation in the control group. Continuous labeling for 24 to 72 hours would yield sufficiently sensitive results in both control and treated groups. This type of approach would also allow for reasonable control values that would permit examination of circumstances that lead to inhibition of cell proliferation (e.g., diet restriction).

In situations where an exogenous labeling agent cannot be administered, such as when using archival samples, immunostaining of PCNA is a reasonable choice for tissues that have a moderate to high cell proliferation rate. The PCNA S-phase LI should be approximately equivalent to a BrdU pulse dose LI. It is always possible to stain for PCNA in situations where the animal has had prolonged exposure to an exogenous labeling agent such as BrdU. In such situations, the BrdU S-phase LI can be acquired from tissues with a slower turnover (e.g., liver, kidney) while the PCNA S-phase LI can be acquired from tissues with a rapid turnover (e.g., intestine, forestomach).

# Methods for Administration of Exogenous Labeling Agents

## SINGLE OR MULTIPLE INJECTIONS
The most common method for administration of labeling agents such as $^3$H-TdR or BrdU is by intraperitoneal injection in a saline vehicle. The labeling agent is rapidly absorbed and incorporated into cells undergoing replicative DNA synthesis. It is fairly traditional for investigators to inject their animals with $^3$H-TdR or BrdU 2 hours prior to necropsy. While this is practical and allows time to complete the injections and prepare for the necropsy, it should not be assumed that there is continuous labeling of S-phase cells during the entire interval between injection and necropsy. The availability of injected $^3$H-TdR or BrdU for incorporation into replicating DNA is approximately 20–30 minutes (Hell-man and Ullberg 1986; Wynford-Thomas and Williams 1986; deFazio et al. 1987; Boswald et al. 1990). Following subcutaneous injection of $^3$H-TdR, the maximum concentration in the blood appears within minutes and subsequently decreases nearly exponentially with a half-life of 10 to 20 minutes (Carlsson et al. 1979). Once labeled, the cells will retain their label for several hours or days in rapidly dividing cells and for months in slowly dividing cells (Ward et al. 1991), with progressively diminished label retention as labeled cells divide into daughter cells. If a somewhat longer interval of labeling is necessary, multiple intraperitoneal injections may be given at selected intervals. Subcutaneous injections also can be used and should result in a somewhat slower absorption of the labeling agent, particularly if the vehicle is corn oil. Recommended injection doses of $^3$H-TdR and BrdU for mice are 1 µCi/g body weight and 50 mg/kg body weight, respectively (Table 5.5).

## OSMOTIC MINIPUMPS
Administration of labeling agents for 24 hours or longer, even up to 2 weeks or longer, can be achieved by using surgically implanted osmotic minipumps. These devices are available in different sizes and with different pumping rates [*http://www.alzet.com*]. They allow for the continuous slow administration of the labeling agent and are ideal for tissues with a low intrinsic rate of cell proliferation, where continuous administration of labeling agent is critical. The use of an anesthetic and the surgical procedure associated with implantation may be accompanied by some unwanted physiological effects (Wyatt et al. 1995) and, thus, may not be appropriate for some research. The recommended concentration for continuous dosing of mice with $^3$H-TdR is 1 mCi/ml with a specific activity ranging from 25 to 90 mCi/mmol, and for continuous dosing of mice with BrdU, 30 mg/ml when the rate of delivery is 1 µl/h (Table 5.5).

In a study comparing the prolonged administration of BrdU by osmotic minipump and slow-release pellets, it was shown that prolonged administration by subcutaneously implanted pellets may be associated with toxic effects that could either increase or decrease cell proliferation rates (Weghorst et al. 1991). The authors suggest that slow-release pellets may not provide a constant rate of BrdU release and suggest that minipump administration is preferable for prolonged BrdU administration. Caution is recommended in interpreting data from prolonged BrdU administration; rigorous preliminary studies are needed to establish nontoxic doses.

## DRINKING WATER ADMINISTRATION
We have recently explored the merits of BrdU administration in the drinking water for toxicology-based cell

**TABLE 5.5.  Recommended dosage of exogenous labeling agents for mice**

|  | [3]H-TdR | BrdU | Colcemid |
|---|---|---|---|
| Pulse dose | 1 µCi/g BW | 50 mg/kg BW | 1–4 mg/kg BW |
| Continuous administration |  |  |  |
|     Osmotic pump | Specific activity of 25–90 mCi/mmol | NA | NA |
|  | Concentration of 1 mCi/mL | Concentration of 30 mg/ml | NA |
|  | Delivery rate of 1 µL/h | Delivery rate of 1 µL/h | NA |
|     Drinking water | NA | Concentration of 0.2 mg/ml | NA |

proliferation analysis in mice (Ton et al. 1997). The periodic drinking habits of rodents, particularly during the evening hours, should provide the opportunity for long-term intermittent labeling of S-phase cells. Under the assumption that drinking habits are relatively consistent between groups, comparison of treated versus controls, or transgenic versus wild-type animals, is possible using dose water for administration of BrdU. Should there be a difference in water consumption between the animal groups being compared, measurement of water consumption will provide an estimate of the amount of BrdU consumed over a finite period of time.

While results from drinking water administration of BrdU are not expected to be quantitatively similar to those of continuous administration via osmotic minipump, the use of dosed water for administration is practical and cost-effective and permits comparison of results between groups of animals (Ton et al. 1997). Thus, relative comparisons would be valid, but an LI from a dosed water study would not be as exact as that from administration by osmotic minipump. Experiments requiring more precise labeling data necessitate use of osmotic minipumps. As a further caution in adopting the dosed water route of delivering BrdU, there is some evidence that metabolism may be sufficiently rapid to preclude accurate labeling of proliferating immune cells (Jecker et al. 1997). The implication here is that rapid metabolism of orally administered BrdU may prevent sufficient labeling agent from reaching lymphoid and bone marrow cells such that BrdU incorporation is below a level necessary for immunohistochemical detection.

## Selecting Doses of Exogenous Labeling Agents

While low levels of [3]H-TdR and BrdU do not apparently interfere with the cell cycle, there is concern that high doses of these agents may be toxic, resulting in enhanced LIs (Maurer 1981; Wynford-Thomas and Williams 1986; Goldsworthy et al. 1992). Recom-

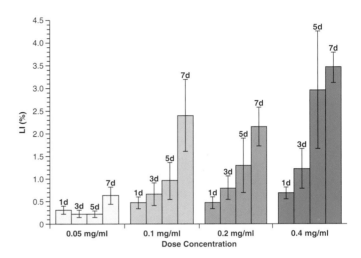

**FIGURE 5.6** The hepatocyte labeling index in mice receiving different concentrations of BrdU in drinking water for 1, 3, 5, or 7 days. Bars represent means. Error bars are standard deviations.

mended doses that do not result in toxicity are presented in Table 5.5.

In an effort to determine the lowest concentration of BrdU in drinking water that will result in acceptable immunostaining, mice were given 0.05, 0.1, 0.2, and 0.4 mg of BrdU/ml of drinking water for up to 1 week. Immunostaining of liver sections and determination of LI are presented in Fig. 5.6. Based on these results, we recommend a concentration of 0.1 to 0.2 mg BrdU per ml for drinking water administration in mice. Ton et al. (1997) compared liver labeling indices following BrdU administration in drinking water with those following osmotic minipump administration.

In studies conducted in our laboratory, aqueous solutions of BrdU were found to be stable for 35 days at room temperature or 4°C at a concentration of 0.05 mg/ml. Samples stored in clear or amber drinking water bottles exposed to light and air for 7 days showed no significant loss of BrdU. The dose analysis method was validated over a concentration range of 0.0409 to 0.50 mg/ml. It is noteworthy that blood and liver samples taken at necropsy at 9 a.m. had minimal to no detectable levels of free BrdU when BrdU was administered in drinking water at 0.05 to 0.4 mg/ml (unpublished observation). However, adequate BrdU immunostaining was observed in liver sections.

## Counting/Measurement of Indices

One of the most important considerations in determining mitotic or labeling indices relates to generation of the denominator data for the calculation:

$$\text{Mitotic index (MI)} = \frac{\text{Number of mitotic cells}}{\substack{\text{Total number of cells examined} \\ \text{(mitotic + nonmitotic)}}}$$

$$\text{Labeling index (LI)} = \frac{\text{Number of labeled cells}}{\substack{\text{Total number of cells examined} \\ \text{(labeled + nonlabeled)}}}$$

The generation of denominator values for the above calculations is labor-intensive but is required for precise estimation of indices, especially when investigating potential dose responses. It is generally acceptable to count 1000 to 2000 cells for estimating LI.

For a relatively solid tissue such as the liver, when the cellular density is similar in all portions of the hepatic lobule, one labor-saving approach in generating an MI is to determine the average number of hepatocytes per microscopic field and then simply to count the number of mitoses per microscopic field and calculate the MI as follows:

$$\text{MI} = \frac{\text{Total number of mitoses in all microscopic fields examined}}{\substack{\text{Number of microscopic fields examined} \\ \times \text{ Average number of hepatocytes} \\ \text{per microscopic field}}}$$

Simply counting mitotic figures per microscopic field without determining the denominator is rapid and may be a reasonable first estimate of relative mitotic rates between groups of animals. If the cellular density per microscopic field of view is essentially identical between the groups of animals being compared, then counting mitotic figures per microscopic field or per square millimeter area for solid tissues is certainly reasonable. Counting mitoses per microscopic field has also been used for decades by pathologists when grading neoplasia (Quinn and Wright 1992). To generate the data, one only has to settle on the number of microscopic fields or the square area to examine. Since the mitotic rate is generally low in most nonneoplastic tissues, it is often necessary to examine many microscopic fields when generating mitotic counts. We recommend counting at least 5000 cells (or the representative number of microscopic fields) to determine a mitotic index.

Although the S-phase LI is traditionally generated by counting both the numerator (labeled cells) and the denominator (total labeled and unlabeled cells) and performing the above calculation, some alternatives to ease the burden of laborious counting have been used in different laboratories and may be applicable in specific situations. One alternative is to count the total number of cells in four to six microscopic fields and to use these counts to calculate the average number of cells per microscopic field. Subsequently, the labeled cells in many microscopic fields can be counted in relatively rapid fashion, and the labeling index can be calculated as follows:

$$\text{Labeling index} = \frac{\text{Number of labeled cells}}{\substack{\text{Total number of microscopic} \\ \text{fields examined} \\ \times \text{ Average number of cells} \\ \text{per microscopic field}}}$$

This approach works well for solid tissues, such as liver or endocrine tissues, where there is uniform density of cells throughout the organ and between the groups being compared. If there were centrilobular hepatocyte hypertrophy in one group, this approach would not be appropriate since the cellular density would vary between successive random microscopic fields and hypertrophy is not expected to be present in the control group.

Another method for estimating the labeling index that is especially useful for mucosal and epidermal surfaces is the unit length labeling index (ULLI). The ULLI is defined as the number of labeled cells per millimeter of lining epithelium. This measurement involves counting the labeled nuclei along a measured length of basement membrane. This methodology has been described in detail for nasal epithelial surfaces (Monticello et al. 1990). ULLI comparisons between animal groups should also take into consideration histopathological alterations that further clarify any quantitative response data. For example, comparison of two basically similar mucosal surfaces (Fig. 5.7A, B) using the ULLI approach is a useful measurement. However, if some of the groups have a hyperplastic or thickened mucosal surface where the proliferating pool of cells extends considerably beyond the basement membrane (Fig. 5.7C) or a dysplastic epithelium (Fig. 5.7D), then simply reporting the ULLI does not adequately reflect the pathophysiological process being observed. Some indication of relevant tissue alterations in the population being counted should accompany the ULLI.

Measurement of cell proliferation in lesions often represents a significant challenge. In some instances the labeling index is so high that accurate counts are difficult (Fig. 5.8). Hyperplastic and neoplastic lesions may

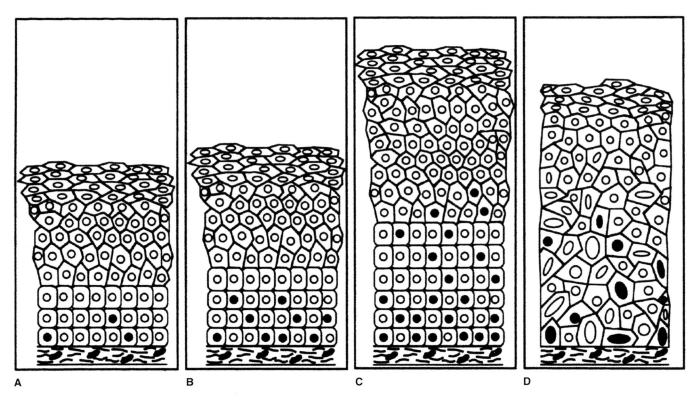

A          B          C          D

**FIGURE 5.7** Diagrammatic representation of normal (A), minimally hyperplastic (B), markedly hyperplastic (C), and dysplastic (D) mucosal surfaces with black nuclei in labeled cells. Comparison of the unit length labeling index (ULLI) between normal and abnormal mucosal surfaces should be accompanied by a description of the histopathologic changes.

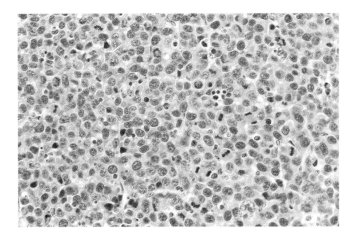

**FIGURE 5.8** Immunohistochemical stain for PCNA in a highly proliferative mouse liver lesion. Over 90 percent of the cells are immunopositive.

be characterized by cellular crowding, pleomorphism, dysplasia, or other tissue alterations (Fig. 5.9), making it difficult to establish uniform guidelines for quantitation of a labeling index. The situation may be further complicated by patchy staining within lesions and lack of a distinct boundary between the hyperplastic/

neoplastic lesion and the surrounding normal parenchyma. When the difference in labeling is dramatic, a photomicrograph may be more communicative of the ongoing process than laboriously obtained LI comparisons between lesions and "nonlesioned" parenchyma. Reporting of any quantitative data on labeling indices should include appropriate documentation of histopathological features of the lesions.

## Variability and Study Design Issues for Cell Proliferation Measurements

Since different tissues have different intrinsic rates of cell turnover (Table 5.4), the target tissue of interest will influence the optimal duration for administering the labeling agent. In general, pulse doses of labeling agent are appropriate for rapidly proliferating tissues. For tissues such as liver or kidney, continuous administration of a labeling agent for approximately 7 days is usually ideal for generating reliable LIs in the absence of proliferative lesions. Administration of labeling agents for 3 to 5 days may also be appropriate for these tissues and possibly for some of the more rapidly proliferating tissues. However, continuous labeling for 3 to 5 days would essentially label all cells in the intestinal tract,

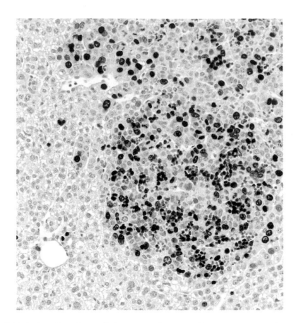
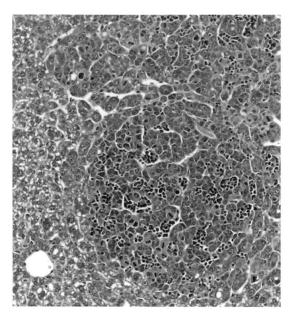

**FIGURE 5.9** A proliferative focus of hepatocytes from a mouse carrying the SV40 large T antigen under the influence of an albumin promoter. The left panel is stained with hematoxylin and eosin, and islands of darkly stained hematopoietic cells are present in the focus of proliferating hepatocytes. In the right panel, stained for BrdU following a pulse labeling dose, determining an LI for hepatocytes is complicated by the presence of the labeled hematopoietic cells.

thereby precluding the possibility of detecting any increase in cell proliferation state. In such a situation, use of a pulse dose of BrdU or employing PCNA immunostaining would be preferred for assessing the intestine, while immunostaining for BrdU following a 3-, 5-, or 7-day continuous administration would be the method for assessing more slowly proliferating tissues.

Cell proliferation is generally cyclical, with important circadian rhythms that could significantly influence study data (Barbason et al. 1995), especially when using pulse doses of labeling agents. Hormonal cyclicity (Fujii et al. 1985; Oishi et al. 1993) is well-known to influence proliferation and cellular differentiation in the reproductive tract and liver. Cyclicity is also influenced by environmental factors such as room lighting, feeding schedules, and fluctuating corticosterone levels (Leduc 1949; Llanos et al. 1971; Schulte-Hermann and Landgraf 1974; Hume and Thompson 1990). Mouse tongue epithelium has a declining S-phase LI from 0900 to 1500 hours and an increase in LI from 2100 to 0300 hours with associated change in duration of S-phase from approximately 6 to 9 hours, respectively (Hume and Thompson 1990).

It is theoretically possible that certain treatment regimens could shift the normal circadian cycle, thereby making valid comparison between treated and control animals dependent on appropriate timing of pulse doses of exogenous labeling agents. Dealing with potential problems associated with cyclicity turns out to be most problematic for those tissues with a relatively rapid

intrinsic rate of proliferation that are being assessed by a pulse dose of labeling agent. Thus, if the maximum rate of cell proliferation in the esophagus, stomach, or intestine, for example, is at 10 a.m., pulse dosing in the late afternoon will miss the peak of the circadian cycle and will result in a lower and less sensitive assessment of the target cell proliferative state. Critical experiments for such tissues may require some preliminary pilot studies to determine the optimal time for pulse dosing. For tissues with lower intrinsic rates of cell proliferation, such as the liver and kidney, continuous administration of labeling agent over a 3- to 5-day period will capture the peaks as well as the valleys of any circadian cyclicity and, thus, will yield sensitive and accurate assessments of cell proliferative states.

Study design factors that influence cell proliferation results include the number of animals used per time point, the age of the animals, and the number of cells counted. Since there is intrinsic biological variability between animals, it is recommended that at least 8 to 10 animals be used per sampling time point. Using fewer animals may result in enough variability to obscure any potential treatment effects, particularly for more subtle increases or decreases in cell proliferation. Younger animals that are still in the rapid growth phase may give more erratic results depending upon whether the individual animals are sampled during a growth burst or if the experimental conditions happen to retard growth. For many situations, the best cell proliferation results in rodents will be obtained from animals that are 10 weeks of age or older. Extremely old animals generally have a constellation of spontaneous degenerative and inflammatory changes that could adversely affect and confound cell proliferation analysis, and their use should be avoided if possible. The National Toxicology Program does not generally perform cell proliferation measurements in rodents older than 18 months for this reason, although exceptions are sometime made depending upon the question being asked. Other variables that should be considered in the design of cell proliferation studies include treatment regimen, route and dose of chemical exposure, species, strain, sex, diet, environment, target cell population, method of quantitation, and statistical approaches (Goldsworthy et al. 1991).

Perturbations in PCNA synthesis may occur as a consequence of cellular transformation. Transformed cells and tumors generally synthesize high but variable levels of PCNA (Matthews 1989; Hall et al. 1990) depending upon the mechanism of transformation. Cells expressing oncogenes of SV40 and adenovirus 5 have been characterized as having "runaway PCNA synthesis" (Matthews 1989). PCNA is involved in DNA repair, and since many tumors have active ongoing DNA repair, PCNA could be up regulated in nonproliferating tumor cells (van Diest et al. 1998).

# APOPTOSIS

Apoptosis is a form of cell death with distinctive morphological features. It has been documented as single-cell death in tissue sections by pathologists for decades but in the past 15 to 20 years has received renewed interest with the publication of information related to the molecular mechanisms of this type of cell death (Corcoran et al. 1994; Uchiyama 1995; Slyuser 1996). Many contemporary references underscore the dynamics of apoptosis during experimental carcinogenesis and the constellation of molecular changes that accompany apoptosis (Goldsworthy et al. 1996a, 1996b; Slyuser 1996; Harmon and Allan 1997; Staunton and Gaffney 1998; Levin et al. 1999; Hall 1999). Apoptosis is a form of active cell death, requiring gene transcription and mRNA production (Staunton and Gaffney 1998). It is an important factor in embryonic organogenesis, in aging, and in the pathogenesis of cancer. The apoptotic process that occurs during embryogenesis is often termed "programmed cell death." The popularity of apoptosis in research and the casual use of this term in recent years has led to considerable confusion over the distinction between necrotic cell death versus apoptotic cell death. Characteristics of apoptosis and differences between apoptosis and necrosis have been reviewed (Columbano 1995; Majno and Joris 1995; Levin et al.

1999). Apoptotic cell death frequently accompanies necrotic cell death and is often elevated in rapidly growing tissues such as neoplasms. The reason that untreated cancers continue to grow despite the presence of ample numbers of apoptotic cells is that the balance between cell proliferation and apoptotic cell death is skewed in favor of cell proliferation. A primary goal in cancer radiation and chemotherapy is induction of tumor regression as a consequence of the cancer cells undergoing apoptotic cell death (Cotter et al. 1992; Glynn et al. 1992; Martin and Green 1994; Anand et al. 1995).

## Morphologic Features of Apoptosis

While there are distinct ultrastructural features characteristic of apoptosis, electron microscopy is often not a practical means for assessing apoptosis in tissues. The criteria for identification of apoptosis have been well defined (Kerr et al. 1972; Wyllie et al. 1980). Histomorphologic features of apoptosis as seen in standard hematoxylin- and eosin-stained sections include deletion of single cells; cell shrinkage with condensation of cytoplasm; condensation of chromatin into crescents, smooth masses, or beads in apposition to the nuclear membrane, followed by nuclear fragmentation; cytoplasmic membrane "blebbing" with ultimate pinching off of pieces of the cell (apoptotic bodies), some of which may contain condensed bits of chromatin; phagocytosis and digestion by adjacent normal cells; and absence of an inflammatory response. Extracellular as well as intracellular phagocytosed apoptotic bodies frequently are surrounded by a narrow clear halo (Staunton and Gaffney 1998). The histomorphologic features of apoptosis vary depending upon the inciting cause, the specific tissue, and the concomitant presence of necrosis. Apoptotic cells and bodies that occur along mucosal and luminal surfaces may be primarily lost by exfoliation. It is noteworthy, however, that delayed fixation for intervals as brief as 15 minutes has been reported to significantly increase the number of visible apoptotic cells (Hall et al. 1994).

## Alternative Methods for Documenting Apoptosis

Alternative methods for assessing apoptotic cell death are all fundamentally based on intrinsic features of tissues. Molecular assays based on demonstrating nucleosome-size fragments of cleaved DNA by electrophoresis (DNA ladders), immunohistochemical staining of growth factors, or in situ end-labeling of fragmented DNA are popular (Goldsworthy et al. 1996b). While clearly defined DNA ladders are reasonable assays if there is extensive apoptosis, they are less satisfactory when there are only a few apoptotic cells in a tissue comprised of predominately normal cells. Furthermore, in situ end-labeling is not specific for apoptosis and has been shown to also occur in necrotic cell death (Grasl-Kraupp et al. 1995; Mundle 1995). Histomorphologic features of apoptotic cells are sufficiently distinctive (see above), and the most widely accepted standard for assessing apoptosis is based on quantitation of apoptotic bodies in histologic sections stained with hema-

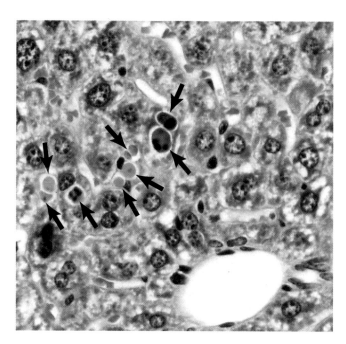

**FIGURE 5.10** Hematoxylin- and eosin-stained mouse liver with numerous apoptotic bodies (*arrows*).

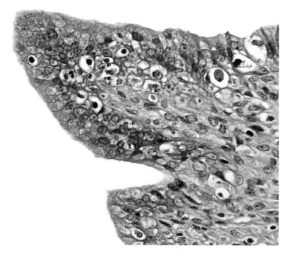

**FIGURE 5.11** Hematoxylin- and eosin-stained mouse uterine mucosa with apoptotic bodies surrounded by clear halos.

toxylin and eosin (Figs. 5.10, 5.11; Potten 1996). Use of in situ end-labeling, use of flow cytometry on cell suspensions, or demonstration of DNA ladders can be helpful in confirming apoptosis observed in standard histological tissue specimens.

## Counting/Measuring Apoptosis

Quantitation of apoptotic indices is labor-intensive because generally large numbers of normal cells need to be examined just to find a few apoptotic cells. It is common to count 5000 to 10,000 hepatocytes just to find a single or a few apoptotic cells in normal mouse liver (Goldsworthy et al. 1996b). Since most investigations require comparison of the relative apoptotic state between treated and control animals, between tissue lesions and normal tissue, or between wild-type and genetically modified mice, a considerable amount of time will be required to generate appropriate apoptotic indices. Furthermore, just as generating cell proliferation counts alone does not adequately address total tissue dynamics, an apoptotic index without a corresponding assessment of cell proliferation may not correctly depict important tissue dynamics.

Quantitation of apoptosis typically involves generation of an apoptotic index (AI). The AI is defined by the number of apoptotic bodies divided by the total number of nuclei counted. Since a single apoptotic cell may give rise to multiple apoptotic bodies, estimation of an apoptotic cell index is based upon the number of apoptotic bodies observed and their proximity to each other. As a rule of thumb in the mouse liver, a maximum of four apoptotic bodies in close proximity would be considered to be derived from a single apoptotic cell, while apoptotic bodies separated from each other by more than two hepatocytes would be considered to be derived from two different apoptotic cells (Goldsworthy et al. 1996b). Similar to the situation with generating LIs, shortcuts to generating denominator value for an AI (e.g., number of apoptotic bodies per square millimeter of tissue, using the average number of cells per field for estimating the denominator) might sometimes be warranted.

## Variability and Study Design Issues for Apoptosis Measurements

Although not as well defined or understood as cell proliferation cyclicity, apoptosis may also be subject to circadian cyclicity (Potten 1996). This cyclicity is dramatically demonstrated in the female mouse reproductive system, where apoptosis is high in ovarian follicles undergoing atresia, or in uterine epithelium during the estrous cycle. In rats, the feeding schedule appears to synchronize apoptosis during the day-night cycle (Bursch et al. 1984, 1986). Sensitive measurement of apoptosis, much like the case for measurement of mitosis, is further compromised by the fact that the duration of morphologically visible apoptosis is relatively short. Visible apoptosis is estimated to last approximately 4 hours (Bursch et al. 1990; Goldsworthy et al. 1996b); however, there is a wide variability in reported duration of visible apoptosis (Potten 1996) with suggested estimates as short as 1 hour (Coles et al. 1993). In some regards, the balance between cell birth and cell death might best be assessed by comparison of the mitotic and apoptotic indices (Arends et al. 1994), since both measures are of relatively similar duration in terms of visibility in stained tissue sections. But even with attempts to achieve both measurements, temporal difference in peak activity may require sampling at different intervals to first measure the increase in cell proliferation and subsequently to measure the peak of apoptosis several hours later.

The interanimal variability in apoptotic indices is likely to be considerably larger than that for some of the more sensitive measures of cell proliferation. This has been demonstrated for mouse hepatocytes (Goldsworthy et al. 1996b) and is expected to be true for other tissues as well. This is probably attributable to the short duration of apoptosis and to the fact that not all animals in a given group will be synchronized with respect to peak apoptosis. Based upon our experience with mouse liver, we recommend that greater than 10 animals per group be used for accurate assessment of apoptosis.

# REFERENCES

Alabi, J. and Alison, M. 1984. Liver cell hyperplasia: on the suitability of using the metaphase-arrest technique. Cell Tissue Kinet. 17:515–523.

Alison, M., Chardry, Z., Baker, J., et al. 1994. Liver regeneration: a comparison of in situ hybridization for histone mRNA with bromodeoxyuridine labeling for the detection of S-phase cells. J. Histochem. Cytochem. 42:1603–1608.

Amati, B. and Land, H. 1994. Myc-Max-Mad: a transcription factor network controlling cell cycle progression, differentiation and death. Curr. Opin. Genet. Dev. 4:102–108.

Anand, S., Verma, H., Kumar, L., et al. 1995. Induction of apoptosis in chronic myelogenous leukemia lymphocytes by hydroxyurea and adriamycin. Cancer Lett. 88:101–105.

Arends, M.J., McGregor, A.H. and Wyllie, A.H. 1994. Apoptosis is inversely related to necrosis and determines net growth in tumors bearing constitutively expressed myc, ras, and HPV oncogenes. Am. J. Pathol. 144:1045–1057.

Barbason, H., Herens, C., Robaye, B., et al. 1995. Importance of cell kinetics rhythmicity for the control of cell proliferation and carcinogenesis in rat liver (Review). In Vivo 9:539–548.

Baserga, R. and Wiebel, F. 1969. The cell cycle of mammalian cells. In: Richter, G.W. and Epstein, M.A. (Eds.), International Review of Experimental Pathology, vol. 7. New York: Academic Press, pp. 1–30.

Baserga, R., Sell, C., Procu, P., et al. 1994. The role of the IGF-I receptor in the growth and transformation of mammalian cells. Cell Proliferation 27:63–71.

Bisconte, J.-C. 1979. Kinetic analysis of cellular populations by means of the quantitative radioautography. Internatl. Rev. Cytol. 57:75–126.

Boswald, M., Harasim, S. and Maurer-Schultze, B. 1990. Tracer dose and availability time of thymidine and bromodeoxyuridine: application of bromode-oxyuridine in cell kinetic studies. Cell Tissue Kinet. 23:169–181.

Bowen, I.D. and Bowen, S.M. 1990. Programmed Cell Death in Tumours and Tissues. London: Chapman and Hall. 260 pages.

Bravo, R., Frank, R., Blundell, P.A., et al. 1987. Cyclin/PCNA is the auxiliary protein of DNA polymerase delta. Nature 326:515–517.

Brodsky, W. and Uryvaeva, I. 1977. Cell Polyploidy: its relation to tissue growth and function. Internatl. Rev. Cytol. 50:275–332.

Bursch, W., Lauer, B., Timmermann-Trosiener, I., et al. 1984. Controlled death (apoptosis) of normal and putative preneoplastic cells in rat liver following withdrawal of tumor promoters. Carcinogenesis 5:453–458.

Bursch, W., Dusterberg, B. and Schulte-Hermann, R. 1986. Growth, regression and cell death in rat liver as related to tissue levels of the hepatomitogen cyproterone acetate. Arch. Toxicol. 59:221–227.

Bursch, W., Paffe, S., Putz, B., et al. 1990. Determination of the length of the histological stages of apoptosis in normal liver and in altered hepatic foci of rats. Carcinogenesis 11:847–853.

Carlsson, J., Johanson, K.J. and Safwenberg, J.O. 1979. Age dependent changes in the metabolism of 3H-thymidine and 3H-uridine in young rats. Growth 43:105–115.

Carriere, R. 1967. Polyploid cell reproduction in normal adult rat liver. Exp. Cell Res. 46:533–540.

Coles, H.S.R., Burne, J.F. and Raff, M.C. 1993. Large-scale normal cell death in the developing rat kidney and its reduction by epidermal growth factor. Development 118:777–784.

Columbano, A. 1995. Cell death: current difficulties in discriminating apoptosis from necrosis in the context of pathological processes in vivo. J. Cell. Biochem. 58:181–190.

Corcoran, G., Fix, L., Jones, D., et al. 1994. Apoptosis: molecular control point in toxicity. Toxicol. Appl. Pharmacol. 128:169–181.

Cotter, T., Glynn, J., Echeverri, F., et al. 1992. The induction of apoptosis by chemotherapeutic agents occurs in all phases of the cell cycle. Anticancer Res. 12:773–780.

deFazio, A., Leary, J.A., Hedley, D.W., et al. 1987. Immunohistochemical detection of proliferating cells in vivo. J. Histochem. Cytochem. 35:571–577.

Eldridge, S.R., Tilbury, L.F., Goldsworthy, T.L., et al. 1990. Measurement of chemically induced cell proliferation in rodent liver and kidney: a comparison of 5-bromo-2′-deoxyuridine and [3H]thymidine administered by injection or osmotic pump. Carcinogenesis 11:2245–2251.

Eldridge, S.R., Butterworth, B.E. and Goldsworthy, T.L. 1993. Proliferating cell nuclear antigen: a marker for hepatocellular proliferation in rodents. Environ. Health Perspect. 101 (Suppl. 5):211–218.

Foley, J., Ton, T., Maronpot, R., et al. 1993. Comparison of proliferating cell nuclear antigen to tritiated thymidine as a marker of proliferating hepatocytes in rats. Environ. Health Perspect. 5:199–205.

Fujii, H., Hayama, T. and Kotani, M. 1985. Stimulating effect of natural estrogens on proliferation of hepatocytes in adult mice. Acta Anat. 121:174–178.

Gelfant, S. 1981. Cycling-noncycling cell transitions in tissue aging, immunological surveillance, transformation, and tumor growth. Internatl. Rev. Cytol. 70:1–25.

Gerlach, C., Sakkab, D.Y., Scholzekn, T., et al. 1997. Ki-67 expression during rat liver regeneration after partial hepatectomy. Hepatology 26:573–578.

Glynn, J.M., Cotter, T.G. and Green, D.R. 1992. Apoptosis induced by Actinomycin D, Camptothecin or Aphidicolin can occur in all phases of the cell cycle. Biochem. Soc. Trans. 20:84S.

Goldsworthy, T., Connolly, R. and Fransson-Steen, R. 1996a. Apoptosis and cancer risk assessment. Mutat. Res. 365:71–90.

Goldsworthy, T., Fransson-Steen, R. and Maronpot, R. 1996b. Importance of and approaches to quantification of hepatocyte apoptosis. Toxicol. Pathol. 24:24–35.

Goldsworthy, T.L., Morgan, K.T., Popp, J.A., et al. 1991. Guidelines for measuring chemically-induced cell proliferation in specific rodent target organs. In: Butterworth, B.E. and Slaga, T.J. (Eds.), Chemically Induced Cell Proliferation: Implications for Risk Assessment. New York: Willy Liss, pp. 253–284.

Goldsworthy, T.L., Dunn, C.S. and Popp, J.A. 1992. Dose effects of bromodeoxyuridine (BRDU) on rodent hepatocyte proliferation measurements. Toxicologist 12:265.

Gong, J., Li, X., Traganos, F., et al. 1994. Expression of G1 and G2 cyclins measured in individual cells by multiparameter flow cytometry: a new tool in the analysis of the cell cycle. Cell Proliferation 27:357–371.

Grasl-Kraupp, B., Ruttkay-Nedecky, B., Koudelka, H., et al. 1995. In situ detection of fragmented DNA (TUNEL assay) fails to discriminate among apoptosis, necrosis, and autolytic cell death: a cautionary note. Hepatology 21:1465–1468.

Greenwell, A., Foley, J.F. and Maronpot, R.R. 1991. An enhancement method for immunohistochemical staining of proliferating cell nuclear antigen in archival rodent tissues. Cancer Lett. 59:251–256.

Greenwell, A., Foley, J.F. and Maronpot, R.R. 1993. Detecting proliferating cell nuclear antigen in archival rodent tissues. Environ. Health Perspect. 101 (Suppl. 5):207–210.

Hall, P.A. 1999. Assessing apoptosis: a critical survey. Endocrine-Related Cancer 6:3–8.

Hall, P.A. and Levison, D.A. 1990. Review: assessment of cell proliferation in histological material. J. Clin. Pathol. 43:184–192.

Hall, P.A., Levison, D.A., Woods, A.L., et al. 1990. Proliferating cell nuclear antigen (PCNA) immunolocalization in paraffin sections: an index of cell proliferation with evidence of deregulated expression in some neoplasms. J. Pathol. 162:285–294.

Hall, P.A., Coates, P.J., Ansari, B., et al. 1994. Regulation of cell number in the mammalian gastrointestinal tract: the importance of apoptosis. J. Cell Sci. 107:3569–3577.

Harmon, B. and Allan, D. 1997. Apoptosis. Adv. Genetics 35:35–56.

Hellman, B. and Ullberg, S. 1986. Rate of incorporation of [3H]thymidine in various tissues of the mouse. Cell Tissue Kinet. 19:183–194.

Hume, W.J. and Thompson, J. 1990. Double labelling of cells with tritiated thymidine and bromodeoxyuridine reveals a circadian rhythm-dependent variation in duration of DNA synthesis and S phase flux rates in rodent oral epithelium. Cell Tissue Kinet. 23:313–323.

Ito, T., Mitui, H., Udaka, N., et al. 1998. Ki-67 (MIB-5) immunostaining of mouse lung tumors induced by 4-nitroquinoline 1-oxide. Histochem. Cell Biol. 110:589–593.

Jecker, P., Beuleke, A., Dressendorfer, I., et al. 1997. Long-term oral application of 5-bromo-2-deoxyuridine does not reliably label proliferating immune cells in the LEW rat. J. Histochem. Cytochem. 454:393–401.

Kerr, J.F.R., Wyllie, A.H. and Currie, A.R. 1972. Apoptosis: a basic biological phenomenon with wide-ranging implications in tissue kinetics. Br. J. Cancer 26:239–257.

Kurki, P., Vanderlaan, M., Dolbeare, F., et al. 1986. Expression of proliferating cell nuclear antigen (PCNA)/Cyclin during the cell cycle. Exp. Cell Res. 166:209–219.

Lanier, T., Berger, E. and Eacho, P. 1989. Comparison of 5-bromo-2-deoxyuridine and [3H]thymidine for studies of hepatocellular proliferation in rodents. Carcinogenesis 10:1341–1343.

Lavin, M. and Watters, D. (Eds.). 1993. Programmed Cell Death: The Cellular and Molecular Biology of Apoptosis. Chur, Switzerland: Harwood Academic Publishers. 325 pages.

Leduc, E.H. 1949. Mitotic activity in the liver of the mouse during inanition followed by refeeding with different levels of protein. Am. J. Anat. 84:397–429.

Levin, S., Bucci, T., Cohen, S., et al. 1999. The nomenclature of cell death: recommendations of an ad hoc committee of the Society of Toxicologic Pathologists. Toxicol. Pathol. (in press).

Levine, A. and Broach, J. 1995. Oncogenes and cell proliferation. Curr. Opin. Genet. Dev. 5:1–4.

Lin, P. and Allison, D. 1993. Measurement of DNA content and of tritiated thymidine and bromodeoxyuridine incorporation by the same cells. J. Histochem. Cytochem. 41:1435–1439.

Llanos, J.M.E., Aloisso, M.D., Souto, M., et al. 1971. Circadian variations of DNA synthesis, mitotic activity, and cell size of hepatocyte population in young immature male mouse growing liver. Virchows Arch. Abt. B Zellpath. 8:309–317.

Loyer, P., Glaise, D., Cariou, S., et al. 1994. Expression and activation of cdks (1 and 2) and cyclins in the cell cycle progression during liver regeneration. J. Biol. Chem. 269:2491–2500.

Majno, G. and Joris, I. 1995. Apoptosis, oncosis, and necrosis. An overview of cell death. Am. J. Pathol. 146:3–15.

Martin, S.J. and Green, D.R. 1994. Apoptosis as a goal of cancer therapy. Curr. Opin. Oncol. 6:616–621.

Matthews, M.B. 1989. The proliferating cell nuclear antigen, PCNA, a cell growth-regulated DNA replication factor. In: Wang, E. and Warner, H.R. (Eds.), Growth Control during Cell Aging. Boca Raton, FL: CRC Press, pp. 89–120.

Maurer, H.R. 1981. Potential pitfalls of [3H]thymidine techniques to measure cell proliferation. Cell Tissue Kinet. 19:179–182.

Monticello, T.M., Morgan, K.M. and Hurtt, M.E. 1990. Unit length as the denominator for quantitation of cell proliferation in nasal epithelia. Toxicol. Pathol. 18:24–31.

Mundle, S. 1995. Correspondence. The two in situ techniques do not differentiate between apoptosis and necrosis but rather reveal distinct patterns of DNA fragmentation in apoptosis. Lab. Invest. 72:611–613.

Oishi, Y., Okuda, M., Takahashi, H., et al. 1993. Cellular proliferation in the anterior pituitary gland of normal adult rats: influences of sex, estrous cycle, and circadian change. Anat. Rec. 235:111–120.

Pederson, T. and Gelfant, S. 1970. G2-population cells in mouse kidney and duodenum and their behavior during the cell division cycle. Exp. Cell Res. 59:32–36.

Piwnica-Worms, H.M. 1994. Regulation of the eukaryotic cell cycle. In: Arias, I.M., Boyer, J.L., Fausto, N., Jakoby, W.B., Schachter, D.A., Shafritz, D.A. (Eds.), The Liver: Biology and Pathobiology. New York: Raven Press, pp. 1557–1562.

Potten, C.S. 1996. What is an apoptotic index measuring? A commentary. Br. J. Cancer 74:1743–1748.

Quinn, C.M. and Wright, N.A. 1992. Mitosis counting. In: Hall, P.A., Levison, D.A., Wright, N.A. (Eds.), Assessment of Cell Proliferation in Clinical Practice. London: Springer-Verlag, pp. 83–91.

Reed, M., Corsa, A., Pendergrass, W., et al. 1998. Neovascularization in aged mice: delayed angiogenesis is coincident with decreased levels of transforming growth factor beta1 and type I collagen. Am. J. Pathol. 152:113–123.

Schulte-Hermann, R. and Landgraf, H. 1974. Circadian rhythm of cell proliferation in rat liver: synchronization by feeding habits. Z. Naturforsch. 29:421–424.

Simpson-Herren, L. 1987. Autoradiographic techniques for measurement of the labeling index. In: Gray, J.W. and Darzynkiewicz, Z. (Eds.), Techniques in Cell Cycle Analysis. Clifton, NJ: Humana Press, pp. 1–30.

Slyuser, M. (Ed.). 1996. Apoptosis in Normal Development and Cancer. London: Taylor and Francis. 303 pages.

Staunton, M. and Gaffney, E. 1998. Apoptosis. Basic concepts and potential significance in human cancer. Arch. Pathol. Lab. Med. 122:310–319.

Stein, G.I. and Kudryavtsev, B.N. 1992. A method for investigating hepatocyte polyploidization kinetics during postnatal development in mammals. J. Theor. Biol. 156:349–363.

Tannock, I.F. 1965. A comparison of the relative efficiencies of various metaphase arrest agents. Exp. Cell Res. 47:345–356.

Tomei, L.D. and Cope, F.O. (Eds.). 1991. Apoptosis: The Molecular Basis of Cell Death. Plainview, NY: Cold Spring Harbor Laboratory Press. 321 pages.

Ton, T., Foley, J., Flagler, N., et al. 1997. Feasibility of administering 5-bromo-2'-deoxyuridine (BRDU) in drinking water for labeling S-phase hepatocytes in mice and rats. Toxicol. Methods 7:123–136.

Uchiyama, Y. 1995. Apoptosis: the history and trends of its studies. Arch. Histol. Cytol. 58:127–137.

van Diest, P.J., Brugal, G. and Baak, J.P.A. 1998. Proliferation markers in tumours: interpretation and clinical value. J. Clin. Pathol. 51:716–724.

Ward, J.M., Henneman, J.R., Osipova, G.Y., et al. 1991. Persistence of 5-bromo-2'-deoxyuridine in tissues of rats after exposure in early life. Toxicology 70:345–352.

Weghorst, C.M., Henneman, J.R. and Ward, J.M. 1991. Dose response of hepatic and renal DNA synthetic rates to continuous exposure of bromodeoxyuridine (BrdU) via slow-release pellets or osmotic minipumps in male B6C3F1 mice. J. Histochem. Cytochem. 39:177–184.

Wilke, M.S., Hsu, B.M. and Scott, R.E. 1988. Two subtypes of reversible cell cycle restriction points exist in cultured normal human keratinocyte progenitor cells. Lab. Invest. 58:660–666.

Wright, N. and Alison, M. 1984. The Biology of Epithelial Cell Populations. Oxford: Clarendon Press. 1247 pages.

Wright, N. and Appleton, D. 1980. The metaphase arrest technique. A critical review. Cell Tissue Kinet. 13:643–663.

Wyatt, I., Coutts, C., Foster, P., et al. 1995. The effect of implantation of osmotic pumps on rat thyroid hormone and testosterone levels in the plasma, an implication for tissue 'S' phase studies. Toxicology 95:51–54.

Wyllie, A.H., Kerr, J.F.R. and Currie, A.R. 1980. Cell death: the significance of apoptosis. Internatl. Rev. Cytol. 68:251–306.

Wynford-Thomas, D. and Williams, E.D. 1986. Use of bromodeoxyuridine for cell kinetic studies in intact animals. Cell Tissue Kinet. 19:179–182.

Zietz, S. and Nicolini, C. 1978. Flow microfluorometry and cell kinetics: a review. In: Valleron, A.J. and Macdonald, P.D.M. (Eds.), Biomathematics and Cell Kinetics. New York: Elsevier, pp. 357–394.

## Web Sites

Immunohistochemistry procedures for PCNA and BrdU
*http://dir.niehs.nih.gov/dirlep/immuno.html*

In situ end-labeling (TUNEL) for apoptosis
*http://dir.niehs.nih.gov/dirlep/ish.html*

Osmotic minipumps
*http://www.alzet.com*

# II

# Embryos

# 6
# Methods for Handling Mouse Embryos for Anatomy Studies: Gross and Microscopic Anatomy of the Mouse Embryo

Matthew H. Kaufman

The mouse is the most commonly employed experimental animal, and much information may be obtained from the analysis of its embryonic and fetal stages. Accordingly, most effort is presently concentrated in attempting to understand the genetic factors that influence its normal development. This is accomplished through analyzing the effect of an abnormal genome on its phenotype. One of the most informative approaches for undertaking such an analysis is through the examination of appropriately fixed material that has been embedded in either paraffin wax or plastic and then serially sectioned in one of several "conventional" planes—usually such material is sectioned in either the *transverse, sagittal,* or *coronal* plane. The most commonly used fixatives are Bouin's solution, 10 percent formalin, and 4 percent paraformaldehyde, but specific stains may need other fixatives. In order to maximally facilitate the interpretation of the sectioned material, the orientation of the embryo in the paraffin or plastic "block" is of critical importance, and every effort should be made to section the embryo both symmetrically and in one or other of the planes indicated above. It is particularly important to

follow exact guidelines during the preparation of this material, as the duration of various stages of preparation is largely dependent on the stage of embryonic/fetal development studied. Most researchers employ the staging system proposed by Theiler. In the interpretation of the histological sections, it is useful, though not absolutely essential, to have a sound knowledge of the anatomical tissues and features likely to be present at the stage being studied, and text-based databases are now available for this purpose. It is also essential to have access to a standard reference manual in which all of the key features on the individual sections are clearly labeled. If a specific system is studied, then a sound knowledge of its embryological development is also of critical importance. The availability in the near future of three-dimensional reconstructions prepared from serially sectioned material from all stages of mouse development will provide an additional important teaching aid for those required to work with morphologically normal material with which they are not familiar, as each of the sections' component tissues will be color-coded. Additionally, to facilitate the recognition of specific tissues, once the developmental stage is established, the "reference" or "standard" reconstructed embryo may be "resectioned" in any orientation so that computer-generated sections may be obtained that match the viewer's own sections. Using this resource, it will soon be possible for researchers to insert (or "paint") domains of gene expression onto these "standard" embryos. Though it has to be appreciated that domains of gene expression may not always adhere strictly to conventional, anatomical domains, it should be possible to use appropriate

The author wishes to thank his Edinburgh colleagues who collaborate on the work described here: J.B.L. Bard, R.M. Brune (anatomy), D.R. Davidson, R.A. Baldock, C. Dubreuil, W. Hill, A. Ross and M. Stark (MRC Human Genetics Unit), K. Lawson and other members of the European Science Foundation (ESF) workshops on the project, and M. Ringwald (Jackson Laboratory). For those who have not been mentioned by name, the author is equally indebted. The work has been supported by the BBSRC, the ESF, and the MRC and Glaxo-Wellcome.

bioinformatics approaches to search such expression databases both spatially and textually. For them to be of maximum value, they will have to be easy to use, comprehensive, and accessible over the Internet.

# METHODOLOGY INVOLVING CONVENTIONAL HISTOLOGY

At the present time, the mouse is the most commonly employed experimental animal, and while there may be compelling medical and scientific reasons why we should study the early stages of human development, there are many reasons why access to these is always likely to be extremely limited. In the foreseeable future, therefore, the mouse is likely to remain the animal model of choice, despite the many limitations involved (Strachan and Lindsay 1997).

The principal aim of this methodology section is to provide baseline information that will allow an individual who has no previous experience working with the mouse to undertake meaningful research involving the histological analysis of serially sectioned mouse embryos. While the techniques involved in the isolation of preimplantation embryos is briefly considered—if, for example, in vitro fertilization is to be carried out, or this material is to be analyzed at the ultrastructural level—histological analysis is almost exclusively the preserve of individuals working with postimplantation mouse embryos. By following the steps indicated below, and with some practice, the novice should be able to obtain histological sections of a publishable quality. Certain of the steps described below require a considerable degree of skill; this can be obtained by following all of the indicated steps meticulously, but much time can be saved by carefully watching someone who is skilled in producing high-quality sections of the stage or stages required.

## Isolation of Mouse Embryos at Specific Stages of Pregnancy

### SPONTANEOUS VERSUS INDUCED OVULATION

The best quality histological sections are usually obtained from embryos isolated from the matings between fertile males and spontaneously cycling females, though large numbers of mating pairs may have to be set up (usually late in the afternoon or during the early evening) in order to obtain a relatively small number of mated females. It is also relatively easy to select females that are in proestrus by vaginal inspection using the criteria outlined by Champlin et al. (1973). This technique tends to be extremely reliable, and well over half of the

females selected in this way normally mate that night. While this may be disadvantageous if large numbers of preimplantation embryos are required, this approach ensures that the embryos that do implant develop normally, with no artifactual changes associated with intrauterine crowding.

Alternatively, females may be induced to ovulate (termed *superovulation*), and to achieve this, they need to be injected (usually intraperitoneally) with exogenous hormones. The dose involved depends on the strain of the female and the number of embryos needed. If preimplantation embryos are to be isolated, then very large numbers may be obtained by increasing the dose of the hormones injected: an injection of PMSG (equivalent to the natural hormone, follicle-stimulating hormone) is followed about 48 hours later by HCG (equivalent to the natural substance, luteinizing hormone). The dose of pregnant mare's serum gonadotropin (PMSG) and human chorionic gonadotropin (HCG) will depend on whether large numbers of embryos are required, for which a higher dose of these agents will be given (e.g., 5 or 10 IU). If a lower dose is given (e.g., 1 or 2.5 IU), then the number of eggs ovulated will approximate the number ovulated in a natural (i.e., noninduced) cycle, when about 9–12 eggs might reasonably be expected to be isolated.

Ovulation occurs about 11–12 hours after the injection of HCG, and it is usual to give these injections at about midday so that ovulation occurs at about midnight, similar to the timing in the natural cycle. There may be critical experimental reasons why ovulation should occur at another time; if this is the case, either the exogenous hormones can be injected at another time, or if spontaneously cycling females are used, the light:dark schedule can be appropriately adjusted. If this is to be the standard practice, then colonies of mice will have to be maintained under these unusual light:dark conditions from about the time of puberty or, preferably, from the time of birth.

## TERMINOLOGY FOR DESCRIBING DEVELOPMENTAL OR GESTATIONAL AGE

As long as the date is noted when the vaginal plug is recognized, it is possible to determine with a reasonable degree of accuracy the stage of development of embryos isolated a specified number of days later. While the duration of pregnancy in the mouse is usually about 19.5–20 days, implantation usually occurs at about 4.5 days postcoitum. Before implantation, cleavage-stage embryos may be isolated by flushing through the female reproductive tract with phosphate-buffered saline or tissue culture medium, initially from the oviduct and uterotubal junction (up to about the 8-cell or early morula stage), and then from the uterus (zona-intact advanced morulae and cavitating blastocysts, or zona-free blastocysts), while all postimplantation stages are isolated from the uterus.

Various "standard" staging systems are available for those who work with mouse embryos. All are equally acceptable, as long as the system employed is clearly stated in the methodology. If this information is not provided, then difficulties will inevitably arise because there can be a difference of at least 12 hours in the degree of embryonic development achieved, depending on which of the various systems is employed. In a breeding colony where mice are retained under a controlled lighting schedule (e.g., a 12 hours:12 hours light:dark or a 10 hours:14 hours light:dark schedule), it is usually assumed that mating occurs close to the middark point, usually set for 2 a.m. All timings are therefore taken from the *assumed* time of mating; this is then referred to as time zero. Using this system, the morning of finding a vaginal plug would therefore be referred to as either *E0.5* (embryonic day 0.5) or *0.5 dpc* (0.5 days post-coitum). Even though the exact time of mating is unclear, this scheme still provides the most accurate means of describing the degree of embryonic development (Copp and Cockroft 1990; Hogan et al. 1994). In another scheme, though now less commonly employed, the day on which the vaginal plug is observed is considered day 1 of pregnancy.

## ISOLATION OF PREIMPLANTATION EMBRYOS FROM THE OVIDUCT

If the pregnant female is sacrificed by an acceptable means, different methods are then employed to isolate various stages of development. If the preimplantation embryos are at any stage between the fertilized 1-cell stage and the early morula stage, it is appropriate to isolate the section of the reproductive tract between the fimbriated os of the oviduct and the distal part of the uterine horn, including the uterotubal junction. The tip of a 32-gauge needle bent to about 135 degrees is carefully inserted into the fimbriated os, and between 0.2 and 0.5 ml of phosphate-buffered saline or tissue culture medium is flushed through the tract in the direction of the uterotubal junction, into a small plastic or glass petri dish. It is easiest to carry out this maneuver under the relatively low magnification of a good quality dissecting microscope, using transmitted light illumination. The embryos may then be handled using a finely drawn Pasteur-pipette with an inner diameter of between 70 and 100 µm, and the movement of the embryos may be controlled using either a rubber bulb or, preferably, a "mouth"-pipette (Hogan et al. 1994)

## ISOLATION OF PREIMPLANTATION EMBRYOS FROM THE UTERUS

In order to isolate morulae and blastocysts, it is necessary to isolate the two uterine horns. The segment of the reproductive tract that needs to be removed is the segment just distal to the cervix and just proximal to the uterotubal junction. If there is any uncertainty with regard to the stage of development to be isolated, it is wise to remove *both* the segment of the tract indicated in the preceding section of this chapter and the remainder of the uterine horn, as indicated here. The uterine segment is then flushed in both directions with about 2.5–5 ml of saline or medium, and if no embryos are isolated, then the segment of oviduct should also be flushed, as indicated in the preceding section of this chapter. If some of the embryos are at the "expanded" blastocyst stage, or are zona free, then a drawn pipette with a slightly larger internal diameter may need to be used.

## ISOLATION OF EARLY POSTIMPLANTATION EMBRYOS FROM THE UTERUS—UP TO THE EARLY SOMITE STAGE (TS12)

If the two entire uterine horns are dissected from the female and stretched out onto blotting paper, or a paper towel, it should next be possible to separate the uterus from the mesometrium, its dorsal mesentery, which also contains its arterial supply and venous drainage. During the early postimplantation period, the embryo is located in the center of the so-called decidual swelling. While it is possible to isolate embryos from the egg cylinder stage (Theiler stage 7 and 8 [TS7 and TS8]) to the stage when the first pairs of somites are recognized (TS12), it is technically quite difficult, particularly if the embryo and its extraembryonic membranes (the amnion and the yolk sac that largely surrounds it) are to be damage free. This condition would be essential if such stages are to be isolated and cultured for 24 to 48 hours in appropriate tissue culture medium (for detailed methodology, see Cockroft 1990). For most purposes, it is only necessary to isolate the intact decidual swelling and process it as a single unit. This is certainly acceptable if *transverse* histological sections are required, but it would not be acceptable if *sagittal* sections are needed. In the latter case, it would be necessary to isolate the embryo and then orientate it in such a way that sections of a particular orientation are obtained (see below, "Orientation of Specimens for Appropriate Sectioning").

## ISOLATION OF DEVELOPMENTALLY MORE ADVANCED POSTIMPLANTATION EMBRYOS FROM THE UTERUS—UP TO THE STAGE JUST BEFORE THE TIME OF BIRTH (TS26)

It is technically considerably easier to isolate embryos from about TS13 to birth than those described in the previous section, though it is still essential to carry out the dissection under the low magnification of a dissecting microscope using sharpened watchmakers' forceps. What is of critical importance, however, is that great care is taken to ensure that the embryo is not damaged in any way. The removal of limb bud embryos (TS15–17) from the uterus and yolk sac can occasionally pose problems. It is essential therefore that the dissection is carefully performed in order to avoid the embryo being severely damaged as it is isolated from what remains of the decidual swelling, as this appears to exert a considerable pressure on the embryo, and any sudden decompression of the embryo will severely damage it.

For most purposes, the embryo should be isolated from its yolk sac, as the yolk sac vasculature can obscure a clear view of the embryo. The amnion may be retained, as this should not interfere with the orientation of the embryo in the paraffin wax block prior to serial sectioning. It would only be useful to retain the embryo with its yolk sac if the relationship between the embryo and its placental and yolk sac circulations is to be investigated. The separation of the embryo from its placental circulation often leads to a considerable degree of bleeding from the cut end of the umbilical cord. To remove the majority of this extravasated blood from the saline solution into which the embryo has been isolated, the embryo will need to be passed through a series of saline washes. To undertake these maneuvers with relatively small embryos, a large-bore pipette with a rubber bulb may be used, though for more advanced stages of development a teaspoon or similar shaped spatula should be used for this purpose.

## Fixation, Dehydration, and Embedding in Paraffin Wax

While a considerable number of fixative agents are available, Bouin's solution generally produces acceptable results, with minimal levels of artifactual damage to the sections. If, for various reasons, this fixative is unsuitable, then 10 percent neutral buffered formalin is a good alternative. The duration in fixative can be of critical importance because the tissue tends to harden, become brittle, and break up during sectioning. It is usually the case that the smaller the embryo, the shorter the time needed in the fixative. Thus, embryos with a crown-rump length (CRL) of about 2 mm or less need only about 1 hour in Bouin's fixative, 3–5 mm CRL embryos require only about 2 hours, 6–10 mm CRL embryos require about 6 hours, and 11–15 mm CRL embryos require about 10 hours, up to a maximum of about 24 hours. The fixed embryos should then be transferred into 70 percent alcohol for long-term storage at room temperature. While the time spent in 70 percent ethanol is relatively unimportant, it is essential that the volume of this solution be large compared with that of the embryo. It is

also important that this solution be changed on at least several occasions.

During the next stage of processing, the material needs to be dehydrated, and this is carried out by taking the material through a graded series of alcohols. Several changes each of 80 percent, 90 percent, 96 percent, and finally 100 percent ethanol will be required, and the duration of each of these steps varies according to the size and developmental age of the embryo. The material is then transferred into a 1:1 mixture of 100 percent ethanol: benzene. General guidelines are available indicating the duration of the various stages involved in the processing of embryos of different ages (Table 6.1). The timing of the individual steps is of critical importance, as overexposure at any stage can result in excessive hardening and disintegration of the material during sectioning. To minimize the risk of damaging the material during handling, it should be placed in a fine wire mesh basket or cassette. The addition of a few drops of eosin into the 90 percent ethanol stage stains the embryo pink and makes it easier to see during the embedding stage. It also allows the orientation of the embryo to be more clearly seen when it is in the wax block. Embryos with a CRL of greater than 6 mm should be transferred into xylene until they become translucent or "cleared," while smaller embryos are cleared with benzene.

## Orientation of Specimens for Appropriate Sectioning

In order to section an embryo serially in a particular orientation, it is necessary to be able to determine its orientation within the wax block with a considerable degree of accuracy. Embryos that are more advanced than Theiler stage 14, and have been removed from the yolk sac, are usually reasonably easy to orientate within the wax block, as they automatically tend to fall onto their side in the wax. What is of importance is to establish in which direction the embryo is facing and the locations of the head and tail regions. These critical landmarks should then be indicated with pins with different colored heads. While smaller embryos that have been isolated from within their extraembryonic membranes tend to be more difficult to orientate, the principles described above also apply. Since the decidual swelling has a pearlike shape, this is relatively easy to orientate within the wax block, and little difficulty is usually encountered when serial transverse sections of the contained embryos are required. Sectioning of the decidual swelling longitudinally produces either sagittal sections (Fig. 6.1), coronal sections, or sections of intermediate obliquity. When working with these early stages, it is often necessary to section a considerable number of decidual swellings in order to obtain sections of embryos

**TABLE 6.1.   Preparation of paraffin-embedded embryos**

| Process | Solution | Crown-rump length of embryo (mm) | | |
| --- | --- | --- | --- | --- |
| | | <2 | 3–5 | >6 |
| Fixation | Bouin's fluid (saturated picric acid, 75 ml; glacial acetic acid, 5 ml; 40% formaldehyde, 25 ml) | 2–24 h | 2–24 h | 2–24 h |
| Storage after fixation | 70% Ethanol | Variable period | Variable period | Variable period |
| Dehydration and clearing | 80% Ethanol | 1 min | 3–5 min | 30 min |
| | 90% Ethanol | 1 min | 3–5 min | 30 min |
| | 96% Ethanol I | 1 min | 3–5 min | 60 min |
| | 96% Ethanol II | — | — | 30 min |
| | 100% Ethanol I | 1 min | 3–5 min | 60 min |
| | 100% Ethanol II | — | — | 30 min |
| | (1:1) 100% Ethanol: benzene[a] | 1 min | 3–5 min | 15 min |
| | Benzene[a] | Until cleared | Until cleared | — |
| | Xylene | — | — | Until cleared |
| Embedding | Paraplast I | 1 min | 3–5 min | Vacuum embed |
| | Paraplast II | 1 min | 3–5 min | Vacuum embed |
| | Paraplast III | 1 min | 3–5 min | Vacuum embed |

Source: From Kaufman 1990, with permission.

[a]With embryos of up to about 5 mm crown-rump length, benzene is preferable to alternatives, such as xylene, toluene, or inhibisol, because it facilitates visualizing when the end point of "clearing" has occurred. The other agents appear to cause increased hardening of the tissues and possible problems with processing because the material is more brittle and consequently difficult to handle. With larger embryos these other agents should be employed instead of benzene for the clearing stage. Since benzene is a particularly dangerous chemical, appropriate safety measures must be taken when this agent is being used.

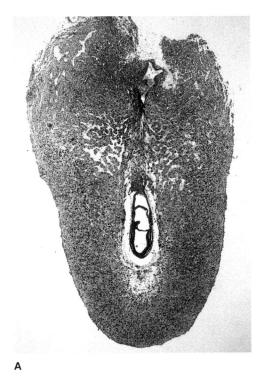

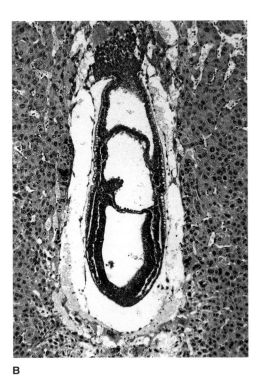

A

B

**FIGURE 6.1**   (**A**) Longitudinal section through a decidual swelling containing a primitive streak–stage embryo, E7 (Theiler stage advanced 10/early 11). (**B**) Enlarged view of primitive streak–stage embryo from decidual swelling illustrated in **A**. The embryo is sectioned in the sagittal plane. The ectoplacental cone is located toward the top of the micrograph.

of the appropriate orientation. For further details of the preparation, trimming, and mounting of the wax block prior to sectioning the embryo, the reader should consult a standard manual of histological techniques (e.g., Bancroft and Stevens 1995; Culling et al. 1985; Drury and Wallington 1980).

For most purposes, embryos are sectioned in one of three standard planes: *transverse, sagittal,* or *coronal.* While it is important to obtain symmetrical sections for ease of analysis of anatomical structures, perfect symmetry is only rarely obtained. It should be remembered that, while sections through the cephalic region may be almost perfectly symmetrical, as the sections progress more caudally, they tend to show less evidence of symmetry. This is inevitable and is clearly related to the lateral curvature of the embryonic axis. This is particularly evident during the limb bud stages of development, as the tail increases in length and usually deviates toward one or other side of the embryo. Specific planes of sectioning are used for different purposes.

Kaufman 1994 displays large numbers of examples of representative black-and-white photomicrographs of intermittent serial sections through mouse embryos at all postimplantation stages of development and sectioned in the transverse and sagittal planes. Kaufman 1994 also includes a few representative coronal sections of the cephalic region of developmentally more advanced embryos. For most purposes it is only necessary to study black-and-white photomicrographs in a reference manual, rather than examples in full color, as it is the anatomical features that need to be recognized so that, for example, mutant and knockout embryos may be assessed for normality.

## TRANSVERSE

Serial sections cut in the transverse plane may be used to analyze all of the components of mouse embryos spanning the entire postimplantation period (Figs. 6.2–6.6). While it is optimal that such sections are symmetrical to facilitate their interpretation, sections that are slightly oblique are relatively easy to interpret and can therefore still be extremely informative. The information that can be gained from the analysis of such sections is far greater than can be obtained from the analysis of sagittal sections (see below), but the effort and skill involved in their preparation is far greater.

## SAGITTAL

Sections in the sagittal plane provide useful information on structures that are exclusively located in the midline (Figs. 6.7–6.13). Such midline sagittal sections provide useful information on a wide range of structures from the pituitary gland to the heart, the liver, and components of the alimentary tract. The great disadvantage of serial sagittal sections is that they are particularly difficult to interpret the farther they get from the midline, and for this reason it is common that only a few sections close to the median plane are ever cut. Equally, the effort involved for the histologist is relatively small. Photomicrographs of median sections are particularly photogenic, but are far less informative than serial transverse sections, for the reasons indicated above.

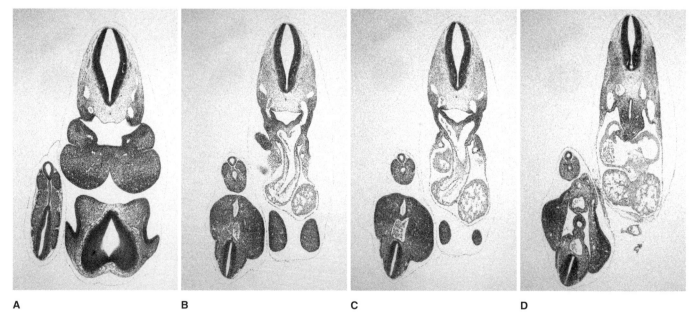

A                    B                    C                    D

**FIGURE 6.2** Representative intermittent transverse sections through the cephalic (**A**) and thoracic regions (**B–D**) of an E10.25–10.5 (TS16–17) embryo.

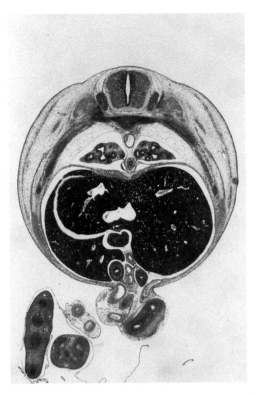

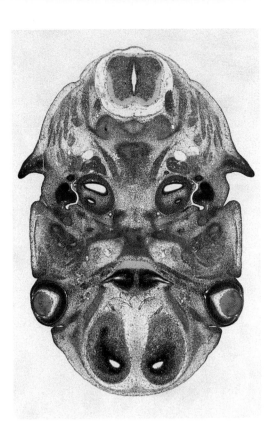

**FIGURE 6.3** Representative transverse section through the lower thoracic and upper abdominal region of an E12.5–13 (TS21) embryo. This section shows an early stage in the development of the physiological umbilical hernia and a large liver cross section.

**FIGURE 6.4** Representative transverse section through the cephalic region of an E13.5 (TS22) embryo. This section is through the olfactory region of the brain, the eyes, and the inner ear apparatus.

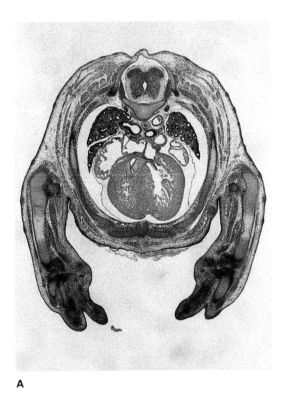

**A**

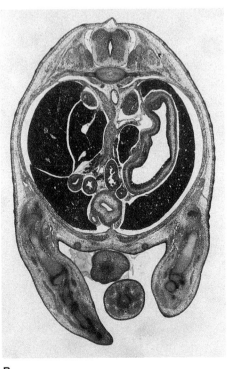

**B**

**FIGURE 6.5** Representative transverse sections through the thoracic and midabdominal regions of an E14.5 (TS22–23) embryo. Note the heart and lungs in **A** and large liver in **B**.

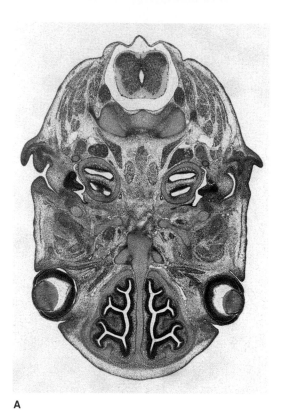

**A**

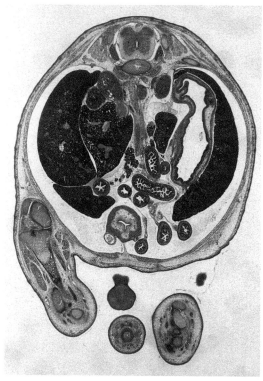

**B**

**FIGURE 6.6**  Representative transverse sections through the cephalic (**A**) and midabdominal (**B**) regions of an E15.5 (TS24) embryo. The cephalic section is through the olfactory region, the eyes, and the inner ear apparatus.

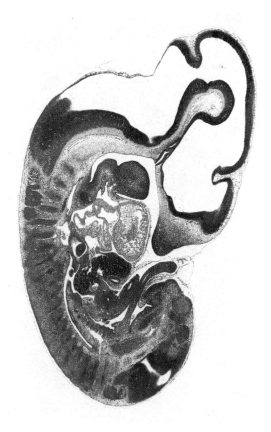

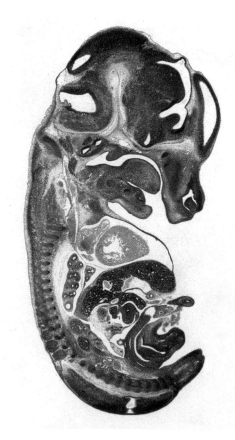

**FIGURE 6.7**  Representative sagittal section through an E11–11.5 (TS18) embryo. Note the large telencephalic vesicle, mesencephalic vesicle, and fourth ventricle.

**FIGURE 6.8**  Representative sagittal section through an E12.5–13 (TS21) embryo. The heart and lungs can be seen.

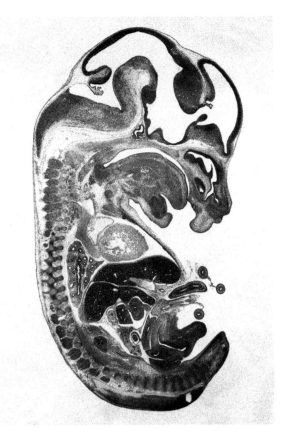

**FIGURE 6.9**    Representative sagittal section through an E13.5 (TS22) embryo. Cervical dorsal root ganglia can be seen.

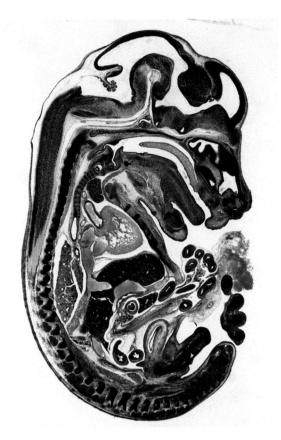

**FIGURE 6.10**    Representative sagittal section through an E14.5 (TS22–23) embryo. Note upper cervical region of spinal cord.

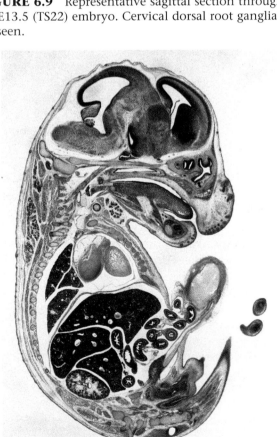

**FIGURE 6.11**    Representative sagittal section through an E15.5 (TS24) embryo. The large liver and smaller kidney are visible.

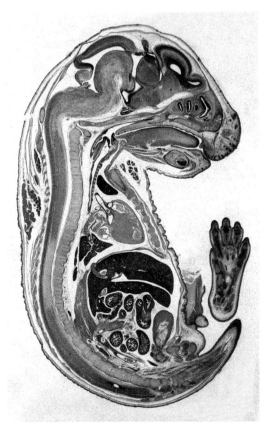

**FIGURE 6.12**    Representative sagittal section through an E16.5 (TS25) embryo. The entire spinal cord is visible.

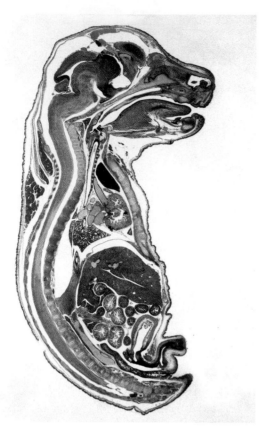

**FIGURE 6.13** Representative sagittal section through an E17.5 (TS26) embryo. The dark thymus and entire spinal cord can be seen.

## CORONAL

Sections in the coronal plane are only rarely of value and are almost exclusively used for examining the cephalic region of mouse embryos from about E14.5–15.5 to term (Fig. 6.14). Such sections, if reasonably symmetrical, allow the brain, in particular, and craniofacial region to be examined in detail. For the analysis of the brain, more information can usually be obtained when sections have been stained with a silver stain and the sections counterstained with, for example, Luxol fast blue. For the examination of the craniofacial region, most conventional stains are satisfactory. If it is necessary to analyze, for example, the degree of differentiation of structures within the distal part of the limb (Fig. 6.15), it is often advantageous to remove the limb and then section it in the coronal plane (see, for example, Chang et al. 1998), and these sections may then be compared with double-stained cleared specimens from littermates (e.g., Chang et al. 1996; see also Patton and Kaufman 1995).

## Serial Sectioning of Embedded Material

For material that has been embedded in paraffin wax, it is usual to cut sections of about 5 μm thickness for the early postimplantation stages and about 7–8 μm for embryos at more advanced stages of development. There are, however, advantages to be gained in embedding the early postimplantation stages in plastic. The material usually needs to be fixed in paraformaldehyde and then prestained with osmium tetroxide before embedding, as this allows the material to be clearly seen in the plastic block, orientated, and sectioned in the desired plane. If the sections are then cut on a conventional ultramicrotome, it is usual to cut sections of between 1 and 2 μm in thickness because, following appropriate staining with, for example, alcian blue, cellular detail is readily seen. Ultrathin sections may also be taken as and when desired, although it is usually necessary to trim down the size of the "face" of the block before ultrathin sections can be taken.

## Choice of Histological Stains

For the histological analysis of all of the postimplantation stages of mouse development, paraffin sections are usually stained with hematoxylin and almost invariably counterstained with eosin, this being the stain combination of choice. This staining regimen is simple to follow (Table 6.2), and the results are usually very reliable. Its greatest weakness is in the clear demonstration of the nervous tissue. For example, it is often difficult to recognize even quite large nerve trunks, and it is certainly not possible to analyze in any detail the brain or spinal cord or to gain information on the innervation of the gut or other structures. For examining nervous tissue, it is necessary to use one of the various silver-based stains (e.g., Linder's stain). To facilitate the interpretation of the anatomical structures present, it is often helpful if the sections are counterstained with, for example, Luxol fast blue (Fig. 6.16).

Histochemical stains have the considerable advantage over conventional stains in their ability to specifically demonstrate evidence of intracellular enzyme activity—for example, the presence of alkaline phosphatase activity in the primordial germ cells, in the apical ectodermal ridge, and in localized regions of the neural tube (Fig. 6.17; Kaufman and Schnebelen 1986; Kaufman 1994, Plate 67, see p. 450). If histochemical stains are to be employed, then care must be taken to use the appropriate fixative solution. In other instances, such stains may only function on material that has been frozen for cryostat sectioning, for which reference to an appropriate manual of histochemical techniques will be required (e.g., Pearce 1980, 1992).

Other techniques may also have to be employed for specific purposes, such as for the analysis of fluorescent-labeled material, but this is beyond the scope of these general observations, and reference should be made to one of the specialist texts. A variety of approaches may be employed to analyze gene expression during early mammalian development. The technique of in situ

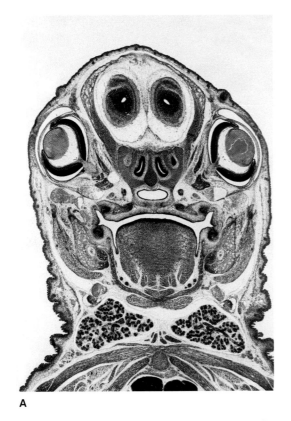

A

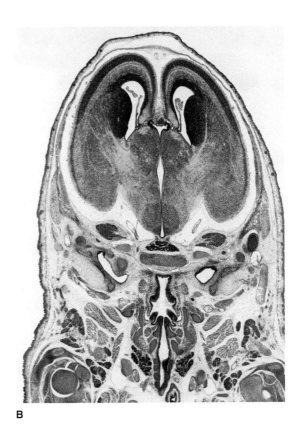

B

**FIGURE 6.14** Representative coronal sections through the cephalic region of an E16.5 (TS25) embryo. (**A**) The eyes with lens and retina are present. (**B**) The bilateral trigeminal ganglia are seen beneath the brain.

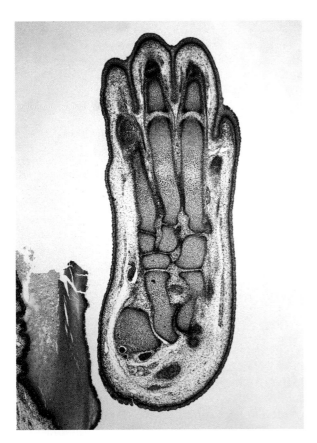

**FIGURE 6.15** Representative "coronal" section through the distal part of the hind limb of an E16.5 (TS25) embryo.

**TABLE 6.2. Staining paraffin sections of embryos**

| Process | Solution | Duration |
|---|---|---|
| Dewaxing | Xylene | 5 min |
| Rehydration | 100% Ethanol | 5 min |
| | 96 % Ethanol | 5 min |
| | 90% Ethanol | 5 min |
| | 70% Ethanol | 5 min |
| | Running tap water | Wash |
| Staining | Hematoxylin (Delafield's or Ehrlich's) | 10 min |
| Differentiating | Acid-alcohol (1% HCl in 70% ethanol) | 15–30 sec |
| | Running tap water | Wash |
| Counterstaining | Eosin (aqueous) | 5 min |
| Dehydration | Ascending alcohols to 100% ethanol | Rapid changes |
| Clearing | Xylene | 2 changes of 5 min each |
| Mounting | Dammar xylene mounting medium | — |

Source: From Kaufman 1990, with permission.

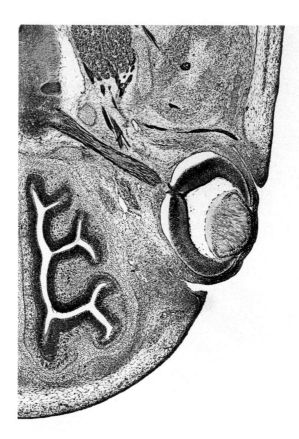

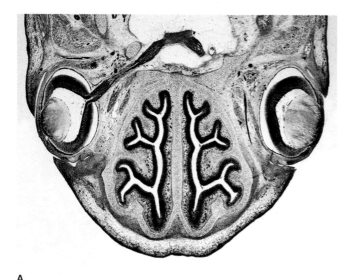

A                                                                              B

**FIGURE 6.16** (**A**) Low-magnification transverse section through the eyes of an E14.5 (TS22–23) embryo. (**B**) Slightly higher magnification section through the left eye of part of the same embryo illustrated in **A**. Lens and retina are shown. Section stained with Linder's silver method and counterstained with Luxol fast blue.

hybridization is now well established, and the detailed protocols well described (Akhurst 1992; Moorman et al. 1993; Wilkinson 1998). Its use for the analysis of gene expression in early human material, however, has only recently been described (Wilson 1997).

## Value of Serial Sections

It is obvious from the information provided above that an enormous amount of extremely detailed information can be gained from the analysis of serially sectioned material. The orientation of the sectioning undertaken depends on what information is required, though for most purposes—with the exception of those areas indicated above, such as the detailed analysis of the brain in near-term embryos—most can be gained from the analysis of serial transverse sections. Unless there is a very good reason why a single section is undertaken, or even intermittent sections, either of these methods will inevitably mean that potentially valuable information is likely to be lost. However, if a similar region in a large number of embryos has to be scanned, then what is possible becomes more important than what is optimal—

unless limitless pairs of hands are available to undertake the histological sectioning.

## Whole-Mount In Situ–Stained Preparations

For most purposes, whole-mount preparations are only undertaken as a preliminary step toward establishing the site of activity of, for example, a particular gene at a specific stage or stages of development. With this information, it is then possible to concentrate on a specific site or sites at one or more stages of development.

## Interpretation of Histology

### ESTABLISHMENT OF DEVELOPMENTAL/ GESTATIONAL AGE OF EMBRYOS WHEN TIMING INFORMATION IS NOT AVAILABLE

Should it ever be of critical importance to establish the exact developmental/gestational age of an embryo, or group of embryos, when the time of mating is not known, it is possible to determine this with a reasonable degree of accuracy by analyzing the pattern of ossification "centers" present in an embryo's long bones. This

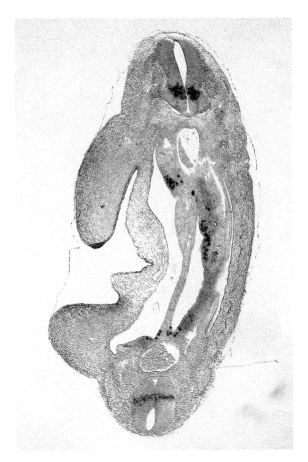

**FIGURE 6.17** Slightly oblique transverse section through a limb-bud stage embryo histochemically stained to demonstrate the presence of intracellular alkaline phosphatase enzyme activity (E10.5, TS17).

technique is, however, only of value after 15.5–16.5 dpc once an adequate number of centers of ossification are present. The technique increases in accuracy with increasing developmental age thereafter and is particularly accurate during the last few days of pregnancy once evidence of ossification is seen in the carpal, metacarpal, and phalangeal bones of the forelimb, and in the tarsal, metatarsal, and phalangeal bones of the hindlimb.

Intact individual embryos from within the same litter as those to be studied histologically may be isolated, fixed in 80 percent ethanol, cleared, and "double-stained" using alcian blue to demonstrate the cartilage models of the individual bones and alizarin red S to demonstrate the pattern of primary and secondary ossification centers within them, using the technique described by Patton and Kaufman (1995). The information obtained by this approach is of particular value, as it provides a basis with which abnormal growth and development can be compared. It has been suggested that alizarin red S is an extremely efficient means of determining early centers of ossification, being slightly

more sensitive than radiography after silver impregnation and only marginally less sensitive than serial sectioning of comparable-staged material (Meyer and O'Rahilly 1958).

## VALUE OF "STANDARD" STAGING SYSTEM

The staging system that has been adopted by all mouse embryologists is the system devised by Theiler (Theiler 1972, reprinted with minor changes 1989). This has largely been based on the classification of Streeter (1942) in his "Developmental Horizons of Human Embryos," a classification that has itself recently been updated by O'Rahilly and Müller (1987). It has been adopted and used in all of the recent standard texts on mouse embryology (Kaufman 1992, reprinted with index, 1994; Kaufman 1997; Kaufman and Bard 1999) and has itself also been recently amended to take into account the minor differences observed during the primitive streak stage of development in a variety of commonly used mouse strains. For a table giving an expanded version of the Theiler system for staging mouse embryos on the basis of their external appearance, see Table 6.3 (see also, [*http://genex.hgu.mrc.ac.uk/*]). To aid identification, the table includes both the morphological features present for the first time and those that are absent until the next stage.

As with the Carnegie staging system used for defining the different stages of human embryonic development, the Theiler staging system principally reflects developmental velocity. The externally observed morphological criteria used to define each stage are those that are considered to be most characteristically recognized in normal embryos at each of these stages. Thus, at the early stages of development, when tissue differentiation is rapidly evolving, each Theiler stage up to about TS20 lasts for about 12 hours. Because of the variability observed between embryos of nominally the same temporal age (see below), there is inevitably some temporal overlap between these stages. During the later stages of development, from TS21 to 26, the intervals between each Theiler stage are closer to 24 hours, and accordingly, there is minimal overlap, and the embryos at each of these stages are more readily distinguished.

It is important to note that, as in all biological systems, some degree of variability exists even in embryos within a single litter; there may be up to about 6–12 hours of growth difference between the least and the most developmentally advanced embryos. Similarly, embryos from different females that have been isolated at an identical gestational time may vary quite considerably in the stage of development achieved. As has already been noted above, it has recently been recognized that minor differences are observed between the embryos of different strains of mice at the primitive streak stage of development, and the original staging system described by Theiler

**TABLE 6.3.  Table of mouse developmental stages**

| Principal features to allow stage identification | Theiler stage | Embryonic age (E)[a] | Size (approx. values, in mm) | Somites (range) |
|---|---|---|---|---|
| One cell (fertilized)—in oviduct. | 1 | 0–1 | | |
| Two cells in oviduct. | 2 | 1–2 | | |
| Cleavage stages; early: 4–8 cells; late: morula (early to fully compacted). | 3 | 2–2.5 | | |
| Blastocyst, zona-intact. Inner cell mass apparent. | 4 | 2.5–3.5 | | |
| Blastocyst, zona-free. | 5 | 3.5–4 | | |
| Attaching blastocyst: decidual reaction domain. | 6 | 4–4.5 | | |
| Early egg cylinder. Ectoplacental cone appears. Embryo implanted, enlarged epiblast, primary endoderm lines mural trophectoderm. | 7 | 4.5–5.5 | | |
| Differentiation of egg cylinder. Proamniotic cavity appears. Reichert's membrane forms. | 8 | 5.5–6 | | |
| Advanced decidual/endometrial reaction. Primitive streak first evident at late-stage.<br>  9. Prestreak (PS), ectoplacental cone invaded by blood, extraembryonic ectoderm, embryonic axis visible.<br>  9a. Early-streak (ES). Gastrulation starts, first evidence of mesoderm. | 9, 9a | 6–6.5 | | |
| Primitive streak and groove. Amnion formation (anterior and posterior amniotic folds—at late-stage). Allantois. Ectoplacental and exocoelomic cavities—at late-stage. Secondary yolk sac (late), Hensen's node.<br>  10.  Midstreak (MS). Amniotic folds start to form.<br>  10a.  Late-streak, no allantoic bud (LSOB). Exocoelomic cavity present.<br>  10b.  Late-streak, early allantoic bud (LSEB). | 10, 10a, 10b | 6.5–7.5 | | |
| Late primitive streak. Neural plate. Cephalic neural (head) folds. Presomite stage. Foregut pocket and cardiogenic plate (late-stage).<br>  11.  Neural plate (NP). Head process developing. Amnion complete.<br>  11a.  Late neural plate (LNP). Elongated allantoic bud (late).<br>  11b.  Early headfold (EHF).<br>  11c.  Late headfold (LHF). Foregut invagination, cardiogenic plate. | 11, 11a–c | 7–7.5 | | |
| "Unturned," headfold stage. Neural folds begin to close in occipital/cervical region. Heart differentiation. Components of first branchial/pharyngeal arch present. Optic placode/pit (early), sulcus (late).<br>  12.  Allantois extends. First branchial arch. Heart starts to form. Foregut pocket visible. Preotic sulcus (2–3 somites present). Cephalic neural crest migrates.<br>  12a.  Allantois contacts chorion (late-stage).<br>*Absent 2nd arch, > 7 somites* | 12, 12a | 7.5–8.5 | | 1–4 (12)<br>5–7 (12a) |
| "Turning." Optic sulcus (well formed). Components of first and second branchial arches. Thyroid primordium. Nephrogenic cord. Early evidence of caudal neuropore.<br>*Absent 3rd arch, >12 somites* | 13 | 8.5–9 | | 8–12 |

**TABLE 6.3. Continued**

| Principal features to allow stage identification | Theiler stage | Embryonic age (E)[a] | Size (approx. values, in mm) | Somites (range) |
|---|---|---|---|---|
| Elevation of cephalic neural folds. Formation and closure of rostral neuropore. Optic vesicle formation. Mandibular and maxillary components of first branchial arch. Components of third branchial arch. Rathke's pouch (pituitary rudiment). Liver rudiment. Pronephros. Forelimb ridge (late-stage). <br> *Absent forelimb bud* | 14 | 8.5–9 | | 13–20 |
| Caudal neuropore diminishing in size. Components of three branchial arches. Optic cup. Otocyst (late). Forelimb bud. Hindlimb ridge. Tracheal diverticulum. Lung bud. Mesonephros. <br> *Absent hindlimb bud* | 15 | 9–9.75 | 1.8–3.3 | 21–29 |
| Caudal neuropore closes. Components of four branchial arches. Lens placode. Otocyst (otic vesicle) separated from surface ectoderm. Olfactory placode/pit. Hindlimb bud. <br> *Absent thin and long tail* | 16 | 9.75–10.25 | 3–4 | 30–34 |
| Deep lens indentation, optic cup. Differentiation of cephalic neural tube. Tail elongates and thins. Umbilical hernia first evident. <br> *Absent nasal pits* | 17 | 10–10.5 | 3.5–5 | 35–39 |
| Formation and closure (late) of lens vesicle, deep nasal pit. Cervical somites becoming indistinct. <br> *Absent auditory hillocks, hand plate* | 18 | 10.5–11 | 5–6 | 40–44 |
| Lens vesicle completely separates from surface. Cervical somites indistinct. Distal part of forelimb bud paddle shaped (i.e., hand plate). Footplate not yet differentiated. Auditory hillocks first evident. <br> *Absent retinal pigmentation and sign of fingers* | 19 | 11–11.5 | 6–7 | 45–47 |
| Earliest signs of fingers. Splayed-out digits. Footplate present. Retinal pigmentation present (only in pigmented strains). Tongue well differentiated. Brain vesicles recognized. <br> *Absent 5 rows of whiskers, indented anterior footplate* | 20 | 11.5–12 | 7–8 | 48–51 |
| Anterior part of footplate indented. Elbow and wrist regions evident. Five rows of whiskers. Umbilical hernia now well defined. <br> *Absent hair follicles, fingers separated distally* | 21 | 12.5–13 | 8–9 | 52–55 |
| Fingers separated distally. Only indentations between toes. Long bones of limbs present. Hair follicles in pectoral, pelvic, and trunk regions. <br> *Absent open eyelids, hair follicles in cephalic region* | 22 | 13.5–14 | 9–10 | 56–60 |
| Toes separated. Hair follicles additionally in cephalic region but not near vibrissae. Eyelids open. <br> *Absent nail primordia, fingers 2–5 parallel* | 23 | 14.5–15 | 10–11.5 | |
| Reposition of umbilical hernia (midgut loop returned to abdominal cavity). Eyelids closing. Fingers 2–5 are parallel. Nail primordia seen on toes. <br> *Absent wrinkled skin, fingers and toes joined together* | 24 | 15.5–16 | 11.5–14 | |
| Skin wrinkled. Eyelids closed. No evidence of umbilical hernia. <br> *Absent ear extending over auditory meatus, long whiskers* | 25 | 16.5–17 | 13.5–16 | |
| Elongated whiskers. Eyes barely visible through closed eyelids. External ear covers auditory meatus. | 26[b] | 17.5–18 | 17–19 | |

Source: Principally from Theiler 1989; Kaufman 1994; Bard et al. 1998. Detailed staging of Theiler stages 9–12 courtesy of K. Lawson (personal communication). The data here are for (C57BL × CBA)F$_1$ hybrid mice. For PO mice, see Downs and Davies 1993.
[a]These figures are for *typical* embryos, although the occasional *viable* embryo may lie outside the figures and timings given here. These timings are based on matings taking place at the middark point (typically 2 a.m.), with vaginal plugs being noted the following morning and embryos being observed at about midday (i.e., the plug day is E0.5).
[b]Mice are typically born at about E19.5.

(1972) has had to be amended to take these strain differences into account. As only a very few strains of mice have been examined in sufficient detail at the histological level at the present time, it is unclear whether other amendments to the original staging system will be required to take these strain differences into account. The studies of Theiler (1972) and Kaufman (1992) both analyzed embryos isolated from the matings between (C57BL × CBA)F$_1$ hybrid male and female mice, while others have studied the early postimplantation stages of development of PO strain mice (Downs and Davies 1993).

## VALUE OF A REFERENCE MANUAL FOR ANATOMICAL TISSUE ANALYSIS

All of the recent references to mouse embryo histology have used the staging system originally developed by Theiler (1972). While his text is detailed and comprehensive, the principal disadvantage of this monograph, from the point of view of the inexperienced researcher, is that it only provides a limited number of photomicrographs of "representative" low-magnification histological sections of embryos at each of his developmental (or Theiler) stages. Even though these micrographs are frequently accompanied by higher-magnification histological sections of organs and tissues from the same or developmentally similar embryos, insufficient micrographs are provided to allow the reader to accurately distinguish the majority of the anatomically defined structures present.

In order to overcome this particular problem, *The Atlas of Mouse Development* (Kaufman 1992, reprinted 1994, with index) contains a large number of plates in which intermittent serial histological sections through embryos at each of the Theiler stages are displayed. The material is particularly comprehensive between Theiler stages 9 and 26, covering the periods of embryogenesis, organogenesis, and postorganogenetic development to full-term, and most of the stages are illustrated with intermittent serial sections cut in both the transverse and sagittal planes. Coronal sections through the cephalic region of a few embryos are also provided, as this plane of sectioning is favored for the analysis of the near-term brain. Diagrams are also provided indicating the locations of the intermittent sections. Each of the sections is comprehensively labeled so that the inexperienced viewer should be able to recognize each of the principal anatomically defined features in their own material. A descriptive account is also provided for each of the Theiler stages, drawing attention not only to the anatomical features that characterize each stage but also indicating which structures have yet to appear. In the second part of the book, the external appearance of intact embryos throughout development is shown, as is the differentiation of all of the specific organs and organ systems, including the spinal cord, eyes, olfactory system, gonads, kidneys, lungs, the placenta and extraembryonic membranes in singleton and multiple pregnancies, and the skeletal system.

## VALUE OF A DESCRIPTIVE TEXT PROVIDING INFORMATION ON THE NORMAL DEVELOPMENT OF EACH OF THE ORGAN SYSTEMS

Until very recently, the only reference text that provided detailed information on the developing mouse embryo was that written by Rugh (1968, reprinted 1990). The book is comprehensive and also covers a wide range of additional topics, including the physiology of the mouse's reproduction. The book's principal limitation, however, is that it tends to be stage specific, so in order to study the development of a particular organ system, it is necessary to read what information is provided at each sequential stage of development. When this was the only reference text available, it was essential to scan textbooks of rat anatomy and embryology (e.g., Hebel and Stromberg 1986) or equivalent texts of human embryology (e.g., Hamilton and Mossman 1972; O'Rahilly and Müller 1987; Larsen 1993) in situations where more detailed information was required. It was then necessary to extrapolate from the information supplied about these other species to the situation in the mouse. In many instances, because of species differences, this was neither easy nor occasionally possible. In most instances, however, if more detailed information was required, it was necessary to refer to the specialist mouse literature.

What was missing therefore was a well-illustrated text that provided a descriptive account of the normal development of all of the major organ systems of the mouse, that would complement, rather than duplicate the material provided in *The Atlas of Mouse Development* (Kaufman 1992). The principal purpose of *The Anatomical Basis of Mouse Development* (Kaufman and Bard 1999) is to try to describe the mechanisms underpinning mouse embryogenesis. The developmental anatomy of each of the major organ systems and their constituent tissues is described in the main body of the text. This section of the book is provided with line diagrams showing how each of the components of the various organs evolves, as well as "wiring diagrams" showing developmental lineages. The text is complemented by a series of indices detailing when individual anatomically defined tissues first appear and which tissues are present in each stage of mouse development (i.e., for each of the 26 Theiler stages) (for details, see the following section).

# COMPUTER-AIDED METHODOLOGIES

An international research exercise involving the collaboration of a number of anatomists, developmental biologists, and computer scientists is beginning to bear fruit. Much of the ongoing work is based in Edinburgh, although scientists from other centers, principally in Europe, have provided special expertise in specific aspects of the project, the eventual aim of which is the preparation of a user-friendly 3-D gene-expression database that is readily accessible to all interested scientists who may wish to gain information from it or interact with it, for example, by inserting their own gene-expression data into it. A description of the various components of this work forms the basis of the second part of this chapter, though it has to be appreciated that to gain the maximum value from this information it is necessary for the reader to be able to interpret efficiently what is observed in his or her own sectioned and stained material.

## Text-Based Anatomical Databases

### INFORMATION ON ANATOMICALLY DEFINED TISSUE COMPONENTS OF MOUSE EMBRYOS AT EACH OF THE 26 THEILER STAGES

The origin of the various indices provided in Kaufman and Bard 1999 was the initial attempt to produce an index for *The Atlas of Mouse Development* (Kaufman 1994). These indices principally contain lists of anatomically defined tissues, with the number indicated at each stage of development increasing dramatically: while there are only 24 tissues listed at Theiler stage 11, there are about 240 indicated at Theiler stage 16, nearly 700 at Theiler stage 22, and about 1000 at Theiler stage 26. The figures presented here are not exact because a considerable number of the tissues are further subdivided, for example: *meninges* (includes arachnoid, dura mater, and pia mater), *heart: valve* (includes aortic, mitral [bicuspid], pulmonary, tricuspid), *radioulnar joint* (includes proximal, distal), *epididymis* (includes caput [head], cauda [tail], corpus [body]). The amount of information listed at each Theiler stage provides a reasonable indication of the increase in the complexity of the mouse embryo during the postimplantation period. In addition to anatomical tissues, the index also contains anatomical landmarks or features, such as the *interventricular groove* and the *sulcus limitans*. Equally, and for the same reason, certain components of the interatrial septum, such as the *foramen primum* and *foramen secundum* are also featured in the list of anatomical terms. These indices are also available on the WWW: [*http://genex.hgu.mrc.ac.uk/*].

## HIERARCHY AND TISSUE GROUPINGS WITHIN THE INDEX

The embryo is divided into its major components, and these are presented in the form of a tree, with larger and smaller branches until the end points (the leaves) are reached, the latter representing the anatomically defined tissues. The embryo at any particular stage of development therefore represents the summation of all of its major organ system–based components, such as the ear, eye, gut, heart, and skeleton, all of which can be readily subdivided into moderate-sized units that can themselves be subdivided into smaller units. In some cases, these can also be further subdivided. As a simple example:

Stage 26, day 17.5

brain
  forebrain
    diencephalon
      epithalamus
        pineal gland (epiphysis)
          stalk (peduncle)
      hypothalamus
        nucleus, lenticular
      internal capsule
      thalamus
        interthalamic adhesion (massa intermedia)
      ganglionic eminence (lateral and medial aspects)
      hippocampus
      telencephalon
        choroid fissure
        choroid invagination (tela choroidea)
        choroid plexus
        corpus striatum
        etc.

Each group therefore represents a collection of linked components. A named tissue, such as a specific muscle, can be located either by its specific name or by passing initially to higher elements in the hierarchy until the name of the desired muscle is eventually located. For example, the *biceps (brachii)* muscle is linked through *forelimb* to *limb* to *muscle*.

It is also possible to use the index to investigate the lineage of a particular tissue to establish information about progenitor and derivative tissues. This is possible because the links can be made across stages. While aspects of this arrangement are in hand, others have yet to be established, and it is hoped that each successive version of the index that is made available in the future will have increasingly sophisticated software to allow the system to be interrogated in greater detail (for details about the WWW interface, the interested reader should refer to Bard et al. 1998a and b or to [*http://genex.hgu.mrc.ac.uk/*]).

## THE PROBLEM OF TISSUE
## DIFFERENTIATION

An attempt has been made to ensure that differentiating tissues are given their new names as and when appropriate, though clearly a decision had to be made, for example, when the "neural tube" should be allowed to *differentiate* to form the "spinal cord," when "ectoderm" should be allowed to *differentiate* into "epithelium" and later into "skin," and when "mesoderm" should be allowed to *differentiate* into "mesenchyme." Although any decisions made would seem to be largely subjective, they were, in fact, based on what seemed to be intuitively reasonable, and where possible, all decisions providing evidence of *differentiation* were based on any guidelines available in the literature.

## HOW SYNONYMS ARE DEALT
## WITH IN THE INDEX

Reference to the literature rapidly revealed that over the years different authors have often referred to the same structure or tissue by a variety of different names, for example: *branchial, aortic, visceral, or pharyngeal arches.* In most cases, the various terms used are well-known and interchangeable. In this regard, the single term was selected that was believed to be either that which is most appropriate or the term that is in most common usage in the current mouse embryological literature as the *prime identifier.* Accordingly, where several synonyms appear in the literature, only the term selected appears in the principal index, while the synonyms appear in parentheses on the first occasion that the selected term appears. If the synonym is selected by a reader, then the reader's attention is drawn to the fact that an *alternative* term is used throughout the index. Occasionally, eponyms have also been included in the index, though on most occasions this information is provided in parentheses. As new information becomes available with research, it is likely that in time a term that is presently located in parentheses, as a synonym, may be transposed with the favored term, or prime identifier. The term that presently appears in the index would accordingly be replaced by the new term and would itself then be relegated into parentheses. Such an index, therefore, must be flexible enough to accommodate changes of this nature. Equally, as new information emerges, new terms will have to be inserted into the index, while others may be amended or, if they are seen to be inappropriate, they will need to be discarded.

## "NOTES" REGARDING DECISION MAKING

In a more complete version of the anatomy database, which will hopefully be released in the near future, information will be provided in the form of "notes" indicating why any particular decision was made.

Equally, after TS12, it was decided, first, to exclude the extraembryonic membranes from the list because embryos are usually dissected out of their membranes in order to expose the embryos so that they may be more readily seen, and second, to replace the term *mesoderm* by that of *mesenchyme.* Where there is obvious left/right symmetry, only a single name is given for the two parts. Only the larger and more readily recognized muscles, arteries, and veins are listed, and this equally applies to a considerable proportion of the bony elements. With regard to the hindlimb, for example, the global terms *metatarsal* and *phalangeal bone* appear, but these are not individually distinguished, nor are the ribs or most of the vertebral units; in the *tarsus,* only the *calcaneus* and *talus* are individually identified.

## THE VOLUMETRIC COMPONENT
## OF THE INDEX

Because many of the anatomical domains in the embryo do not have distinguishing names, an arrangement has had to be made to accommodate this problem, as in the 3-D database the *complete volume* of the embryo has to be capable of being labeled. To achieve this end, pseudonames have had to be devised. Thus, the different domains of the mesenchyme of the early embryo have had to be given names in order to ensure volumetric completeness so that at TS11 the head mesenchyme is subdivided into *i. mesenchyme,* derived from head mesoderm, and *ii. mesenchyme,* derived from neural crest; in other anatomic locations, it has been necessary to refer to them as simply "un-named part of structure A or structure B."

This text-based index, which represents the first comprehensive attempt to produce a systematic standard anatomical nomenclature for the developing mouse embryo, is of considerable value in that, when linked with the spatial coordinates of the "digital" atlas, or gene-expression database (see below), it provides a means not only of labeling all of the various components of the embryo but also of accessing data electronically and therefore providing a means of probing the genetic basis of development. It is only possible to undertake such an exercise when there are unambiguous names for individual anatomically defined tissues.

## POTENTIAL DIFFICULTIES ASSOCIATED
## WITH A TEXT-BASED ANATOMICAL INDEX

The principal disadvantage of a text-based anatomical index relates to the fact that embryos nominally isolated at the same *temporal age* are not necessarily uniform in their *developmental age* and inevitably show some degree of natural variation. Equally, the stage at which a tissue first appears, and is thus so designated in the index, depends to a considerable degree on how closely the histological sections are examined. Equally, it is of critical importance to be able to indicate when a particular tissue is no longer present, for example, because it has differentiated to form another anatomically defined tissue or several anatomically defined tissues.

Different histologists will almost inevitably use different criteria when assessing whether a particular tissue has appeared or has yet to appear. Clearly, there is a considerable subjective element involved in preparing such a tissue index, and it is most unlikely that all viewers will be in exact agreement with all of the information provided. Still, it is unlikely that the information provided for any specific tissue is going to be more than one, or hopefully at most two, Theiler stages different than is published in our index. The index was prepared by the careful analysis of serially sectioned material stained with hematoxylin and eosin, and the possibility clearly exists that if the histological sections had been stained specifically to demonstrate certain tissues, that these tissues may have been observed at slightly earlier stages than they are indicated in the index.

## VALUE OF A TEXT-BASED ANATOMY DATABASE IN THE CONTEXT OF PREPARING A 3-D GENE-EXPRESSION DATABASE

There is now an Internet-accessible database of mouse developmental anatomy that currently holds a hierarchy of the names, and many of the synonyms, of the majority of the anatomically defined tissues present during all stages of mouse development between fertilization and birth, that is, covering all of the 26 Theiler stages indicated above. For a more detailed description of the underlying principles involved in establishing an Internet-accessible database of mouse developmental anatomy, see Bard et al. 1998b.

The availability of a text-based database of mouse developmental anatomy represents a useful first step in that it provides the essential unambiguous anatomical terminology needed before progress can be made in the preparation of a gene-expression database. The second step requires the construction of a further text database for accepting and accessing the gene-expression data, and this aspect of the project is being undertaken by scientists at the Jackson Laboratory (Ringwald et al. 1994, 1997). Before the 3-D gene-expression database can be realized, it is essential that a computer-generated 3-D database of mouse developmental anatomy be prepared. This work is progressing satisfactorily, and the work involved is discussed in the next section. In the long term it is proposed that the text descriptions of gene expression being prepared at the Jackson Laboratory will be superimposed onto the high-resolution 3-D embryo

reconstructions that are presently being prepared in Edinburgh. In the final phase of this exercise, the viewer will be able to undertake direct mapping of his or her own gene-expression domains onto the standard 3-D embryo reconstructions that will also display the gene-expression domains derived from the literature.

## ADDITIONAL ROLES OF THE ANATOMY DATABASE

It is proposed that the present database will eventually have links to other databases, including those of other mammalian and nonmammalian species, and for this reason alone, it is critical that the terminology used allows, as far as is technically possible, interoperability between the various systems. Clearly, despite the fact that many nonmammalian species have their own unique features, it should still be possible to investigate a wide range of questions relating to the more general aspects of vertebrate and even possibly invertebrate development.

# 3-D Reconstructions Prepared from Serially Sectioned Mouse Embryos

## COMPUTER-AIDED 3-D RECONSTRUCTIONS OF SERIALLY SECTIONED MOUSE EMBRYOS AT "STANDARD" STAGES OF DEVELOPMENT

It is now possible to make 3-D reconstructions from the gray-level voxel images of serially sectioned mouse embryos by a process of digitization, image alignment and review, image warping, and finally restacking (Baldock et al. 1992; Kaufman et al. 1997, 1998). In this way it is possible to produce so-called digital mice. The computer technology involved is complex and initially involves the "capturing" of each of the sequential images of the serial histological sections to produce a computer-generated gray-level image of each section, with each image having a resolution of about 10 μm.

The captured images then need to be accurately stacked, for which a "warping" program is used in order to achieve almost perfect alignment (Guest and Baldock 1995). During the process of sectioning and subsequent histological processing, systematic and random distortions are introduced into each section. These need to be eliminated so that the arbitrary sections through the digitized image do not show the ragged edges of misaligned image features. Because of the accuracy of the alignment of the sections, it is then possible to "resection" the reconstructed embryo in any plane so that the computer-generated histological sections simulate as near as possible an exact match on the computer screen to any conventional sectioned plane, or even the viewer's own sectioned material. Thus if the "standard" embryo was originally sectioned in the transverse plane,

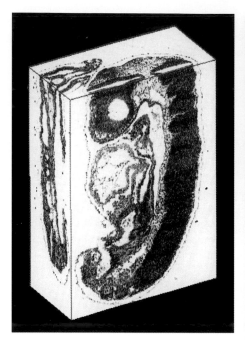
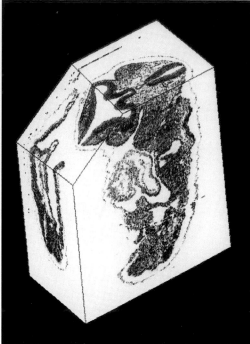
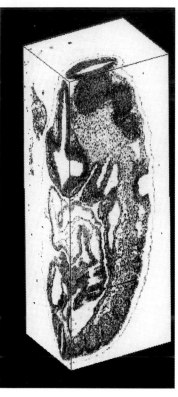

**FIGURE 6.18** Three 3-D reconstructions of the intact Theiler stage 14 mouse embryo viewed as though still within its solid block of paraffin wax. Sections have been removed from different faces of the block to reveal gray-level images that closely resemble histological sections. In these examples, the sections through the upper face of the block reveal the gray-level images that closely resemble the orientation of the original transverse sections that were captured, aligned, and warped, being the first stage in the 3-D reconstruction exercise. (From Kaufman et al. 1997, Fig. 6.1, with permission)

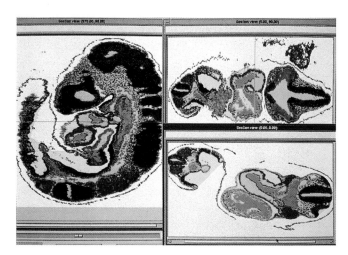

**FIGURE 6.19** Figure with three orthogonally cut, "painted" sections from the Theiler stage 14 mouse embryo. The transverse section closely resembles the orientation of the original transverse section, while the sagittal and coronal sections are computer-generated images. The anatomically defined tissues have been delineated in these sections.

it is possible to view computer-generated images of the same embryo as though it were sectioned in either the sagittal or coronal plane, or indeed in any orientation that is desired. In this way, as long as the viewer knows the developmental age of his or her own material, he or she initially needs only to access the appropriate "standard" embryo of the same developmental age and then to resection it until sections are obtained that closely resemble those viewed down the microscope.

Three-dimensional reconstructions of a series of "standard" mouse embryos (mostly the same embryos as those illustrated in *The Atlas of Mouse Development* [Kaufman 1994]) are presently being prepared (Figs. 6.18, 6.19), though for embryos up to TS12, computer-generated models are being reconstructed from 2 μm thick plastic serial sections stained with alcian blue. In the sections isolated from these plastic-embedded embryos, it is also possible to display details of tissue structure at the cellular level. This is an ongoing exercise, and most of the stages between fertilization (TS1) and TS14 (an embryo with about 17 pairs of somites, about 9 dpc) have already been reconstructed. Work is presently in progress with a TS20 embryo (about 12.5 dpc) and a TS26 embryo (in collaboration with Glaxo-Wellcome). Ideally, at least one representative 3-D reconstructed embryo will be prepared for each of the 26 Theiler stages. Because of the strain differences that have recently been observed during the early postimplantation period, it is proposed that computer-generated reconstructions of representative embryos for each of the substages of TS9–11 will eventually be prepared.

## THE PAINTING PROGRAM

Special software has been developed to facilitate the manual delineation, or "painting," of anatomically defined structures. While some of this work can now be undertaken automatically, by the recognition of well-defined tissue boundaries and the propagation of delineated images from one section to the next, much of the work still has to be undertaken manually. In order to increase the accuracy of this critical component of the exercise, the user can view his or her progress and delineate structures in any arbitrary plane. The painted structures can also be viewed in 3-D as the work progresses. In the early program, up to five different features could be delineated on a particular section at a time, each being individually color-coded. In the more advanced program currently employed, there is technically no limit to the number of colors that can be employed to delineate the anatomically defined tissues.

Sections occasionally display cracks or other imperfections. With the methodology that is presently available, it is now possible to propagate a small part of the complete image from either the former or the successive section into the area with the imperfection in order to fill in the missing or damaged part. The only alternative available is to leave the damaged region. While this might be acceptable under certain circumstances, in the case of the reconstructions of the "standard" embryos, an attempt has been made to remove the imperfections by this means.

As indicated above, these embryos may be resectioned in any orientation so that computer-generated images of sections that closely match the viewer's own sections may be interrogated by the viewer. As all of the anatomically defined tissues in each of the sections are color-coded, this has additional advantages: its principal value is as a teaching resource to facilitate the recognition of anatomically defined tissues and organs in the viewer's own material. Furthermore, all of the images can be manipulated by the viewer so that the viewer can display only those structures that he or she is interested in. By this means, the viewer will be able to follow the

configurational changes that occur in association with gastrulation, neurulation, and somitogenesis, as well as observe the increasing complexity of the heart and cardiovascular system that occurs during embryonic development. As a natural extension of this component of the exercise, it will soon be possible to observe the sequential changes that occur in, for example, the heart or cardiovascular system during development. But first, appropriate "morphing" technology will have to be applied to the images that are presently available.

## MATCHING THE COMPUTER-GENERATED IMAGES WITH THE VIEWER'S OWN SECTIONED MATERIAL

One of the most important features of the 3-D "digital" embryo is that the viewer may resection it in any orientation until the computer-generated image on the screen matches the histological section of his or her own material viewed through the microscope. More importantly, because in the "standard" embryo all of the anatomically defined domains have been individually "painted" in different colors, isolated domains, or groups of domains, may then be selected and formally identified by appropriately querying the textual database. Appropriately delineated tissues may also be shown as a transparent overlay on the computer-generated histological sections. The advantage of this facility is that it can act as an additional aid for the identification of all of the anatomical structures encountered in the sectioned material.

## VIEWING ANATOMICALLY DEFINED TISSUES IN ISOLATION AND IN COMBINATION WITH OTHER TISSUES

Anatomically defined tissues can also be viewed as 3-D images without the histological background. This exercise in itself is extremely informative in that it allows individual components of an embryo to be visualized either in isolation or in the context of other components of the embryo. In this way, it is now technically possible to dissect components out of the embryo but without them being deformed by the dissection process. By this means, it is now becoming increasingly possible to understand the complex relationships that exist within the early embryo.

It is now possible, for example, to view the 3-D relationship between the outflow tract of the heart, the first and second arch arteries, the paired dorsal aortae and the umbilical artery, and the primitive alimentary tract in a TS14 mouse embryo. For certain purposes, it may also be advantageous initially to view these elements of the vascular system and the alimentary tract within the ghostlike outline of the surface contours of the whole embryo, then to delete the latter as it tends to obscure the principal images being analyzed (Fig. 6.20). As an additional

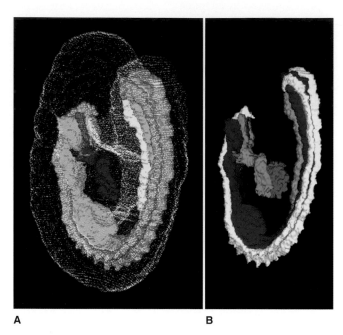

**A**　　　　　　　　　　　　　　**B**

**FIGURE 6.20** Two views showing reconstructions of the outflow tract of the heart, the first and second arch arteries, and the paired dorsal aortae and the umbilical artery to show their relationship to the primitive alimentary tract. In **A**, a faint ghostlike image of the outline of the intact embryo has been included (from Kaufman et al. 1997, Fig. 6.4a, with permission), while in **B**, the outline of the intact embryo has been removed (from Kaufman et al. 1998, Fig. 6.6e, with permission).

feature, when the computer graphics–derived images are combined with 3-D glasses, it is now possible for the viewer to see the object under analysis in stereo. This can be particularly helpful in drawing attention to topological relationships that had not previously been readily noted.

One facility that is now readily available is the ability to analyze the topological changes that take place during the process of "turning," or axial rotation, in which inversion of the germ layers occurs. This is a process that is exclusively observed in the early embryos of the mouse and its closely related species. During this process, the embryonic endoderm, which is initially on the outer aspect of the embryo, comes to line the gut tube, while the embryonic ectoderm, which is initially located on the inner aspect of the embryo, eventually gives rise to the skin and neural tube. The configurational changes that take place in the embryo during this period also alter the relationship that exists between the embryo and its extraembryonic membranes. The conformational changes that occur during the process of turning allow the mouse embryo to achieve the characteristic fetal position and thus to adopt the same configuration observed by all other chordates (for further details of this process, see Snell and Stevens 1966; Kauf-

man 1992). The sequential changes that occur when the mouse embryo "rolls into its membranes" are illustrated in Figure 6.21.

As one indicator of the configurational changes that occur during this period, it is informative to observe the appearance of the endothelial lining of the various anatomically defined components of the heart and vascular system of the mouse embryo at TS12, 13, and 14 (Fig. 6.22). The TS12 embryo, which possesses about 8 pairs of somites, has barely initiated the process of turning, the TS13 embryo, which has about 12 pairs of somites, is progressing through this process, while the TS14 embryo, which has about 17 pairs of somites, has almost completed the turning sequence.

## Gene-Expression Databases

### PROGRESS REGARDING THE PREPARATION OF A GRAPHICAL GENE-EXPRESSION DATABASE OF MOUSE DEVELOPMENTAL ANATOMY

Because of the very large amounts of gene-expression data that are already available, although only a small proportion of this information has been published in the appropriate literature, the data are now already too extensive to be stored in any format other than that of a database. Furthermore, the only way that this enormous volume of information can be stored is in a three-dimensional graphical format because this material is by its nature three-dimensional and its boundaries only occasionally map directly to specific anatomical domains, as, for example, occurs with regard to the *Hox-2* gene, which is specifically expressed in rhombomeres 1 and 2 (Wilkinson et al. 1989), while other genes (indeed the majority that have so far been mapped, for example, *Msx1* and *Msx2*) appear to be expressed over complex epithelial and mesenchymal domains (Houzelstein et al. 1997). Because of the complexities involved, it is now recognized that text alone cannot adequately describe all gene-expression patterns. The particular difficulty is that although these signals eventually determine specific structures, the relationship between gene-expression and the structures that are formed is very rarely obvious. More often than not, various cell types interact with each other through complex intercellular signals and feedback loops, which are only now beginning to be understood.

While the technical difficulties of producing a graphical gene-expression database are clearly considerable, the eventual aim of this exercise is to prepare a developmentally sequential and complete gene-expression database for all of the species that are studied by developmental biologists, including the pre- and postimplantation human embryo (preimplantation study: Daniels

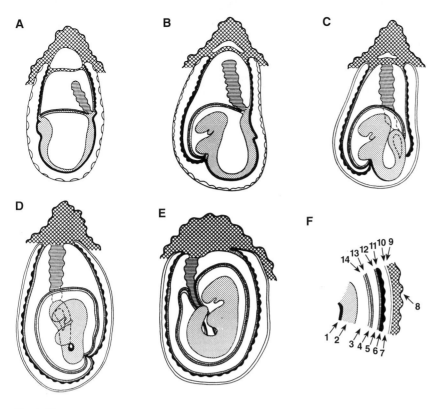

**FIGURE 6.21** Simplified diagrammatic sequence to illustrate changes in the conformation of the embryo and the way in which the extraembryonic membranes surround it as it undergoes the process of "turning." The following stages are illustrated: (**A**) presomite headfold stage, E7.5–8; (**B**) embryo with 8–10 pairs of somites, about E8.5; (**C**) embryo with 10–12 pairs of somites, about E8.75; (**D**) embryo with 12–14 pairs of somites, about E9; (**E**) embryo with 15–20 pairs of somites, about E9.5; (**F**) embryonic layers, extraembryonic tissues, and cavities encountered in the embryo illustrated in **E**. (From Kaufman 1990, with permission)

Key to (F)
1. embryonic endoderm
2. embryonic ectoderm + mesoderm
3. amniotic cavity
4. amnion
5. exocoelomic cavity
6. yolk sac
7. yolk sac cavity
8. ectoplacental cone and trophectoderm derivatives
9. Reichert's membrane
10. parietal (extraembryonic) endoderm
11. visceral (extraembryonic) endoderm
12. extraembryonic mesodermal component of yolk sac
13. mesodermal component of amnion
14. ectodermal component of amnion

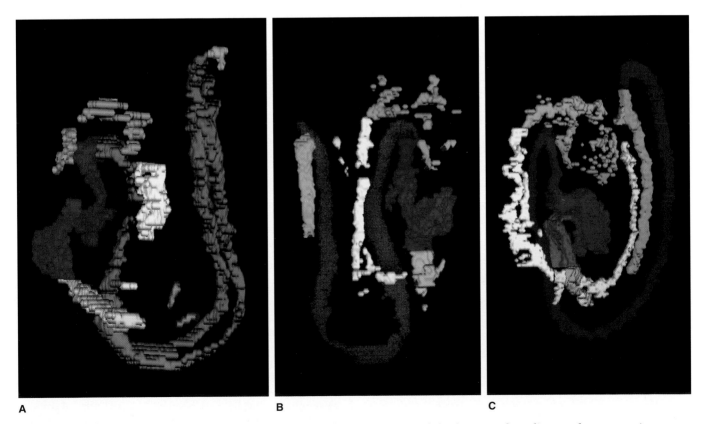

**FIGURE 6.22.** Sequence of reconstructions of the endothelial lining of the heart and cardiovascular system in isolation as observed at TS12 (**A**), TS13 (**B**), and TS14 (**C**). (From Kaufman et al. 1998, Figs. 4d, 5c, 6d, with permission)

85

and Monk 1997; postimplantation studies: Boncinelli and Thorogood 1997; Lindsay et al. 1997; Wilson 1997). Indeed, information gained from the preparation of the mouse gene-expression database suggests that it should be technically feasible to establish a similar gene-expression database of human development (Davidson and Baldock 1997). Using standard bioinformatics approaches, it should, at least in theory, be possible to search these gene-expression databases to increase our understanding of the genetic/molecular factors that control embryonic development in each of these species (Bard et al. 1998a, b).

At the present time, the gene-expression databases that are available are all text based, but work is in progress, in a collaborative project between the Edinburgh-based group and scientists at the Jackson Laboratory, to establish a graphical gene-expression database of the mouse, the eventual aim being to build a complete picture of all aspects of gene function during the development of this species. Accordingly, the computer-generated three-dimensional reconstructions of mouse embryos that have been prepared, or are in the process of being prepared, from the reconstruction of serially sectioned "standard" mouse embryos will act as graphical templates onto which domains of gene expression may be mapped (Davidson et al. 1997, 1998).

In the longer term, with the availability of text-based anatomical databases of, for example, *Caenorhabditis elegans, Drosophila*, puffer fish, rats, and humans, as well as the increasing availability of developmental databases of individual organ systems, it should eventually be possible to interrogate these databases to obtain information on the (possibly common) genetic factors that control the development of similar organ systems in a wide variety of different species (for a list of the key web sites for these and other developmental databases, see Bard et al. 1998a, b). It is likely that when, in the long term, 3-D gene-expression databases of a wide range of vertebrate and invertebrate species are readily available, it will eventually be possible to establish software systems that will allow interoperability between these various databases.

## How the 3-D Gene-Expression Database Will Be Used

It is proposed that researchers will, in the near future, obtain CD-ROMs of the 3-D reconstructions of computer-generated "digital" mouse embryos at "standard" stages of development. Each will then be accessed on its own computer screen, while the gene-expression database will be maintained at a single host site. The two will then be linked over the Internet so that researchers will be able to submit their own data which, once reviewed

(in much the same way that an article submitted to a refereed journal is reviewed), and if considered acceptable, will then be inserted onto the database. Researchers will also have the facility to query the database.

## REFERENCES

Akhurst, R.J. 1992. Localisation of growth factor mRNA in tissue sections by *in situ* hybridization. In Growth Factors. A Practical Approach, ed. I. McKay and I. Leigh, pp. 109–132. Oxford: IRL, Oxford University Press.

Baldock, R., Bard, J., Kaufman, M.H., and Davidson, D. 1992. A real mouse for your computer. BioEssays 14: 501–502.

Bancroft, J.D. and Stevens, A. 1995. Theory and Practice of Histological Techniques. 4th edition. Edinburgh and London: Churchill Livingstone.

Bard, J.B.L., Baldock, R.A., and Davidson, D.R. 1998a. Elucidating the genetic networks of development: a bioinformatics approach. Genome Res. 8: 859–863.

Bard, J.B.L., Kaufman, M.H., Dubreuil, C., Brune, R.M., Burger, A., Baldock, R.A., and Davidson, D.R. 1998b. An Internet-accessible database of mouse developmental anatomy based on a systematic nomenclature. Mech. Dev. 74: 111–120.

Boncinelli, E. and Thorogood, P. 1997. The expression of *Hox* genes in postimplantation human embryos. In Molecular Genetics of Early Human Development, ed. T. Strachan, S. Lindsay, and D.I. Wilson, pp. 171–192. Oxford: Bios Scientific Publishers.

Champlin, A.K., Dorr, D.L., and Gates, A.H. 1973. Determining the stage of the estrus cycle in the mouse by the appearance of the vagina. Biol. Reprod. 8: 491–494.

Chang, H.H., Schwartz, Z., and Kaufman, M.H. 1996. Limb and other postcranial skeletal defects induced by amniotic sac puncture in the mouse. J. Anat. 189: 37–49.

Chang, H.H., Tse, Y., and Kaufman, M.H. 1998. Analysis of interdigital spaces during mouse limb development at intervals following amniotic sac puncture. J. Anat. 192: 59–72.

Cockroft, D.L. 1990. Dissection and culture of postimplantation embryos. In Postimplantation Mammalian Embryos. A Practical Approach, ed. A.J. Copp and D.L. Cockroft, pp. 15–40. Oxford: IRL Press.

Copp, A.J. and Cockroft, D.L. 1990. Postimplantation Mammalian Embryos. A Practical Approach. Oxford: IRL Press.

Culling, C.F.A., Allison, R.T., and Barr, W.T. 1985. Cellular Pathology Technique. 4th edition. London: Butterworths.

Daniels, R. and Monk, M. 1997. Gene expression in human preimplantation embryos. In Molecular Genetics of Early Human Development, ed. T. Strachan, S. Lindsay, and D.I. Wilson, pp. 155–170. Oxford: Bios Scientific Publishers.

Davidson, D. and Baldock, R. 1997. A 3-D atlas and gene-expression database of mouse development: implications for a database of human development. In Molecular Genetics of Early Human Development, ed. T. Strachan, S. Lindsay, and D.I. Wilson, pp. 239–260. Oxford: Bios Scientific Publishers.

Davidson, D., Bard, J., Brune, R., Burger, A., Dubreuil, C., Hill, W., Kaufman, M., Quinn, J., Stark, M., and Baldock, R. 1997. The mouse atlas and graphical gene-expression database. Sem. Cell and Dev. Biol. 8: 509–517.

Davidson, D., Baldock, R., Bard, J., Kaufman, M., Richardson, J.E., Eppig, J.T., and Ringwald, M. 1998. Gene expression databases. In In Situ Hybridization: A Practical Approach, 2nd edition, ed. D.G. Wilkinson, pp. 189–214. Oxford: Oxford University Press.

Downs, K.M. and Davies, T. 1993. Staging of gastrulating mouse embryos by morphological landmarks in the dissecting microscope. Development 118: 1255–1266.

Drury, R.A.B. and Wallington, E.A. 1980. Carleton's Histological Technique. 4th edition. Oxford: Oxford University Press.

Guest, E. and Baldock, R.A. 1995. Automatic reconstructions of serial sections using the finite element method. Bioimaging 3: 154–167.

Hamilton, W.J. and Mossman, H.W. 1972. Hamilton, Boyd and Mossman's Human Embryology. Prenatal Development of Form and Function. 4th edition. Cambridge: W. Heffer and Sons Limited.

Hebel, R. and Stromberg, M.W. 1986. Anatomy and Embryology of the Laboratory Rat. Wörthsee, FRG: BioMed Verlag.

Hogan, B., Beddington, R., Constantini, F. and Lacy, E. 1994. Manipulating the Mouse Embryo. A Laboratory Manual. 2nd edition. New York: Cold Spring Harbor Laboratory.

Houzelstein, D., Cohen, A., Buckingham, M.E., and Robert, B. 1997. Insertional mutation of the mouse Msx1 homeobox gene by an nlacZ reporter gene. Mech. Dev. 65: 123–133.

Kaufman, M.H. 1990. Morphological stages of postimplantation embryonic development. In Postimplantation Mammalian Embryos: A Practical Approach, ed. A.J. Copp and D.L. Cockroft. Oxford: IRL Press, pp. 81–91.

Kaufman, M.H. 1992. The Atlas of Mouse Development. London: Academic Press.

Kaufman, M.H. 1994. The Atlas of Mouse Development. 2nd printing, with index. London: Academic Press. 525 pp.

Kaufman, M.H. 1997. Mouse and human embryonic development: a comparative overview. In Molecular Genetics of Early Human Development, ed. T. Strachan, S. Lindsay, and D.I. Wilson, pp. 77–110. Oxford: Bios Scientific Publishers.

Kaufman, M.H. and Bard, J.B.L. 1999. The Anatomical Basis of Mouse Development. San Diego: Academic Press.

Kaufman, M.H. and Schnebelen, M.T. 1986. The histochemical identification of primordial germ cells in diploid parthenogenetic mouse embryos. J. Exp. Zool. 238: 103–111.

Kaufman, M.H., Brune, R.M., Baldock, R.A., Bard, J.B.L., and Davidson, D. 1997 Computer-aided 3-D reconstruction of serially sectioned mouse embryos: its use in integrating anatomical organization. Int. J. Dev. Biol. 41: 223–233.

Kaufman, M.H., Brune, R.M., Davidson, D.R., and Baldock, R.A. 1998. Computer-generated 3-D reconstructions of serially sectioned mouse embryos. J. Anat. 193: 323–336.

Larsen, W.J. 1993. Human Embryology. New York: Churchill Livingstone.

Lindsay, S., Bullen, P., Lako, M., Rankin, J., Robson, S.C., and Strachan, T. 1997. Expression of Wnt genes in human postimplantation embryos. In Molecular Genetics of Early Human Development, ed. T. Strachan, S. Lindsay, and D.I. Wilson, pp. 193–212. Oxford: Bios Scientific Publishers.

Meyer, D.B. and O'Rahilly, R. 1958. Multiple techniques in the study of the onset of prenatal ossification. Anat. Rec. 132: 181–193.

Moorman, A.F.M., De Boer, P.A.J., Vermeulen, J.L., and Lamers, W.H. 1993. Practical aspects of radio-isotopic in situ hybridization. Histochem. J. 25: 251–266.

O'Rahilly, R. and Müller, F. 1987. Developmental Stages in Human Embryos. Washington, DC: Carnegie Inst. Pub. Number 637.

Patton, J.T. and Kaufman, M.H. 1995. The timing of ossification of the limb bones, and growth rates of various long bones of the fore and hindlimbs of the prenatal and early postnatal laboratory mouse. J. Anat. 186: 175–185.

Pearce, A.G.E. 1980. Histochemistry: Theoretical and Applied. 4th edition, volume 1. Preparation and Optical Technology. Edinburgh and London: Churchill Livingstone.

Pearce, A.G.E. 1992. Histochemistry: Theoretical and Applied. 4th edition, volume 3. Enzyme Histochemistry. Edinburgh and London: Churchill Livingstone.

Ringwald, M., Baldock, R., Bard, J., Kaufman, M., Eppig, J.T., Richardson, J.E., Nadeau, J.H., and Davidson, D. 1994. A database for mouse development. Science 265: 2033–2034.

Ringwald, R., Davis, G.L., Smith, A.G., Trepanier, L.E., Begley, D.A., Richardson, J.E., and Eppig, J.T. 1997. The mouse gene expression database GXD. Semin. Cell Dev. Biol. 8: 489–497.

Rugh, R. 1968. The Mouse. Its Reproduction and Development. Minneapolis: Burgess Publishing Company.

Rugh, R. 1990. The Mouse. Its Reproduction and Development. Oxford: Oxford University Press.

Snell, G.D. and Stevens, L.C. 1966. Early embryology. In Biology of the Laboratory Mouse, ed. E.L. Green, pp. 205–245. New York: McGraw-Hill.

Strachan, T. and Lindsay, S. 1997. Why study human embryos? The imperfect mouse model. In Molecular Genetics of Early Human Development, ed. T. Strachan, S. Lindsay, and D.I. Wilson, pp. 13–26. Oxford: Bios Scientific Publishers.

Streeter, G.L. 1942. Developmental horizons in human embryos. Description of age group XI, 13–20 somites, and age group XII, 21–29 somites. Contr. Embryol. 30: 211–245.

Theiler, K. 1972. The House Mouse: Development and Normal Stages from Fertilization to 4 Weeks of Age. Berlin: Springer-Verlag.

Theiler, K. 1989. The House Mouse: Atlas of Embryonic Development. New York: Springer-Verlag.

Wilkinson, D.G. 1998. The theory and practice of *in situ* hybridization. In In Situ Hybridization. A Practical Approach, 2nd edition, ed. D. Wilkinson, pp. 1–21. Oxford: Oxford University Press.

Wilkinson, D.G., Bhatt, S., Cook, M., Boncinelli, E., and Krumlauf, R. 1989. Segmental expression of *Hox-2* homeobox-containing genes in the developing mouse hindbrain. Nature 341: 405–409.

Wilson, D.I. 1997. Approaches used to study gene expression in early human development. In Molecular Genetics of Early Human Development, ed. T. Strachan, S. Lindsay, and D.I. Wilson, pp. 111–127. Oxford: Bios Scientific Publishers.

# 7

# Induced Mutations Affecting Development of the Mouse Embryo

Colin L. Stewart

The technological advances of today's genetics allows the manipulation of the murine genome and the derivation of mice carrying a specific mutation in any endogenous gene. In turn, this has revolutionized the analysis of gene function in mammals. Gene targeting by homologous recombination in murine embryonic stem (ES) cells is the primary method used to study the role of gene products in mammalian biology. Mice derived by this methodology have been useful in determining the role of genes in embryonic development, the derivation of mouse models of human congenital diseases, cancer, and the susceptibility to more complex polygenic traits such as atherosclerosis, obesity, and hypertension. Emphasis has often been placed on deriving mouse lines that can act as disease models; this objective has frequently proven to be more difficult since mice carrying the mutated gene as gene deletions die in utero, frustrating the investigators' intentions.

Other chapters in this book review the effects that induced mutations have on specific tissues in adult or newborn mice. This chapter reviews the consequences of mutations on embryonic development. It is not intended to be an exhaustive review covering every induced mutation that affects development because the number of new mutations reported is increasing almost weekly. Specific examples will be used to illustrate particular stages at which embryos die and the tissues affected by the mutation. For additional references, there is an excellent web site in BioMednet (The Mouse KnockOut Database, [*http://www.biomednet.com/*

*db/mkmd*]) that lists the existing mutations under a variety of categories and is updated regularly.

## DEVELOPMENT OF THE MOUSE EMBRYO

In the mouse following fertilization, most maternal RNAs in the zygote are degraded (Schultz 1993), and thus early development is not dependent on maternally inherited transcripts. Transcriptional activation of the zygote genome starts at the early 2-cell stage, which is relatively rapid compared with other mammalian species where activation starts as late as the 8- to 16-cell stage (Telford et al. 1990). It was anticipated that such early transcriptional activation would result in many early-acting lethals, particularly in those genes encoding so-called household functions, such as ubiquitous transcription factors. Surprisingly, mutations in genes such as *c-fos* and *c-jun* (which are both components of the AP-1 transcriptional complex) and the ubiquitous transcription factor SP-1 don't affect development until a relatively late stage (Hilberg et al. 1993; Marin et al. 1997; Wang et al. 1992). The earliest-acting lethals, resulting in death of the embryo at the 2- to 4-cell stage, are mutations in genes regulating DNA replication/proofreading/excision repair and RNA metabolism (Fig. 7.1). Examples of the former are the xeroderma pigmentosa D gene *Xpd* (de Boer et al. 1998b), *Rad51*, and the Alzheimer precursor protein *Aplp2* (Rassoulzadegan et al. 1998; Tsuzuki et al. 1996). Those affecting RNA metabolism include the *Smn* (survival motor neuron) gene (Schrank et al. 1997) and Raly, an RNA-binding protein, the gene of which is mutated by

I wish to thank Anne Wang for her comments and Cheri Rhoderick in the preparation of this chapter. Research sponsored by the National Cancer Institute, DHHS, under contract with ABL.

fusion to the agouti locus ($A^y$ lethal yellow) (Duhl et al. 1994; Michaud et al. 1993). Other early-acting mutations are in genes affecting chromosome segregation, such as *Cenpc* (centromere C protein) (Kalitsis et al. 1998) and oligosyndactyly (*Os*), where the gene is unidentified but the mutation results in mitotic arrest at the late morula/blastocyst stage (Magnuson and Epstein 1984). Other genes in which loss of function results in early lethality are *Npat*, a gene of unknown function that was inactivated by retroviral insertion (Di Fruscio et al. 1997); the nuclear pore complex protein *Can/Nup214* (van Deursen et al. 1996); and the phospholipase-C β gene (*Plc-β*), which regulates cellular fluctuations in calcium levels and activation of heterodimeric G proteins (Wang et al. 1998a).

As the preimplantation embryo undergoes successive rounds of cleavage divisions, genes regulating cell adhesion and cell-to-cell interactions become critical. By the end of the fourth day of development, the mouse embryo has formed the blastocyst, consisting of a hollow epithelial sphere of trophectoderm (or trophoblast) enclosing the inner cell mass (ICM). The trophectoderm, during subsequent development, contributes to the formation of the placenta, whereas the ICM forms the embryo proper and part of the allantoic placenta. With the formation of the ICM and trophectoderm, the viability and continued development

of these two tissues become mutually dependent. Loss of either E-Cadherin, the homodimeric cell surface adhesion molecule, or of α E-Catenin, an intracellular protein involved in integrating signal transduction from E-Cadherin to the cellular cytoskeleton, results in embryonic arrest at the blastocyst stage due to the lack of epithelial trophectoderm formation (Larue et al. 1994; Riethmacher et al. 1995; Torres et al. 1997). Although not specifically cell lethal, as cell lines can be established from these null embryos, the embryos die in vivo because loss of the trophectoderm results in the failure of embryo implantation.

The trophectoderm acts as the epithelial interface with the maternal environment, regulating the availability of nutrients and the ionic composition of the blastocoele, within which the ICM is located. In turn, the ICM supports the growth and cell proliferation of the trophoblast (Gardner and Johnson 1972). The proliferative effect of the ICM on the trophectoderm is mediated through the expression of fibroblast growth factor 4 (Fgf4), which activates the Fgf2 receptor. Induced mutations in the genes of both factors result in failure of blastocyst development and implantation (Arman et al. 1998; Feldman et al. 1995). The requirement for Fgf4 was recently shown by the in vitro establishment of trophectoderm cell lines whose growth was dependent on, among other factors, exogenously added Fgf4 (Tanaka

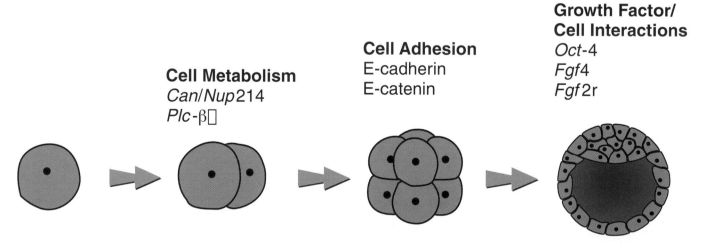

**Growth Factor/
Cell Interactions**
*Oct*-4
*Fgf*4
*Fgf*2r

**Cell Adhesion**
E-cadherin
E-catenin

**Cell Metabolism**
*Can/Nup*214
*Plc*-β

*Xpd*   Xeroderma Pigmentosa D (DNA helicase-transcription/nucleotide excision)
*Aplp*2   Alzheimer precursor protein (replication segregation)
*Smn*   Survival motor neuron RNA metabolism Gem association
*Rad*51   Homologous recombination DNA repair
*Cnpc*   Centrosome C protein mitotic segregation
$A^y$   Fusion between Agouti locus and Raly, an RNA binding protein
*Os*   Oligosyndactyly causes mitotic arrest

**FIGURE 7.1**   Summary of known mutations affecting preimplantation development.

et al. 1998). Likewise, Fgf4 is produced by the ICM under control of the POU transcription factor Oct-4, where its expression is restricted to the ICM and subsequent pluripotent lineages. Loss of Oct-4 also results in developmental arrest at the blastocyst stage (Nichols et al. 1998).

## PERI-IMPLANTATION DEFECTS

All mammalian embryos establish an intimate physical contact with the maternal reproductive tract at implantation. Such contact is necessary to sustain the continued development of the embryo. Implantation is a potential developmental bottleneck in mammalian reproduction because not only must embryonic development be proceeding normally but also the uterine tissues, to which the developing embryo will attach, must be in both a physiologically and anatomically receptive state.

Physiologically, implantation is dependent on uterine expression of Lif. Lif (leukemia inhibitory factor) is a secreted cytokine of the interleukin-6 family. Lack of Lif does not affect development to the blastocyst stage. However, in Lif-deficient females, the uterus is unresponsive, as Lif is required to stimulate the uterine luminal epithelium to respond to signals from the embryo at implantation (Stewart et al. 1992). The uterine response to the implanting embryo is also dependent on cyclooxygenase-2 (Cox-2) for the localized synthesis of prostaglandins that appear to be essential for decidualization of the uterus (Lim et al. 1997).

Anatomically, uterine development is dependent on expression of two homeotic genes, Hoxa-10 and Hoxa-11. Loss of Hoxa-10 results in homeotic transformation of the proximal one-third of the uterus into oviduct (Satokata et al. 1995). Expression of both gene products is regulated during the reproductive cycle by the steroid hormones estrogen and progesterone and may, therefore, be required physiologically to bring the uterus into a state of receptivity; Hoxa-11–null mice don't express Lif in the endometrial glands at implantation (Gendron et al. 1997). Deficiency in another homeobox gene, Hmx-3, results in no overt structural transformation to the uterus, but as with the Hox mutants, implantation frequencies were reduced in null mutants (Wang et al. 1998b).

At implantation, a variety of embryonic gene products are essential for continued development (Fig. 7.2). The cell adhesion molecules, the β-integrins, are required for maintaining the integrity and viability of the ICM (Stephens et al. 1995). Likewise, desmoplakin, a component of the desmosome that links this adhesive structure

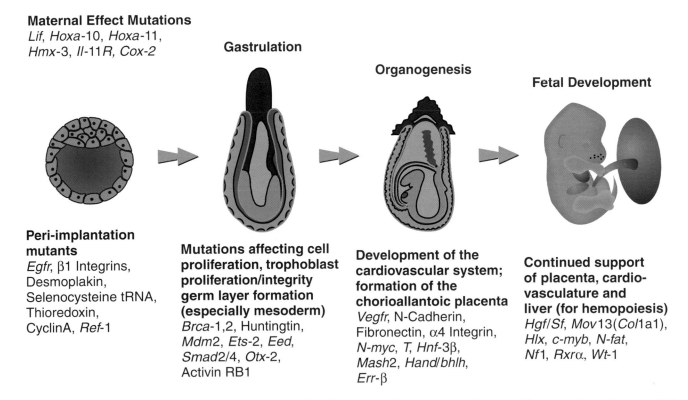

**FIGURE 7.2** Summary of some of the mutations affecting postimplantation development from implantation to ~E14.

to the cellular intermediate filament network, is necessary for sustaining growth of the trophectoderm and for the cellular organization of the ICM as it proliferates to form the epiblast (Gallicano et al. 1998).

Intriguingly, mutations in three genes, all involved in regulating the cellular reduction/oxidation (redox) state, result in developmental failure at or shortly after implantation. These genes are the selenoproteins and selenocysteine tRNA, which is required by selenoproteins for their incorporation of selenocysteine (Bosl et al. 1997). The selenoproteins, such as thioredoxin, mediate the intracellular redox status (Matsui et al. 1996). Thioredoxin translocates into the nucleus where it regulates the expression of various genes involved in cell proliferation through the dual redox factor, redox factor-1 (Ref-1). Ref-1 is a DNA repair protein/apurinic endonuclease that modulates activity of the transcription factor *Ap-1* (Xanthoudakis et al. 1996). Why selenocysteine tRNA, thioredoxin, and Ref-1 are critical at this stage is obscure. It may reflect a change in embryonic cellular physiology at implantation as the embryo undergoes transition from developing in a relatively simple salt and amino acid solution during preimplantation growth to becoming dependent on the more complex range of factors present in maternal serum. Other genes that, when mutated, result in peri-implantation lethality are *CyclinA2*, which regulates $G_1/S$ and $G_2/M$ transition points in the cell cycle (Murphy et al. 1997), and the Egf receptor, although the lethal effect of the latter is strain dependent, as its loss in some strains does not affect viability till later stages in embryogenesis or even in postnatal stages (Threadgill et al. 1995).

# MUTATIONS AFFECTING DEVELOPMENT AT GASTRULATION

Following implantation, the embryo embarks on a rapid series of cell divisions. In the ICM, which now is called the epiblast, the total number of cells increases from ~120 at implantation to ~4500 some 36 hours later (equivalent to day 7 of gestation). With this increase in cell number, over such a short period of time, it is estimated the mean cell cycle time in the epiblast decreases from 11.5 hours to 4.5 hours. In the rat embryo at an equivalent stage, the cell cycle length is estimated as being as short as 3.5 hours in the primitive streak (Mac Auley et al. 1993). During this same period, the epiblast undergoes differentiation with formation of the primitive streak, which defines the future anterior-posterior embryonic axis, together with the appearance of the mesoderm, which will give rise to many somatic tissues, including the cardiovascular system (for an excellent review on the molecular basis of these events

see Beddington and Robertson 1989). Thus, two essential processes are occurring simultaneously over this period: a rapid increase in cell number and cellular differentiation into different lineages.

Some 60 genes have been identified to date that, when mutated, result in lethality at this stage of embryogenesis (Fig. 7.2). One of those that affect cell viability/proliferation is *huntingtin*. This gene, when mutated in humans by the amplification of CAG repeats, results in the degenerative neurological disease Huntington's chorea. In mice, ablation of this gene results in developmental arrest at 7.5 days of gestation (Duyao et al. 1995; Nasir et al. 1995; Zeitlin et al. 1995). The cause of arrest/death is unknown, as is the function of the protein, although it has been suggested that it may protect cells against apoptosis. Similarly, mutation of *Mdm2*, which regulates *p53*—a factor critical to regulating cell proliferation arrest/apoptosis and is induced by cell stress or DNA damage—is lethal at this stage (Jones et al. 1995; Montes de Oca Luna et al. 1995). Intriguingly, loss of *p53* function is not, in itself, an embryonic-lethal event (Donehower et al. 1992). Other genes whose products are essential at this stage of development are the breast carcinoma susceptibility genes, *Brca1* (Hakem et al. 1997; Ludwig et al. 1997; Suzuki et al. 1997) and *Brca2* (Sharan et al. 1997). The functions of these two proteins are not fully understood, but both appear to be required for DNA repair.

Recent evidence has shown that differentiation of the epiblast, with formation of the anterior/posterior embryonic axis, formation of the primitive streak, and organization of the mesoderm, is dependent on signaling interactions between the epiblast and the surrounding visceral endoderm. The Egf-related factor *Cripto* is required to establish the anterior-posterior axis in the pregastrulation embryo; *Cripto* is expressed in the epiblast in a proximo-distal gradient (Ding et al. 1998). Mutations in the transcription factor *Hnf3-β* (Ang and Rossant 1994) result in failure of the primitive streak to elongate as *Hnf3-β* is expressed in the visceral endoderm, notochord, and floorplate. Similarly, mutations in both the activin receptor *ActRIB* and the *Smad-2* transcriptional activator that is induced by the TGF-β family of receptors result in failure of mesoderm formation and organization (Gu et al. 1998; Nomura and Li 1998; Waldrip et al. 1998). These mutations can be rescued, to varying degrees, by replacing the mutant visceral endoderm with wild-type endoderm. Further evidence that mesoderm formation is critical to continued embryonic development is revealed by deletion of the Polycomb group gene *eed*. Loss of function of this gene results in failure of the embryonic mesoderm to proliferate and organize properly, although extraembryonic mesoderm formation contributing to the amnion and yolk sac appears normal (Faust et al. 1998).

These developmental stages continue to depend on a functional interaction between the uterine tissues and trophoblast, as shown by the mutation of the *Ets2* transcription factor that results in failure of trophoblast proliferation (Yamamoto et al. 1998). Similarly, proper response of the maternal uterine tissues to the implanting embryo is revealed by the loss of interleukin-11 receptor (*Il-11r*) function. This causes a defect of decidual proliferation resulting in small deciduae. Consequently, trophoblast proliferation and its uterine invasion are increased, with resulting failure to maintain proper interactions between the embryo and uterus and followed by embryonic death at embryonic day (E) 7.5 (Bilinski et al. 1998; Robb et al. 1998).

# ORGANOGENESIS AND FETAL DEVELOPMENT

With the establishment of the embryonic axis and germ layers at E7.5, the major organ rudiments, such as the central nervous system, somites (which will give rise to most of the skeletal and muscular systems), and gut begin to form. With the increase in embryonic size and formation of the major organs, the supply of nutrients and oxygen, up to this point sustained by the diffusion from the uterus, become limiting factors. The embryo therefore must develop a circulatory system to transport oxygen and nutrients to its tissues. An early circulatory system is first formed in the yolk sac where blood islands form both hematopoietic and endothelial cells. The embryonic heart is also developing at this time, and it initiates a functional circulation. However, once the embryo has reached a certain size (E9.5), the yolk sac circulation becomes insufficient to sustain further development. Hence, a more direct link between the fetal and maternal circulation via the fusion of the allantois and chorion to form the chorioallantoic placenta is established. The allantois also forms the umbilical artery and vein. A variety of gene products have been shown to be critical around this time. The vascular endothelial growth factors (Vegf) and their receptors (Vegfr), when mutated, result in lethality due to disorganized development of the vascular system (Dumont et al. 1998; Ferrara et al. 1996; Lin et al. 1998). In addition to these factors, disruption of the genes encoding *N-Cadherin* and *N-myc* result in embryonic lethality via defects in heart development (Moens et al. 1993; Radice et al. 1997). Despite expression commencing at the blastocyst stage, loss of the extracellular matrix protein fibronectin does not result in lethality till E9, with lethality being due to widespread abnormalities in mesodermally derived tissues, particularly in the heart and vasculature (George et al. 1993, 1997). The continued dependence of the embryo on a properly functioning trophectoderm/placenta is revealed by mutations in the genes of the basic helix-loop-helix (bHLH) nuclear proteins that regulate the differentiation of a variety of cells. Mutations in *Mash2* and *Hand1/Thing1* result in abnormal differentiation of the trophoblast and placental failure (Guillemot et al. 1994; Kraut et al. 1998; Riley et al. 1998). Similarly, loss of the adhesion molecule α4-integrin prevents the allantois from fusing with the chorion, resulting in placental failure together with abnormal cardiac development (Yang et al. 1995).

From E12 to birth, embryonic development is dependent on the function of three tissues: the cardiovascular system, placenta, and liver (Copp 1995). Inefficient pumping by the heart and abnormal heart development result in circulatory failure at various stages, as illustrated by the loss of function mutations in the retinoic acid α receptor (*Rxr* α) (Sucov et al. 1994), the Wilms tumor gene, *Wt-1* (Kreidberg et al. 1993), and neurofibromatosis (*Nf*) genes (Brannan et al. 1994). Furthermore, structural instability of the blood vessel walls results in hemorrhage and death as shown in the retroviral insertion mutation *Mov-13*, which disrupts the α 1(I) procollagen gene (Lohler et al. 1984; Schnieke et al. 1983). Continued reliance on proper placental development and function is also apparent as mice lacking hepatocyte growth factor (*Hgf*) develop placental abnormalities (Bladt et al. 1995) (for a more detailed description of mutations affecting this tissue, see Chap. 12). Of the principal internal organs, the liver must function normally to sustain development to term since the major site of hematopoiesis shifts from the yolk sac to the liver at E13. Mutations in genes such as *c-myb*, *Sek/MKK4*, mitogen-activated protein kinase, and the *Hlx* homeobox gene affect liver development, which, in turn, results in hematopoietic failure and anemia (Hentsch et al. 1996; Mucenski et al. 1991; Yang et al. 1997). Embryonic viability does not appear to depend on the formation of other internal organs. This is illustrated by the mutations shown in Figure 7.3. Loss of *Lim1* results in a failure of head development (Shawlot and Behringer 1995). Deficiency in either glial-derived growth factor (*Gdnf*)or its receptor, *Ret*, causes a lack of kidney formation (Moore et al. 1996; Pichel et al. 1996a, 1996b; Sanchez et al. 1996; Schuchardt et al. 1995). Mutation in fibroblast growth factor 10 (*Fgf10*) results in limb and lung deficiency (Sekine et al. 1999), and lastly, simultaneous loss of *MyoD* and *Myf5*, the muscle specific transcription factors, results in the absence of all skeletal muscles and ribs (Rudnicki et al. 1993). In mutants lacking these major organs, the embryos develop to term but die at birth.

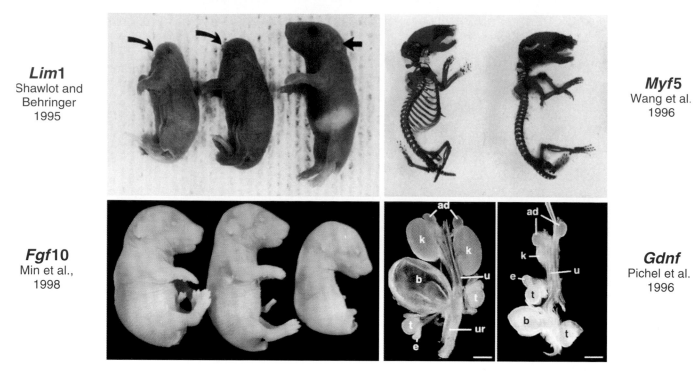

**Lim1**
Shawlot and
Behringer
1995

**Myf5**
Wang et al.
1996

**Fgf10**
Min et al.,
1998

**Gdnf**
Pichel et al.
1996

**FIGURE 7.3** Four mutations affecting development of some of the principal organs in embryos. *Lim1* deficiency results in an absence of head structures. *Myf5/Myod* results in loss of all skeletal muscle and ribs. *Fgf10* deficiency results in a failure of lungs, limbs, and lower abdomen development. *Gdnf/Ret* deficiency results in loss of kidneys. All these mutations develop to term but die at birth. (*Lim1*, Shawlot and Behringer 1995; *Fgf10*, Min et al. 1998; *Myf5*, Wang et al. 1996; *Gdnf*, Pichel et al. 1996a, b)

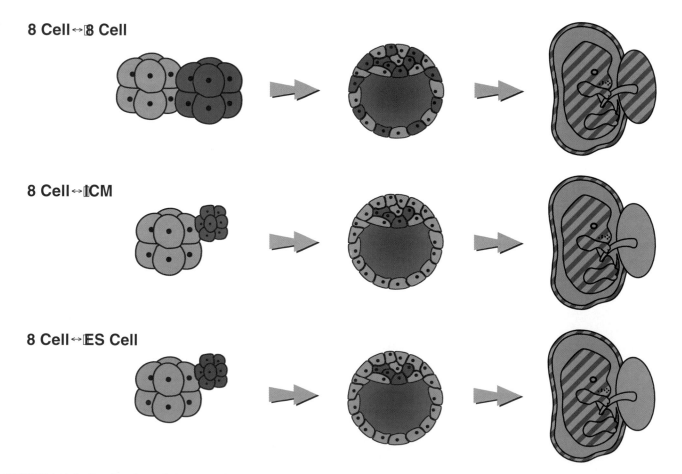

**8 Cell↔8 Cell**

**8 Cell↔ICM**

**8 Cell↔ES Cell**

**FIGURE 7.4** Production of chimeras by aggregation. The embryonic tissues used to make the chimera affects the distribution of their descendants in the resulting chimera, as shown by the differences in shading.

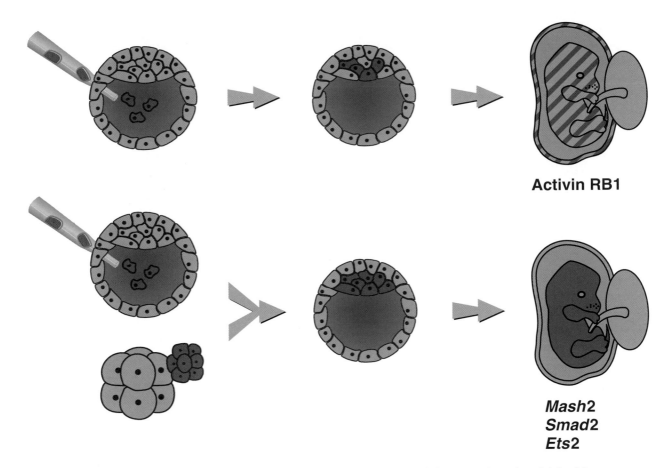

**Activin RB1**

**Mash2**
**Smad2**
**Ets2**

**FIGURE 7.5**    Production of chimeras by blastocyst injection and some of the mutations in which chimera production was used to test the effect of the mutations on cell fate. Injection of ES or ICM cells, or aggregation with 8-cell–stage embryos, into blastocysts restricts their eventual contribution to the embryonic compartment and exclusion from the trophoblast and yolk sac compartments.

# ALTERNATIVE ROUTES TO GENERATING AND ANALYZING INDUCED MUTATIONS

The phenotype of the embryo resulting from the induced mutation is frequently complex, and it is often difficult to determine which tissue is primarily affected by loss of the gene in question. Furthermore, many mutations have been induced in genes with the original intention being to determine the requirement of the genes in adult or later stages of development, but this is impossible if the embryo dies. Consequently, investigators have developed a variety of techniques, both molecular and embryological, to address and circumvent these problems (Rossant and Spence 1998).

The principal embryological technique for analyzing complex mutations has been to produce chimeras by intermingling embryonic cells of the mutant embryo with those of a wild-type embryo. By tracing the contribution of either genotype in the chimera to particular tissues, deductions can be made as to which tissue(s) is(are) affected by the particular mutation. Frequently, one or other of the embryos is genetically marked so as to distinguish its cellular progeny from those of the other. Currently, the most commonly used marker is the *Escherichia coli* β-galactosidase gene; it is either incorporated into the gene of interest or can be used as an independent marker, as in the Rosa-26 line of mice where it is constitutively expressed in all cells (Zambrowicz et al. 1997).

Embryonic chimeras are usually made using preimplantation embryos, although postimplantation chimeras have been generated using embryos cocultured in vitro or by the injection of cells into midgestation embryos in utero (Jaenisch 1985; Tam and Zhou 1996). The various routes to making preimplantation chimeras are shown in Figures 7.4 and 7.5, with each method offering different advantages. Aggregation of embryos at the 8-cell stage results in both genotypes being able to contribute to all lineages, both embryonic and extraembryonic (trophoblast, parietal and yolk sac endoderm).

Such chimeras were instrumental in showing that parthenogenetic embryos could contribute to all lineages at the onset of development. Yet, as embryogenesis progressed, parthenogenetic derivatives were first lost from the extraembryonic tissues and subsequently from most somatic cell lineages, with the exception of parts of the central nervous system and the germline (Fundele et al. 1989; Nagy et al. 1989).

Aggregation of or injection of 8-cell–stage embryos or blastocysts, respectively, with mutant ICM or ES cells exploits the latter's developmental restriction in that the ICM or ES cells contribute only to the embryonic lineages (Beddington and Robertson 1989). Conversely, aggregation or injection of wild-type ES cells with mutant 8-cell–stage embryos or blastocysts can achieve the reverse, with the resulting embryonic lineages being composed of a mixture of wild-type and mutant cells. For example, embryos lacking the activinRB1 (*ActRIB*) receptor show disorganization of the epiblast and extraembryonic ectoderm with developmental arrest at E6.5, before mesoderm formation. Injection of *ActRIB*-null ES cells into wild-type embryos resulted in their contribution to mesoderm and neural ectoderm, with many chimeric embryos developing to E9.5 (Gu et al. 1998). This demonstrated that cells lacking the receptor were not intrinsically incapable of forming mesoderm but failed to do so because development of the null embryos was arrested before mesoderm formation.

The most effective means of separating chimeric contributions to embryonic and extraembryonic lineages has been to inject ICM or ES cells into tetraploid blastocysts. Tetraploid embryos can develop to term; however, when combined with diploid cells, the tetraploid cells almost always segregate to the extraembryonic lineages of the trophectoderm and visceral endoderm. Thus, the entire embryonic lineage is derived from the injected ICM or ES cells. This approach has been particularly effective in analyzing trophectodermal and placental mutants. For example, the transcription factors *Mash2* and *Ets2* are essential only to trophoblast development. Aggregation of *Mash2*- or *Ets2*-null embryos with wild-type tetraploid embryos results in both null embryos developing to adulthood, whereas the nonaggregated null embryos died around E9.5 due to trophoblast failure (Guillemot et al. 1994; Yamamoto et al. 1998).

Similarly, investigations into the role of the visceral endoderm in regulating both mesoderm formation and epiblast differentiation in the early postimplantation embryo have also benefited from using the tetraploid rescue approach. Embryos null for the *Smad-2* transcription factor die before gastrulation with poor and disorganized mesoderm formation. Injection of *Smad-2*–null ES cells into wild-type tetraploid embryos resulted in embryo development to E10.5 with mesoderm and axis formation, although

other defects, such as a failure of embryo turning and cyclopia, were evident (Heyer et al. 1999). Conversely, injection of wild-type ES cells into *Smad-2*–null embryos failed to rescue the early postimplantation lethality, with the embryos forming yolk sac–like structures with disorganized mesoderm (Waldrip et al. 1998). From these results, it was concluded that *Smad-2* is first required by the visceral endoderm to regulate mesoderm and embryonic axis formation in the epiblast. It is also required in later stages of development for turning of the embryo and proper formation of the anterior neuronal structures.

## MOLECULAR APPROACHES TO MANIPULATING EMBRYONIC DEVELOPMENT

Recently, a molecular approach to generating induced mutations, either in a specific tissue or at a specific time during the life cycle of the mouse, has emerged. The Cre/loxP system mediates site-specific DNA recombination and is being increasingly utilized to study gene function in vivo (Fukushige and Sauer 1992; Lakso et al. 1996). This system is principally directed to disrupting gene function in a single cell type or tissue, allowing the analysis of the physiological and pathological consequences of mutating a particular gene in that specific cell type or tissue. This procedure relies on the properties of the bacterial *Cre* recombinase to recognize specific nucleotide sequences, the lox-P sites, and to delete the intervening nucleotide sequences between flanking lox-P sequences. The deletions can be as short as a few bases to many megabases. A particularly clear example of the applicability of this technique is illustrated by the tissue-specific deletion of the insulin receptor in the pancreatic β cells. Disrupting the insulin receptor (IR) in all tissues results in perinatal lethality of the homozygous null mice (Accili et al. 1996). Viable mice were, however, derived by specifically targeting the deletion to the pancreatic β cells so that only the insulin-producing cells were defective in expressing the insulin receptor. This was achieved by introducing lox-P sites so that they flanked a critical exon of the insulin receptor gene. In this state, the insulin receptor was still functional. Subsequent mating of mice homozygous for the floxed IR gene with a separate line of transgenic mice expressing Cre recombinase under control of the insulin promoter resulted in offspring in which the insulin receptor was only deleted in the pancreatic β cells. These mice were unable to respond to increased glucose levels by the secretion of insulin and eventually developed a form of Type 2 diabetes characterized by a progressive glucose intolerance (Kulkarni et al. 1999).

Other attempts have been directed toward temporally regulating Cre expression during embryogenesis. In one such experiment, the Cre recombinase gene was placed under the combined control of a mutated estrogen receptor responsive only to the estrogen analogue tamoxifen. When combined with the *Wnt1* enhancer, Cre is expressed within regions of the CNS and floorplate in which *Wnt1* is also normally expressed. A single injection of tamoxifen into the pregnant females resulted in Cre activation only within regions of the embryonic CNS where *Wnt1* is expressed (Danielian et al. 1998).

Such examples of tissue-specific and temporal regulation of Cre open up the possibility of modulating gene expression at specific times during embryogenesis. This permits the study of gene function at stages of development subsequent to those in which initial expression of the gene results in developmental abnormalities or lethality. The technology is still at an early stage with a variety of approaches being used to improve its applicability. Much of its success will depend on the identification of a range of promoters whose activity is restricted to specific cells or tissues.

Finally, other techniques are being used to avoid embryonic lethality, particularly with regard to deriving mice that can serve as models for human congenital diseases. In many of the initial attempts to derive such mice, the entire function of the gene was ablated. The majority of human congenital diseases, however, are due to hypomorphic mutations of the gene resulting in a reduction of gene activity rather than complete loss of function. Only by introducing a more subtle mutation into the murine gene, homologous to the mutation seen in the human gene, has it been possible to produce viable mice that then develop symptoms characteristic of the disease. A recent example of this approach is illustrated by mutations in the xeroderma pigmentosa D gene described earlier in this chapter. Total loss of function of this gene results in one of the earliest embryonic lethals, with death occurring at the 2- to 4-cell stage (de Boer et al. 1998b). However, viable mice were produced by redesigning the targeting vector such that the gene function was left largely intact, with the exception of the carboxy terminus of the protein, which was replaced with the equivalent human region carrying the specific point mutation (Fig. 7.6). These mice developed trichothiodystrophy (brittle hair) and exhibited increased sensitivity to UV light, both symptoms of xeroderma pigmentosa D–deficiency found in humans (de Boer et al. 1998a).

In conclusion, mouse embryos are susceptible to induced mutations throughout development from shortly after fertilization to E14 and beyond. The majority of lethal mutations described to date cluster around the peri-implantation and early postimplantation period (E5–7). This probably reflects the substantial changes in gene expression occurring at these stages. This is the time in which the embryo undergoes a profound increase

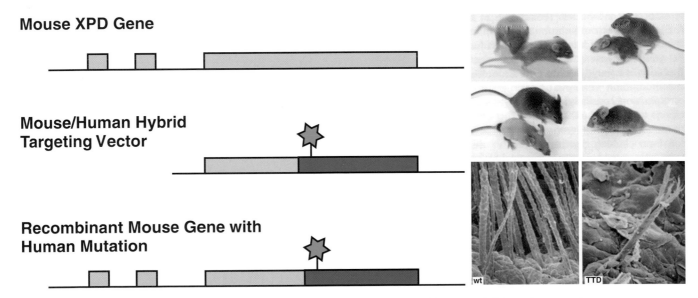

**FIGURE 7.6** An example (xeroderma pigmentosa D gene mutations) of how modifying the targeting construct to introduce the mutation into the germline affects the development of the embryo. Deletion of the entire *Xpd* gene results in lethality at the 2- to 4-cell stage. A subtle point mutation results in viable mice exhibiting a phenotype similar to that of patients with *Xpd* point mutations where "brittle hair" and UV sensitivity is characteristic. Figures show wild-type mouse with normal hair on left and mouse with brittle hair on right and scanning electron micrographs of the hair [bottom right images]. (Modified from de Boer et al. 1998b)

in cell proliferation and is coincident with the onset of many developmental processes, such as establishment of the embryonic axes, germ layer formation, and gastrulation—all essential to establishing the future body plan. Furthermore, trophoblast and subsequent placental development is critical and vulnerable to mutations in genes specific to that development (e.g., *Mash2*). Similarly, some genes are also essential to proper uterine function during pregnancy. However, it has been particularly surprising, as first pointed out by Copp (1995), that, following implantation and gastrulation, embryogenesis is critically dependent on only three tissues: a placenta, cardiovascular system, and liver. Mutations resulting in loss of function of the other major organ systems, such as the brain, kidneys, lungs, limbs, and skeletal musculature, are not essential to embryogenesis and are probably not a cause for embryonic lethality, at least until birth.

The number of mutations affecting embryogenesis will continue to increase, and this will result in a more detailed description of the requirement of individual gene products in development. Complementing this, the emerging technology of manipulating gene expression, both temporally and in a cell/tissue-specific manner, will result in a more accurate understanding of the role of particular genes throughout the animal's life span.

# REFERENCES

Accili, D., Drago, J., Lee, E.J., et al. 1996. Early neonatal death in mice homozygous for a null allele of the insulin receptor gene. Nat Genet 12:106–109.

Ang, S.L. and Rossant, J. 1994. HNF-3 beta is essential for node and notochord formation in mouse development. Cell 78:561–574.

Arman, E., Haffner-Krausz, R., Chen, Y., et al. 1998. Targeted disruption of fibroblast growth factor (FGF) receptor 2 suggests a role for FGF signaling in pregastrulation mammalian development. Proc Natl Acad Sci USA 95:5082–5087.

Beddington, R.S. and Robertson, E.J. 1989. An assessment of the developmental potential of embryonic stem cells in the midgestation mouse embryo. Development 105:733–737.

Bilinski, P., Roopenian, D., and Gossler, A. 1998. Maternal IL-11Ralpha function is required for normal decidua and fetoplacental development in mice. Genes Dev 12:2234–2243.

Bladt, F., Riethmacher, D., Isenmann, S., et al. 1995. Essential role for the c-met receptor in the migration of myogenic precursor cells into the limb bud [see comments]. Nature 376:768–771.

Bosl, M.R., Takaku, K., Oshima, M., et al. 1997. Early embryonic lethality caused by targeted disruption of the mouse selenocysteine tRNA gene (Trsp). Proc Natl Acad Sci USA 94:5531–5534.

Brannan, C.I., Perkins, A.S., Vogel, K.S., et al. 1994. Targeted disruption of the neurofibromatosis type-1 gene leads to developmental abnormalities in heart and various neural crest-derived tissues [published erratum appears in Genes Dev, 1994 Nov 15, 8(22):2792]. Genes Dev 8:1019–1029.

Copp, A.J. 1995. Death before birth: clues from gene knockouts and mutations [see comments]. Trends Genet 11:87–93.

Danielian, P.S., Muccino, D., Rowitch, D.H., et al. 1998. Modification of gene activity in mouse embryos in utero by a tamoxifen-inducible form of Cre recombinase. Curr Biol 8:1323–1326.

de Boer, J., de Wit, J., van Steeg, H., et al. 1998a. A mouse model for the basal transcription/DNA repair syndrome trichothiodystrophy. Mol Cell 1:981–990.

de Boer, J., Donker, I., de Wit, J., et al. 1998b. Disruption of the mouse xeroderma pigmentosum group D DNA repair/basal transcription gene results in preimplantation lethality. Cancer Res 58:89–94.

Di Fruscio, M., Weiher, H., Vanderhyden, B.C., et al. 1997. Proviral inactivation of the Npat gene of Mpv 20 mice results in early embryonic arrest. Mol Cell Biol 17:4080–4086.

Ding, J., Yang, L., Yan, Y.T., et al. 1998. Cripto is required for correct orientation of the anterior-posterior axis in the mouse embryo. Nature 395:702–707.

Donehower, L.A., Harvey, M., Slagle, B.L., et al. 1992. Mice deficient for p53 are developmentally normal but susceptible to spontaneous tumours. Nature 356:215–221.

Duhl, D.M., Stevens, M.E., Vrieling, H., et al. 1994. Pleiotropic effects of the mouse lethal yellow (Ay) mutation explained by deletion of a maternally expressed gene and the simultaneous production of agouti fusion RNAs. Development 120:1695–1708.

Dumont, D.J., Jussila, L., Taipale, J., et al. 1998. Cardiovascular failure in mouse embryos deficient in VEGF receptor-3. Science 282:946–949.

Duyao, M.P., Auerbach, A.B., Ryan, A., et al. 1995. Inactivation of the mouse Huntington's disease gene homolog Hdh. Science 269:407–410.

Faust, C., Lawson, K.A., Schork, N.J., et al. 1998. The Polycomb-group gene eed is required for normal morphogenetic movements during gastrulation in the mouse embryo. Development 125:4495–4506.

Feldman, B., Poueymirou, W., Papaioannou, V.E., et al. 1995. Requirement of FGF-4 for postimplantation mouse development. Science 267:246–249.

Ferrara, N., Carver-Moore, K., Chen, H., et al. 1996. Heterozygous embryonic lethality induced by targeted inactivation of the VEGF gene. Nature 380:439–442.

Fukushige, S. and Sauer, B. 1992. Genomic targeting with a positive-selection lox integration vector allows highly reproducible gene expression in mammalian cells. Proc Natl Acad Sci USA 89:7905–7909.

Fundele, R., Norris, M.L., Barton, S.C., et al. 1989. Systematic elimination of parthenogenetic cells in mouse chimeras. Development 106:29–35.

Gallicano, G.I., Kouklis, P., Bauer, C., et al. 1998. Desmoplakin is required early in development for assembly of desmosomes and cytoskeletal linkage. J Cell Biol 143:2009–2022.

Gardner, R.L. and Johnson, M.H. 1972. An investigation of inner cell mass and trophoblast tissues following their isolation from the mouse blastocyst. J Embryol Exp Morphol 28:279–312.

Gendron, R.L., Paradis, H., Hsieh-Li, H.M., et al. 1997. Abnormal uterine stromal and glandular function associated with maternal reproductive defects in Hoxa-11 null mice. Biol Reprod 56:1097–1105.

George, E.L., Georges-Labouesse, E.N., Patel-King, R.S., et al. 1993. Defects in mesoderm, neural tube and vascular development in mouse embryos lacking fibronectin. Development 119:1079–1091.

George, E.L., Baldwin, H.S., and Hynes, R.O. 1997. Fibronectins are essential for heart and blood vessel morphogenesis but are dispensable for initial specification of precursor cells. Blood 90:3073–3081.

Gu, Z., Nomura, M., Simpson, B.B., et al. 1998. The type I activin receptor ActRIB is required for egg cylinder organization and gastrulation in the mouse. Genes Dev 12:844–857.

Guillemot, F., Nagy, A., Auerbach, A., et al. 1994. Essential role of Mash-2 in extraembryonic development. Nature 371:333–336.

Hakem, R., de la Pompa, J.L., Elia, A., et al. 1997. Partial rescue of Brca1 (5–6) early embryonic lethality by p53 or p21 null mutation. Nat Genet 16:298–302.

Hentsch, B., Lyons, I., Li, R., et al. 1996. Hlx homeo box gene is essential for an inductive tissue interaction that drives expansion of embryonic liver and gut. Genes Dev 10:70–79.

Heyer, J., Escalente, D., Stewart, C.L., et al. 1999. Postgastrulation Smad2 deficient embryos show defects in embryo turning and anterior morphogenesis. Proc Natl Acad Sci USA, 96:12595–12600.

Hilberg, F., Aguzzi, A., Howells, N., et al. 1993. c-jun is essential for normal mouse development and hepatogenesis [published erratum appears in Nature, 1993 Nov 25, 366(6453):368]. Nature 365:179–181.

Jaenisch, R. 1985. Mammalian neural crest cells participate in normal embryonic development on microinjection into post-implantation mouse embryos. Nature 318:181–183.

Jones, S.N., Roe, A.E., Donehower, L.A., et al. 1995. Rescue of embryonic lethality in Mdm2-deficient mice by absence of p53. Nature 378:206–208.

Kalitsis, P., Fowler, K.J., Earle, E., et al. 1998. Targeted disruption of mouse centromere protein C gene leads to mitotic disarray and early embryo death. Proc Natl Acad Sci USA 95:1136–1141.

Kraut, N., Snider, L., Chen, C.M., et al. 1998. Requirement of the mouse I-mfa gene for placental development and skeletal patterning. EMBO J 17:6276–6288.

Kreidberg, J.A., Sariola, H., Loring, J.M., et al. 1993. WT-1 is required for early kidney development. Cell 74:679–691.

Kulkarni, R.N., Bruning, J.C., Winnay, J.N., et al. 1999. Tissue-specific knockout of the insulin receptor in pancre-

atic beta cells creates an insulin secretory defect similar to that in type 2 diabetes. Cell 96:329–339.

Lakso, M., Pichel, J.G., Gorman, J.R., et al. 1996. Efficient in vivo manipulation of mouse genomic sequences at the zygote stage. Proc Natl Acad Sci USA 93:5860–5865.

Larue, L., Ohsugi, M., Hirchenhain, J., et al. 1994. E-cadherin null mutant embryos fail to form a trophectoderm epithelium. Proc Natl Acad Sci USA 91:8263–8267.

Lim, H., Paria, B.C., Das, S.K., et al. 1997. Multiple female reproductive failures in cyclooxygenase 2-deficient mice. Cell 91:197–208.

Lin, Q., Lu, J., Yanagisawa, H., et al. 1998. Requirement of the MADS-box transcription factor MEF2C for vascular development. Development 125:4565–4574.

Lohler, J., Timpl, R., and Jaenisch, R. 1984. Embryonic lethal mutation in mouse collagen I gene causes rupture of blood vessels and is associated with erythropoietic and mesenchymal cell death. Cell 38:597–607.

Ludwig, T., Chapman, D.L., Papaioannou, et al. 1997. Targeted mutations of breast cancer susceptibility gene homologs in mice: lethal phenotypes of Brca1, Brca2, Brca1/Brca2, Brca1/p53, and Brca2/p53 nullizygous embryos. Genes Dev 11:1226–1241.

Mac Auley, A., Werb, Z., and Mirkes, P.E. 1993. Characterization of the unusually rapid cell cycles during rat gastrulation. Development 117:873–883.

Magnuson, T. and Epstein, C.J. 1984. Oligosyndactyly: a lethal mutation in the mouse that results in mitotic arrest very early in development. Cell 38:823–833.

Marin, M., Karis, A., Visser, P., et al. 1997. Transcription factor SP1 is essential for early embryonic development but dispensable for cell growth and differentiation. Cell 89:619–628.

Matsui, M., Oshima, M., Oshima, H., et al. 1996. Early embryonic lethality caused by targeted disruption of the mouse thioredoxin gene. Dev Biol 178:179–185.

Michaud, E.J., Bultman, S.J., Stubbs, L.J., et al. 1993. The embryonic lethality of homozygous lethal yellow mice (Ay/Ay) is associated with the disruption of a novel RNA-binding protein. Genes Dev 7:1203–1213.

Minn, H., Danilenko, D.M., Scully, S.A., et al. 1998. Fgf is required for both limb and lung development and exhibits striking functional similarity to Drosophila branchless. Genes Dev 12:3156–3161.

Moens, C.B., Stanton, B.R., Parada, L.F., et al. 1993. Defects in heart and lung development in compound heterozygotes for two different targeted mutations at the N-myc locus. Development 119:485–499.

Montes de Oca Luna, R., Wagner, D.S., and Lozano, G. 1995. Rescue of early embryonic lethality in mdm2-deficient mice by deletion of p53. Nature 378:203–206.

Moore, M.W., Klein, R.D., Farinas, I., et al. 1996. Renal and neuronal abnormalities in mice lacking GDNF. Nature 382:76–79.

Mucenski, M.L., McLain, K., Kier, A.B., et al. 1991. A functional c-myb gene is required for normal murine fetal hepatic hematopoiesis. Cell 65:677–689.

Murphy, M., Stinnakre, M.G., Senamaud-Beaufort, C., et al. 1997. Delayed early embryonic lethality following disruption of the murine cyclin A2 gene. Nat Genet 15:83–86.

Nagy, A., Sass, M., and Markkula, M. 1989. Systematic non-uniform distribution of parthenogenetic cells in adult mouse chimaeras. Development 106:321–324.

Nasir, J., Floresco, S.B., O'Kusky, J.R., et al. 1995. Targeted disruption of the Huntington's disease gene results in embryonic lethality and behavioral and morphological changes in heterozygotes. Cell 81:811–823.

Nichols, J., Zevnik, B., Anastassiadis, K., et al. 1998. Formation of pluripotent stem cells in the mammalian embryo depends on the POU transcription factor Oct4. Cell 95:379–391.

Nomura, M. and Li, E. 1998. Smad2 role in mesoderm formation, left-right patterning and craniofacial development [see comments]. Nature 393:786–790.

Pichel, J.G., Shen, L., Sheng, H.Z., et al. 1996a. Defects in enteric innervation and kidney development in mice lacking GDNF. Nature 382:73–76.

Pichel, J.G., Shen, L., Sheng, H.Z., et al. 1996b. GDNF is required for kidney development and enteric innervation. Cold Spring Harb Symp Quant Biol 61:445–457.

Radice, G.L., Rayburn, H., Matsunami, H., et al. 1997. Developmental defects in mouse embryos lacking N-cadherin. Dev Biol 181:64–78.

Rassoulzadegan, M., Yang, Y., and Cuzin, F. 1998. APLP2, a member of the Alzheimer precursor protein family, is required for correct genomic segregation in dividing mouse cells. EMBO J 17:4647–4656.

Riethmacher, D., Brinkmann, V., and Birchmeier, C. 1995. A targeted mutation in the mouse E-cadherin gene results in defective preimplantation development. Proc Natl Acad Sci USA 92:855–859.

Riley, P., Anson-Cartwright, L., and Cross, J.C. 1998. The Hand1 bHLH transcription factor is essential for placentation and cardiac morphogenesis. Nat Genet 18:271–275.

Robb, L., Li, R., Hartley, L., et al. 1998. Infertility in female mice lacking the receptor for interleukin 11 is due to a defective uterine response to implantation. Nat Med 4:303–308.

Rossant, J. and Spence, A. 1998. Chimeras and mosaics in mouse mutant analysis. Trends Genet 14:358–363.

Rudnicki, M.A., Schnegelsberg, P.N., Stead, R.H., et al. 1993. MyoD or Myf-5 is required for the formation of skeletal muscle. Cell 75:1351–1359.

Sanchez, M.P., Silos-Santiago, I., Frisen, J., et al. 1996. Renal agenesis and the absence of enteric neurons in mice lacking GDNF. Nature 382:70–73.

Satokata, I., Benson, G., and Maas, R. 1995. Sexually dimorphic sterility phenotypes in Hoxa10-deficient mice. Nature 374:460–463.

Schnieke, A., Harbers, K., and Jaenisch, R. 1983. Embryonic lethal mutation in mice induced by retrovirus insertion into the alpha 1(I) collagen gene. Nature 304:315–320.

Schrank, B., Gotz, R., Gunnersen, J.M., et al. 1997. Inactivation of the survival motor neuron gene, a candidate gene for human spinal muscular atrophy, leads to massive cell death in early mouse embryos. Proc Natl Acad Sci USA 94:9920–9925.

Schuchardt, A., D'Agati, V., Larsson-Blomberg, L., et al. 1995. RET-deficient mice: an animal model for Hirschsprung's disease and renal agenesis. J Intern Med 238:327–332.

Schultz, R.M. 1993. Regulation of zygotic gene activation in the mouse. Bioessays 15:531–538.

Sekine, K., Ohuchi, H., Fujiwara, M., et al. 1999. Fgf10 is essential for limb and lung formation. Nat Genet 21:138–141.

Sharan, S.K., Morimatsu, M., Albrecht, U., et al. 1997. Embryonic lethality and radiation hypersensitivity mediated by Rad51 in mice lacking Brca2 [see comments]. Nature 386:804–810.

Shawlot, W. and Behringer, R.R.. 1995. Requirement for Lim1 in head-organizer function [see comments]. Nature 374:425–430.

Snow, M.H. 1981. Growth and its control in early mammalian development. Br Med Bull 37:221–226.

Stephens, L.E., Sutherland, A.E., Klimanskaya, I.V., et al. 1995. Deletion of beta 1 integrins in mice results in inner cell mass failure and peri-implantation lethality. Genes Dev 9:1883–1895.

Stewart, C.L., Kaspar, P., Brunet, L.J., et al. 1992. Blastocyst implantation depends on maternal expression of leukaemia inhibitory factor [see comments]. Nature 359:76–79.

Sucov, H.M., Dyson, E., Gumeringer, C.L., et al. 1994. RXR alpha mutant mice establish a genetic basis for vitamin A signaling in heart morphogenesis. Genes Dev 8:1007–1018.

Suzuki, A., de la Pompa, J.L., Hakem, R., et al. 1997. Brca2 is required for embryonic cellular proliferation in the mouse. Genes Dev 11:1242–1252.

Tam, P.P. and Zhou, S.X. 1996. The allocation of epiblast cells to ectodermal and germ-line lineages is influenced by the position of the cells in the gastrulating mouse embryo. Dev Biol 178:124–132.

Tanaka, S., Kunath, T., Hadjantonakis, A.K., et al. 1998. Promotion of trophoblast stem cell proliferation by FGF4. Science 282:2072–2075.

Telford, N.A., Watson, A.J., and Schultz, G.A. 1990. Transition from maternal to embryonic control in early mammalian development: a comparison of several species. Mol Reprod Dev 26:90–100.

Threadgill, D.W., Dlugosz, A.A., Hansen, L.A., et al. 1995. Targeted disruption of mouse EGF receptor: effect of genetic background on mutant phenotype. Science 269:230–234.

Torres, M., Stoykova, A., Huber, O., et al. 1997. An alpha-E-catenin gene trap mutation defines its function in preimplantation development. Proc Natl Acad Sci USA 94:901–906.

Tsuzuki, T., Fujii, Y., Sakumi, K., et al. 1996. Targeted disruption of the Rad51 gene leads to lethality in embryonic mice. Proc Natl Acad Sci USA 93:6236–6240.

van Deursen, J., Boer, J., Kasper, L., et al. 1996. G2 arrest and impaired nucleocytoplasmic transport in mouse embryos lacking the proto-oncogene CAN/Nup214. EMBO J 15:5574–5583.

Waldrip, W.R., Bikoff, E.K., Hoodless, P.A., et al. 1998. Smad2 signaling in extraembryonic tissues determines anterior-posterior polarity of the early mouse embryo. Cell 92:797–808.

Wang, S., Gebre-Medhin, S., Betsholtz, C., et al. 1998a. Targeted disruption of the mouse phospholipase C beta3 gene results in early embryonic lethality. FEBS Lett 441:261–265.

Wang, W., Van De Water, T., and Lufkin, T. 1998b. Inner ear and maternal reproductive defects in mice lacking the Hmx3 homeobox gene. Development 125:621–634.

95. Wang, Z.Q., Ovitt, C., Grigoriadis, A.E., et al. 1992. Bone and haematopoietic defects in mice lacking c-fos. Nature 360:741–745.

Wang, Y., Schnegelsberg, P.N., Dausman, J. 1996. Functional redundancy of the muscle-specific transcription factors Myf5 and myogenin. Nature 379:823–825.

Xanthoudakis, S., Smeyne, R.J., Wallace, J.D., et al. 1996. The redox/DNA repair protein, Ref-1, is essential for early embryonic development in mice. Proc Natl Acad Sci USA 93:8919–8923.

Yamamoto, H., Flannery, M.L., Kupriyanov, S., et al. 1998. Defective trophoblast function in mice with a targeted mutation of Ets2. Genes Dev 12:1315–1326.

Yang, D., Tournier, C., Wysk, M., et al. 1997. Targeted disruption of the MKK4 gene causes embryonic death, inhibition of c-Jun NH2-terminal kinase activation, and defects in AP-1 transcriptional activity. Proc Natl Acad Sci USA 94:3004–3009.

Yang, J.T., Rayburn, H., and Hynes. R.O. 1995. Cell adhesion events mediated by alpha 4 integrins are essential in placental and cardiac development. Development 121:549–560.

Zambrowicz, B.P., Imamoto, A., Fiering, S., et al. 1997. Disruption of overlapping transcripts in the ROSA beta geo 26 gene trap strain leads to widespread expression of beta-galactosidase in mouse embryos and hematopoietic cells. Proc Natl Acad Sci USA 94:3789–3794.

Zeitlin, S., Liu, J.P., Chapman, D.L., et al. 1995. Increased apoptosis and early embryonic lethality in mice nullizygous for the Huntington's disease gene homologue. Nat Genet 11:155–163.

# 8

# Gestational Mortality in Genetically Engineered Mice: Evaluating the Extraembryonal Embryonic Placenta and Membranes

Jerrold M. Ward and Deborah E. Devor-Henneman

When trying to evaluate developmental errors, whether induced or spontaneous, the origin and function of extraembryonic tissues are often forgotten. Because of the degree of interdependence between the fetus and its supporting structures, failure in one usually results in failure of the other. It may be impossible to determine the real cause of embryonic death if a vital component of the conceptus is ignored. In fact, while many cases of spontaneous embryonal mortality have been reported (Hirning-Folz et al. 1992), the etiology of most resorptions usually remains undetermined and the concommitant state of the supporting membranes is not described. When investigated, embryonic death is found to lead to placental regression and atrophy, but placental dysplasia as a cause of embryonic death is not usually reported.

Extraembryonic tissues include not only the trophoblastic derivatives of the placenta proper but also the various tissues comprising the yolk sac, allantois, amnion, and, in rodents, Reichert's membrane. These structures, although extraembryonic, are initiated by the conceptus and can rightly be considered aggressively embryonal in origin. The maternal contribution, while environmentally essential, appears to be more hormonally/immunologically permissive and cooperative. These support tissues share subsets of critical growth factors, often expressed in an elegant, temporal pattern, with the tissues of the developing fetus (Dumont et al. 1995). An extraembryonic failure, especially in early gestation,

is commonly fatal for the embryo. Conversely, a lethal defect in the embryo proper, especially affecting the germ layer differentiation or cardiovascular development, commonly results in failure of the extraembryonic (placental) tissues.

Embryonic deaths and resorptions are natural and of common occurrence in placental mammals, and probably in other orders of the animal kingdom as well. It has been shown in the mouse that the rate of normal intrauterine mortality varies with strain, commonly occurring in 5–20 percent of litters (Peters et al. 1997; Heinecke 1972; Muralidhara and Natasimhamurthy 1995; Copp 1995; Lyon et al. 1996), and can be modified by age, nutrition, and husbandry practices.

In manipulations of the mouse genome, as with transgene insertions or so-called gene knockouts (targeted mutants), the first indication of possible embryo lethality is reduction in normal litter size or the absence of pups of an expected phenotype/genotype according to Mendelian inheritance. Before concluding that a small litter is due to genetic manipulation, it is critical to determine (1) if the parents are fertile, (2) *when* fetuses are being lost (postpartum cannibalization is always a possibility when births are not actually observed), and (3) if the never-to-be-born are exclusively of the missing phenotype or if all phenotypes are represented. To evaluate the possible causes of embryonic lethality, first evaluate pregnant uteri at 9 or 10 days postcoitum (dpc), common gestation days for placental developmental defects to result in embryonic death. At 10 dpc, the yolk sac should be vascularized and functioning, and the embryo should be developing its cardiovascular system and be large enough to see, with or without a dissecting scope. In addition, pregnancy often becomes grossly obvious to the trained eye at 10 dpc, which answers the basic fertility question. If everything seems normal at this point, work forward. If dead embryos or resorption sites are noted, work backward. Large numbers of animals are not needed to answer these basic questions. Determining when embryos are dying in utero can help identify the underlying cause(s).

## ORIGIN AND EMBRYONIC DEVELOPMENT OF THE MOUSE PLACENTA

At some point before blastocyst formation, the cells of the conceptus become committed to one of two primary lineages. One of these gives rise to many of the extraembryonic membranes and the fetal component of the placenta, and the other to the embryo proper. What exactly determines which cell is committed to which lineage is not known with any certainty. It has been suggested that imprinting is responsible (i.e., that paternal genes drive the development of extraembryonic tissues, while maternal genes direct embryonic differentiation). An alternative and more widely held theory is that the relative position of cells in relation to others determines their fates (i.e., lineage diversion is a result of cell-cell and cell-environment interactions) (Brown 1994; Cross et al. 1994).

In the mouse, growth and differentiation of the two lineages have been fairly well elucidated. By 4 dpc, the still free-floating blastocysts are distinctly separated into the physical manifestations of divergent paths: the trophoblast and the inner cell mass (ICM) or embryoblast. The spherical-to-cuboidal cells of the ICM are clustered at one end of the blastocyst and bulge slightly into the blastocoele. The more flattened epithelioid cells of the trophoblast (trophectoderm) cover and are continuous with the outer edges of the ICM and provide the "limiting membrane" of both ICM and blastocoele. Implantation begins when the blastocyst slips into a crypt formed by the thickened uterine walls and the trophoblast comes in contact with maternal epithelium. This commonly occurs at about 4.5 dpc in mice. Contact triggers a transformation of the flattened trophoblast cells into *primary giant cells,* which form long cytoplasmic processes, invading the epithelium and essentially eroding and dissolving the adjacent endometrium. The trophoblast cells above and in contact with the ICM, referred to as the polar trophectoderm (Tanuka et al. 1998), migrate apically and pile upon one another to form a somewhat

compact cap, the *ectoplacental cone* (EC), which, in turn, gives rise to the *labyrinth* and *spongiotrophoblast* layers of the mature placenta (Cross et al. 1994). At the same time the ecto- and endodermal cells of the ICM itself enlarge and project even farther into the blastocoele.

By 6 dpc, the erstwhile blastocyst has become an egg cylinder with the ICM elongating and showing a small continuous indentation around its periphery that will initially divide the cylinder into extraembryonic and embryonic compartments (Fig. 8.1). A small cavity forms in the embryonic portion and extends into the extraembryonic; this is the *proamniotic cavity.* All around the trophoblast-derived primary giant cell layer, the uterine endometrial cells are swelling into large glycogen-laden *decidual cells,* which will become the maternal component of the placenta. At the EC, trophoblast cells migrate unevenly up into the eroding endometrium. This forms small spaces that anastomose with other adjacent spaces and fill with maternal blood leaking from the damaged maternal capillaries. This area enlarges and forms the *placental labyrinth,* where the major nutrient and gas exchange between fetus and dam occurs. In addition to the migrating trophoblasts, some peripheral EC trophoblasts enlarge to become the so-called *secondary giant cells.* Others remain as stem cell precursors of the *chorionic plate* ectoderm (or ectoplacental plate) (Theiler 1989).

Until 6 dpc, the developing embryo has been composed of the primitive ectoderm of the trophoblast and the ectoderm and endodermal derivatives of the ICM. Primitive mesoderm makes its appearance at approximately 6.5 to 7 dpc during gastrulation. Cells from the region of the primitive streak (parietal endoderm) migrate to the lumenal or basal surface of the trophoblast layer and secrete *Reichert's membrane,* which functions as an acellular basement membrane between ectoderm and endoderm (Fig. 8.1). These tissues, including trophoblast giant cells, Reichert's membrane, and parietal endoderm, make up the *parietal yolk sac,* which is the earliest structure functioning in a placental capacity. Mesoderm develops basal to the endodermal layer, and the *visceral yolk sac* is born. The mesodermal layer gives rise to the blood islands and the development of the primitive circulatory system (Cross et al. 1994; Kaufman 1992; Rugh 1968; Theiler 1989).

The *amnion* makes its first appearance around 7 dpc as a series of folds in ICM-derived extraembryonic ectoderm that unite to form a continuous medial constriction of the egg cylinder (Fig. 8.1). Fusion of the folds at about 7.5 dpc effectively delineates the new amniotic cavity, leaving an ectoplacental cleft, or cavity, proximally. In the mesodermal layer beneath the ectoderm of the most prominent posterior amniotic fold, the exocoelomic cavity develops from coalescing spaces arising between mesodermal cells. The egg cylinder now contains three separate lumens: the ectoplacental cavity, the exocoelom, and the amniotic cavity. The latter two structures will progress and enlarge, compressing the ectoplacental cavity such that the opposing layers of extraembryonic ectoderm fuse into the bilaminar *chorionic plate* (Kaufman 1992).

At the same time that the amnion is closing, a small bulge in the mesodermal lining of the exocoelom is extending farther into that cavity. This is the rudimentary *allantois,* which will eventually form the umbilical connection to the placenta (Fig. 8.1). The allantois continues to grow and elongate upward toward the EC. The tip of the allantois pierces through the thin mesothelial lining of the exocoelom to come in contact and fuse with the ectoderm of the chorion above; this fusion generally occurs prior to turning of the embryo at 8 to 9 dpc. The distal portion of the allantois becomes a loose network of cells in which endothelial cells form and differentiate into the umbilical vasculature.

Since implantation, the embryo itself has been concurrently developing in the lower half of the egg cylinder below the now distinct amniotic cavity; development is especially rapid in the early circulatory system. While the yolk sac is still the main organ of nutrition, nutrient and gas exchange is being accomplished primarily via diffusion. The vasculature of the yolk sac at 7 to 7.5 dpc is rudimentary, made up of the blood islands developed, as previously mentioned, from the mesoderm and completely separate from the embryo (Fig. 8.3, mature blood island). However, at about 8 dpc, the differentiating embryo starts to remedy this situation. A paired set of *vitelline vessels* develops in the area of the posterior gut near the burgeoning allantois. The pair eventually fuses into one vessel that will be connected to the bilateral dorsal aortae forming to either side of the trunk somites. The aorta will also form a connection with the umbilical vessels of the allantois. As the blood islands coalesce into a vascular network, the vitelline vessels from the embryo anastomose with it to form a direct and more efficient link to the maternal environment (Theiler 1989). Later, different connections to the aorta will be formed as the umbilical vessels take prominence.

The rodent embryo undergoes a unique process of "turning" somewhere between 8 and 9 dpc when it is at the 6–8 somite stage. In turning, the embryo not only inverts the germ layers by reversing the curvature of the primitive trunk region but it also rolls into the amnion and yolk sac such that these membranes now surround the developing fetus. The somewhat stationary point about which the rotation occurs is the umbilical ring, where the membranes, particularly the yolk sac stalk and allantois, and embryo are essentially continuous (Kaufman 1992). This is the area at which the umbilicus becomes attached to the fetus. At the other end of the allantois, at the now fused *chorioallantoic plate,* the

true placenta is taking shape. Materno-fetal exchange is still the function of the now well-vascularized yolk sac/vitelline circulation, and this remains the case until its rupture before birth, although its physiological importance is dwarfed by that of the mature placenta proper (Muntener and Hsu 1977; Jollie 1990; Kirby and Bradbury 1965; Pijnenborg et al. 1981).

The allantoic vessels, once formed, invade as well as traverse the chorioallantoic plate by 10 dpc. Just proximal to the plate, on the decidual side, the ectoplacental tissues have developed into the labyrinth. The yolk sac (Figs. 8.2, 8.3) (i.e., both parietal and visceral layers) maintains communication here via continuance with intralabyrinthine sinuses and the margins of the chorioallantoic plate (the intraplacental yolk sac or sinus of Duval) (Ogura et al. 1998). Between the labyrinth and the maternal decidua, the spongiotrophoblast, a layer of large cells of variable thickness, through which run maternal blood vessels, has developed (Figs. 8.4, 8.5). The cells of this layer have been implicated as a source of steroid hormones and other factors necessary for chemical communication between dam and conceptus; they have also been shown to be phagocytic for maternal RBCs, which may be a mechanism for iron transport to the fetus (Fig. 8.6) (Kaufman 1992). The spongiotrophoblast is separated from the decidua by another layer of trophoblast-derived giant cells that are also a likely source of hormones and signaling factors important for fetal development (Fig. 8.5). The decidua actually surrounds the developing conceptus but becomes distinctly divided in gross and microscopic appearance. While the decidua basalis, lying in the mesometrial side above the spongiotrophoblast layer, is heavily vascularized and is the part commonly associated with the placenta proper, it is continuous with the thinning and less vascularized capsularis over the antimesometrial embryonic pole (Fig. 8.2). Here the trophoblast giant cells are the boundary between maternal tissue and Reichert's membrane/yolk sac. In the small space between Reichert's membrane and cells of the capsularis, the giant cells extend cytoplasmic fingers into the maternal tissues. This area is known as the *perivitelline meshwork*, the interdigitating spaces being filled with maternal blood. The meshwork probably supplies the diffusion media for nutrient transport and waste exchange across the yolk sac vital for preplacental survival (Muntener and Hsu 1977; Jollie 1990).

The placenta proper is fully formed and functional by 12 dpc (Fig. 8.2). The volume of the labyrinth increases to a little more than half of the total placental volume between 12 and 17 dpc, while the trophoblast giant cells tend to decrease after 14 dpc. Although there are some degenerative changes apparent from about 14.5 or 15 dpc on, the yolk sac continues to function to some extent in an auxiliary placental role until rupture

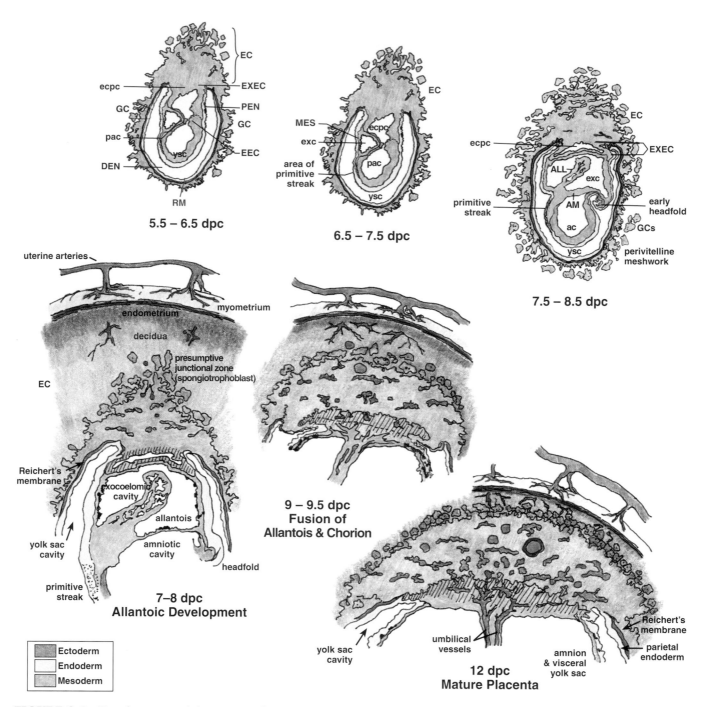

**FIGURE 8.1**  Development of the mouse placenta.

*5.5-6.5 dpc, pregastrulation.* In the differentiating egg cylinder, the ICM has elongated and is dividing into embryonic and abembryonic poles. Both are comprised of primitive ectoderm and endoderm. Trophoblast cells from the ectoplacental cone (which is, itself, a product of migratory trophoblast) interdigitate between maternal decidual and endometrial cells, forming small spaces into which seeps maternal blood from disrupted capillaries. Reichert's membrane, only seen in rodents, is secreted by the distal endoderm and lies between the endoderm and trophectoderm.

*6.5-7.5 dpc, gastrulation.* Gastrulation is marked by the appearance of the third germ layer, the mesoderm, which forms between the ectoderm and endoderm in the primitive streak. Mesodermal cells migrate apically and distally, eventually lining the expanding exocoelomic cavity within the posterior amniotic fold and giving rise to, among other structures, the allantois and the blood islands of the visceral yolk sac. The amniotic cavity is also forming during this time period. The posterior amniotic fold bulges into the proamniotic cavity in the area above the posterior end of the

*(legend continued on next page)*

**FIGURE 8.1 Continued.**

primitive streak and reaches toward the smaller lateral folds. The folds will meet and fuse to form the amniotic membrane, separating the amniotic cavity from the exocoelomic cavity above. The ectoplacental cone continues to invade the decidua, forming marked trabecular processes and resultant sinuses filled with maternal blood. An additional irregular apical layer of giant cells is forming, which will give rise to the spongiotrophoblast (junctional zone).

*7.5-8.5 dpc, allantois and chorion + headfold.* The amniotic folds have met and fused to form the amnion and the amniotic cavity. The exocoelomic mesoderm bulges out to form the allantois, which projects up across the exocoelomic cavity and eventually contacts and fuses with the chorionic plate. This fusion initiates the development of the chorioallantoic placenta. The ectoplacental cavity, compressed by the exocoelomic expansion during allantois growth, will be obliterated. Fusion of its opposing surfaces forms the bilaminar chorionc plate (chorion). Above the fusing chorion, the ectoplacental cone continues to differentiate into an identifiable labyrinth of sinuses, in which now mixes both maternal RBCs and fetal erythrocytes produced by the blood islands of the visceral yolk sac. The early headfold in the embryonic tissues forms in the germ layers opposite the primitive streak. "Turning" of the early embryo, a rodent inversion/rotation phenomenon necessary for proper germ layer and embryo orientation, will soon commence and is usually completed by 9 dpc.

*9-12 dpc, development and maturation of chorioallantoic placenta.* While the embryo below turns and begins the business of organogenesis, the chorioallantoic placenta takes on its final form and function. The allantois, containing the developing umbilical vessels, reaches across the exocoelomic cavity to contact and spread across the chorion. The labyrinthine layer above the chorion is thickening as the decidua thins and is developing an intricate and profuse system of sinuses and lacunae where maternal/fetal blood mixing for major nutrient/waste exchange is already occurring. The maternal circulation is supplied by relatively large decidual and labyrinthine arteries modified for the increasing demands. The spongiotrophoblast is now much more of a distinct cell layer. By 12 dpc, the fusion of the allantois and chorion is complete, and large umbilical vessels entering through the structure connect embyro and dam via the interchange of fetal and maternal blood in the labyrinth. The spongiotrophoblast layer is now a distinct belt of giant cells of variable thickness. Although the chorioallantoic placenta carries the burden of embryo support, the visceral yolk sac will continue to function in a minor placental capacity until a short time prior to birth, when it ruptures over the amnion.

*ac* = amniotic cavity
*ALL* = allantois
AM = amniotic membrane
*DEN* = distal (parietal) endoderm (ICM-primitive endoderm)
*EC* = ectoplacental cone (trophoblast-trophectoderm)
*ecpc* = ectoplacental cavity
*EEC* = embryonic ectoderm (ICM-primitive ectoderm)
*exc* = exocoelomic cavity
*EXEC* = extraembryonic ectoderm (trophoblast-trophectoderm)

*GC* = giant cell(s) (trophoblast)
*MES* = mesoderm
*pac* = proamniotic cavity
*PEN* = proximal (visceral) endoderm (ICM-primitive endoderm)
*RM* = Reichert's membrane (ICM-primitive endoderm)
*ysc* = yolk sac cavity
*dashed line* = delineation between abembryonic (proximal→placental) and embryonic (distal) division

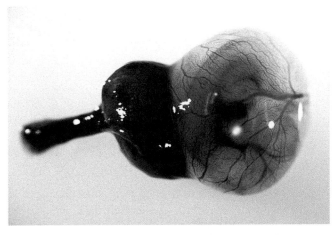

**FIGURE 8.2** Gross appearance of the yolk sac containing the mouse embryo 12 dpc and placenta (left side) with decidua capsularis removed and shown on the left side.

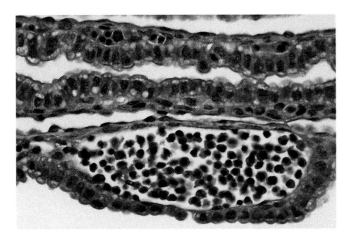

**FIGURE 8.3** Normal yolk sac and mature blood island at 12 dpc. Note tall columnar endodermal layer and nucleated embryonic erythrocytes within blood vessels.

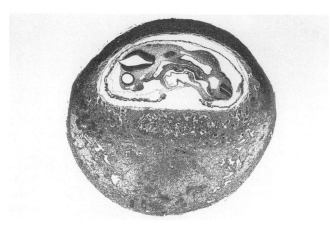

**FIGURE 8.4** Cross section through an entire mouse placenta and embryo. Note the large decidua (bottom of figure), darker labyrinth in middle of figure beneath the embryo, and thin yolk sac surrounding the embryo. 10 dpc.

of Reichert's membrane over most of the sac shortly prior to birth. The membrane remains intact, however, over the greater part of the surface of the chorioallantoic placenta (Kaufman 1992).

## GENE EXPRESSION IN THE PLACENTA AND EMBRYO

It is an important concept to understand that embryonic and/or placental failure may occur if the gene being manipulated is normally expressed within the embryo, placenta, or associated membranes at critical stages in embryonic development. The gene must have an important function that effects tissue development or differentiation. However, if a gene is normally expressed in a specific tissue or cell, it does not definitively suggest that a null mutation will produce failure of that tissue or cell. Gene redundancy can rescue a null mutant, and specific gene functions may not be critical for survival at that embryonic stage. If no expression of the gene of interest is seen in the placenta at the critical 9–12 dpc period, it is unlikely that primary placental failure will occur due to a null mutation in that gene.

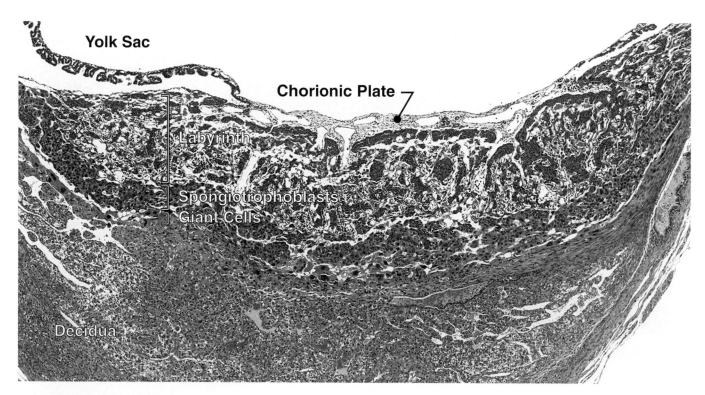

**FIGURE 8.5** A normal mouse placenta showing all layers. Only the decidua is completely composed of maternal tissue. The yolk sac is embryonal, while the labyrinth contains mostly embryonal labyrinth trophoblasts, embryonal endothelium-forming blood vessels, and erythrocytes and maternal blood cells. The spongiotrophoblasts and giant cell trophoblasts are of embryonal origin. 11.5 dpc.

Often a gene is expressed in both placental and embryonic tissues (Fig. 8.7) at 9-12 dpc and also in the placenta (Fig. 8.8; Dumont et al. 1995; Senior et al. 1988). Gene expression may be determined by Northern blotting, in situ hybridization, and other methods.

Gene expression can be observed in placentas and embryos by evaluating LacZ/β-galactosidase expression when LacZ is used as a reporter gene in the construct (Dumont et al. 1998; Tanaka et al. 1997). Wild-type mice will have no enzyme expression, while mutants (–/–) and heterozygous mice (+/–) will show expression. The placenta of the heterozygous mothers will show expression reflecting enzyme levels in decidua and maternal blood cells in the labyrinth.

A variety of antibodies and gene probes have been used to identify specific cellular layers of the mature placenta. They may be used to characterize the specific anatomical defect induced by a null mutation. These include macrophage antigens for decidual cells (Fig. 8.9), prolactin (Fig. 8.10), and Pl-I for giant trophoblasts, 4311 and Sos1 for spongiotrophoblasts (Fig. 8.8), and MECA-32 (Pharmingen, San Diego, CA) for labyrinth endothelial cells (Fig. 8.11; Kraut et al. 1998; Ward unpublished).

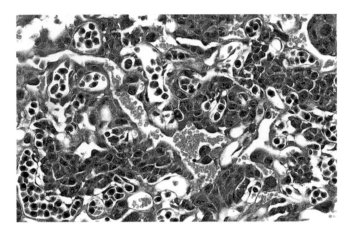

**FIGURE 8.6** The labyrinth is composed of embryonic labyrinthine trophoblasts, embryonic blood vessels lined by embryonal endothelium, nucleated erythrocytes within these vessels, and maternal mature erythrocytes (the eosinophilic cells without nuclei) within spaces lined by embryonal labyrinth trophoblasts.

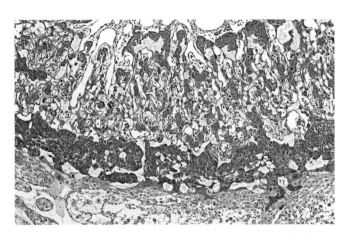

**FIGURE 8.8** Immunohistochemistry showing high expression (brown) of an antigen within spongiotrophoblasts and lower expression within labyrinth trophoblasts.

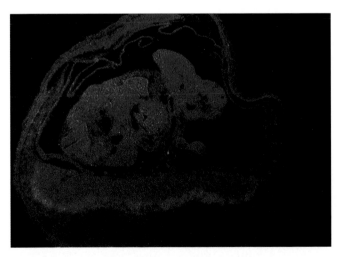

**FIGURE 8.7** High expression (mRNA) of a gene within various tissues of the embryo (top) and placenta (spongiotrophoblasts and less expression in labyrinth trophoblasts). In situ hybridization using $S^{35}$-labeled probe, dark-field.

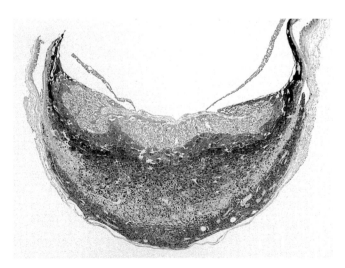

**FIGURE 8.9** Mac2 expression within maternal decidual cells. ABC immunohistochemistry.

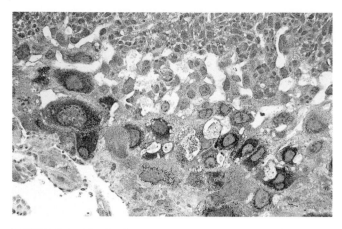

**FIGURE 8.10**  Prolactin expression in giant cell trophoblasts. ABC immunohistochemistry.

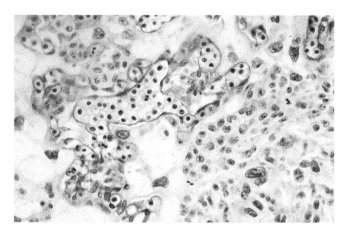

**FIGURE 8.11**  Endothelial cells in the placental labyrinth express MECA-32. Nucleated erythrocytes are seen within the vessels. The spongiotrophoblast layer contains no immunoreactive endothelium. Ethanol fixation, ABC immunohistochemistry.

# CLASSIFICATION OF PLACENTAL AND EXTRAEMBRYONIC MEMBRANE LESIONS IN MICE

In reviewing publications, we identified more than 50 knockout mice reported to have placental or extraembryonic membrane defects. They may also occur for any type of embryonic lethality but have been reported in the most detail in knockout mice. From these publications and our own experience, we have classified placental and membrane lesions into the following categories (Tables 8.1–8.3). Multiple defects often occur. We found 15 with extraembryonic membrane defects that

**TABLE 8.1.  Potential causes of embryonic death from 9 to 12 dpc**

1. Placental failure (trophoblast dysplasia, hemorrhage, vascular agenesis/dysplasia)
2. Extraembryonic membrane abnormalities (yolk sac dysplasia, erythroid hypoplasia, vascular agenesis)
3. Cardiovascular abnormalities (heart developmental defects, abnormal vasculogenesis)
4. Abnormal erythropoiesis (in yolk sac or elsewhere, none or decreased)
5. Loss of normal cell cycle controls (increased apoptosis/necrosis)
6. Cell adhesion/germ layer defects

**TABLE 8.2.  Classification of developmental defects and other lesions in extraembryonic embryonal tissues of the mouse**

Yolk sac and vitelline vessels
    Vitelline vessel dysgenesis/agenesis
    Agenesis of blood vessels
    Dysplastic blood vessels
    Lack of erythropoiesis
    Mesodermal defects
    Abnormal endoderm
Chorion/allantois
    Lack of or abnormal fusion
    Mesodermal abnormalities
    Allantoic ballooning
    Chorionic ectodermal abnormalities
Placenta
    Labryrinth
      Vasculogenesis, lack of or deficient
      Labyrinth trophoblasts, degeneration, dysplasia
    Spongiotrophoblasts, degeneration, dysplasia
    Giant cell trophoblasts, degeneration, dysplasia
Decidua
    Agenesis, dysplasia

probably led to embryonic death, 14 with critical placental defects only, and 26 with fatal embryonic defects that also had some membrane or placental lesion. Often embryonic defects and placental or membrane defects occur together (Chang et al. 1999).

Primary embryonic failure can be due to a variety of causes including failure of the heart to beat (cardiac contractility), lack of normal blood vessel formation in the embryo or yolk sac, loss of normal cell cycle control (e.g., increased embryonic apoptosis), improper turning, craniofacial and neural tube defects, or cell adhesion/germ layer defects (especially in embryos from 6 to 9 dpc) (Table 8.1). Secondary embryonic death may occur from a failure of normal development of the extraembryonic membranes and/or the placenta. It is important to determine if embryonic death is secondary to placental or membrane failure.

**TABLE 8.3.  Critical mouse developmental events demonstrated by the occurrence of embryo-lethal defects in knockout mice**

| Event | Dpc | Gene | Reference |
|---|---|---|---|
| PREPLACENTATION (early gestational period, <8 dpc) | | | |
| Blastocyst formation | 3–3.5 | *txn* | Matsui et al. 1996 |
| | | *E-cadherin* | Larue et al. 1994 |
| Implantation | 4–5 | *LIF* | Stewart et al. 1992 |
| | | *IL-11Rα* | Bilinski et al. 1998 |
| Egg cylinder formation and gastrulation | 6 | *BMP-4* | Winnier et al. 1995 |
| | | *BRCA1* | Hakem et al. 1996 |
| | | *NF2* | McClatchey et al. 1997 |
| | | *Ets2* | Yamamoto et al. 1998 |
| Formation of yolk sac, blood islands, and vitelline circulation | 6 | *TF* | Carmeliet et al. 1996b; Bugge et al. 1996 |
| | | *fibronectin* | George et al. 1993 |
| | | *Hand 1* | Firulli et al. 1998 |
| | | *scl* | Robb et al. 1995 |
| | | *VEGF* | Ferrara et al. 1996; Carmeliet et al. 1996a |
| | | *VEGFR-3* | Dumont et al. 1998 |
| | | *Flk-1* | Shalaby et al. 1995 |
| | | *Flt-1* | Fong et al. 1995 |
| | | *c-myc* | Davis et al. 1993 |
| | | *MEF2C* | Lin et al. 1998 |
| | | *α-5 integrin* | Yang et al. 1993 |
| | | *tie-2/tek* | Dumont et al. 1994; Sato et al. 1995 |
| | | *TFPI* | Huang et al. 1997 |
| | | *JunB* | Schorpp-Kistner et al. 1999 |
| | | *Smad5* | Chang et al. 1999 |
| | | *Mash-2* | Guillemot et al. 1994 |
| | | *ERR-β* | Luo et al. 1997 |
| | | *FII (75%)* | Sun et al. 1998 |
| | | *BRCA2* | Suzuki et al. 1997 |
| Development of primitive streak, mesoderm; amnion, allantois, and chorionic plate formation | 7 | *Mash-2* | Guillemot et al. 1994 |
| | | *ERR-β* | Luo et al. 1997 |
| | | *FII (75%)* | Sun et al. 1998 |
| | | *BRCA2* | Suzuki et al. 1997 |
| PLACENTATION (midgestational period, 8.5–12 dpc) | | | |
| Chorioallantoic fusion; labyrinth and spongiotrophoblast development | 9–10 | *α-4 integrin* | Yang et al. 1995 |
| | | *I-mfa (C57BL/6)* | Kraut et al. 1998 |
| | | *VCAM1* | Gurtner et al. 1995 |
| | | *VHL* | Gnarra et al. 1997 |
| | | *EGFR (129/Sv)* | Threadgill et al. 1995; Sibilia and Wagner 1995 |
| | | *Mash-2* | Guillemot et al. 1994 |
| | | *ARNT* | Kozak et al. 1997 |
| | | *HGF-SF* | Uehara et al. 1995 |
| | | *Tfeb* | Steingrimsson et al. 1998 |
| | | *ERR-β* | Luo et al. 1997 |
| | | *RBP-J$_k$* | Oka et al. 1995 |
| | | *LIFR* | Ware et al. 1995 |
| | | *Mek-1* | Giroux et al. 1999 |
| Establishment of materno-fetal circulation; endothelial integrity | 9–12 | *TGFβ-1* | Dickson et al. 1995 |
| | | *TFPI* | Huang et al. 1997 |
| | | *PDGFRα* | Ogura et al. 1998 |

*(continued)*

**TABLE 8.3.    Continued**

| Event | Dpc | Gene | Reference |
|---|---|---|---|
| | | **ORGANOGENESIS** | |
| Primitive streak formation (7 dpc) through birth formation of heart and vascular system | 7– | VEGF | Carmeliet et al. 1996a; Ferrara et al. 1996 |
| | | VEGFR-3 | Dumont et al. 1998 |
| | | Flk-1 | Shalaby et al. 1995 |
| | | Flt-1 | Fong et al. 1995 |
| | | tie-2/tek | Sato et al. 1995; Dumont et al. 1994 |
| | | α-4 integrin | Yang et al. 1995 |
| | | α-5 integrin | Yang et al.1993 |
| | | FII | Sun et al. 1998 |
| | | n-myc | Stanton et al. 1992 |
| | | fibronectin | George et al. 1993 |
| | | TGFβ-1 | Dickson et al. 1995 |
| | | Braf | Wojnowski et al. 1997 |
| | | PDGFα | Soriano 1997 |
| | | TFPI | Huang et al. 1997 |
| | | Hand 1 | Firulli et al. 1998 |
| | | RXRα | Sapin et al. 1997 |
| | | MEF2C | Lin et al. 1998 |
| | | Smad5 | Chang et al. 1999 |
| Hepatic hemopoieses | 11.5 | K-ras | Johnson et al. 1997 |
| | | MTP | Raabe et al. 1998 |
| | | apo B | Huang et al. 1995 |
| Cell proliferation and differentiation | 7 | BRCA1 | Hakem et al. 1996; Gowen et al. 1996 |
| | | BRCA2 | Suzuki et al. 1997 |
| | | Sp1 | Marin et al. 1997 |
| | | DNA ligase IV | Barnes et al. 1998 |
| | | p130 | LeCouter et al. 1998 |

Note: Times (dpc) noted are those at which listed events are taking place; the death of the conceptus/embryo itself (with the null mutation of the gene indicated) follows some hours or days afterward. Note that some genes, especially those such as *VEGF* and its ligands (which are heaviliy implicated in vascular development), are expressed in both extraembryonic and embryonic tissues, although expression may peak at different times in different structures. This coexpression reinforces the fact that early gestational failure frequently involves defects in both placenta and embryo, making cause of death difficult to assess if both components are not analyzed routinely.

Lesions of the yolk sac, chorion/allantois, vitelline vessels, and placenta have been described (Table 8.2). The normal histology of these structures (Figs. 8.2–8.6) must be compared with the histology found in the genetically engineered mouse under study. In some cases, no normal structures are found, while in others, abnormal development, indicated by histological changes and functional collapse, are seen. In chorioallantoic defects, lack of adhesion or fusion have been commonly described, but in scant detail.

For the yolk sac, lack of blood vessels, defective erythropoiesis, abnormal blood vessel development, mesodermal defects, and abnormal endoderm have been reported. The morphology of the endoderm may be atypical, hyperplastic, or degenerative. Blood islands may be lacking, or erythroid precursors within the vessels may be deficient. The placenta commonly shows abnormalities in cases of primary or secondary embryo lethality. It may be difficult, however, to distinguish the two processes based on the histological changes in the placenta. If lesions are found within the placenta and/or its membranes prior to initial embryonic necrosis, this is evidence for primary placental failure inducing embryonic death. Labyrinth collapse with hemorrhage characteristically results in death of the embryo and occurs as an end stage of diverse abnormal processes (Figs. 8.12–8.17) (Table 8.2). Several critical genes expressed in the labyrinth, especially in the labyrinth trophoblasts, and in the spongiotrophoblasts and giant cell trophoblasts have been identified. Disruptions of these gene functions have been correlated to trophoblast dysplasia evidenced by abnormal trophoblasts with morphological degenerative changes including pleomorphism, vacuolation, eosinophilic granulation (Figs. 8.16, 8.17), and formation of abnormal multinucleated syncytial giant cells in zones where giant cell trophoblasts are not normally found (Fig. 8.15). The eosinophilic droplets in the three types of placental trophoblasts can be seen in normal placenta, but dramatic increases in the numbers of trophoblasts with these granules is often seen in various stages of primary or secondary placental failure. The granules resemble nonnucleated maternal erythrocytes

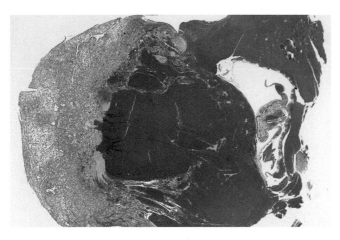

**FIGURE 8.12** Massive hemorrhage and total anatomical destruction in the placenta resulting from abnormal development of the labyrinth leading to disruption. Note necrotic embryo in the right portion of the figure.

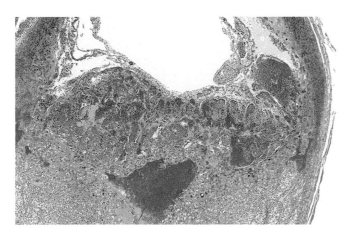

**FIGURE 8.13** Hemorrhage in the labyrinth of the placenta. The labyrinth is dysplastic (irregular). A portion of a dead embryo can be seen in upper right portion of the figure.

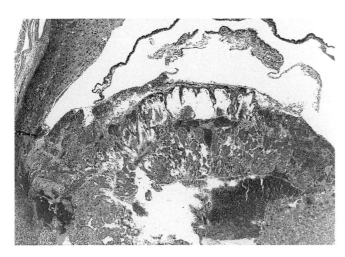

**FIGURE 8.14** Hemorrhagic and disrupted placenta and necrotic embryo (top). The entire labyrinth has lost its normal structure.

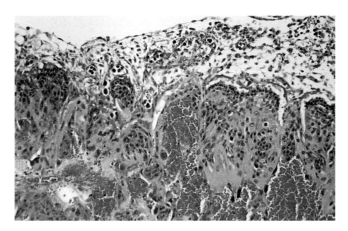

**FIGURE 8.15** Disruption of the maternal vascular spaces in the labyrinth. Note disorganized labyrinth trophoblasts and lack of embryonal vascular invasion from the chorionic plate. Multinucleated labyrinth trophoblasts can be seen.

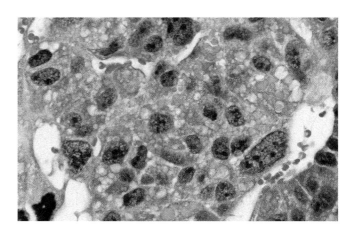

**FIGURE 8.16** Degenerative labyrinth trophoblasts with eosinophilic hyaline droplets.

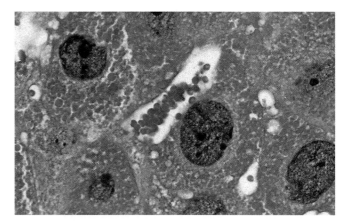

**FIGURE 8.17** Eosinophilic granular degeneration of trophoblast giant cells.

seen in adjacent vascular spaces containing maternal erythrocytes or in areas of placental hemorrhage.

Other genes have been shown to be heavily involved in the process of vasculogenesis, especially in the labyrinth. Vasculogenesis of the labyrinth from the chorion mesoderm is an important step in placental development and survival. Several genes have been shown to slow or prevent vasculogenesis of the labyrinth (*EGFR, JunB, Mash-2, Mek-1, Tfeb, VEGF, VHL*). Embryonic blood vessels, containing embryonic nucleated erythroid cells, can be seen within the chorionic plate but not within the labyrinth (Fig. 8.15) or may not be present at all. Maternal vessels, containing mature nonnucleated erythrocytes, can be readily observed in the labyrinth (Fig. 8.15). Lack of normal placental vasculogenesis leads to embryonic death due directly to impaired nutrition/oxygen supply.

Even though the decidua is composed of maternal tissues, signaling from embryonic tissues is important in its normal development and survival. Decidual abnormalities are rare but have been reported in *IL-11Rα* knockout mice (Bilinski et al. 1998). These knockouts showed reduced cell proliferation of decidual cells and degeneration of maternal decidua leading to defects in trophoblasts and placenta.

Cell cycle regulation is obviously important for the placenta and the embryo. Genes important in cell cycle regulation may theoretically interfere with normal cell growth and cell death of the embryo and placenta. Some mutant null mice (*DNA ligase IV, Rb-related p130, Brca1, Brca2, Braf, K-ras, ski, rad51*) have been reported to die at 6.5 dpc and later due to increased apoptosis. In some cases, the placenta was not examined histologically, and placental failure could not be ruled out as a cause of increased embryonic apoptosis in the embryo. It is often difficult to distinguish apoptosis from early embryonic necrosis due to placental failure. Apoptotic bodies can be normally seen throughout the normal growth period of the embryo, most commonly in some tissues including dorsal root ganglion (Figs. 8.18, 8.19) or due to specific gene inactivation (Figs. 8.20–8.22; Takuma et al. 1998). Necrosis starts in small foci in the embryo (Fig. 8.23), becomes multifocal, and spreads into large areas of the embryo (Fig. 8.24). Early changes of necrosis may resemble normal apoptosis seen in embryonic tissues (Figs. 8.18, 8.23, 8.25). Even with use of special immunohistochemical procedures that are supposed to distinguish between apoptosis and necrosis, it may be difficult to do so. For example, in an embryo dying due to placental failure, you can see widespread immunohistochemical reactivity in the TUNEL assay (Fig. 8.24), but this finding does not distinguish between apoptosis and necrosis (Levin et al. 1999).

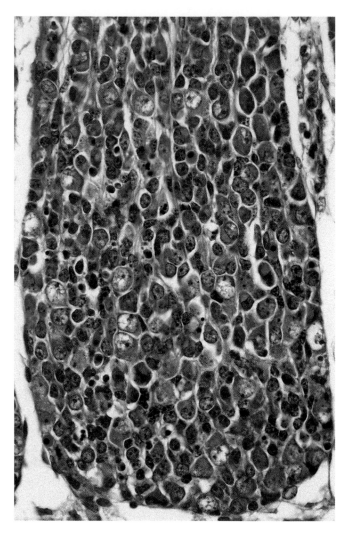

**FIGURE 8.18** The dorsal root ganglion has prominent apoptotic bodies (dark dots).

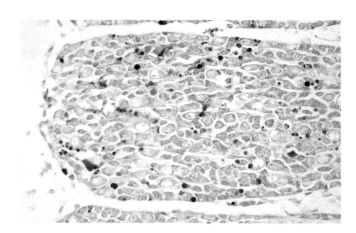

**FIGURE 8.19** Apoptosis in normal mouse embryonic dorsal root ganglion at 12 dpc. Note many positive apoptotic bodies (brown). TUNEL method, methyl green counterstain.

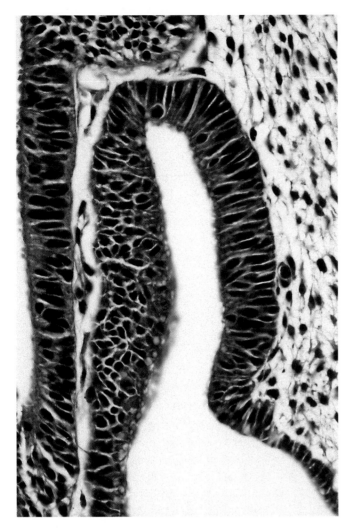

**FIGURE 8.20** Normal Rathke's pouch shows several cell layers and no apoptotic bodies.

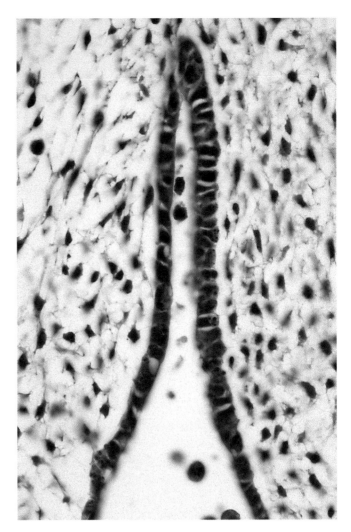

**FIGURE 8.21** Rathke's pouch in a T/ebp –/– mouse showing a thin layer of cells and prominent apoptosis.

# DIFFERENTIATING BETWEEN NATURAL AND INDUCED INTRAUTERINE DEATH

As previously stated, the first indication an investigator may have that his or her genetically engineered mice (GEM) are showing embryo lethality is reduction in total litter size (compared with the wild-type breedings of the normal strain) and/or few or no pups of an expected genotype at birth. How do you show this is due to genetic manipulation and not to normal spontaneous aberrations (lethal mutations, metabolic lethality, etc.) in the strain?

Using a gene knockout scenario and assuming simple Mendelian inheritance for the engineered gene mutation, the mating of heterozygous (+/–) parents would be expected to produce a ratio of 25 +/+: 50 +/–: 25 –/– offspring. If the observed reduction in litter size is produced by underrepresentation of +/– and –/– pups, some embryo lethality associated with the disrupted gene is likely, but chance spontaneous intrauterine death cannot be ruled out. If no homozygous null (–/–) animals are produced, it is highly likely that the null mutation is embryo-lethal, but the true incidence, cause, and developmental stage at the time of death cannot be determined unless the embryos are examined and genotyped.

The natural death/resorption rate, at least for mice of the 129/Sv and C57BL/6 strains, has been reported to be average for between 5 and 20 percent of conceptuses/pregnancy at 9–12 dpc (Peters et al. 1997; Heinecke 1972; Muralidhara and Natasimhamurthy 1995). It is certain that other strains have varying rates, as each strain carries its own complement of endogenous genetic loci that, in some random combinations, are potentially lethal.

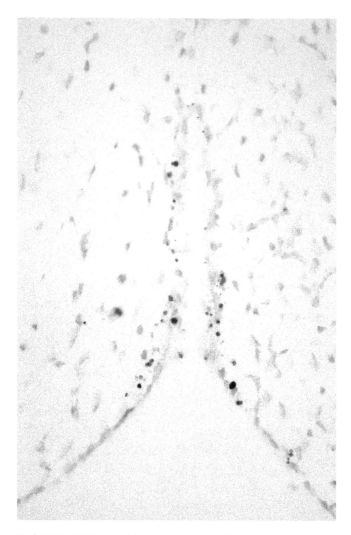

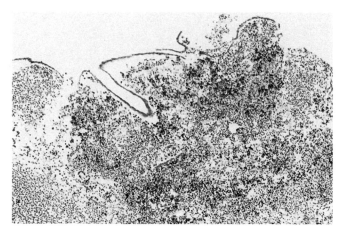

**FIGURE 8.24**   Necrotic mouse embryo at 12 dpc showing diffuse positive brown staining by TUNEL method. The positive staining is due to necrosis and not apoptosis. The method used apparently cannot distinguish between the two modes of cell death. (Levin et al. 1999)

**FIGURE 8.22**   Rathke's pouch in a T/ebp –/– mouse reveals apoptotic bodies (brown stain). TUNEL, methyl green counterstain.

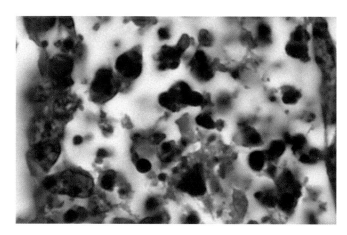

**FIGURE 8.25**   Necrosis of embryonic cells is seen. Note nuclear fragmentation similar to that seen in apoptotic cells; hyperchromatic nuclei and nuclei from live cells in left portion.

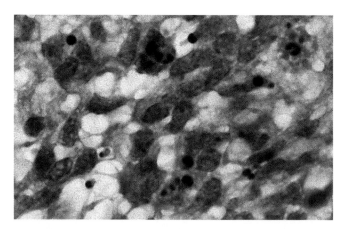

**FIGURE 8.23**   Early necrosis in embryonic brain showing individual and clusters of dead and dying cells resembling apoptotic bodies.

As a result of histopathology and genotyping of the normal and abnormal embryos, it was demonstrated that although disruption of the *VHL* gene is truly lethal in the null state from 9 to 12 dpc, some dead or dying embryos (Fig. 8.26) were found to be *VHL* + /+ or +/– (Gnarra et al. 1997). Induced intrauterine death can be grossly overestimated—and probably underestimated, as well—if there is no detailed investigation prior to birth. The following sections detail some of the methods necessary to dissect and phenotype mouse embryos.

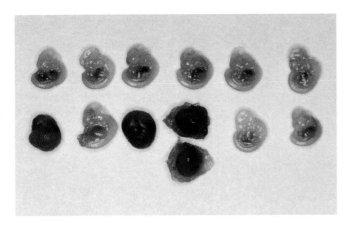

**FIGURE 8.26** Gross appearance of 12 dpc mouse embryos from *VHL +/– × VHL +/–* pairing. Three implantation sites are hemorrhagic.

# DISSECTION OF THE PREGNANT UTERUS, PLACENTA, AND EMBRYO

This section is not a definitive "how to" on embryo dissection. There are a number of excellent dissection manuals on the subject (Kaufman 1992; Hogan et al 1994). Instead, this is a section on what to look for in initially evaluating the uterus, placental site, and conceptus and how to gather pertinent background information in preparation for a more thorough investigation, if required.

After a period of trial and error, we have designed a method that works fairly well (although it's under constant improvement and revision) for embryos at 9 through 14 or 15 dpc. Prior to 8 dpc, individual dissection can be very tedious, and for these earlier stages we like to deal with entire uterine horns and embryos left in situ, when possible. Beyond 15 dpc, the fetus itself, although small, is amenable to detailed gross examination by standard methods. Older placentas and fetal membranes, however, tend to thin and often have to be handled with more care than at earlier phases. We would like to emphasize that this method is one that we have found extremely useful. It has allowed us to sort out and answer many questions that have frustrated us and others in the past, such as

1. Did the reproductive tract look healthy?
2. Was there a horn preference for the resorption sites?
3. What was the total number of viable/nonviable conceptuses?
4. Were there external indications of internal problems?

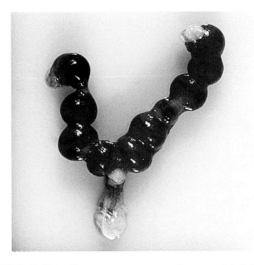

**FIGURE 8.27** Gross appearance of normal wild-type uterus showing nine normal placental sites and one darker, smaller placental site. This site is a spontaneous resorption.

5. Was there any abnormal bleeding seen internally, or were there signs of above-normal amniotic fluid pressure?
6. In the absence of conceptuses or resorption sites, were placentation/decidual scars seen?
7. Were corpora lutea present in cases of nonpregnancy?

## Dissection of the Mouse Uterus

A standardized tissue layout and necropsy (dissection, autopsy) form is used to minimize human-induced variability. It is important to have all the tools, solutions, and objectives on hand before starting.

Place the deeply anesthetized or freshly sacrificed dam on her back, and soak the entire belly with 70 percent ethanol. Open the dam ventrally, using a large H-shaped incision from sternum to pubic symphysis, and reflect the skin (with hair) back such that the introduction of hair into the whole process is minimized or eliminated. Locate the ovaries and the urinary bladder, and cut them away *with* the uterus (Fig. 8.27). Ovaries and bladder become reference points, especially when dealing with large litters and multiple abnormalities. In addition, since the urinary bladder lies on the ventral side of the uterine body, left and right horns can be identified even if the ovaries are inadvertently lost.

Lay the uterus out on a flat surface, and label the fetal compartments (the system we use is just one method). Keep the entire organ moist by periodically dribbling phosphate-buffered saline (PBS) or physiologic saline over the working surface. These tissues dry out rapidly, and dessication of tissues adds a whole new set of artifacts that can seriously confuse interpretations. You

## *In utero* Embryo/fetal evaluation record

Date 10/26/98
Experiment/gene: BYOBβ
Dam ID & genotype T+/- (x +/-)          Investigator Kluess
Gestational day 12.5 dpc to 13 dpc

(diagram gravid uterus, if applicable)       No. embryos right horn = 4
                                                       left horn = 5

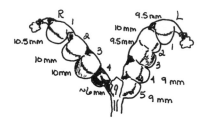

Gross observations:

R4 Probable resorption

L2 May have increased intra-yolk sac
          fluid pressure

| PHL No. | Embryo ID | Crown-to rump length | wt./comments | Placenta size | wt/comments |
|---|---|---|---|---|---|
| | R1 | 10 mm | normal | 8.5 x 6 x 2 mm | full; good color |
| | R2 | ~10 mm | normal | 8.5~6x2mm | " " " |
| | R3 | 9.5 mm | Rel. pale but good heartbeat and umbilical flow | 8X6X2mm | " " " |
| | R4 | 3 mm | Resorbing: fetal remains shapeless, necrotic yellow. Yolk sac still intact - ½ frozen for genotyping | 4x5x~2mm | Hemorrhagic, consolidated and somewhat friable |
| | | | | | |
| | L1 | 10 mm | normal | 8x7x~2mm | normal |
| | L2 | 8.5 mm | Embryo smaller than previous, but definite heartbeat. Somewhat anemic w/poss. mild distension of pericardium. + amniotic fluid | 7.5x7x2mm | Slightly pale chorionic plate & seems less tightly adhered to labyrinth |
| | L3 | 9.5mm+ | normal | 7.5x7.5x2mm | normal |
| | L4 | 9.5 mm | " | 8x7.5x2mm | " |
| | L5 | 9.5mm+ | " (saw whole-body contraction) | 8x7x~2mm | " |
| | | | | | |

Comments: 1st litter out of 3 matings (different ♂ each pairing)

**FIGURE 8.28** An example of a gross necropsy sheet that can be used to record gross findings when dissecting the uterus, placenta, and embryo.

should note the relative sizes of the swellings as well as their overall appearance. It's a good idea to record this data using a specialized necropsy sheet (Fig. 8.28). With nonpregnant dams, preserve the reproductive tract for histological and/or immunohistological evaluation. There are a number of maternal factors that are not conducive to pregnancy that can be evaluated in a nongravid uterus.

Choose a horn, and separate an intact individual uterine swelling (i.e., the embryo and placenta enclosed in the uterine wall). Work with one embryo at a time, maintaining the numbering system through preserving each placenta/embryo in individual vials. You can use a

dissecting microscope (one with a mounted camera is very helpful) or dissect with the naked eye and move the subject to a scope for more detailed work. Check for viability via color and heartbeat.

## Dissection of the Placenta and Embryo

While working on an individual embryo, keep the remainder of the uterus and conceptuses in cooled PBS or saline to avoid dessication and to delay autolysis. Start the dissection by sliding the tips of fine sharp scissors (iris scissors work well) through the narrow uterine lumen at the slightly broader antimesometrial pole of the conceptus and gently pulling the uterine covering from the placenta. If inserted too deeply, the scissors will knick the decidua capsularis, and the yolk sac will bulge out. It is also common to pierce the yolk sac itself, in which case the embryo will pop out. Neither scenario is critical. You will have to use some skill and patience to retrieve the sac for examination.

## Evaluation of the Yolk Sac and Placenta

Once the placenta-yolk sac-embryo entity is removed from the uterus, examine the yolk sac for vascularity and integrity in relation to the placenta and embryo (Fig. 8.2). Check the placenta for color and plumpness. Some obvious observations that can indicate something is wrong include

1. A pale, contracted (small), or brittle placental disk
2. A yolk sac that is pale or in which vessels cannot be delineated
3. A flaccid yolk sac, or one adhering tightly to the embryo (make sure this is not an artifact of dissection), or the opposite case of an overdistended sac
4. No or poor connection of yolk sac/embryo to the placenta
5. Blood free within the yolk sac or amniotic cavities indicating hemorrhage
6. An amorphous "blob" of tissue with little or no definition of placenta, embryo, or membranes (Fig. 8.30)

Since the yolk sac is of embryonic, as opposed to maternal, origin, it can be used for DNA extraction and genotyping of the embryo. A good section of the sac should also be preserved for histological examination. Most of the placenta is also embryo derived, but it is a chimeric organ containing vascular and tissue components and blood from both embryo and dam and should not be used for genotyping. The placenta should always, however, be preserved. After fixation of the intact placenta, we normally make a good cross section through each placenta to check for overall thickness as well as the presence and relative depth of the chorioallantoic plate, labyrinth, spongiotrophoblast layer, and maternal decidua.

## Evaluation of the Embryo

After evaluating the external appearance of the yolk sac and placenta, rupture the sac and turn your attention to the gross appearance of the embryo. It is important to note that, at times, you may have to compare embryos among and between litters to confirm true abnormalities.

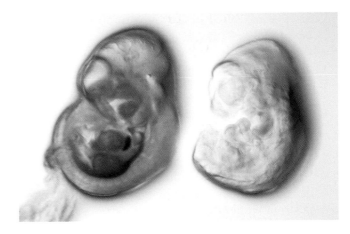

**FIGURE 8.29** On the left is a viable 12 dpc embryo, while on the right is a dying embryo that has lost its normal structures and is smaller. It also had no heartbeat. Transmitted light.

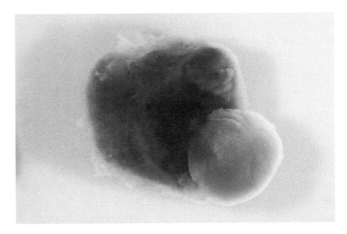

**FIGURE 8.30** Gross appearance of advanced necrotic embryo in the remaining placental cavity.

Recording descriptions and identifications of each embryo can help identify individual subjects. A good atlas of embryonic development (Kaufman 1992), or a readily available developmental biologist, is an important reference. With an atlas, however, make sure that you are comparing live embryos to live embryos or that you have some reference of conversion since shrinkage occurs after fixation; additionally the atlas should state if weight or crown-to-rump measurements were recorded before or after fixation. Common gross observations include

1. Overall embryonic morphology (surface features and internal organs) based on gestational age. It should be noted, however, that there could be as much as a 0.5-day (12-hour) difference in development within a normal litter.
2. Color and consistency. Dead embryos are more translucent and fragile (Figs. 8.29-8.30).

3. Size, as measured in crown-to-rump length, again based on gestational age (you could also weigh embryos, but for some reason, this is not done as often as taking the length). Dead or developmentally retarded embryos will be noticeably smaller than their normal littermates (Figs. 8.29, 8.30).

4. Cardiovascular development—heart contractility (beating), which is usually evident in day 9 embryos, and the formation of portions of the aorta and vitelline vessels.

5. "Turning," which should have been completed by day 9. The embryo is in its typically inward curled position within the amnion.

6. Size and functionality of the umbilicus. Can you see it? Does it bleed when cut?

## Fixation and Processing of the Placenta and Embryo

Embryos are generally fixed whole (in toto) and subsequently embedded according to the histological orientation desired (sagittal, transverse, or coronal). Occasionally, fixed embryos are trimmed prior to embedding, but because of the compaction of internal organs and the normal body curvature, such sectioning is often anatomically off center and physically disruptive if not done with care and experience (Kaufman 1992; Chap. 6). Commonly preferred and generally useful fixatives include 10 percent neutral buffered formalin (NBF), Bouin's fixative, and 4 percent paraformaldehyde (PF). Each solution has its advantages and disadvantages. It has been recommended that Bouin's is best for mouse embryo histology (Kaufman 1992), but prolonged fixation in Bouin's solution causes tissues to become brittle and difficult to use for sectioning. Many immunohistochemical and in situ hybridization studies work best with PF. Bouin's and NBF provide optimal preservation of cell and tissue morphology and are preferred for routine hematoxylin and eosin staining; they also give good results with many diverse special stains. NBF-fixed tissues have been found to work in some immunohistochemistry procedures using antigen-retrieval methods, and tissues can be stored in NBF for long periods. It is a time- and tissue-saving exercise to determine what your endpoints are likely to be before you choose a fixative. Dehydration and embedding should be done in the method recommended by Kaufman (Chap. 6 and 1992). Collaboration with a pathologist for embryo and placental tissue processing, staining, and evaluation is advised.

## REFERENCES

Barnes, D.E., Stamp, G., Rosewell, I., et al. 1998. Targeted disruption of the gene encoding DNA ligase IV leads to lethality in embryonic mice. Curr. Biol. 8:1395–1398.

Bilinski, P., Roopenian, D., and Gossler, A. 1998. Maternal IL-11Rα function is required for normal decidua and fetoplacental development in mice. Genes Dev. 15:2234–2243.

Brown, N.A. 1994. Normal Development. Mechanisms of Early Embryogenesis. In Developmental Toxicology, second edition, ed. C.A. Kimmel and J. Buelke-Sam. New York: Raven Press.

Bugge, T.H., Xiao, Q., Kombrinck, K.W., et al. 1996. Fatal embryonic bleeding events in mice lacking tissue factor, the cell-associated initiator of blood coagulation. Proc. Natl. Acad. Sci. USA 93:6258–6263.

Carmeliet, P., Ferreira, V., Breier, G., et al. 1996a. Abnormal blood vessel development and lethality in embryos lacking a single VEGF allele. Nature 380:435–439.

Carmeliet, P., Mackman, N., Moons, L., et al. 1996b. Role of tissue factor in embryonic blood vessel development. Nature 383:73–75.

Chang, H., Huylebroeck, D., Verschueren, K., et al. 1999. Smad5 knockout mice die at mid-gestation due to multiple embryonic and extraembryonic defects. Development 126:1631–1642.

Copp, A.J. 1995. Death before birth: clues from gene knockouts and mutations. TIG 11:87–93.

Cross, J.C., Werb, Z., and Fisher, S.J. 1994. Implantation and the placenta: key pieces of the development puzzle. Science 266:1508–1518.

Davis, A.C., Wims, M., Spotts, G.D., et al. 1993. A null c-myc mutation causes lethality before 10.5 days of gestation in homozygotes and reduced fertility in heterozygous female mice. Genes Dev. 7:671–682.

Dickson, M.C., Martin, J.S., Cousins, F.M., et al. 1995. Defective haematopoiesis and vasculogenesis in transforming growth factor-β1 knock out mice. Development 121:1845–1854.

Dumont, D.J., Gradwohl, G., Fong, G.-H., et al. 1994. Dominant-negative and targeted null mutations in the endothelial receptor tyrosine kinase, tek, reveal a critical role in vasculogenesis of the embryo. Genes Dev. 8:1897–1909.

Dumont, D.J., Fong, G.H., Puri, M.C., et al. 1995. Vascularization of the mouse embryo: a study of flk-1, tek, tie, and vascular endothelial growth factor expression during development. Dev. Dyn. 203:80–92.

Dumont, D.J., Jussila, L., Taipale, J., et al. 1998. Cardiovascular failure in mouse embryos deficient in VEGF receptor-3. Science 282:946–949.

Ferrara, N., Carver-Moore, K., Chen, H., et al. 1996. Heterozygous embryonic lethality induced by targeted inactivation of the VEGF gene. Nature 380:439–442.

Firulli, A.B., McFadden, D.G., Lin, Q., et al. 1998. Heart and extra-embryonic mesodermal defects in mouse embryos lacking the bHLH transcription factor Hand1. Nat. Genet. 18:266–270.

Fong, G-H., Rossant, J., Gertsenstein, M., et al. 1995. Role of the Flt-1 receptor tyrosine kinase in regulating the assembly of vascular endothelium. Nature 376:66–70.

George, E.L., Georges-Labouesse, E.N., Patel-King, R.S., et al. 1993. Defects in mesoderm, neural tube and vascular development in mouse embryos lacking fibronectin. Development 119:1079–1091.

Giroux, S., Tremblay, M., Bernard, D., et al. 1999. Embryonic death of Mek1-deficient mice reveals a role for this kinase in angiogenesis in the labyrinth region of the placenta. Curr. Biol. 9:369–372.

Gnarra, J.R., Ward, J.M., Porter, F.D., et al. 1997. Defective placental vasculogenesis causes embryonic lethality in VHL-deficient mice. Proc. Natl. Acad. Sci. USA 94:9102–9107.

Gowen, L.C., Johnson, B.L., Latour, A., et al. 1996. *Brca1* deficiency results in early embryonic lethality characterized by neuroepithelial abnormalities. Nat. Genet. 12:191–194.

Guillemot, F., Nagy, A., Auerbach, A., et al. 1994. Essential role of *Mash-2* in extraembryonic development. Nature 371:333–336.

Gurtner, G.C., Davis, V., Li, H., et al. 1995. Targeted disruption of the murine *VCAM1* gene: essential role of VCAM-1 in chorioallantoic fusion and placentation. Genes Dev. 9:1–14.

Hakem, R., de la Pompa, J.L., Sirard, C., et al. 1996. The tumor suppressor gene *Brca1* is required for embryonic cellular proliferation in the mouse. Cell 85:1009–1023.

Heinecke V.H. 1972. Embryologische parameter verschiedener mausestamme. Z. Versuchstierk 14:154–171.

Hirning-Folz, U., Winking, H., and Hameister, H. 1992. Aberrant *myc* expression in the murine trisomy 15 syndrome is correlated with prolonged proliferation in spongiotrophoblast cells of the placenta. Cytogenet. Cell Genet. 61:289–294.

Hogan B., Beddington R., Costantini F., et al. 1994. In Manipulating the Mouse Embryo. A Laboratory Manual, second edition. Cold Spring Harbor: Cold Spring Harbor Laboratory Press, p. 487.

Huang, L-S., Voyiaziakis, E., Markenson, D.F., et al. 1995. Apo B gene knockout in mice results in embryonic lethality in homozygotes and neural tube defects, male infertility, and reduced HDL cholesterol ester and apo A-1 transport rates in heterozygotes. J. Clin. Invest. 96:2152–2161.

Huang, Z-F., Higuchi, D., Lasky, N., et al. 1997. Tissue factor pathway inhibitor gene disruption produces intrauterine lethality in mice. Blood 90:944–951.

Johnson, L., Greenbaum, D., Cichowski, K., et al. 1997. *K-ras* is an essential gene in the mouse with partial functional overlap with *N-ras*. Genes Dev. 11:2468–2481.

Jollie, W.P. 1990. Development, morphology, and function of the yolk-sac placenta of laboratory rodents. Teratology 41:361–381.

Kaufman, M.H. 1992. In The Atlas of Mouse Development. London: Academic Press, p. 512.

Kirby, D.R.S. and Bradbury, S. 1965. The hemo-chorial mouse placenta. Anat. Rec. 152:279–282.

Kozak, K.R., Abbott, B., and Hankinson, O. 1997. ARNT-deficient mice and placental differentiation. Dev. Biol. 191:297–305.

Kraut, N., Snider, L., Chen, C.-M.A., et al. 1998. Requirement of the mouse *I-mfa* gene for placental development and skeletal patterning. EMBO J. 17:6276–6288.

Larue, L., Ohsugi, M., Hirchenhain, J., et al. 1994. E-cadherin null mutant embryos fail to form a trophoectoderm epithelium. Proc. Natl. Acad. Sci. USA 91:8263–8267.

LeCouter, J.E., Kablar, B., Whyte, P.F.M., et al. 1998. Strain-dependent embryonic lethality in mice lacking the retinoblastoma-related p130 gene. Development 125:4669–4679.

Levin, S., Bucci, T.J., Cohen, S.M., et al. 1999. The nomenclature of cell death: recommendations of an ad hoc committee of the Society of Toxicologic Pathologists. Tox. Pathol. 27:484–490.

Lin, Q., Vanagisawa, H., Webb, R., et al. 1998. Requirement of the MADS-box transcription factor MEF2C for vascular development. Development 125:4565–4574.

Luo, J., Sladek, R., Bader, J.-A., et al. 1997. Placental abnormalities in mouse embryos lacking the orphan nuclear receptor ERR-β. Nature 388:778–782.

Lyon, M.F., Rastan, S., and Brown, S.D.M. (eds.) 1996. In Genetic Variants and Strains of the Laboratory Mouse, third edition, volume 1. Oxford: Oxford University Press, p. 854.

Marin, M., Karis, A., Visser, P., et al. 1997. Transcription factor Sp1 is essential for early embryonic development but dispensable for cell growth and differentiation. Cell 89:619–628.

Matsui, M., Oshima, M., Oshima, H., et al. 1996. Early embryonic lethality caused by targeted disruption of the mouse thioredoxin gene. Dev. Biol. 178:179–185.

McClatchey, A.I., Saotome, I., Ramesh, V., et al. 1997. The *Nf2* tumor suppressor gene product is essential for extraembryonic development immediately prior to gastrulation. Genes Dev. 11:1253–1265.

Muntener, M. and Hsu, Y-C. 1977. Development of trophoblast and placenta of the mouse. Acta. Anat. 98:241–252.

Muralidhara, N. and Natasimhamurthy, K. 1995. Incidence of spontaneous post implantation deaths in CFT-Swiss mice: its suitability to access dominant lethal mutations. Lab. Anim. 30:138–142.

Ogura, Y., Takakura, N., Yoshida, H., et al. 1998. Essential role of platelet-derived growth factor receptor α in the development of the intraplacental yolk sac/sinus of duval in mouse placenta. Biol. Reprod. 58:65–72.

Oka, C., Nakano, T., Wakeham, A., et al. 1995. Disruption of the mouse *RBP-J* gene results in early embryonic death. Development 121:3291–3301.

Peters, J.M., Taubeneck, M.W., Keen, C.L., et al. 1997. Di(2-ethylhexyl)phthalate induces a functional zinc deficiency during pregnancy and teratogenesis that is independent of peroxisomal proliferator-activated receptor-α. Teratology 56:311–316.

Pijnenborg, R., Robertson, W.B., Brosens, I., et al. 1981. Trophoblast invasion and the establishment of haemochorial placentation in man and laboratory animals. Placenta 2:71–92.

Raabe, M., Flynn, L.M., Zlot, C.H., et al. 1998. Knockout of the abetalipoproteinemia gene in mice: reduced lipoprotein secretion in heterozygotes and embryonic lethality in homozygotes. Proc. Natl. Acad. Sci. USA 95:8686–8691.

Robb, L., Lyons, I., Li, R., et al. 1995. Absence of yolk sac hematopoiesis from mice with a targeted disruption of the *scl* gene. Proc. Natl. Acad. Sci. USA 92:7075–7079.

Robb, L., Li, R., Hartley, L., et al. 1998. Infertility in female mice lacking the receptor for interleukin 11 is due to a defective uterine response to implantation. Nat. Med. 4:303–308.

Rugh, R. 1968. In The Mouse: Its Reproduction and Development. Minnesota: Burgess Publishing Company, p. 430.

Sapin, V., Dolle, P., Hindeland, C., et al. 1997. Defects of the chorioallantoic placenta in mouse RXRα null fetuses. Dev. Biol. 191:29–41.

Sato, T.N., Tozawa, Y., Deutsch, U., et al. 1995. Distinct roles of the receptor tyrosine kinases Tie-1 and Tie-2 in blood vessel formation. Nature 376:70–71.

Schorpp-Kistner, M., Wang, Z.Q., Angel, P., et al. 1999. JunB is essential for mammalian placentation. EMBO J. 18:934–948.

Senior, P.V., Critchley, F.R., Beck, F., et al. 1988. The localization of laminin mRNA and protein in the postimplantation embryo and placenta of the mouse: an *in situ* hybridization and immunocytochemical study. Development 104:431–446.

Shalaby, F., Rossant, J., Yamaguchi, T.P., et al. 1995. Failure of blood-island formation and vasculogenesis in Flk-1-deficient mice. Nature 376:62–66.

Sibilia, M. and Wagner, E.F. 1995. Strain-dependent epithelial defects in mice lacking the EGF receptor. Science 269:234–238.

Soriano, P. 1997. The PDGFα receptor is required for neural crest cell development and for normal patterning of the somites. Development 124:2691–2700.

Stanton, B.R., Perkins, A.S., Tessarollo, L., et al. 1992. Loss of *N-myc* function results in embryonic lethality and failure of the epithelial component of the embryo to develop. Genes Dev. 6:2235–2247.

Steingrimsson, E., Tessarollo, L., Reid, S.W., et al. 1998. The bHLH-Zip transcription factor *Tfeb* is essential for placental vascularization. Development 125:4607–4616.

Stewart, C.L., Kaspar, P., Brunet, L.J., et al. 1992. Blastocyst implantation depends on maternal expression of leukaemia inhibitory factor. Nature 359:76–79.

Sun, W.Y., Witte, D.P., Degen, J.L., et al. 1998. Prothrombin deficiency results in embryonic and neonatal lethality in mice. Proc. Natl. Acad. Sci. USA 95:7597–7602.

Suzuki, A., de la Pompa, J.L., Hakem, R., et al. 1997. *Brca2* is required for embryonic cellular proliferation in the mouse. Genes Dev. 11:1242–1252.

Takuma, N., Sheng, H.Z., Furuta, Y., et al. 1998. Formation of Rathke's pouch requires dual induction from the diencephalon. Development 125:4835–4840.

Tanaka, M., Gertsenstein, M., Rossant, J., et al. 1997. Mash2 acts cell autonomously in mouse spongiotrophoblast development. Dev. Biol. 190:55–65.

Tanuka, S., Kunath, T., Hadjantonakis, et al. 1998. Promotion of trophoblast stem cell proliferation by FGF4. Science 282:2072–2075.

Theiler, K. 1989. In The House Mouse. Atlas of Embryonic Development. New York: Springer-Verlag, p. 178.

Threadgill, D.W., Dlugosz, A.A., Hansen, L.A., et al. 1995. Targeted disruption of mouse EGF receptor: effect of genetic background on mutant phenotype. Science 269:230–234.

Uehara, Y., Minowa, S., Mori, C., et al. 1995. Placental defect and embryonic lethality in mice lacking hepatocyte growth factor/scatter factor. Nature 373:702–705.

Ware, C.B., Horowitz, M.C., Renshaw, B.R., et al. 1995. Targeted disruption of the low-affinity leukemia inhibitory factor receptor gene causes placental, skeletal, neural and metabolic defects and results in perinatal death. Development 121:1283–1299.

Winnier, G., Blessing, M., Labosky, P.A., et al. 1995. Bone morphogenetic protein-4 is required for mesoderm formation and patterning in the mouse. Genes Dev. 9:2105–2116.

Wojnowski, L., Zimmer, A.M., Beck, T.W., et al. 1997. Endothelial apoptosis in Braf-deficient mice. Nat. Genet. 16:293–297.

Yamamoto, H., Flannery, M.L., Kupriyanov, S., et al. 1998. Defective trophoblast function in mice with a targeted mutation of Ets2. Genes Dev. 12:1315–1326.

Yang, J.T., Rayburn, H., and Hynes, R.O. 1993. Embryonic mesodermal defects in $\alpha_5$ integrin-deficient mice. Development 119:1093–1105.

Yang, J.T., Rayburn, H., and Hynes, R.O. 1995. Cell adhesion events mediated by $\alpha_4$ integrins are essential in placental and cardiac development. Development 121:549–560.

# 9

# Normal Brain Development and Gene Discovery in the Embryo

David M. Jacobowitz, Louise C. Abbott, Abraham T. Kallarakal, Chihiro Tohda, Francis C. Lau, and John W. Gillespie

The mouse is currently acknowledged to be the species of choice in developmental studies, particularly with respect to investigation of gene expression during development. The vast amount of information already accumulated relative to gene expression in the mouse, and the rapid rate of new information being added almost on a daily basis, make the mouse one of the most useful models for the study of mammalian development. Study of spontaneous and induced mouse mutants and the relative ease of producing transgenic and gene-knockout mice have increasingly focused attention on this species in the study of gene function. Teratological studies in the mouse have provided invaluable information concerning administration of various drugs and other experimental manipulations that may alter embryonic and fetal central nervous system development.

*Chemoarchitectonic Atlas of the Developing Mouse Brain* (Jacobowitz and Abbott 1998) provides a resource of information that allows research scientists to more accurately identify major anatomical structures of the developing murine brain. It is the first complete color atlas of the brain. Several different antisera used as immunocytochemical markers and a histochemical stain, acetylcholinesterase (AChE), are utilized to identify discrete regions of the developing brain. The combination of chemical neuroanatomy with classical cytoarchitectonic criteria yields a powerful source of information providing state-of-the-art brain cartography. This chemoarchitectonic atlas will help brain research scientists to more accurately map anatomical structures in the developing brain as well as the adult brain. This prenatal mouse chemoarchitectonic atlas has been assembled at progressive stages of brain development. It consists of a collection of color photomicrographs at gestational ages E (embryonic day) 11/12, E13/14, E15/16, E17/18, and P0 (newborn). These five representative ages were selected to illustrate the major, currently known, structural features of the developing murine brain. At each of the five ages examined, the presented coronal plane of sectioning is approximately equivalent to the plane of sectioning in one or more of the major, conventional, modern-day adult rodent atlases (König and Klippel 1963; Sidman et al. 1971; Slotnick and Leonard 1975; Paxinos and Watson 1986; Swanson 1992; Kruger et al 1995).

Four different antisera were used to produce this chemoarchitectonic atlas, including antisera to tyrosine hydroxylase (TH), 5-hydroxytryptamine (5-HT, serotonin), calretinin (CR), and calbindin (CB). These four antigens were selected for their known usefulness in specific labeling of important and distinct areas within the developing and adult rodent brain. Use of TH, an enzyme important in catecholamine neurotransmitter production; 5-HT, a biogenic amine neurotransmitter; and two different calcium-binding proteins (CR and CB) known to be highly expressed in the CNS, but not significantly overlapping in their labeling pattern, provides an enormous amount of information concerning the location and first appearance of specific cell bodies and/or intensely staining neuronal processes. In addition to the antisera used, the histochemical stain for AChE was also employed in this atlas. All chemical markers used in this atlas were selected because of their early expression in the developing murine brain. Finally, the Nissl stain, thionin, served its classic, conventional function of revealing gross morphological features of neuronal cell body accumulations, as well as the presence of axonal bundles. Use of multiple chemical markers, such as those displayed in this atlas, goes far beyond classical cytoarchitecture, and using such chemoarchitecture will help to refine structural boundaries in the developing murine brain.

# METHODS FOR IDENTIFYING MAJOR ANATOMICAL STRUCTURES

## Embryo Timing

Mice of the inbred strain C57BL/6J were originally obtained from the Jackson Laboratory (Bar Harbor, ME). Breeding mice were housed in an AALAC-approved animal facility at Texas A&M University. This specific strain was selected as the subject of this atlas due to its relative genetic uniformity and wide use in a variety of experimental studies. Ten- to 36-week-old male and female breeding mice were housed in a constant temperature (23–24°C), constant humidity (45–50 percent) room, with a 12-hour light/12-hour dark cycle and access to commercial rodent chow and water ad libitum.

All embryos, fetuses, and newborn pups used to prepare this atlas were obtained from timed pregnant C57BL/6J dams by placing one male mouse in each cage with two or three female mice at the beginning of the dark cycle. At the beginning of the light cycle, the male mice were removed from the females' cages, and each female was checked for the presence of a copulation plug, which was considered to indicate the beginning of gestation. The gestational ages are given as a range (e.g., E11/12) in order to accommodate the two major methods of calculating gestational ages in rodents. With the first method, the day the copulation plug is observed can be considered day 0; the gestational age based on this method represents the first date in the range (E11). However, because copulation usually occurs shortly after the dark cycle begins, in the second method the morning the copulation plug is observed is considered to be approximately 12 hours past copulation, and thus one-half of the first day has already taken place. The second date in the range (E12) represents the date based on this method for calculating gestational age. Both ages are given for all prenatal specimens.

## Dissection and Fixation of the Embryo Brain

Between 2 and 6 p.m. on the appropriate day of gestation (E11/12 through E17/18), each dam was injected with ketamine/xylazine anesthetic, given intraperitoneally (ip). Embryos or fetuses were removed from the uterus, and their crown-rump lengths (CRLs) recorded. Specimens of the following average CRLs were selected for inclusion in the atlas: E11/12, 7 mm; E13/14, 9 mm; E15/16, 13 mm; and E17/18, 20 mm. Embryos varying more than ±1.5 mm in CRL for E15/16 and E17/18 fetuses, were not included. The CRLs for postnatal pups

(postnatal day/newborn, P0/NB; CRL 24 mm) were recorded between 2 and 6 p.m. on the day of birth. P0/NB pups were taken between 12 and 18 hours after birth, and pups that varied more than ±2 mm in CRL were not used. All embryos, fetuses, and pups were closely examined for any obvious external defects. Only individuals that appeared completely normal were used in this study. E11/12 and E13/14 embryos were immersion fixed at 4°C for 36 hours in 4 percent paraformaldehyde buffered with 0.1M phosphate buffer (PB, pH 7.4). E15/16 and E17/18 fetuses and P0/NB pups were fixed by cardiac perfusion. First, each fetus or pup was anesthetized with ketamine/xylazine (ip) and pinned onto a wax plate. The ventral chest wall was opened, and then the heart was perfused using a 28- or 30-gauge needle attached to fine polyethylene tubing on the end of a 20 cc syringe. The abdominal aorta was cut to allow the perfusate to leave the circulatory system during the perfusion process. Each fetus or pup was briefly perfused with physiologic saline in 0.1M PB (pH 7.4) followed by 4 percent paraformaldehyde with 0.1M PB (pH 7.4). The fetuses and pups were then stored in fresh paraformaldehyde fixative at 4°C for 24–36 hours. The heads of the perfused P0/NB pups were removed from the bodies, and the skin over the calvaria was removed to facilitate penetration of the fixative. All specimens were transferred to 0.1M PB containing 20 percent sucrose for cryoprotection and stored at 4°C for 2–3 days until they were embedded in gelatin/albumin and frozen.

## Sectioning of the Brain

We had originally embedded formalin-fixed embryo brains in paraffin. We deparaffinized the sections and processed them for immunocytochemistry using the calretinin antiserum. We also compared these results with formalin-fixed fresh frozen cryostat sections. Unfortunately, the paraffin sections revealed a much reduced density of staining, whereas the cryostat sections demonstrated excellent immunostains. We concluded that, although paraffin sections clearly produced superior hematoxylin and eosin (H&E) and Nissl stains, the drastic conditions of heat and solvents compromised the antigen reaction with certain antisera. We therefore used only cryostat sections.

Each cryoprotected whole embryo, fetus, or head of the postnatal pups was embedded in an albumin/gelatin block to facilitate sectioning. A mixture of 22 percent bovine serum albumin (BSA) and 6–7 percent gelatin, which was made with sterile phosphate-buffered saline (PBS; pH 7.4), was placed in a peel-away paraffin mold and heated to 40°C, at which temperature the mixture was liquid. The block was allowed to cool slightly, and then the specimen was positioned into the still liquid solution that was then allowed to solidify. The albumin/gelatin block containing the specimen was trimmed to a square approximately 2–3 mm larger than the size of the specimen. The albumin/gelatin block was then quickly frozen using powdered dry ice and stored at –70°C until sectioning.

Serial sections, in either the coronal or sagittal planes, were cut at 20 μm on a cryostat. Prior to sectioning the olfactory bulbs, coronal sections were first oriented according to the nasal passages. Left-right and dorsal-ventral orientations were adjusted as needed. Final adjustments to the orientation were made in the region of the striatum and prefrontal cortex; then the orientation was maintained for the remaining sections. The serial sections were thaw-mounted onto chrom-alum/gelatin-coated slides in sets of four slides. Once the sections had dried onto the slides, they were immediately stored in a slide box on dry ice during sectioning and then stored at –70°C until they were stained.

## Immunocytochemical Staining Procedure

All antisera were generated in rabbits. Slides were incubated for 24 hours in the antisera diluted in sterile PBS with 2 percent goat serum, using a streptavidin-peroxidase immunocytochemistry procedure (Shi et al. 1988). The antisera used were calretinin (CR) (Chemicon, Temecula, CA), 1:2500; calbindin (CB) (Swant, Bellinzona, Switzerland), 1:10,000; serotonin (5-HT) (Eugene Tech, Allandale, NJ), 1:10,000; and tyrosine hydroxylase (TH) (Pel Freeze, Rogers, AR), 1:2000.

Slides were removed from the –70°C freezer, warmed to room temperature, and then placed in the following solutions, with extensive washing (30 minutes/wash) with PBS between each step:

1. Triton-X-100, 0.3 percent, in PBS for 1 hour at room temperature
2. Five percent normal goat serum (NGS) in PBS for 1 hour at room temperature
3. Antiserum in PBS with 2 percent NGS for 24 hours at 4°C
4. Biotinylated goat antirabbit immunoglobulin G (Vector, Burlingame, CA) 1:400 in PBS for 2 hours at room temperature
5. Streptavidin-peroxidase (Kirkegaard and Perry Lab, Gaithersburg, MD) 1:5000 in PBS for 2 hours at room temperature
6. Tissue-bound peroxidase activity was visualized with 0.024 percent 3,3'-diaminobenzidine ([DAB] Sigma Chemical Co., St. Louis, MO), 0.6 percent nickel ammonium sulfate, 0.006 percent hydrogen peroxide in 0.05M Tris-HCl buffer (pH 7.6), and a timed exposure of 3 minutes before the DAB reaction was terminated by transferring the slides to PBS.
7. After stopping the DAB reaction, slides were dehydrated through a series of alcohols and xylene and coverslipped using Permount.

## Acetylcholinesterase Histochemistry

Frozen sections were stained for AChE by the thiocholine method of Koelle (1955) with minor modifications (Jacobowitz and Creed 1983) as follows:

1. The frozen sections on slides were brought to room temperature and then incubated in PBS for 20 minutes at 37°C in a Coplin jar.
2. Slides were then placed for 30 minutes in a 75 ml Coplin jar containing a freshly prepared preincubation solution of 67.5 ml of 26.7 percent $Na_2SO_4$ (aqueous), 4.8 ml of diluted Iso-OMPA, and 2.7 ml of distilled water, prewarmed to 37°C. The diluted Iso-OMPA was freshly prepared by adding a 1.5 ml aliquot of stock Iso-OMPA (Sigma) (5.34 mg of anhydrous tetraisopropylpyro-phosphoramide dissolved in 100 ml distilled water) to 13.5 ml of distilled water.
3. The preincubation solution was discarded, and the Coplin jar containing the slides was filled with the substrate solution, prepared fresh, as follows:

   *Part A:* To 58.5 ml of 30.8 percent $Na_2SO_4$ with 0.1M $MgCl_2$ (dissolve 77 g anhydrous $Na_2SO_4$ and 2.59 g $MgCl_2·6H_2O$ in 250 ml distilled water; heat to facilitate dissolving; store at 37°C), add 3 ml, of 0.05M copper glycine (3.75 g anhydrous glycine and 2.5 g $CuSO·5H_2O$ in 100 ml distilled water; refrigerate) and 7.5 ml of 0.5M maleate buffer (9.6 g monosodium maleic acid-$3H_2O$ in 52.2 ml of 1 N NaOH; bring to final volume of 100 ml with distilled water; refrigerate). Add a small pinch of copper thiocholine.

   *Part B:* Dissolve 115.0 mg of acetylthiocholine iodide in 6 ml of the diluted Iso-OMPA. To this solution add 2 ml of 0.1M $CuSO_4·5H_2O$ (this addition should be made no more than 5 minutes prior to adding Part B to Part A). Add 6 ml of Part B, dropwise, to Part A while stirring. This combined solution will turn murky brown with copper precipitation. After adding Part B to Part A, titrate to pH 6.0 with concentrated HCl, and filter the solution into a Coplin jar; warm to 37°C. Incubate the slides in this solution for 90 minutes at 37°C.

4. The slides were transferred to a Coplin jar containing 20 percent $Na_2SO_4$ for 5 minutes at room temperature.
5. The 20 percent $Na_2SO_4$ solution was discarded, and the Coplin jar filled with 10 percent $Na_2SO_4$. It was left for 1 minute at room temperature.

6. The slides were washed by dipping five times in distilled water.

7. The stain was developed by transferring slides to a Coplin jar containing 45 ml buffered ammonium sulfide in a hood (4 ml ammonium sulfide [NH4]$_2$S was added to 96 ml PBS and titrated to pH 6.0 with concentrated perchloric acid; it was filtered into a Coplin jar while in a fume hood). This was left for 1 minute.

8. The slides were washed by dipping five times in distilled water.

9. The stain was fixed by transferring slides to a Coplin jar containing 10 percent buffered formalin.

10. The slides were washed by transferring to a Coplin jar containing distilled water and were left for 1 minute at room temperature.

11. The stain was intensified or toned by transferring slides to a Coplin jar containing 0.2 percent gold chloride (Sigma Chemical Co., St. Louis, MO). The slides were left for 5 minutes at room temperature. (After toning, the gold chloride was returned to the stock solution after filtering.)

12. The slides were washed by dipping 10 times in distilled water.

13. The toner was developed by transferring slides to a Coplin jar containing 5 percent sodium thiosulfate (prepared fresh). The slides were left for 5 minutes at room temperature.

14. The slides were washed by transferring to a Coplin jar containing distilled water and were left for 5 minutes at room temperature.

15. Dehydration was begun with 50 percent ethanol for 3 minutes; 80 percent ethanol for 3 minutes; 1 percent eosin in 80 percent ethanol for about 30 seconds; 80 percent ethanol for 10 seconds; 95 percent ethanol for 10 seconds; 100 percent ethanol for 2 minutes (two times); and xylene for at least 5 minutes.

16. Slides were coverslipped with Permount (Fisher).

## Computer Scanning of Stained Sections

After the stained sections were coverslipped and examined, the sections of interest were scanned into a Power Macintosh 8500/200 computer using a Leaf Lumina digital scanning camera mounted on a Nikon microscope. Exposure was optimized via Lumina 2.2 software; resolution was set to 335.65 dpi. Each image file was rendered in Adobe Photoshop 3.0 software, where it was adjusted as needed to achieve uniform presentation across all images. The images were imported into Adobe Illustrator 6.0 software, where text information was placed on each image and the plate layouts were finalized. We found that the resolution achieved with digitized color images was sufficient to match photographic reproductions.

# CORONAL BRAIN SECTIONS

*Chemoarchitectonic Atlas of the Developing Mouse Brain* (Jacobowitz and Abbott 1998) is the first all-color brain atlas and first chemical architecture atlas that covers the entire brain for five developmental ages. The classic Nissl stain and five chemical markers help to reveal the location of specific subpopulations of cell bodies and axonal projections. On each plate there is a Nissl-stained (thionin) sagittal section that clearly marks the location of the coronal section. A whole coronal section on each plate provides information about surrounding landmarks associated with the head. The plates are clearly labeled and contain an abbreviation key that makes it easy to find and identify structures. An example is provided of a whole page display of E13/14 (Fig. 9.1).

## Time Sequence

A chemoarchitectonic atlas has the advantage of allowing one to follow the development of a neurochemical (e.g., tyrosine hydroxylase, serotonin) in a discrete nucleus or brain region. Examples of the development of tyrosine hydroxylase are presented in the substantia nigra (Fig. 9.2) and the locus coeruleus (Fig. 9.3). The tyrosine hydroxylase enzyme is a marker for the catecholaminergic neurons dopamine (substantia nigra), norepinephrine (locus coeruleus), and epinephrine.

The sequence of development of serotonergic cells is observed in Figure 9.4. Serotonin is contained within raphe nuclei.

The enzyme acetylcholinesterase is a good marker for cholinergic neurons. An example of developing AChE-containing neurons in the caudate-putamen is shown in Fig. 9.5. However, AChE histochemical stain is not considered the best marker for cholinergic neurons since there are a few major exceptions, such as the locus coeruleus and the substantia nigra cells, which stain for AChE. The best marker for cholinergic cells is the antibody for choline acetyltransferase (ChAT), the enzyme responsible for the synthesis of acetylcholine. We found this marker to be ineffective for photographic display in the developing mouse atlas; therefore, the AChE stain was the marker of choice. Adult brain maps for ChAT are available (Satoh, Armstrong, and Fibinger 1983). Regardless of the lack of 100 percent specificity, the AChE stain itself provides a marker for the noncholinergic cells of the locus coeruleus and substantia nigra pars compacta.

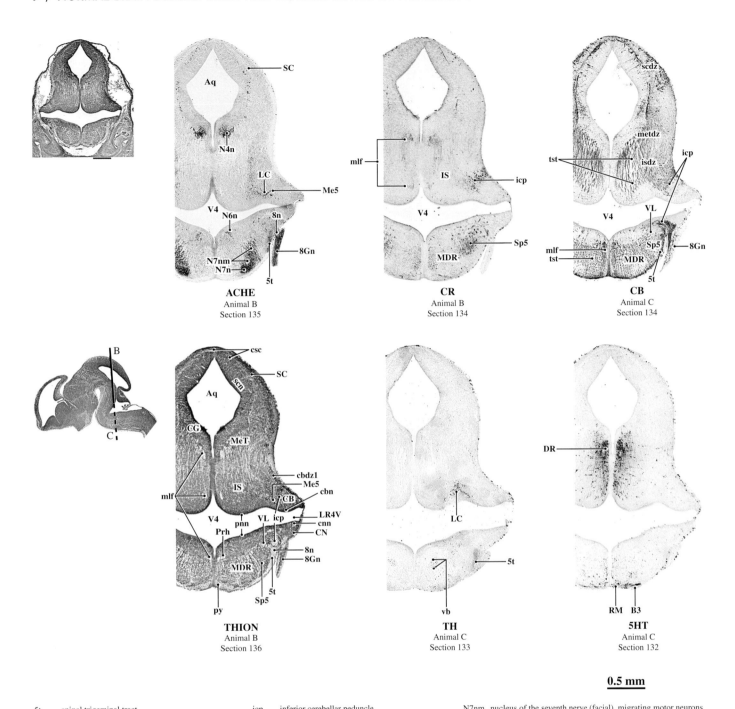

| | | |
|---|---|---|
| 5t | spinal trigeminal tract | icp | inferior cerebellar peduncle | N7nm | nucleus of the seventh nerve (facial), migrating motor neurons |
| 8Gn | vestibular ganglion (Scarpa) | IS | isthmus | pnn | pontine neuroepithelium |
| 8n | vestibular nerve | isdz | isthmal differentiating zone | Prh | prepositus hypoglossal nucleus |
| Aq | aqueduct | LC | locus coeruleus (A6, noradrenergic cell bodies) | py | pyramidal tract |
| B3 | B3 serotonergic cell bodies | LR4V | lateral recess fourth ventricle | RM | raphe magnus nucleus |
| CB | cerebellum | MDR | medullary reticular formation | SC | superior colliculus |
| cbdz1 | cerebellar deep neurons, first differentiating zone | Me5 | mesencephalic trigeminal nucleus of the fifth nerve | scdz | superior colliculus, differentiating zone |
| cbn | cerebellar neuroepithelium | | | scn | superior colliculus, neuroepithelium |
| CG | central gray | MeT | mesencephalic tegmentum | Sp5 | spinal trigeminal nucleus |
| CN | cochlear nuclei | metdz | mesencephalic tegmentum, differentiating zone | tst | tectospinal tract |
| cnn | cochlear nuclei, neuroepithelium | mlf | medial longitudinal fasciculus | V4 | fourth ventricle |
| csc | commissure of the superior colliculus | N4n | nucleus of the fourth nerve (trochlear) | vb | ventral noradrenergic bundle |
| DR | dorsal raphe | N6n | nucleus of the sixth nerve (abducens) | VL | lateral vestibular nucleus (Deiter's) |
| | (B7 serotonergic cell bodies) | N7n | nucleus of the seventh nerve (facial) | | |

**FIGURE 9.1** Coronal brain sections from *The Chemoarchitectonic Atlas of the Developing Mouse Brain*. In the upper left-hand corner is a "thumbnail" that gives an indication of surrounding landmarks. A large-scale bar has been placed beneath the thumbnail. On the left is a sagittal section with a line drawn to indicate the approximate level of the brain sections. The sections are usually derived from two (or, infrequently, three) mouse brains labeled *A–C*. (Jacobowitz and Abbott 1998)

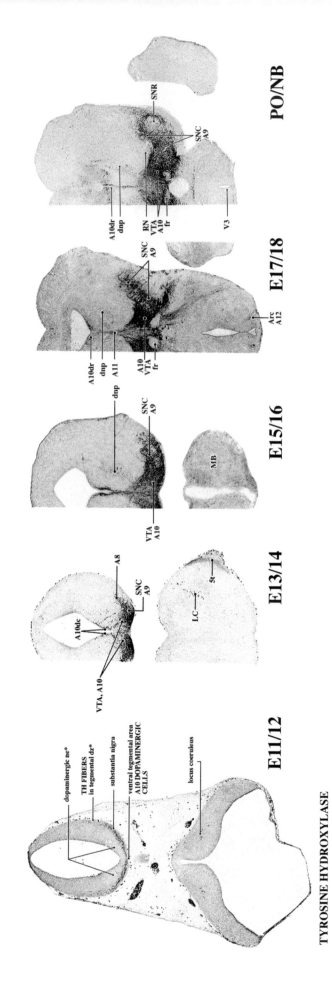

**TYROSINE HYDROXYLASE**

**FIGURE 9.2** The development of tyrosine hydroxylase in the substantia nigra at E11/12, E13/14, E15/16, E17/18, and P0/NB. (Jacobowitz and Abbott 1998)

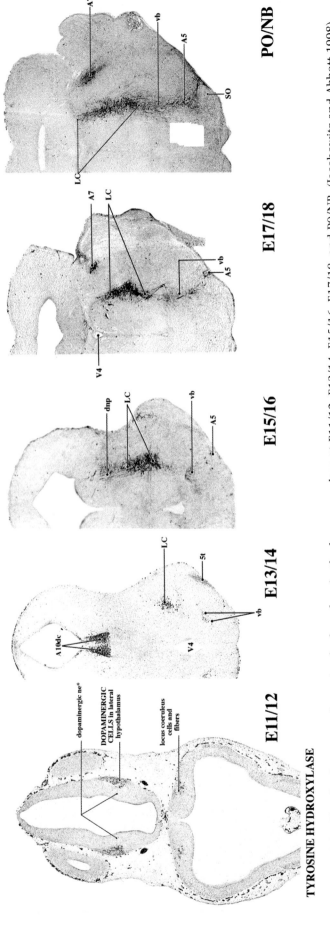

**TYROSINE HYDROXYLASE**

**FIGURE 9.3** The development of tyrosine hydroxylase in the locus coeruleus at E11/12, E13/14, E15/16, E17/18, and P0/NB. (Jacobowitz and Abbott 1998)

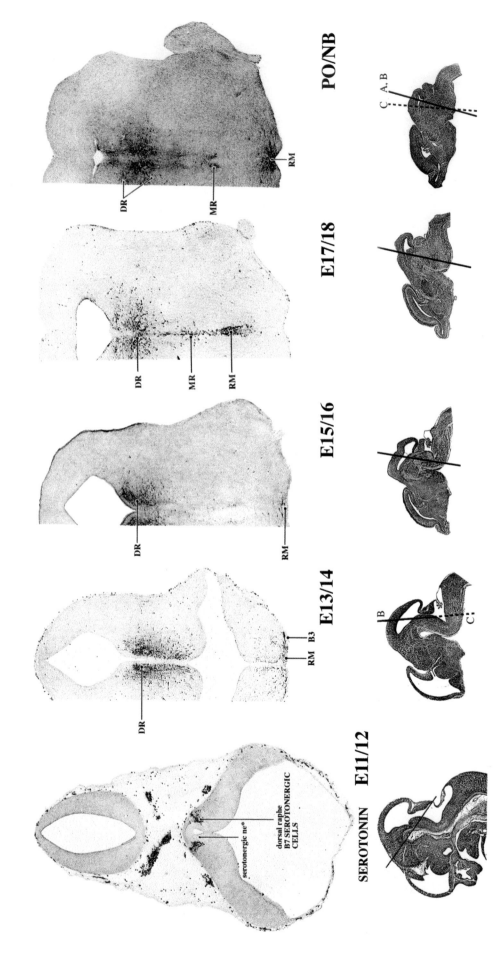

**FIGURE 9.4** The development of serotonin-containing dorsal raphe cells at E11/12, E13/14, E15/16, E17/18, and PO/NB. (Jacobowitz and Abbott 1998)

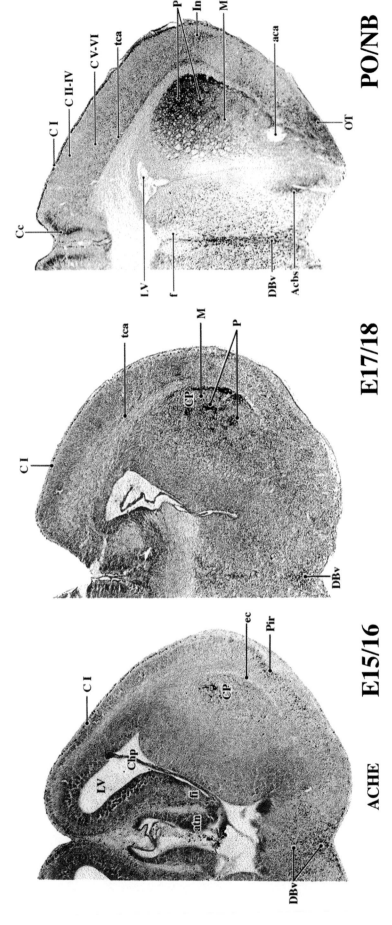

**FIGURE 9.5** Developing cholinergic (ACHE-containing) neurons in the caudate-putamen at E15/16, E17/18, and PO/NB. (*M*—striatal matrix, *P*—striatal patch). (Jacobowitz and Abbott 1998)

# GENE DISCOVERY IN THE EMBRYO BRAIN

Because of a combination of a unique expertise in the chemical anatomy of the developing mouse embryo brain and expertise in laser capture microdissection, we have embarked on a new initiative to discover genes in the substantia nigra neuroepithelium. We believe that the developing substantia nigra may contain valuable unknown growth factors that may prove clinically relevant in the protection of dopaminergic nerves that degenerate in Parkinson's disease. The laser capture microscope was recently developed (Emmert-Buck et al. 1996).

In the first step of the study, our specific aim was to identify differentially expressed cDNAs obtained by laser capture microdissection and differential display of mouse embryo neuroepithelium prior to differentiation of the substantia nigra compacta/ventral tegmental area and subsequently to use the information to analyze the substantia nigra of the human brain. This was done by a variety of molecular biology techniques that include (1) extraction of total RNA, (2) differential display RT-PCR, (3) cloning of differentially expressed cDNAs (4) sequencing the inserted cDNA and comparing with the published DNA database, and (5) confirmation of the differentially displayed cDNA by reverse dot blot.

## Laser Capture Microdissection of the Mouse Embryo Substantia Nigra Neuroepithelium

Laser capture microdissection of the substantia nigra neuroepithelial cells was performed in the E12 mouse embryo brain. Figure 9.6 shows that a 20 μm cryostat section fixed in 70 percent alcohol, stained with eosin, and dehydrated in a series of alcohols followed by xylene allowed us to laser microdissect the neuroepithelial cells that are in the process of migrating to the site of the substantia nigra pars compacta where differentiation takes place as indicated by positive tyrosine hydroxylase staining. Following bilateral laser capture of four sections from one brain, the tissue adhering to the membrane on the base of the cap on the tissue section was placed in a microfuge tube containing guanidine/EDTA solution.

Total RNA was then extracted and quantified spectrophotometrically, and purity was confirmed by RT-PCR for GAPDH. Reverse transcription for differential display was carried out using a GeneHunter Kit (RNA Image Kit 1). A 40-cycle PCR was carried out with anchored primer (HT11G, A or C) and eight arbitrary primers in the presence of $^{32}$P dATP.

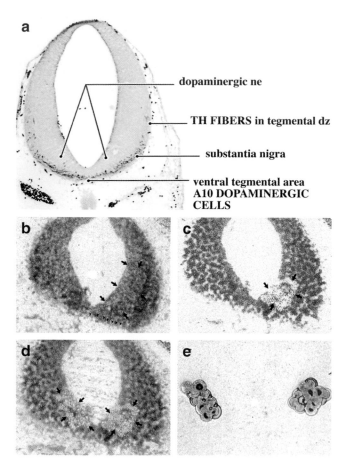

FIGURE 9.6   Laser capture microdissection of the substantia nigra neuroepithelial cells in the E12 mouse embryo. (**a**) Area of the neuroepithelium (dopaminergic ne) and region of the differentiated substantia nigra. (**b**) Neuroepithelial areas prior to laser capture microdissection. (**c, d**) Right and left neuroepithelial areas after laser capture microdissection. (**e**) The captured tissue from both sides. (*ne*—neuroepithelium, *dz*—differentiation zone; *A10 dopaminergic cells*—dopamine cells in the ventral tegmental area).

Differential display was run by comparing embryonic substantia nigra neuroepithelium with a control region (tectum) without dopamine cells. A denaturing polyacrylamide DNA-sequencing gel was run with a total of 32 samples, with each anchored primer and eight arbitrary primers, in duplicate. Differentially expressed cDNAs were excised from the gels and reamplified by PCR using the same set of primers used in the initial PCR. The cDNA was inserted into a T/A cloning vector (pGEM-TEasy; Promega). The ligated product was used to transform *Escherichia coli* cells that were plated on agarose plates. Colonies were picked and checked for cDNA insertion in the vector by colony PCR.

**TABLE 9.1.  Differentially expressed cDNAs in the neuroepithelial cells of mouse embryos**

| Number | Size (bases) | ID | Percentage identity (amino acids) | Comments |
|---|---|---|---|---|
| 1 | 199 | CAG repeat | 96 (191/199) | Expressed in SN |
| 2 | 395 | Acetylcholine regulator (putative) | 54 (75/137) | Expressed in SN |
| 3 | 380 | ODC antizyme inhibitor | 97 (145/149) | Expressed in SN |
| 4 | 370 | Lactobacillus L-lactate dehydrogenase | 64 (62/140) | Expressed in SN |
| 5 | 380 | Mouse mitochondrial tRNA, 12S and 16S ribosomal RNA | 97 (256/263) | Expressed in SN |

Note: ODC = ornithine decarboxylase; SN = substantia nigra.

Recombinant plasmids were sequenced using an M13 forward-sequencing primer on an ABI Prism 377 (Perkin Elmer) sequencer with a Big Dye Terminator Cycle Sequencing Ready Reaction Kit. The sequences of the inserted cDNA thus obtained are then used as queries in searching the nonredundant DNA database using the homology-searching program BLAST. This search revealed four known and one unknown cDNA (Table 9.1).

One of the cDNAs that is expressed more in the neuroepithelium has 84 percent sequence homology with 90 bases to a known gene, a CAG (glutamine) trinucleotide repeat of the human brain. A recent publication on this gene stated that trinucleotide repeat expansion mutations are known to cause 12 diseases, most with neuropsychiatric features (Margolis et al. 1997). There is indirect evidence that CAG expansion has been detected in heterogeneous populations of patients with bipolar affective disorder and schizophrenia. Also, several neurodegenerative disorders, including spinocerebellar ataxia and familial Parkinson's disease (PD), are phenotypically similar to the type I expansion mutation disorders.

The screening for CAG repeat with total mRNA from the substantia nigra of one PD, two PD/ Alzheimer's disease (AD), and an age-matched control brain revealed a differential expression pattern (unpublished results). The PD brain had the highest expression of CAG repeat relative to the control, while the expression was lowest in PD/AD samples. We also sequenced the CAG repeat region as well as the 3' untranslated region of the CAG repeat cDNA obtained from these samples and found them to be similar to the wild type.

Another interesting differentially expressed cDNA obtained from the neuroepithelium has 97 percent sequence homology with 149 bases to ornithine decarboxylase antizyme inhibitor. This protein is involved in the regulation of intracellular polyamine levels, which in turn plays a crucial role in cell proliferation and dif-

ferentiation (Steglich and Scheffler 1981; Pegg 1988). The expression pattern and role of this protein in the human substantia nigra is not known.

Thus, a knowledge of the differentially expressed genes in the neuroepithelium of the developing mouse brain could be extrapolated to study the mechanisms of nerve degeneration in Parkinson's disease.

# REFERENCES

Emmert-Buck, M.R., Bonner, R.F., Smith, P.D., et al. 1996. Laser capture microdissection. Science 274:998–1001.

Jacobowitz, D.M. and Abbott, L.C. 1998. Chemoarchitectonic Atlas of the Developing Mouse Brain. Boca Raton, FL: CRC Press.

Jacobowitz, D.M. and Creed, G.J. 1983. Cholinergic projection sites of the nucleus of tractus diagonalis. Brain Res. Bull. 10:365–371.

Koelle, G.B. 1955. The histochemical identification of acetylcholinesterase in cholinergic, adrenergic, and sensory neurons. J. Pharmacol. Exp. Ther. 114:167.

König, J.F.R. and Klippel, R.A. 1963. The Rat Brain. A Stereo-taxic Atlas of the Forebrain and Lower Parts of the Brain Stem. Baltimore, MD: Williams and Wilkins.

Kruger, L., Saporta, S., and Swanson, L.W. 1995. Photographic Atlas of the Rat Brain. The Cell and Fiber Architecture Illustrated in Three Planes with Stereotaxic Coordinates. Cambridge: Cambridge University Press.

Margolis, R.L., Abraham, M.A., Gatchell, S.B., et al. 1997. CDNAs with long CAG trinucleotide repeats from human brain. Hum. Genet. 100:114–122.

Paxinos, G. and Watson, S. 1986. The Rat Brain in Stereotaxic Coordinates, second edition. San Diego, CA: Academic Press.

Pegg, A.E. 1988. Polyamine metabolism and its importance in neoplastic growth and as a target for chemotherapy. Cancer Res., 48:759–774.

Satoh, K., Armstrong, D.M., and Fibiger, H.C. 1983. A comparison of the distribution of central cholinergic neurons as demonstrated by acetylcholinesterase pharmacohistochemistry and choline acetyltransferase immuno-histochemistry. Brain Res. Bull. 11:693–720.

Shi, A-R., Itzkowitz, S.H., and Kim, Y.S. 1988. A comparison of three immunoperoxidase techniques for antigen detection in colorectal carcinoma tissues. J. Histochem. Cytochem. 36:317–322.

Sidman, R.L., Angevine, Jr., J.B., and Taber Pierce, E. 1971. Atlas of the Mouse Brain and Spinal Cord. Cambridge: Harvard University Press.

Slotnick, B.M. and Leonard, C.M. 1975. A Stereotaxic Atlas of the Albino Mouse Forebrain. Washington, DC: DHEW Publication No.75–100. U.S. Government Printing Office.

Steglich, C. and Scheffler, I.E. 1981. An ornithine decarboxylase-deficient mutant of Chinese hamster ovary cells. J. Biol. Chem. 257:4603–4609.

Swanson, L.W. 1992. Brain Maps: Structure of the Rat Brain. Amsterdam: Elsevier.

# III

# General Pathology

# 10
# Genetic Background Effects on the Interpretation of Phenotypes in Induced Mutant Mice

Joel F. Mahler

Animal models are essential to our understanding of disease mechanisms, development of therapeutic strategies, and assessment of the safety of drugs or chemicals in the environment. Mice have long served as the mammal of choice for animal modeling due to practical considerations such as small size, ease of handling, and reproductive performance, as well as the enormous experimental database that has accumulated for this species. In particular, a century of mouse inbreeding with strain and genetic characterization has resulted in an extensive mouse genetics database and the availability of numerous inbred and inbred mutant strains with which to study the genetic basis of disease (Sundberg 1991, 1992). Historically, spontaneous mouse mutations formed an important part of the foundation for this database. More recently, mouse genetic engineering techniques that have arisen during the past two decades have greatly expanded that database and accelerated the production of new mouse models for specific applications. For basic research, the promise of genetic engineering has been to reveal the in vivo function of the product of the gene of interest. The fulfillment of that promise has resulted in an explosive growth in the number of published reports providing descriptions of mutant phenotypes, often showing homology to human diseases (for reviews, see Bedell et al. 1997; Shastry 1994, 1995, 1998; Smithies 1993).

Yet with this ability to manipulate the genome to test hypotheses concerning gene function, unexpected results have often been obtained. Most surprising have been instances in which gene disruption has resulted in mice with minimal or normal phenotypes (Shastry 1994), invoking theories of genetic or functional redun-

dancy and compensation. Variability of phenotypes among mice with the same targeted gene is also being reported with increasing frequency. Such variation may be simply due to differences in the gene-targeting strategy yielding essentially different mutants, such as the various intestinal tumor phenotypes of the three adenomatous polyposis coli (*Apc*) gene mutants published to date (Fodde et al. 1996). Environmental variables and the timing of observations may also contribute to phenotype variability between laboratories of mice with the same disrupted gene (Lahvis and Bradfield 1998). However, perhaps the greatest source of variability in such experiments is the genetic background of the mutant mouse. Dissecting out the primary effects of engineered gene mutations requires confidence that observed phenotypes are not the result of genes other than the targeted one. Therefore, considerable attention has been given recently to identification of polymorphism in the genetic background of induced mutants and how the polymorphism might make the results of gene-targeting studies difficult to interpret. A discussion of some of the variables that may need to be considered follows.

## DESIGN AND TECHNOLOGICAL CONSIDERATIONS

### Mouse Strain Selection

A fundamental premise of experimental design is to reduce potential sources of variability such that the effect

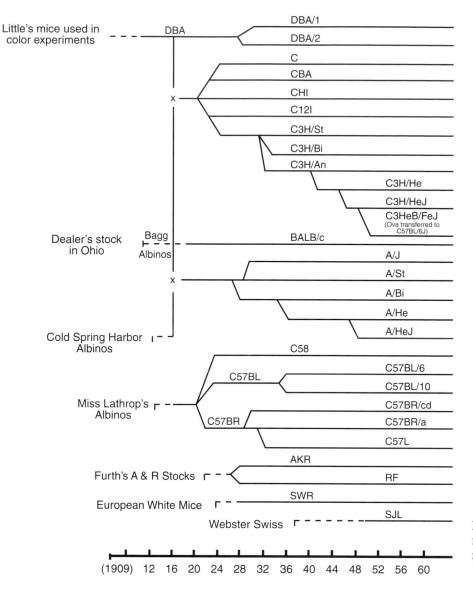

**FIGURE 10.1** Origins and relationships of common inbred mouse strains. (Fox and Witham 1997)

of experimental manipulation can be more precisely detected and characterized. Controlling for sources of variability allows for more stable and reproducible responses and greater precision with smaller numbers of animals. In regard to test animals, it is generally accepted that the use of genetically defined stocks is critical to achieve uniformity of responses. Yet it should be realized that even within a single species such as the laboratory mouse, a century of inbreeding has resulted in tremendous genetic diversity even among inbred strains. The genetic relatedness between different strains can generally be ascertained by knowledge of these origins (Fig. 10.1). For example, characteristics of the C57BL/6 mouse are often contrasted with those of the DBA/2 strain because of their many genetic differences (Fox and Witham 1997). This diversity of genotype is reflected by strain-dependent characteristics; members

of an inbred strain share a set of traits that are often unique, including differences in development, anatomy, behavior, life span, immunological responses, reproductive performance, and the type and frequency of neoplasms. Some traits are determined exclusively by the genotype, while others are influenced by diet and environmental conditions. Genetic and phenotypic details of specific mouse strains are voluminous and may be found in published compilations (e.g., Lyon et al. 1996) or by electronic access to various databases such as the Mouse Genome Informatics [*http://informatics.jax.org/*]. Because of the strain-dependent variation in both spontaneous and experimentally induced diseases, genetic factors are therefore perhaps the largest potential source of variability in biological experiments. For applications such as toxicity and carcinogenicity testing, the ideal animal is one in which the genetic variance is reduced so that the effect of the test substance on the animal can be attributed to dose, route, or exposure duration. Similarly, interpreting the effect of genetic changes requires putting the variable (mutation) on a defined genetic background. Historically, the concept of creating congenic strains, in which a mutant gene can be transferred by breeding onto another inbred strain background, was introduced by George Snell, leading to the creation of the Mouse Mutant Resource at the Jackson Laboratory by Snell and Elizabeth Russell (Silvers 1995).

The mouse strain of choice for any given research application is often determined by empirical or practical considerations. For toxicological studies, it is based in large part on historical acceptance and an extensive and established experimental database. For mouse mutant studies, the historical precedent for use of the C57BL/6J mouse was established by the work of Snell and Russell, as described above, who created congenic strains on this inbred background. With the advent of transgenic technology, the FVB mouse became the strain of choice for production of transgenic mice by the DNA microinjection procedure due to the reproductive vigor of this strain as well as the characteristic of large zygote pronuclei that facilitates the microinjection procedure (Taketo et al. 1991). C57BL/6 strain mice have also been commonly used as embryo donors for transgenic production because of the large number of high-quality embryos that can be obtained. Most recently, targeted mutagenesis has become the major methodology for generation of engineered mice; this method utilizes the almost exclusive use of embryonic stem (ES) cells from the 129 strain (Simpson et al. 1997), due to the relative ease of deriving germline competent ES cell lines from this strain, and the well-characterized C57BL/6 strain, which has become a "general purpose" recipient for targeted ES cells. Therefore, once again, creation of congenic strains on the C57BL/6 inbred background has become the method of choice for evaluating mouse genetic mutations. However, it can be expected that mouse modeling will increasingly involve placing induced mutations on other background strains that have specifically desired characteristics, or, alternatively, lack certain undesirable traits, in order to test the specific hypotheses of individual investigators.

## Targeted Mutation Methods and the Problems of Hybrid Mice

While a pure genetic background is desired for the evaluation of effects of gene targeting, the current procedures to generate these mice actually produces genetically heterogenous mice that are hybrids of two strains, the ES cell donor strain (typically 129) and the host strain (often C57BL/6), as diagrammed in Figure 10.2. The breeding strategy depicted is designed to produce

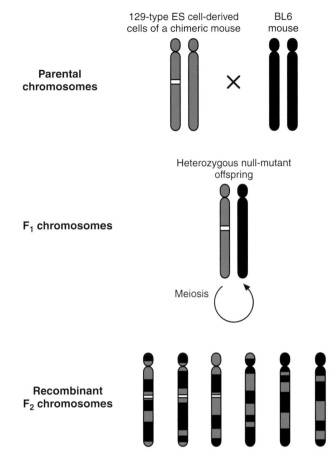

**FIGURE 10.2** Genetic heterogeneity generated by gene targeting. (Modified from Gerlai 1996)

mice that are homozygous mutant, heterozygous mutant, and wild type for the targeted locus, but in the process, $F_2$ littermates are also produced that have highly divergent background genotypes due to random segregation of parental genes during meiosis in the $F_1$ mouse. In order to purify the genetic background, backcrosses to an inbred strain are performed such that the contribution of genetic material from the donor (ES cell) strain decreases logarithmically with each successive generation (Fig. 10.3) until "congenic" status is achieved (i.e., when all loci except for the target locus and a linked segment of chromosome are considered identical, usually considered to require at least 10 generations of backcrossing). Until that point, however, there is the probability (greatest during early backcross generations) that mutant mice are still segregating for genes from both the donor and host strains and that any phenotype variation may be due to differences in the individual genetic backgrounds. Therefore, the generation of hybrid mice is an experimental variable that is a direct result of the gene-targeting technology itself and a potential source of genetic background variability that must be considered when comparing the phenotypes of

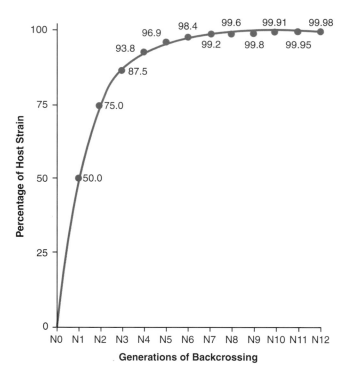

**FIGURE 10.3** The effect of backcrossing on the genetic composition of hybrid mice. (Fox and Witham 1997)

separate null mutant experiments. While it may be informative and useful in some situations to put a targeted allele on a mixed strain background (Doetschman 1999), congenic strains are usually generated for initial gene characterizations, a situation in which hybrid backgrounds are clearly a confounding variable.

There are other consequences of the genetic mixture found in mice generated by "knockout" technology that are relevant to experimental design and interpretation. These include (1) the choice of appropriate controls and (2) the potential problems of ES cell variability and linkage.

## Choice of Appropriate Controls

In the interpretation of mutant effects, detection of early phenotypes such as embryonic lethality or marked abnormalities in very young animals may be relatively straightforward. However, delayed expression of phenotypes is often found; expression may not become apparent until some critical threshold of loss of function is reached, or it may not become apparent until another critical intrinsic or extrinsic factor is present such as may be the case with neoplastic transformation. In such instances of delayed or age-related phenotypes, comparison with age- and sex-matched controls and weight of evidence factors are essential for interpretation of phenotypic effect. Unlike other experiments in which untreated animals of the same strain, age, and sex are the appro-

priate controls, littermates that are wild type at the targeted locus become the preferred control for induced mutant effects. However, from the above discussion, it is apparent that even littermates that are wild type at the targeted locus may be only approximate controls, since alleles at other loci may be different, particularly if there has not been extensive backcrossing. If wild-type littermates are not available, $F_2$ mice from crosses of the donor and host strains may be the control of choice because the genetic mix in these mice at least mimics that generated by knockout strategies. The $F_1$ hybrid is a less appropriate control because all $F_1$ mice are genotypically identical and do not mimic the genetic mixture found as a result of gene segregation from the $F_1$ hybrid parents.

## 129 ES Cell Variability

As stated above, most induced mutations are derived within the 129 strain genome due to the ease of derivation and manipulation of ES cell lines from this strain. However the history of the 129 strain and its substrains is complex and confusing. Considerable genetic diversity has been shown to exist among 129 substrains and the ES cells derived from them. This has led to some uncertainties regarding experimental design and the need for more stringent ES cell subline characterization and use (reviewed by Simpson et al. 1997). If the mutation is to be maintained on a 129 background, a noteworthy precaution arising from 129 ES cell variability is to backcross to a substrain matched to the one from which the ES cells were derived. The most appropriate genetically matched controls would also be of this substrain.

## ES Cell Linkage

Regardless of the strain from which the ES cells for targeted mutagenesis are derived, a potential problem relevant to genetic background is one of ES cell linkage. This problem relates to the technique itself and the genetic recombination that occurs between the ES cell donor strain and the host strain on which the mutation is to be maintained (Fig. 10.2). In the process of backcrossing to the host strain, the amount of donor strain genetic material decreases rapidly with each generation (Fig. 10.3). However, since the probability of recombination is inversely related to the distance between loci, this is not the case with the ES cell–derived DNA immediately flanking the target locus, and there is a linkage disequilibrium in which these donor genes are preferentially retained (Fig. 10.4). Estimates have been made that even after years of backcrossing, hundreds of ES cell genes linked to the target locus may still remain in the genome of the mutant animal (Gerlai 1996). The obvious concern is that any observed phenotype may be

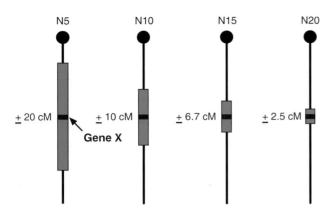

**FIGURE 10.4** The effect of backcrossing on donor strain DNA linkage. (Fox and Witham 1997)

dependent on the flanking loci from the donor strain and not necessarily a direct result of the disrupted gene of interest. This has been of particular concern for induced mutant models in the field of behavior and neuroanatomy, given the fact that most ES cells are of 129 strain origin, a strain considered to have a number of behavioral and neuroanatomical peculiarities (Gerlai 1996; McNamara et al. 1998).

As a result of the potential problems of ES cell linkage and hybrid genetic backgrounds, as well as the disadvantageous features of the 129 strain in particular as ES cell donor, efforts have been made to find germline competent ES cells from strains other than the 129. This approach could provide the least complicated way to generate nonhybrid mutant mice (i.e., to breed ES cell–derived chimeras with the strain from which the ES cells originated and to select those mice having the mutated allele). Gene targeting and successful germline transmission has been accomplished in ES cells from the C57BL/6 and other strains (Kawase et al. 1994; Lemckert et al. 1997), although widespread application awaits further technical advances.

# TARGET GENE/BACKGROUND GENE INTERACTIONS

## Modifier Loci

In the preceding discussion, diversity in the genetic background was presented as a potentially confounding variable in the interpretation of gene function from evaluation of induced single-gene mutants. However, most normal and pathological phenotypes are under the control of multiple genetic loci, and exploiting genetic diversity is an important research tool that can be used to dissect out the genetic interactions known to occur in these processes. The polygenic control of particular phe-

notypes is perhaps best exemplified in studies of individual cancer risk due to combinations of inherited resistance and susceptibility alleles, for which mice have served as useful models (Balmain and Nagase 1998). Crossing of tumor-resistant and -sensitive strains can provide information on the dominant or recessive nature of resistance, the number of genes involved, and the genes' approximate location in the genome, as has been done for numerous tumor resistance and susceptibility modifier loci in the mouse (Balmain and Nagase 1998; Fijneman et al. 1996; Manenti et al. 1994; Moen et al. 1996).

Table 10.1 gives selected examples of phenotype variability, presumably due to modifiers in the genetic background. A particularly illustrative example of tumor phenotype modulation by background modifier loci is provided by studies of induced mutants of the *Apc* gene. Three *Apc* mutants have been described with distinctive intestinal tumor phenotypes (Fodde et al. 1996); a strong dependence on strain background for the particular phenotype has been demonstrated for two of these mutants. With the ethylnitrosourea-induced *Min* mutation (Moser at al. 1990), a strong phenotype (as many as 100 tumors per intestinal tract) is observed on a C57BL/6 background. However, breeding of the *Min* mutation onto the AKR/J strain resulted in a markedly reduced tumor multiplicity, a finding that led to the identification of *Mom-1*, a major modifier of the *Min* locus (Dietrich et al. 1993). It is noteworthy that the same strain susceptibility to *Min*-induced intestinal tumorigenesis is seen with chemically induced colon carcinogenesis (Rosenberg and Liu 1995). In contrast to *Apc^{Min}*, the *Apc*1638N model develops only approximately five intestinal tumors per animal on the C57BL/6 background, but similar to *Apc^{Min}*, intestinal tumor multiplicity is reduced by *Mom-1* and possibly other modifier loci (van der Houven van Oordt et al. 1999). The genetic background does not seem to affect the incidence of other tumor types in *Apc*1638N mice.

Phenotypes other than neoplasia, such as embryonic lethality and severity of nonneoplastic disease, may be similarly modified by interactions between the target and background genes (Table 10.1). Importantly, phenotype variation due to genetic background has been seen in several newly developed models of human disease such as atherosclerosis and cystic fibrosis, emphasizing again the importance of genetic modifier loci on the penetrance of mutant phenotypes and the utility of genetically engineered animals to gain insights into the phenotypic heterogeneity of inherited disease. In general, given the polygenic nature of most diseases, it has become clear that producing better mouse models of those diseases involves not only inserting the right mutation but also placing the mutation by breeding onto a genetic background with the most appropriate

**TABLE 10.1.   Selected examples of induced mutant phenotype variation due to genetic background modifiers**

| Mutant | Phenotype variation | Reference |
|---|---|---|
| $Apc^{Min}$ | Tumor multiplicity | Dietrich et al. 1993 |
| Apc1638N | Tumor multiplicity | van der Houven van Oordt et al. 1999 |
| p53 disruption | Tumor spectrum | Donehower et al. 1995 |
| TGFα overexpression | Tumor incidence | Takagi et al. 1992 |
| c-Ha-ras expression | Tumor spectrum | Nielsen et al. 1995 |
| Tgfβ1 disruption | Embryonic lethality | Bonyadi et al. 1997 |
| Egfr disruption | Embryonic lethality | Sibilia and Wagner 1995 |
| Tcr disruption | Disease severity | Mombaerts et al. 1993 |
| mK8 disruption | Disease severity | Baribault et al. 1994 |
| Cftr disruption | Disease severity | Rozmahel et al. 1996 |
| Ahr disruption | Disease severity | Lahvis and Bradfield 1998 |
| Hprt disruption | Neurochemical level | Jinnah et al. 1999 |

modifier genes (Erickson 1996). A mutation may need to be evaluated against several genetic backgrounds to optimize its phenotype for a particular application, and modeling a human disease may be possible on one background but not another (Smithies 1993).

## Compensatory Phenotypes

The purpose of gene engineering is to reveal the in vivo function of the gene of interest. However, a major issue in interpretation of mutant phenotypes is the possible compensation by other genes for the missing or overexpressed gene in knockout and transgenic mice (Crawley 1996). In fact, the functional relevance of gene targeting has often been questioned because any mutation is likely to lead to a cascade of compensatory up- or down-regulation of related gene products, particularly since the gene is missing through development, allowing the opportunity for another gene in a related pathway to take over the function of the disrupted one. One possible consequence is a complex array of phenotypes that may or may not be the primary effects of the target gene manipulation. Another consequence may be a silent or "minimal" phenotype (Shastry 1994), indicating either that the gene has no function in that particular tissue or that the function is compensated by another member of the gene family. For highly conserved and presumably critical proteins, it is difficult to accept that there is no function, and therefore genetic compensation and functional redundancy is usually the default interpretation. Such an explanation has been made to explain the viable phenotypes observed after disruption of the genes for retinoic acid receptor and p53, critical regulators of embryogenesis and the cell cycle respectively (Donehower et al. 1992; Li et al. 1993). There is now experimental support for the compensation/redundancy theory that comes from observations in mice with multiple gene disruptions, in which a single deletion of either of

two related genes has produced minimal phenotypes whereas mice lacking both have more severe phenotypes (Shastry 1998). It should be noted that an alternative explanation for the lack of an expected phenotype may be that there is little redundancy in the genome and that the apparent lack of a phenotype more likely reflects our inability to identify it (Doetschman 1999). New genetic engineering technologies are on the horizon with which to further dissect these complex biological processes.

## TARGET GENE–INDEPENDENT, STRAIN-DEPENDENT PHENOTYPES

Previous discussion has focused on the ways in which the linked genes of the ES cell donor strain or the genetic background of the host strain may influence or modulate the phenotype of the induced mutation. However, the investigator also needs to be aware of changes that may be completely unrelated to the mutation but rather are characteristics of the particular host strain on which the mutation is carried. This is particularly true when delayed onset phenotypes such as neoplasia are expected, since spontaneous natural disease of the aging host may either mask a mutant effect or erroneously be interpreted as a mutant phenotype. Distinguishing mutation-specific changes from strain-dependent ones requires close comparison to wild-type mice, and therefore the need for appropriate controls mentioned previously in this chapter bears repeating in regards to strain-dependent phenotypes. Wild-type littermates are the preferred controls, particularly for targeted mice with mixed or segregating genetic backgrounds. Age- and sex-matched $F_2$ mice from crosses between ES cell donor and host strains (e.g., B6,129 $F_2$) may also approximate the mixed genetic background in some mutants, while the inbred host strain would be a more appropriate control for congenic strains. Obviously it is also critical that the timing and extent of evaluations be matched between control and mutant animals in order for results to be comparable. Unlike toxicology studies in which large historical control databases are established and frequently used for interpretation of results, the investigator working with induced mutants should not rely on the literature for control data due to the possible variability of the age and genetic backgrounds of wild-type mice from various references as well as the variability of the evaluations conducted.

The number of parental inbred strains currently in use for induced mutation studies is relatively limited, primarily the 129, C57BL/6, and FVB/N strains. The 129 and C57BL/6 are relatively well-known and -characterized strains, and specific traits of these and other established inbred mice may be found in various information resources such as the Mouse Genome Informatics [*http://informatics.jax.org/*]. The FVB/N is a more recently derived and characterized strain (Taketo et al. 1991; Mahler et al. 1996). Knowledge of the spontaneous diseases in these strains is essential to phenotype interpretation. For example, the occurrence of malignant teratomas in a mutant on a 129 background must be interpreted in light of the modest incidence of this tumor in most of the 129 substrains (Donehower et al. 1995). Lymphoma is a common tumor observed in several mutants on a partial C57BL/6 background (e.g., Donehower et al. 1995; Serrano et al. 1996); however, lymphoma is not an uncommon natural tumor in the C57BL/6 and other strains, and therefore incidences and latency in mutants must always be interpreted with caution and in comparison with age- and sex-matched wild-type mice. Similarly, a lung tumor phenotype or abnormal neurobehavior in a transgenic mouse may merely be a reflection of the predisposition to lung neoplasia and seizure activity that has been reported in the parental FVB/N strain (Goelz et al. 1998; Mahler et al. 1996). On the other hand, occurrence of unusual tumor types, such as osteosarcomas and soft tissue sarcomas in p53-deficient mutants (Donehower et al. 1995; Serrano et al. 1996) or odontogenic tumors in activated *ras*-expressing Tg.AC transgenics (Mahler et al. 1998) will be more indicative of a mutation-specific and strain-independent effect.

## SUMMARY

Quite obviously, genetic engineering is a powerful new tool to investigate single-gene defects and multigenic disease. However, by their very nature, studies are par-

**TABLE 10.2. Potential genetic background variables in induced mutant mice**

ES cell (129 substrain) variability
ES cell "linked" genes
Mixed donor/host strain backgrounds
Modifier loci
Compensatory phenotypes
Strain-dependent phenotypes

ticularly prone to genetic background effects. It is not expected that experiments using genetically engineered mice will be rigidly standardized to any degree, given the variety of hypotheses to be tested, strategies employed, and phenotypes examined. It therefore will be incumbent upon the investigator to be vigilant of the potential sources of variability with this new technology (Table 10.2) that he or she needs to keep in mind when either evaluating phenotypic effects from individual experiments or comparing the phenotypes of different mutants with the same targeted gene but with different targeting and breeding histories.

While the simplistic goal of these studies may be to detect single-gene functions, the dynamic interaction between the introduced or disrupted DNA and the background genes cannot be ignored. Given this awareness, interpretation of phenotypes may be challenging but potentially even more revealing of the complexity of both single-gene and multigenic disorders.

## REFERENCES

Balmain, A. and Nagase, H. 1998. Cancer resistance genes in mice: models for the study of tumor modifiers. Trends Genet. 14:139–144.

Baribault, H., Penner, J., Iozzo, R., and Wilson-Heiner, M. 1994. Colorectal hyperplasia and inflammation in keratin 8-deficient FVB/N mice. Genes Dev. 8:2964–2973.

Bedell, M.A., Largaespada, D., Jenkins, N., and Copeland, N. 1997. Mouse models of human disease. Part II: recent progress and future directions. Genes Dev. 11:11–43.

Bonyadi, M., Rusholme, S., Cousins, F., et al. 1997. Mapping of a major genetic modifier of embryonic lethality in TGFβ1 knockout mice. Nat. Genet. 15:207–211.

Crawley, J.N. 1996. Unusual behavioral phenotypes of inbred mouse strains. Trends Neurosci. 19:181–182.

Dietrich, W.F., Lander, E., Smith, J., et al. 1993. Genetic identification of *Mom-1*, a major modifier locus affecting *Min*-induced intestinal neoplasia in the mouse. Cell 75:631–639.

Doetschman, T. 1999. Interpretation of phenotype in genetically engineered mice. Lab. Anim. Sci. 49:137–143.

Donehower, L.A., Harvey, M., Slagle, B., et al. 1992. Mice deficient for p53 are developmentally normal but susceptible to spontaneous tumors. Nature 356:215–221.

Donehower, L.A., Harvey, M., Vogel, H., et al. 1995. Effects of genetic background on tumorigenesis in p53-deficient mice. Mol. Carcinog. 14:16–22.

Erickson, R.P. 1996. Mouse models of human genetic disease: which mouse is more like a man? BioEssays 18:993–998.

Fijneman, R.J.A., de Vries, S., Jansen, R., and Demant, P. 1996. Complex interactions of new quantitative trait loci, Sluc1, Sluc2, Sluc3, and Sluc4, that influence susceptibility to lung cancer in the mouse. Nat. Genet. 14:465–467.

Fodde, R., Smits, R., Breukel, C., et al. 1996. Genotype-phenotype correlations in intestinal carcinogenesis: the lessons from the mouse models. In Hereditary Cancer, ed. R. Scott and H.J. Muller, Basel: Karger.

Fox, R.R. and Witham, B.A. (eds.). 1997. *Handbook of Genetically Standardized JAX Mice*. Bar Harbor, ME: The Jackson Laboratory.

Gerlai, R. 1996. Gene-targeting studies of mammalian behavior: is it the mutation or the background genotype? Trends Neurosci. 19:177–181.

Goelz, M.F., Mahler, J., Harry, J., et al. 1998. Neuropathologic findings associated with seizures in FVB mice. Lab. Anim. Sci. 48:34–37.

Jinnah, H.A., Jones, M., Wojcik, B., et al. 1999. Influence of age and strain on striatal dopamine loss in a genetic mouse model of Lesch-Nyhan disease. J. Neurochem. 72:225–229.

Kawase, E., Suemori, H., Takahashi, N., et al. 1994. Strain difference in establishment of mouse embryonic stem (ES) cell lines. Int. J. Dev. Biol. 38:385–390.

Lahvis, G.P. and Bradfield, C.A. 1998. Ahr null alleles: distinctive or different? Biochem. Pharmacol. 56:781–787.

Lemckert, F.A., Sedgwick, J., and Korner, H. 1997. Gene targeting in C57BL/6 ES cells. Successful germ line transmission using recipient BALB/c blastocysts developmentally matured *in vitro*. Nucleic Acids Res. 25:917–918.

Li, E., Sucov, H., Lee, K.-F., et al. 1993. Normal development and growth of mice carrying a targeted disruption of the $\alpha$-1 retinoic acid receptor gene. Proc. Natl. Acad. Sci. 90:1590–1594.

Lyon, M.F., Rastan, S., and Searle, A. (eds.). 1996. Genetic Variants and Strains of the Laboratory Mouse. 3rd ed. Oxford: Oxford University Press.

Mahler, J.F., Stokes, W., Mann, P., et al. 1996. Spontaneous lesions in aging FVB/N mice. Toxicol. Pathol. 24:710–716.

Mahler, J.F., Flagler, N., Malarkey, D., et al. 1998. Spontaneous and chemically induced proliferative lesions in Tg.AC transgenic and p53-heterozygous mice. Toxicol. Pathol. 26:501–511.

Manenti, G., Binelli, G., Gariboldi, M., et al. 1994. Multiple loci affect genetic predisposition to hepatocarcinogenesis in mice. Genomics 23:118–124.

McNamara, R.K., Stumpo, D., Morel, L., et al. 1998. Effect of reduced myristoylated alanine-rich C kinase substrate expression on hippocampal mossy fiber development and spatial learning in mutant mice: transgenic rescue and interactions with gene background. Proc. Natl. Acad. Sci. USA 95:14517–14522.

Moen, C.J.A., Groot, P., Hart, A., et al. 1996. Fine mapping of colon tumor susceptibility (Scc) genes in the mouse, different from the genes known to be somatically mutated in colon cancer. Proc. Natl. Acad. Sci. USA 93:1082–1086.

Mombaerts, P., Mizoguchi, E., Grusby, M., et al. 1993. Spontaneous development of inflammatory bowel disease in T cell receptor mutant mice. Cell 75:275–282.

Moser, A.R., Pitot, H., and Dove, W. 1990. A dominant mutation that predisposes to multiple intestinal neoplasia in the mouse. Science 247:322–324.

Nielsen, L.L., Gurnani, M., Catino, J. and Tyler, R. 1995. In *wap-ras* transgenic mice, tumor phenotype but not cyclophosphamide-sensitivity is affected by genetic background. Anticancer Res. 15:385–392.

Rosenberg, D.W. and Liu, Y. 1995. Induction of aberrant crypts in murine colon with varying sensitivity to colon carcinogenesis. Cancer Lett. 92:209–214.

Rozmahel, R., Wilschanski, M., Matin, A., et al. 1996. Modulation of disease severity in cystic fibrosis transmembrane conductance regulator deficient mice by a secondary genetic factor. Nat. Genet. 12:280–287.

Serrano, M., Lee, H.-W., Chin, L., et al. 1996. Role of the INK4a locus in tumor suppression and cell mortality. Cell 85:27–37.

Shastry, B.S. 1994. More to learn from gene knockouts. Mol. Cell Biochem. 136:171–182.

Shastry, B.S. 1995. Genetic knockouts in mice: an update. Experientia 51:1028–1039.

Shastry, B.S. 1998. Gene disruption in mice: models of development and disease. Mol. Cell Biochem. 181:163–179.

Sibilia, M. and Wagner, E.F. 1995. Strain-dependent epithelial defects in mice lacking the EGF receptor. Science 269:234–238.

Silvers, L.M. 1995. *Mouse Genetics. Concepts and Applications*. New York: Oxford University Press, pp. 44–50.

Simpson, E.M., Linder, C., Sargent, E., et al. 1997. Genetic variation among 129 substrains and its importance for targeted mutagenesis in mice. Nat. Genet. 16:19–27.

Smithies, O. 1993. Animal models of human genetic diseases. Trends Genet. 9:112–116.

Sundberg, J. 1991. Inherited mouse mutations: animal models and biochemical tools. Lab. Anim. Sci. 20:40–65.

Sundberg, J. 1992. Conceptual evaluation of animal models as tools for the study of diseases in other species. Lab. Anim. Sci. 21:48–51.

Takagi, H., Sharp, R., Hammermeister, C., et al. 1992. Molecular and genetic analysis of liver oncogenesis in transforming growth factor $\alpha$ mice. Cancer Res. 52:5171–5177.

Taketo, M., Schroeder, A., Mobraaten, L., et al. 1991. FVB/N: an inbred mouse strain preferable for transgenic analyses. Proc. Natl. Acad. Sci. USA 88:2065–2069.

van der Houven van Oordt, C.W., Smits, R., Schouten, T., et al. 1999. The genetic background modifies the spontaneous and X-ray-induced tumor spectrum in the Apc1638N mouse model. Genes Chromosomes Cancer 24:191–198.

# 11
# Clinical Evaluation of Genetically Engineered Mice

Deborah E. Devor-Henneman

There seems to be some unspoken premise that genetically engineered mice (GEM) are an alien species, that they look, behave, or react to various biological or chemical agents differently than do their wild-type counterparts, and therefore, different and as yet unidentified criteria must be applied in their clinical appraisal. The premise is false. There may well be unusual phenotypic aberrations in GEM, but the means used to assess these aberrations are no different than for conventional mice. The problem, as highlighted by the explosion in GEM production and research, is really a lack of knowledge as to what constitutes the spectrum of "normal" (Brownstein 1998). Misinterpretations of the effects of genomic manipulation are highly likely when endogenous factors are also something of a mystery. This chapter is an attempt to familiarize the reader with "normal" and to make it easier to systematically detect abnormal in genetically altered as well as conventional mice. The following sections also clarify the process of differentiating spontaneous physiological effects from those that may be induced by targeted gene mutations.

The means of clinical evaluation listed and described in the following sections are not startlingly new or developed specifically for mutant mouse populations. All animals have to abide by the rules of physiology; the players may have been altered somewhat, but the game remains the same. This chapter deals with assessing only postnatal populations. Methods of examining developmental effects of gene manipulation in the embryo and fetus are described in Chapters 6 and 8.

## ROUTINE EVALUATION PARAMETERS

It is extremely rare that an investigator has access to a technical staff, animal facility, autopsy laboratory, and/or clinical chemistry laboratory dedicated to him or her as an individual. Resources are generally shared, technicians work on many different studies under time and management constraints, and not everyone, including the investigators, are at the same level of knowledge when it comes to the biology of a particular species/strain. Therefore, a set of commonly used clinical parameters for the collection of elemental data is divided into the measurably objective in Table 11.1 and the more subjective and observational in Table 11.2.

A word of caution here to all study directors, primary investigators, and technicians: Data should be used as a tool; the *interpretation* of the data—*within the context of the phase of the animal's life, its specific strain and sex, and the experimental design*—is what counts. And while it may seem an insult to the intelligence to state an obvious fact, you have to take the time to *see* what the mouse is trying to tell you. Shifting mice from dirty cage to clean does not constitute a clinical observation.

## INTERPRETING THE DATA

Some of the criteria used to clinically assess both standard and transgenic animals (Tables 11.1 and 11.2) may need to be looked at more closely if the evaluations are to be further refined. For instance, let's assume that you have a population of transgenic mice whose only distinguishing physical characteristic is that they are 10–15 percent lighter in body weight than their wild-type littermates at age-matched time points. The transgenic animals appear healthy—they just don't weigh as much. Are they consistently lighter throughout their lifetimes, or does the difference disappear at some point? Is the weight differential due to less body fat, or is their skeletal framework proportionally smaller? Are their bones or muscles any less dense than those of the control

145

TABLE 11.1.  Commonly used and measurable (objective) data for clinical evaluation

| Parameter | Specifics | Normal/abnormal |
|---|---|---|
| Body weight<br>NOTE: *Animals losing 1g/wk or more should be closely monitored; losing 10% body weight within a short time is serious, and euthanasia may be justified, especially when weight loss is accompanied by other adverse clinical signs. However, mild weight loss, especially if transient, should not be used as the* sole *criteria for sacrifice, unless there is a precedent.* | Variable, dependent on growth phase and desired information: collected daily, weekly or biweekly, or monthly by individual, cage, or group | In normal growth phase, gains follow a rapid but not necessarily smooth curve up to a plateau at maturity. At maturity, the plateau phase should show steady to marginal weight increases in nonbreeding populations based on strain and sex.<br><br>*Unusual weight gain*<br>Unexpected pregnancy (check your sexes)<br>Ascites<br>Edema<br>Organ enlargement<br>Tumor development<br>Overfeeding<br><br>*Unusual weight loss*<br>Physical inability to eat, as with malocclusion or deformities of teeth<br>Competition<br>Unpalatable feed/inability to reach feed<br>Dehydration (Suspect this if using automatic watering and an entire cage has lost weight.)<br>Metabolic disturbances or nutritional deficiencies<br>Disease, including but not limited to cancer or injury<br>Pituitary tumors |
| Food/water consumption | Measured most accurately via the use of metabolism cages; fair estimations can be done using daily or weekly measures of a gram of food (or milliliter of water) consumed subtracted from amounts provided. | Data are most useful when used in dosed-feed or dosed-water studies to ensure animals are receiving the proper concentration of test agent. Also used to determine consumption parameters for a population. In many cases, however, it is difficult to separate waste and consumption. |
| Tumor development<br>NOTE: *Palpation or external inspection should not be used as the sole evaluation criterion; each is a tool to be used in conjunction with other clinical signs.* | Visual inspection and/or palpation; performed weekly at a minimum and more frequently for rapidly growing neoplasms and those for which latency and/or rate of progression is/are parameters.<br>Palpation is only effective for dermal, subcutaneous, and intraperitoneal lesions; intrathoracic, CNS, and many PNS lesions will escape detection if other means of evaluation are not used. | A solid knowledge of anatomy is a prerequisite for both palpation and visual inspection—full stomachs, distended bladders, and unsuspected pregnancies can mimic intraperitoneal tumors. Be aware that tumors behave according to their individual biology and location—generalizations about their past progression or effects will cost you animals. |

**TABLE 11.1.  Continued**

| Parameter | Specifics | Normal/abnormal |
|---|---|---|
| Appearance of urine/feces<br>  *NOTE: Urination and defecation should be effortless. If there is straining with voiding, with or without vocalization, something is wrong. Rectal prolapses are also blatant signs of large bowel problems, including parasites.* | Metabolism cages are needed for accurate measurements of output; frequency of bedding changes and relative appearance of bedding are indirect measures. | Fecal pellets should be formed and reasonably firm, although diet will influence color, consistency, and amount; pellets are usually dark olive to brown when fresh, drying to black.<br><br>*Not normal*<br>  Yellow feces may indicate fat (normal in nursing pups).<br>  Soft to watery feces (diarrhea) are indicative of parasites, toxicity, and GI disease/absorptive disturbances.<br>  Tarry black feces are likely to contain blood from lesions in or emptying into the GI tract.<br>  Heavy mucus coating the pellets may indicate colitis of various etiologies.<br>  Scant, extremely dry feces indicate constipation. |
| *The conditions listed here for urine abnormalities are largely indications of kidney and/or urinary bladder problems. Keep in mind that the kidney is also affected by metabolic disturbances in other organs. Gross observations of urine cannot be used to answer all questions about problems elsewhere; you might need to invest in some urine chemistry if you suspect other organs are involved.* | | Urine is normally a clear shade of yellow; males have more potent urine than females. Picking up a mouse usually results in enough urination to judge appearance. Or place the mouse on a white, waterproof surface and wait.<br><br>*You DO NOT want to see*<br>  Cloudy urine (pus, sediment)<br>  Blood (liquid or clotted)<br>  Particulate matter (tissue, sand—also check the fur around the urogenital area)<br>  Colorless urine<br>  Urine of an odd color (orange, green, brown, etc.)<br>  Urine retention or abdominal distension with edema<br>  Excessive urination |

mice? Is their development delayed or accelerated? Do they appear to breed later than usual?

Before jumping to the conclusion that an aberration is caused by genomic interference, step back and cross off the simple possibilities first. For example, a cohort of knockout animals is weaned, and changes are noted in the appearance of the animals' feces. Was there a change in the diet or the drinking water? Were they moved to another location? Was a new caretaker or technician assigned to the room? Are the husbandry routines the same? Perhaps a technician points out a decline in the reproductive rate of a previously fertile transgenic breeding population. What time of year is it? How old are the breeders, and have they been continuously paired with the same partner(s)? Has anything changed in the handling, husbandry, or light cycle? Are the room/facility noise levels about the same as previously?

In addition, other medical diagnostic methods can be used as needed to back up clinical observations and autopsy findings or to refine the interpretation of effect. These include analyses of blood, urine, feces, and other bodily fluids to detect changes in body chemistry and metabolism in representatives of both normal and abnormal populations.

**TABLE 11.2.  More subjective criteria for clinical evaluation**

| Parameter | Specifics | Normal/abnormal |
|---|---|---|
| Overall condition | Eyes<br>  Quality of exposed eye (bright, dull, cloudy, etc.)<br>  Size and symmetry<br>  Color<br>  Condition of membranes, eyelids, and adjacent skin<br>  Presence and type of discharge<br><br>  *Note: There are some fairly common defects that are often genetically determined and are not, by themselves, cause for drastic action:*<br>    *Microphthalmia (small eye), anophthalmia (lack of eye)*<br>    *Cataract (lens opacity)* | The eyes of an animal can tell you a lot. They should be clear, moist, and symmetrical in size and shape and show no discharges or swellings of membranes or lids. Abnormalities worth noting:<br>  *Protruding eye* indicates pressure from within (infection, glaucoma, fluid imbalance) or externally (Harderian gland, bone, or nerve lesions).<br>  *Discharges* milky white are associated with Harderian abnormalities; clear, with irritation; and green or yellow purulent, with infection.<br>  *Opacities* or *scars* from injuries or infections<br>  *Inflammation* (often accompanied by loss of hair) around the eye can mean irritation from parasites, allergies, treatments, or exposure to chemicals and is common in some viral infections.<br>  *Change in color* (anemia in albino or dilute animals, also scarring) or *dulling* of the eye (dehydration, pain, disease)<br>  *Retraction of eye into socket (sunken eyes)* accompanies emaciation disease and/or pain; can also be a sign of dehydration. |
|  | Skin and coat<br>  Keep in mind that problems with the skin and coat can be due to parasites, autoimmune diseases, nutritional and/or metabolic disorders, and environmental factors (e.g., humidity, housing) as well as to any treatment or genetic manipulation.<br>  "Barbering" is another phenomenon that is sometimes confused with alopecia but appears to be a dominance behavior, especially among females. The hair from subordinates is chewed or plucked in a localized pattern. Hair may also be broken off around the nose and muzzle from abrasion from poking through cage/lid holes.<br><br>  *Note: Healthy animals spend a significant amount of time grooming themselves and cagemates. As animals become older, they may groom less often or less fastidiously due to decreased flexibility, less energy, or developing cognitive disorders.* | The coat should be complete and lay smooth with a sheen. Healthy skin is elastic and supple, pale pink or off-white, and without breaks or flaking. Look out for:<br>  *Dryness or dehydration*<br>  *Alopecia* (hair loss, not to be confused with barbering)<br>  *Wounds,* which can be self-inflicted<br>  *Dermatitis* (inflammation), especially if it progresses over the body or turns ulcerative<br>  *Piloerection* of the coat, often seen with subcutaneous/dermal edema, low body temperature, and many diseases<br>  *Matting* or *excessive oiliness* |

**TABLE 11.2.  Continued**

| Parameter | Specifics | Normal/abnormal |
|---|---|---|
| Posture | How does the animal hold itself during normal activity? <br> Is the posture appropriate for that activity? | Some postures that are normal in some instances but not in others: <br> *Kyphosis* is a pronounced hunching that protects the abdominal organs in defense situations but indicates pain in a lab setting. <br> *Lordosis* is an elevation of the pelvis normally seen in females receptive to mating; outside of breeding, it may indicate difficulty in urinating or passing feces. <br> *Arching* or *walking on tips of the toes* (when the animal is not simply stretching) can signal foot/leg/joint pain. <br> *Defensive postures* (e.g., backing into corners with tail rattling, rising up on the hind legs), especially when the animal is not being threatened, is often seen during seizures and with other neurological conditions. |
| Movement/use of limbs | How freely does the animal move? <br> Are all limbs engaged equally? <br> Do all limbs have complete functional range of motion? <br> Is any joint or limb swelling or redness present? | Changes in gait or flexibility are symptomatic of musculoskeletal problems, injury, or neurological impairments. They can be local (i.e., at the site affected) or originate in the spinal column or nerves. Any of the following are serious: <br> *Joint inflammation* and *swelling* or *malformation* can occur from joint disease (natural or exogenously induced), injury or dislocation from rough handling, or nutritional deficiencies (not common). <br> *Broken bones* (These are usually found as a result of poor handling techniques or mechanical accidents; the tails of rodents are especially prone to breaks.) <br> *Paresis* (weakness and reduced function) or outright *paralysis* (no function) likely has, in the absence of noticeable skeletal disorders or known accidents, a PNS and/or CNS pathology. |
| General behavior <br> When looking at behavior and behavior patterns, consider the housing and breeding status, and compare equivalent populations. While CNS defects frequently manifest themselves in perturbed behavior, there are also hormonal and environmental causes. | Patterns <br><br> Appropriate context | Changes in behavior patterns are extremely important as indicators of disease processes and progression. <br><br> Some behaviors that should throw up red flags: <br> *Excessive aggression* <br> *Excessive or exaggerated activity* <br> *Isolation/no social interaction* <br> *Lack of interest in opposite sex* <br> *No maternal behavior* <br> *Lack of or delayed response to stimuli/inappropriate response to stimuli* |

*(continued)*

**TABLE 11.2.   Continued**

| Parameter | Specifics | Normal/abnormal |
|---|---|---|
| Respiration<br>The vast majority of respiratory distress cases involve obstruction of the airways. The obstruction need not be solid, nor is it always within the respiratory organs themselves. Obstructions can be caused by fluids, inhaled particles, tumors, and distension of surrounding tissues (including abdominal organs) that effectively limit bronchial or lung expansion. Other causes of respiratory distress are lesions within the breathing centers in the CNS and PNS and, in rare cases, biochemical abnormalities in oxygen uptake/exchange. | Effort | *Normal respiration* is effortless, inaudible, and even. |
| | Rate | The respiration rate varies with exertion, but regardless of activity level, the color of the extremities should remain healthy and pinkish, indicating adequate oxygenated blood flow. The ribcage is elastic; much of the associated movement appears to be abdominal or in the flank. The lungs fill and empty equally. |
| | Type | There are varying degrees of *respiratory abnormalities* that encompass:<br>    Increased effort upon exertion<br>    *Cyanosis,* exacerbated by increased activity<br>    *Noisy breathing*<br>    *Behaviors that accompany breathing,* such as peculiar postures, pawing at the nose, repetitive sneezing<br>    *Rigidity of the ribcage* with increased abdominal effort<br>    *Mouth breathing* (gasping)<br>    *Preoccupation with breathing,* such that breathing itself interferes with eating, drinking, and other activities |
| | Location of the obstruction | The breathing pattern and behavior of an animal in respiratory distress can frequently indicate the anatomic location of the problem. Lesions and obstructions can occur anywhere around and in the respiratory tree, from the brain and nasal cavities/pharynx down to the lung parenchyma/alveoli and below the diaphragm. To look only at the lungs at necropsy may lead to missing causative factors. |
| Vocalization<br>*Note: As a general rule of thumb,* investigate vocalizations; *it can save damage from fighting, tails and toes caught in caging, and lost or hungry newborns as well as pinpoint animals in need of analgesia or euthanasia.* | Type | Mice vocalize to other mice for various communicative reasons, and much of their "vocabulary" is beyond the normal range of human hearing. However, with experience, the differences between squeaks of irritation, anger, fear, and the peeping noises of newborns become apparent. |
| | Occurrence | Although many suffer in silence, mice will also vocalize when in pain, and this is a distinctive sound. Seizures commonly invoke vocalizations of various sorts. If an animal starts to vocalize in situations where it was previously silent (e.g., routine handling, palpation, or why singly housed), it is a sign that something is wrong. |

# ELEMENTAL CONSIDERATIONS IN ANIMAL STUDIES

There are only two outcomes in most bioassays, be they concerned with toxicology, carcinogenesis, or genetic manipulation: (1) the animals are seemingly unaffected by any exogenous treatments or exposures, or (2) there *is* an effect, and life spans are shortened or seriously compromised, or an abnormal (and not necessarily lethal) phenotype is produced. Elemental considerations, then, involve determining if or when

1. The clinical condition, natural or induced, is significant.
2. The effect has reached its maximal development.
3. The result will be fatal without preemptive intervention.

While it is important to be able to detect an effect, a second and equally important aspect is knowing when an effect has reached the point where the animal should be euthanized and autopsied to give the most and/or the most useful information (i.e., the point or points when the disease process might be best identified and characterized). Animals found dead provide relatively limited information, but discarded animals give none. From a purely economical standpoint, animals allowed to die on their own are an expensive waste. From a purely analytical standpoint, too many "noninformative" deaths may result in total study invalidation. Statistical analyses suffer if surviving populations are too small, and no amount of creative number crunching is going to turn a poor study into a good one. The autolytic changes that occur in dead tissues can significantly cloud histological interpretation, and furthermore, any clinical information not recorded is priceless, especially if it could have been applied to the still-at-risk. There are also ethical and regulatory issues (Hamm 1995), as well as the adverse effects that repetitive unexplained deaths may have on caretaking and technical staff (Halpern-Lewis 1996).

There is no argument that extra effort is required to avoid excessive losses in experimental populations. Because each study has its own built-in variables and experimental questions, it might seem a difficult job to address generalities; however, in the absence of a protocol outlining specific parameters, knowing when you've found an effect and knowing when to send individual test subjects to necropsy is not all that mystifying if you use basic biological principles and common sense concerning the test subjects. Overall, if the sum of clinical observations points to a continual decline in quality of life, or if there are factors such as compromising tumors/lesions in critical organs, obvious pain (Keefe et al. 1991), or significant bleeding, and the protocols do not call for remedial methods, euthanasia is warranted.

# CRITICAL PERIODS IN THE POSTNATAL LIFE SPAN OF GEM

It should come as no surprise to find out that patterns in GEM clinical pathology generally parallel patterns in normal mice. What may shift is the phenotypic developmental timeframe, the severity of pathological phenotypes, and/or the multiplicity of pathological phenotypes. Histopathology is occasionally a very different story. Depending on the background strain genetics (Doetschman 1999), the mode of inheritance, the degree of penetrance and expression, and the particular function of the manipulated gene, mice heterozygous for the altered gene may show no unusual phenotype or phenotypes intermediate to wild-type and homozygous animals.

Assuming that the targeted mutation did not result in death at some point during gestation (see Chap. 7), postnatal GEM pathology can be broadly divided into acute and chronic. Acute effects generally show up early (i.e., in the neonatal period through early adulthood) or present suddenly at some critical transition period in the animals' development—such as weaning, puberty, pregnancy, or parturition—with severe or fatal consequences. Chronic effects may or may not be apparent at birth; often there are compensatory mechanisms that allow for a normal, or something approaching a normal, life span for the strain. This is particularly true in cases of minor aberrations in the musculoskeletal and immune systems. Tumorigenesis is generally a phenomenon of older animals in wild-type populations. In GEM, however, disruptions of genes concerned with tumor suppression, intercellular communication, or growth factors commonly result in acceleration of neoplastic development and/or expansion of the spectrum of neoplasias in much younger animals.

*Neonatal deaths* are frequently encountered in manipulations of genes involved with critical physiology. The newborn has to breath, nurse, metabolize nutrients, and eliminate wastes. It must be able to move and demonstrate appropriate behaviors that allow it to find nourishment and warmth and elicit maternal care. The proper growth factors, receptors, and inter-/intracellular message and transport systems have to be operational to allow tissue function and maturation. Abnormalities of the respiratory system may arguably be the most common immediate cause of unexplained neonatal death in GEM. It's worth wondering if the closer attention paid to the birth of genetically altered offspring doesn't skew the data so that the incidence of respiratory failure is ignored in conventional neonates.

At *weaning*, the digestive system must adapt to solid food, and the immune system must become competent. The young mouse must perfect acceptable social behaviors and responses to stimuli. It is still in a growth and maturation phase requiring considerable energy and metabolic efficiency. Genes that have a particular influence on growth hormones, energy metabolism, and the components of the immune system may produce specific phenotypes at this point.

At *puberty*, a surge of new hormones elicits sexual behavior, acts upon several organ systems to initiate the estrous and spermatogenic cycles, and fosters functional maturation of the mammary and reproductive organs.

*Pregnancy and parturition* comprise other potentially critical periods for the female in that there are several profound changes in the reproductive organs, in the immune and hormonal milieus, and in energy needs. Logically, the effects of mutations in genes that may function, directly or indirectly, in, for example, the reproductive processes, the synchrony or optimal expression of hormones, the proper suppression of the maternal immune system, steroidogenesis, and germ cell maturation may be expressed as delays in sexual maturation, infertility or reduced fertility, difficulties in the birth process, and poor maternal behavior.

# THE FRAMESHIFT IN DISEASES AND DISEASE ONSET IN GEM

Conventional mouse strains are prone to strain-specific aging lesions, the incidence and severity of which, when coupled with environmental factors, determine the average life span for the population. The same is true for GEM, but as was previously stated, the effect of the targeted mutation may markedly affect the life span, disease spectrum, and onset of symptoms (see Chap. 12 for comparisons of the general time frames of disease type and onset between conventional mice and GEM).

Some generalizations about GEM can be made that are fairly consistent. Assessing newborns is both difficult, because of size and the wide array of possible problems, and easy, because they are almost transparent and you can see internal structures to a large extent. A stillbirth or death within the first 48 hours of the perinatal period often occurs as a result of developmental or functional defects in the heart, CNS, or respiratory and alimentary tracts (see previous section, "Critical Periods in the Postnatal Life Span of GEM"). Very severe primary cardiac abnormalities usually result in intrauterine death since the heart is a critical organ in fetal development, but for those pups who make it to birth, the increased demands of life outside the uterus are often fatal when heart function is compromised. Malformations of the palate and epiglottis may prohibit breathing and/or suckling and masquerade as a respiratory defect, making it of some importance to look for milk in the stomach of dead or moribund newborns. Renal insufficiency may take up to several days to kill, unless there is outright atresia of urinary structures. Runting can indicate many abnormalities, both anatomical and metabolic, and is not always fatal; in some cases, it is also reversible with time.

Inflammatory and immune-mediated diseases frequently manifest themselves once pups have lost the immunities provided by the dam's milk (i.e., around weaning—unless the dam's milk is itself antibody deficient as a result of gene targeting). This is related to another facet of GEM evaluation: the delineation of direct and indirect effects of the targeted mutation, especially if there is mutation expression in the heterozygous dam involving placental exchange or lactation. If it is suspected that the dam may be contributing to pup mortality, embryo transfer or fostering litters to a wild-type female may be required.

Other hallmarks of GEM pathology are the acceleration of chronic degenerative diseases, early development of conditions and tumors associated with aging, and/or development of unusual or multiple neoplasias. These are occasionally pronounced in animals in which more than a single gene has been disrupted, a transgene insertion occurred at a particularly sensitive or reactive site, cooperation between genes is destroyed, or there is overexpression of one or more factors controlled by the targeted gene.

An increasing number of reports indicate increased tumor yields in heterozygote as well as homozygous null (knockout) mutants. However, too many of these studies lack information on the condition of equivalent wild-type control animals. This is one area (that of appropriate controls) where the study of GEM should not differ from carcinogenesis and toxicity assays. Concurrent age- and sex-matched controls are absolutely essential to validate any claims of effect. Historical controls are of limited value in light of the strain mixtures employed in the making of GEM. Neither do historical controls or data obtained on controls from another lab reflect the exact conditions under which *your* animals are being held. An all-too-common practice among investigators is to disregard or flatly discard heterozygote and wild-type littermates. Often rationalized as a cost-saving measure, it usually is a costly mistake. These animals provide information to confirm data, redirect studies, and indirectly answer mechanistic questions when the production of null mutants is low or impossible.

# CONFOUNDING FACTORS AFFECTING GEM EVALUATION

The animals are not behaving as you thought they would. You've spent countless hours in independent current research on what the gene does or may do, you've gotten other researchers' opinions and anecdotal recommendations, you trust the integrity of the technology and the data collected. Everything seems to have been done correctly, but the experiment is going in an unexpected direction. Welcome to the Dark Side, wherein are contained all the factors never explained that can obviously confound the best of plans. Rather than panic and start blaming others for ineptitude, or relegating the exercise to the circular file, or considering a career change, step back and look at some of the variables that may have played a part in your scientific life crisis.

1. The gene construct may not have heeded your instructions and randomly inserted elsewhere within the genome (heterologous recombination) with unexpected influence. The construct may also have been unstable in vivo (Thompson et al. 1998) or caused a separate mutation as a technical artifact (Lyon et al. 1996).

2. Animals never read protocols. If they could, the protocols would not make an impression. Your effect may be due to a naturally occurring genetic glitch or the modification of a natural mutation by your construct. In addition, genetic drift resulting from natural mutations is an ongoing phenomenon, as Darwin pointed out, and can be a real problem. The two-volume *Genetic Variants and Strains of the Laboratory Mouse* (Lyon et al. 1996) is a recommended reference for known endogenous mutations that occur in commonly used mouse strains and lists the basic phenotype(s) and chromosomal location, if mapped.

3. For as much as we think we know, we still don't have the mechanics of genetics nailed. Nature has built amazing redundancy into the genome and has also taken measures to eliminate seriously detrimental mutations through in utero and early neonatal mortality or through infertility. Probably of even more significance is the interaction of genes and gene products. An indirect effect of your gene manipulation, far upstream or downstream of the actual mutation, may have more serious consequences than the specific insertion or targeted mutation.

4. You may be the victim of a typographical error when it comes to the supposed mouse strain or embryonic stem (ES) cell lineage used. A case in point is the current concern over substrain/subline variability in the oft-used 129/Sv mouse ([*http://www.taconic.com*]; [*http://www.informatics. jax.org*]; Lyon et al. 1996). Humans are notoriously bad at record keeping and transcribing information. Unfortunately, since mouse strains and sublines of those strains can show marked variations in gene expression, having the "correct" animal to work with is crucial.

5. Technically, things may not have been as perfect as they initially seemed to be. This is really difficult to prove, in most cases, and occasionally results in confrontations between the principal investigator and the technician/caretaker. An unbelievable number of mistakes are made in breeding, animal identification, and consistent data collection. It is extremely difficult to maintain stringent and consistent research conditions when time, workload, and possibly unrealistic expectations become overriding factors.

6. You may be extrapolating largely in vitro data to an in vivo system. Consider yourself a pioneer, and take a lesson from carcinogenicity testing. Cell culture imposes conditions that may show effects not always reproducible in intact animals. Frequently the whole is greater and much different than the sum of its parts.

7. Technical or environmental factors (or both) may be having an effect on your GEM. The technologies used in GEM creation are very rough on the organisms and capable of inducing many abnormalities in and of themselves (Brownstein 1998). This is notably true in implantation and gestation, in the immediate postnatal period where maternal support is crucial, in mutations involving nutritional requirements or utilization, and in mutations that involve seizure conditions exacerbated by noise, handling, or abrupt changes in light. And if you are trying to reproduce the results obtained by another lab, environmental and procedural variabilities may make it difficult or impossible to do so.

# REFERENCES

Brownstein, D.G. 1998. Genetically engineered mice: the holes in the sum of the parts. Lab. Anim. Sci. 48:121–122.

Doetschman, T. 1999. Interpretation of phenotype in genetically engineered mice. Lab. Anim. Sci. 49:137–143.

Halpern-Lewis, J.G. 1996. Understanding the emotional experiences of animal research personnel. Cont. Topics Lab. Anim. Sci. 35:58–60.

Hamm, T.E. 1995. Proposed institutional animal care and use committee guidelines for death as an endpoint in rodent studies. Cont. Topics Lab. Anim. Sci. 34:69–71.

Keefe, F.J., Fillingim, R.B., and Williams, D.A. 1991. Behavioral assessment of pain: nonverbal measures in animals and humans. ILAR News 33:3–13.

Lyon, M.F., Rastan, S., and Brown, S.D.M., eds. 1996. Genetic Variants and Strains of the Laboratory Mouse, 3rd ed., volumes 1 and 2. New York: Oxford University Press.

Thompson, K.L., Rosenzweig, B.A., and Sistare, F.D. 1998. The evaluation of the hemizygous transgenic Tg.AC mouse for carcinogenicity testing of pharmaceuticals. II. A genotypic marker that predicts tumorigenic responsiveness. Tox. Pathol. 26:548–555.

# 12
# Pathology Phenotyping of Genetically Engineered Mice

Jerrold M. Ward

After a new genetically engineered mouse (GEM), either targeted mutant (TM), transgenic (Tg), or other types or combinations of GEM, is developed, the phenotypic characteristics (clinical and pathological) must be determined to characterize the new mouse as a model of a human disease or for studying mechanisms of disease and/or function of a gene. The mutant phenotype may be defined as the clinical and/or pathological manifestation of a specific natural or induced genotype. It should be defined functionally, pathologically, and, if applicable, as a human counterpart. Presently, there are thousands of GEM ([*http://www.biomednet.com/db/mkmd*]; Brandon et al. 1995a, 1995b, 1995c). Much time and money is spent producing new mice. It is important to thoroughly evaluate each new mutant mouse line to ensure that it is used properly as a research tool. For evaluation of mouse embryonic death, see Chapter 8.

A new genetically engineered mouse line should be verified as to its genotype. Because many GEM are developed on the same genetic background and maintained in the same room, their genotype should be verified by DNA analysis prior to characterizing of the phenotype.

## CRITERIA FOR SACRIFICE AND NECROPSY OF MICE

Necropsies also should be performed on clinically normal GEM of different ages to characterize the gross pathology and histopathology of spontaneous and early lesions in important tissues. In addition, when mice show clinical signs, they should be necropsied. These signs include general conditions (progressive body weight loss, hunched appearance, comatose/moribund condition), tumors (a large progressively growing tumor, an ulcerated and/or hemorrhagic tumor), severe skin lesions that are ulcerated or infected, signs of internal disease (nervous system disorder including head tilt, paralysis, circling, ataxia, abdominal distention, palpable internal tumors), respiratory distress, persistent diarrhea, persistent rectal prolapse, or other undesirable clinical conditions. The necropsy should aim to discover the cause(s) of the clinical signs.

## THE NECROPSY

Much has been published on necropsy/autopsy of animals and humans. We have prepared a virtual mouse necropsy web site [*http://www.ncifcrf.gov/vetpath/necropsy.html*]. It includes links to other sites and references on the subject (Devor et al. 1994; Feldman and Seely, 1988; Sundberg and Boggess 1999). The first series of necropsies for a new mouse should be complete screens of all tissues grossly and microscopically on selected mice. Often specific lesions found in the new mice are unanticipated. All tissues should be surveyed histologically. After lesions are found in specific tissues, other specialized pathology methods should be used including histochemistry, electron microscopy, confocal microscopy, immunohistochemistry, in situ hybridization, and quantitative pathology. Examples of these methods are given in other chapters in this book.

## ANCILLARY STUDIES

The basic necropsy should be supported by other veterinary medical diagnostic methods, when necessary. They include evaluation of blood and bone marrow for hematological changes and evaluation of serum, plasma, and urine for clinical chemistry parameters. Serum or plasma can be used to measure hormones, enzymes, and other parameters of normality.

# PATTERNS OF DISEASE

Conventional mice have general life spans of 21–24 months and death due to the types of age-related lesions they develop (Mohr et al. 1996). Some mouse strains, such as AKR, die prior to 1 year of age from thymic lymphomas. Most strains, however, survive over 20 months. Common spontaneous lesions causing death include tumors of many types, renal disease, and, in nonspecific pathogen–defined mice, infectious disease. Mice with targeted mutations in a specific gene (–/–) or with over-expression of a specific gene often develop unique clinical and pathological syndromes that differ greatly from those seen in conventional mice or mice on their wild-type (+/+) backgrounds. The clinical and pathological appearance of the new mouse depends on gene expression in specific cells, tissues, and organs. Inactivation of a gene or overexpression of the gene and its protein may cause changes in cell function, tissue and organ development, and cell and tissue differentiation (Fig. 12.1). These changes can produce abnormalities in clinical

appearance and gross and microscopic pathology. These abnormalities may produce a specific mouse phenotype.

Often, genetically engineered mice develop phenotypes with gross and histological lesions that were not expected. These findings are particularly common for targeted mutant mice. For example, one may produce a new TM mouse with inactivation of a gene thought to be responsible for a specific brain developmental abnormality at birth. At birth, the mouse may be normal, only to develop a completely unexpected disease later in life, not related to the brain. Obviously, gene functional redundancy plays an important role in the phenotype expressed. Scientists should be prepared for the unexpected. In attempting to produce a mouse model for specific specialized research, the result may be a mouse that develops a disease or condition unrelated to the specific expertise of the laboratory. If that situation occurs, collaborators with relevant expertise should be found who can help with investigating the utility of the potential new model. The appropriate phenotypic characterization of the GEM would be a necessary first step in such a situation.

A generalized scheme of life for genetically engineered mice is shown in Figure 12.2. Depending on the gene inactivated or overexpressed, the mice may develop clinical syndromes and die much earlier than conventional mice.

# EMBRYONIC MORTALITY

Embryonic death can result from some basic defects involving implantation, early embryonic development, placental development, or organogenesis. A common cause of embryonic lethality of knockout mice appears to be placental failure. It is discussed in detail in Chapter 8. Defects in organogenesis appear to be less common but may include heart and brain developmental

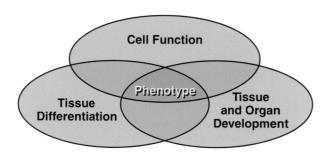

**FIGURE 12.1** Changes in normal gene expression induced by gene targeting or transgene insertion can produce changes in cell function, tissue and cell differentiation, and tissue and organ development. These changes produce the mouse phenotype.

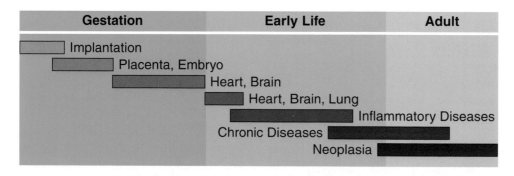

**FIGURE 12.2** The scheme of life showing stages where the results of gene manipulation may manifest in target organs or conditions.

defects occurring prior to birth. These and others are discussed in Chapter 7.

# NEONATAL AND PERINATAL MORTALITY

Death at birth (neonatal period) or in the perinatal period (a few days after birth) often occurs from developmental or functional defects in heart, brain, or lungs. Other tissues may be affected, as well. Newborn mice should nurse soon after birth and have milk visible in their stomachs. They should breathe normally and be active. Severe anatomical or structural cardiac lesions can result in congestive heart failure (CHF) at birth (Tullio et al. 1997). During mid- to late gestation, heart failure is usually evident by generalized edema. After birth, CHF is often manifested by dark livers, ascites, and enlarged hearts. Often the effects of brain defects occurring in utero do not show up until birth (Kimura et al. 1996). Misshapen heads, large domed skulls, and death are often seen. Lung failure due to anatomical developmental defects (Kimura et al. 1996) or potential biochemical defects also appear at birth (Pineau et al. 1995). Several mutants that breathe at birth, but die soon thereafter, have been found to have fully formed and histologically normal lung parenchyma. These mutants should be candidates for studying pulmonary surfactant physiology and physiology of other biochemical mechanisms required for proper oxygen consumption. Specific biochemical metabolic defects in neonatal mutant lungs are not usually studied or described but probably occur in the mutant neonates that breathe and die on day 1.

# MORTALITY IN YOUNG ADULTS

Decreased growth after weaning (3–4 weeks of age) or later often indicates an internal disorder that may not be initially apparent clinically. We have observed three basic patterns of abnormal body weight growth that are associated with several types of histopathologic lesions (Fig. 12.3). Runting is slowed growth (body weight gain) as compared with wild-type littermates. Runting can develop from numerous causes. We have seen it typically in mice with some storage diseases (Lei et al. 1996) and inflammatory/immune disorders (Kulkarni et al. 1993). Its cause(s) often leads to death by 1–4 weeks of age.

Young adult mortality can occur from inflammatory or immune-mediated diseases since the immune system begins functioning after 6-7 days of age. The transforming growth factor β1 targeted mutant, which develops an autoimmune vasculitis (Kulkarni et al. 1993), is an example. The only clinical sign is decreased body weight gain (runting).

# MICE WITH GENETIC STORAGE DISEASES SIMILAR TO THOSE IN HUMANS

Targeted mutant mice have been developed with storage disorders similar and identical to those in humans with the same inactivated gene (mouse models of human genetic disorders) (Bedell et al. 1997; Roths et al. 1999). These include deficiencies in glucose-6-phosphatase (von Gierke's disease), acid α-glucosidase (glycogen storage disease Type II), α-galactosidase A (Fabry's Disease), hexosaminidase A (Tay-Sachs disease), and acid sphingomyelinase (Niemann-Pick disease) (Raben et al. 1998; Lei et al. 1996; Ohshima et al. 1997). Inactivation of the gene results in single-enzyme deficiencies leading to a storage disease. Inactivation of the genes

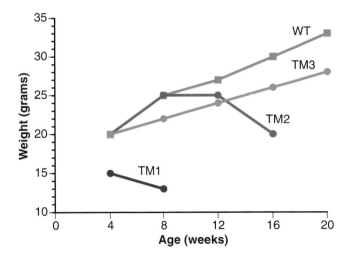

**FIGURE 12.3** Body weight gain patterns in genetically engineered male mice on a B6,129 background. *TM1* shows severe "runting" from a young age that occurs as a result of marked organ/tissue lesions. *TM2* shows weight gain depression due to tumors or chronic lesions developing later in life. *TM3* illustrates a uniform, mild body weight depression throughout life, sometimes due to abnormal, but not life-threatening, physiologic changes in critical organs. (*WT* = wild-type mice)

noted here has produced mice with an almost identical syndrome to that found in humans with mutations in these same genes. The mice develop clinical signs of runting, and tissue lesions can be almost identical to those in humans. They appear to be ideal models for gene therapy. Initial gene therapy studies with these mice have produced encouraging results.

# MICE WITH CHRONIC DEGENERATIVE DISEASES

GEM have been produced with chronic brain (Aguzzi et al. 1996), kidney, liver, and other organ-specific diseases. They may develop body weight gain changes if the condition becomes moderate-severe (Fig. 12.3). These diseases are discussed in specific organ chapters in Section IV. These lesions can produce mice that develop chronic wasting diseases.

# MICE WITH TUMORS

There is an increasing number of single- and double-gene targeted mutant mice that develop tumors at high incidence early in life, usually by 6–10 months of age when no tumors are found in wild-type controls. Usually their body weights are normal until the tumors appear (Fig. 12.3). Lymphomas are by far the most common tumors found in young targeted mutant mice. These TM mice have included mice with mutant *p53*, *Brca-2*, *E2A*, *Ku70*, *Atm*, *INK4a*, *Msh2*, *Pten*, and *Mlh1* genes. Thymic lymphomas are the usual occurrence, but other lymphomas are found including splenic B cell marginal zone lymphomas and B cell follicular center lymphomas. They are discussed in detail in Chapter 24. A variety of other tumors are found in various types of targeted mutant mice including intestinal tumors, endocrine tumors (pituitary, thyroid, adrenal), and sarcomas (undifferentiated sarcomas, hemangiosarcomas). TM mice with nonlymphoid tumors have included mice with mutant *Rb*, *INK4a*, *p53*, *Msh2*, *Pten*, *Mlh1*, *E2F*, *Nf1*, *Tsc2*, α-inhibin, *lats1*, *c-mos*, *p27*, *inhibin*, *XPA*, *Apc*, and *smad3*. Often tumors found in GEM less than 1 year of age are unique in morphological, biological, and molecular features as compared with spontaneous tumors in older wild-type mice. Some types of transgenic mice develop high incidences of preneoplastic and neoplastic lesions in the lung (Maronpot et al. 1991). The entire lung may become involved. It is important to characterize the preneoplastic lesions and tumors found in these genetically engineered mice in order to understand mechanisms of their tumorigenesis.

There is an increasing number of reports of elevated tumor incidence in aging TM or heterozygous mice past 1 year of age. These reports often lack important information on controls, preferably wild-type mice of the same sex and age. They often describe what appears to be slightly higher incidences of spontaneous tumors than found in the wild-type or background controls. Although the tumors in GEM may appear similar in origin and morphology to those in wild-type mice, they can arise in different but adjacent tissues. For example, it is easy to confuse salivary gland tumors with mammary tumors unless one studies the origin of the tumors. Therefore, it is critical to maintain equal numbers of sex- and age-matched wild-type mice to compare the origins of tumors and tumor incidences with those in TM or heterozygous mice. Statistics must be utilized to compare tumor incidences. Often, investigators quickly jump to conclusions when they observe a few extra tumors in a knockout or heterozygous group. They may be unaware of statistical variation of tumor incidences, especially those occurring spontaneously. Statistics must be utilized to compare tumor incidences.

Recently, there has been an increasing number of reports of tumors developing in double-targeted mutants or heterozygous mice. The cooperation of two genes, often involving genes important in the cell cycle or tumor suppression, is obviously of importance (Burns et al. 1999). Some examples of these cooperative genes include *Rb/p53* (Coxon et al. 1998), *BRCA-1/p53*, *Mlh1/Apc1638N*, *Dpc4/Apc*, *Tgfβ1/p21*, and others (Burns et al. 1999).

Transgenic mice often have high incidences of multiple preneoplastic, precancerous, and neoplastic lesions (adenomas, carcinomas) in tissues controlled by an organ-specific promoter. In this book, these tumors are discussed in detail in specific organ chapters in Section IV.

## Mammary Tumors

Mammary tumors have been found in many types of genetically engineered mice. Examples of transgenes used in mice to produce mammary tumors include genes involved as growth factors, receptors, cell cycle control, and cell and tissue differentiation (Munn et al. 1995). Some examples of transgenes inducing mammary tumors are *Wnt1*, *c-myc*, *TGFα*, *c-erB2*, *WAP*, *hgf*, *int3*, *C(3)1*, and *ras*. The tumors may be of alveolar or ductular origin. An excellent web site provides information on the many mouse models of mammary gland carcinoma: [*http://mammary.nih.gov/*]. Procedures for evaluation of the mammary gland are also given on that web site [*http://mammary.nih.gov/tools/index.html*] and also on our virtual mouse necropsy site [*http://www.ncifcrf.gov/vetpath/necropsy.html*]. Recently, a pathology committee has provided a new classification of mouse mammary tumors and hyperplastic lesions, especially in GEM (Tardiff et al. in press).

# NONLETHAL PHENOTYPES AND NORMAL MUTANT MICE WITH FUNCTIONAL DEFECTS

GEM that show no clinical or pathological abnormalities (phenotypes) often occur but are not well reported or may not be reported on at all. For example, mice with immune defects often live normally and are often not studied histologically (Lovik 1997; Ryffel 1997). Their abnormal immune responses to infectious agents and antigens, however, are often reported. Affected mice may be more susceptible to infectious agents. Many of the other apparently "normal" GEM (i.e., normal in clinical behavior, histopathology, and survival) show important functional deficiencies not normally observed in mice with an intact functional gene. For example, a functional defect for those genes involved in xenobiotic metabolism, including *CYP1A2* and *CYP2E1,* can only be observed when a xenobiotic is given to the mouse and its metabolism is studied (Lee et al. 1995). Receptor-deficient mice, such as *Ahr* and *PPARα,* often appear normal but also respond abnormally to xenobiotics (Fernandez-Salguero et al. 1996; Lee et al. 1995). After 1 year of age, however, the Ahr TM mice develop tumors and other lesions that lead to illness (Fernandez-Salguero et al. 1997). Finally, some TM mice appear clinically normal, but their body weight gain is depressed (Fig. 12.3). They are sometimes found to have endocrine or other physiologic abnormalities.

# THE ULTIMATE TASK

Establishing phenotypic features of GEM is dependent upon appropriate longitudinal studies of the mice in question in comparison with age-matched littermates with normal genotypes. These studies require relevant necropsy and tissue protocols for tissue sampling and sampling intervals, as well as active participation of veterinary and other pathologists with expertise in normal rodent gross and microscopic anatomy and pathology.

# REFERENCES

Aguzzi, A., Brandner, S., Marino, S., et al. 1996. Transgenic and knockout mice in the study of neurodegenerative diseases. J. Mol. Med. 74:111–126.

Bedell, M.A., Largaespada, D.A., Jenkins, N.A., et al. 1997. Mouse models of human disease. Part II: Recent progress and future directions. Genes Dev. 11:11–43.

Brandon, E.P., Idzerda, R.L., and McKnight, G.S. 1995a. Targeting the mouse genome: a compendium of knockouts (part I). Curr. Biol. 5:625–634.

Brandon, E.P., Idzerda, R.L., and McKnight, G.S. 1995b. Targeting the mouse genome: a compendium of knockouts (part II). Curr. Biol. 5:758–765.

Brandon, E.P., Idzerda, R.L., and McKnight, G.S. 1995c. Targeting the mouse genome: a compendium of knockouts (part III). Curr. Biol. 5:873–881.

Burns, A., Mikkers, H., Krimpenfort, P., et al. 1999. Identification and characterization of collaborating oncogenes in compound mutant mice. Cancer Res. 59:1773s–1777s.

Coxon, A.B., Ward, J.M., Geradts, J., et al. 1998. RET cooperates with RB/p53 inactivation in a somatic multi-step model for murine thyroid cancer. Oncogene 17:1625–1628.

Devor, D.E., Henneman, J.R., Kurata, Y., et al. 1994. Pathology procedures in laboratory animal carcinogenesis studies. In Waalkes, M. P. and Ward, J. M. (eds.), Carcinogenesis, New York: Raven Press, pp. 429–466.

Feldman, D.B. and Seely, J.C. 1988. Necropsy of Rodents and the Rabbit. Boca Raton: CRC Press.

Fernandez-Salguero, P.M., Hilbert, D.M., Rudikoff, S., et al. 1996. Aryl-hydrocarbon receptor deficient mice are resistant to TCDD (2,3,7,8-tetracholorodibenzo-*p*-dioxin) induced toxicity. Toxicol. Appl. Pharmacol. 140:173–179.

Fernandez-Salguero, P.M., Ward, J.M., Sundberg, J.P., et al. 1997. Lesions of aryl-hydrocarbon receptor deficient mice. Vet. Pathol. 34:605–614.

Kimura, S., Pineau, T., Fernandez-Salguero, P., et al. 1996. The *T/ebp* null mouse: thyroid-specific enhancer-binding protein is essential for the organogenesis of the thyroid, lung, ventral forebrain, and pituitary. Genes Dev. 10:60–69.

Kulkarni, A.B., Huh, C.-G., Beckler, D., et al. 1993. Transforming growth factor $\beta_1$ null mutation in mice causes excessive inflammatory response and early death. Proc. Natl. Acad. Sci. USA 90:770–774.

Lee, S.S., Pineau, T., Drago J., et al. 1995. Targeted disruption of the alpha isoform of the peroxisome proliferator-activated receptor gene in mice results in abolishment of the pleiotropic effects of peroxisome proliferators. Mol. Cell Biol. 15:3012–3022.

Lei, K.J., Hungwen, C., Pan, C.J., et al. 1996. Glucose-6-phosphatase dependent substrate transport in the glycogen storage disease type-1a mouse. Nat. Genet. 13:203–209.

Lovik, M. 1997. Mutant and transgenic mice in immunotoxicology: an introduction. Toxicology 119:65–76.

Maronpot, R.R., Palmiter, R.D., Brinster, R.L., et al. 1991. Pulmonary carcinogenesis in transgenic mice. Exp. Lung Res. 17:305–320.

Mohr, U., Dungworth, D.L., Ward, J.M., et al. 1996. Pathobiology of the Aging Mouse, Volumes 1 and 2. Washington DC: ILSI Press, pp. 505, 527.

Munn, R.J., Webster, M., Muller, W.J., et al. 1995. Histopathology of transgenic mouse mammary tumors (a short atlas). Cancer Biol. 6:153–158.

Ohshima, T., Murray, G.J., Swaim, W.D., et al. 1997. Alpha-galactosidase A deficient mice: a model of Fabry disease. Proc. Natl. Acad. Sci. USA 94:2540–2544.

Pineau, T., Fernandez-Salguero, P., Lee, S.S.T., et al. 1995. Neonatal lethality associated with respiratory distress in mice lacking cytochrome P450 CYP1A2. Proc. Natl. Acad. Sci. USA 92:5134–5138.

Raben, N., Nagaraju, K., Lee, E., et al. 1998. Targeted disruption of the acid α~glucosidase gene in mice causes an illness with the critical features of both infantile and adult human Glycogen Storage Disease Type II. J. Biol. Chem. 273:19086–19092.

Roths, J.B., Foxworth, W.B., McArthur, M.J., et al. 1999. Spontaneous and engineered mutant mice as models for experimental and comparative pathology: history, comparison, and developmental technology. Lab. Anim. Sci. 49:12–34.

Ryffel, B. 1997. Impact of knockout mice in toxicology. Crit. Rev. Toxicol. 27:135–154.

Sundberg, J.P. and Boggess, B. 1999. Systematic approach to evaluation of mouse mutations. Boca Raton: CRC Press, p. 199.

Tardiff, R. D., Anver, M. R., Gusterson, B. A., et al. 2000. The mammary pathology of genetically engineered mice: The consensus report and recommendations from the Annapolis meeting. Oncogene 19:968–988. Classification of mouse mammary tumors. Oncogene.

Tullio, A.N., Accili, D., Ferrans, V.J., et al. 1997. Nonmuscle myosin II-B is required for normal development of the mouse heart. Proc. Natl. Acad. Sci. USA 94:12407–12412.

# 13
# Pathology of Mice Commonly Used in Genetic Engineering (C57BL/6; 129; B6,129; and FVB/N)

Jerrold M. Ward, Miriam R. Anver, Joel F. Mahler, and Deborah E. Devor-Henneman

Only a few mouse strains are currently used in the development of genetically engineered mice; these include the various sublines of the C57BL/6, 129, and FVB strains. Backcrosses of the resulting chimeric offspring to one or the other of the contributing strains (predominately C57BL/6 but occasionally 129) are then performed to "fix" the genetic background. Each of these inbred strains provides certain characteristics that have been found to be advantageous in individual aspects of transgenic and targeted mutation experiments. With refinement of the techniques themselves, there may eventually be a wider range of strains that can be used.

One of the basic requirements for genetic engineering, particularly targeted gene disruption or "knockout" techniques, is the establishment of embryonic stem (ES) cells, which, for practical reasons, are most frequently derived from 129 strain sublines. ES cell lines are more easily established from 129 sublines than from other strains investigated (Stevens 1973; Simpson et al. 1997; Festing 1996). ES cell clones positive for the desired mutation are microinjected into blastocysts, most commonly retrieved from C57BL/6 females.

C57BL/6 blastocysts appear to be particularly hardy and survive microinjection and reimplantation into receptive dams much better than those of other strains. In addition, females of both strains have a high response to superovulation (Silver 1995).

In creating transgenic animals, the direct inter- or intraspecific transfer of altered DNA requires a means of delivering the foreign DNA intracellularly. Development of transgenic mice usually involves the direct injection of DNA into the pronuclei of fertilized ova. The FVB is a desirable strain and the gold standard in this methodology because its characteristically large pronuclei provide a bigger target for microinjection. This is also a very fertile strain that produces many ova without chemical superovulation. In addition, survival of injected and reimplanted zygotes is high (Taketo et al. 1991).

All strains of mice have a spectrum of naturally occurring lesions that arise through the aging process. Offspring of crosses sometimes show intermediate phenotypes, but they may also demonstrate reduced, enhanced, or completely new phenotypes as a result of natural genomic segregation and spontaneous mutations (genetic drift). Therefore, the investigator using these strains should be aware of the basic characteristics of these mice and have access to relevant databases in order to separate natural from induced lesions. This chapter reviews some broad features of the aging pathology of the C57BL/6, the FVB/N, one 129 subline commonly used, and the B6 backcrosses. Many of the

The authors are grateful for the help of Drs. Jeffrey Peters, Frank Gonzalez, Shioko Kimura, Susan Perkins, and Diana Haines, as well as Christine Perella, Darlene Green, Kunio Nagashima, and Barbara Kasprzak. This project has been funded, in part, with federal funds from the National Cancer Institute, NIH, under contract no. NO1-CO-56000.

**TABLE 13.1.   Tumors in C57BL/6 mice**

| Tumor | C57BL/6N[a] (M/24 mo)[e] | C57BL/6J[b] (M/23 mo)[e] | C57BL/6J[b] (F/23 mo)[e] | C57BL/6[c] (M/25 mo)[e] | C57BL6[d] (M/>26 mo)[e] | C57BL6[d] (F/>26 mo)[e] |
|---|---|---|---|---|---|---|
| Histiocytic sarcoma | 3/36 (8.3) | 5/220 (2.3) | 12/220 (5.5) | NR | 29/50 (58) | 12/37 (32.4) |
| Lymphoma | 7/36 (19.4) | 45/220 (20.5) | 69/220 (31.3) | 14/72 (19.4) | 4/50 (8) | 10/37 (27) |
| Hemangioma/ hemangiosarcoma | NR | 6/220 (2.7) | 7/220 (3.2) | NR | 4/50 (8) | 0/37 (0) |
| Lung adenoma or carcinoma | 6/36 (17) | 13/214 (6.1) | 6/216 (2.8) | NR | 3/50 (6) | 1/37 (2.7) |
| Liver adenoma or carcinoma | 5/36 (13.9) | 10/215 (4.7) | 5/216 (2.3) | NR | 6/50 (12) | 1/37 (2.7) |
| Mammary carcinoma | NR | NR | 0/199 (0) | NR | NR | NR |
| Pituitary adenoma | 1/36 (2.8) | 1/154 (0.7) | 20/175 (11.4) | NR | 0/50 (0) | 21/37 (56.8) |
| Harderian Gl tumors | NR | 7/207 (3.4) | 10/205 (4.9) | NR | 4/50 (8) | 1/37 (2.7) |

Note: Figures represent number of mice with lesion/number of mice examined (percentage). NR = not reported or incomplete pathology protocols.

[a]Ward et al. 1975.

[b]Frith et al. 1983. Includes scheduled deaths at 12, 18, and 25 months of age, incidence at >500 days of age (in virgins).

[c]Volk et al. 1994. This source only reported lymphoma incidence.

[d]Blackwell et al. 1995.

[e]Sex/age. Age = allowed to live until this age or mean survival time.

lesions found are similar to those generated in other mouse lines (Frith and Ward 1988; Maronpot et al. 1999; Mohr et al. 1996; Smith et al. 1973; Turusov and Mohr 1994), but some appear to be unique to or are far more common in these strains or stocks.

# C57BL/6 (B6)

This substrain of the C57BL is generally considered to be the most commonly used in biomedical research in the United States today. Lyon et al. (1996) report that 14 percent of all known studies with an inbred mouse strain use the B6 strain. The excellent Jackson Laboratory informatics web site [*http://www.informatics.jax. org/external/festing/mouse/STRAINS.shtml*] provides considerable information on the B6 strain.

The reasons for the popularity of the B6 mouse outside of targeted mutation studies have not been specifically categorized. It is a relatively good breeder (there are substrain variabilities) and easy to handle, although a comparatively active mouse. It has an average longevity of 18–30 months under standard housing conditions (Pinkerton et al. 1996; Sheldon et al. 1996; Zurcher et al. 1982).

Until recently, there were few detailed studies on the naturally occurring lesions found in the strain. Tables 13.1 and 13.2 review by sex the tumor type and inci-

**TABLE 13.2.   Contributing causes of death of male and female C57BL/6 mice**

| Cause of death | Males | Females |
|---|---|---|
| Lymphoma/histiocytic sarcoma | 97/161 (60) | 67/117 (57) |
| Hemangioma/sarcoma | 8/161 (5) | 3/117 (3) |
| Liver tumor | 10/161 (6) | 2/117 (2) |
| Pituitary adenoma | 0/161 (0) | 10/117 (9) |
| Nephropathy | 10/161 (6) | 3/117 (3) |
| Heart thrombosis | 4/161 (3) | 3/117 (3) |
| Inflammation | 9/161 (6) | 6/117 (5) |
| Other causes | 7/161 (4) | 12/117 (10) |
| Unknown causes | 16/161 (10) | 11/117 (9) |

Source: Blackwell et al. 1995.

Note: Figures represent number of mice with lesion/number of mice examined (percentage).

dence, as well as the reported causes of death, in C57BL/6 mice from various sources (Blackwell et al. 1995; Frith et al. 1983; Volk et al. 1994; Ward et al. 1975). Overall, the B6 mouse has a low spontaneous liver and mammary tumor incidence; the primary neoplastic lesions noted are B cell lymphomas (follicular center cell type) and histiocytic sarcomas (Frith et al. 1983, 1996; Frith and Ward 1988; Maronpot et al. 1999). Histiocytic sarcomas are sometimes associated with hyaline droplet formation in the kidneys of various mouse strains, and hyaline droplets have been found in the kidneys of B6 and B6,129 mice with his-

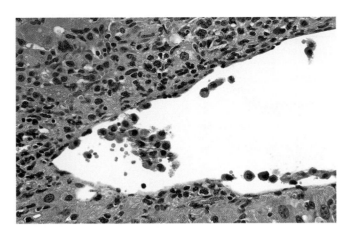

**FIGURE 13.1** Liver with histiocytic sarcoma invading vessel wall and adherent intravascular histiocytic sarcoma tumor cells.

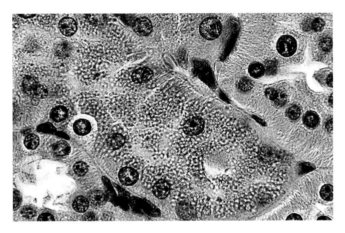

**FIGURE 13.2** Hyaline droplets in the renal tubules of a 129 mouse with histiocytic sarcoma. They represent lysozyme from the tumor cells.

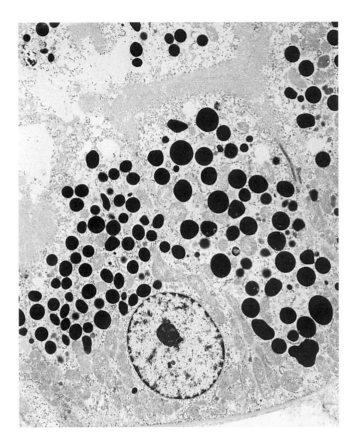

**FIGURE 13.3** Ultrastructure of renal hyaline droplets showing large electron-dense lysosomes.

## STRAIN 129

Several different sublines (substrains) of the 129 mouse have been used to generate various ES cell lines, and because each subline is different in its genetic makeup, particular attention must be paid as to the exact lineage of the ES cells utilized (Stevens 1973; Simpson et al. 1997). The nomenclature for delineating each of these sublines is under constant revision, and the reader is referred to the previously mentioned Jackson Laboratory informatics web site and to the technical notes of individual suppliers, as well as to the report by Threadgill et al. (1997).

The strain has a common origin with the 101 mouse, and the coat color varies by subline from albino to a yellow chinchilla dilute to common agouti. In 1948, three major sublines—129/Re, 129/RrJ, and 129/Sv-*ter*/+—were recognized (Lyon et al. 1996), from which at least a dozen new variants have been produced, frequently as a result of accidental genetic contamination with other strains (Threadgill et al. 1997; The Jackson Laboratory web page). There appears to be very little written on the aging lesions seen in any 129 subline, aside from the incidence of spontaneous teratomas that resulted in the development of the Sv-*ter*/+ lineage. This line is briefly

tiocytic sarcoma (Figs. 13.1–13.3; Hard and Snowden 1991). Glomerulonephritis is a common finding in the B6 mouse, although it is usually incidental (as a minimal, mild, or moderate lesion) and not a cause of death (Porter et al. 1973). Microphthalmia and anophthalmia are seen in 4 to 12 percent of C57BL/6 and C57BL/10 populations (Smith et al. 1994; Smith and Sundberg 1996), and the C57BL strain is also prone to an ulcerative dermatitis that occurs at an incidence as high as 21 percent (Sundberg et al. 1996). Another condition, and one that can be fatal, is mouse urologic syndrome (MUS); this is an obstructive urinary condition of no single definitive cause that crops up in many strains but is especially prevalent in B6C3F$_1$ and ICR mice (approximately 40 percent) (Bendele and Carlton 1998). Mouse urologic syndrome occurs, at a much lower rate, in the parental B6 and can be of either acute or chronic duration.

**TABLE 13.3.  Tumors in aging male and female 129S4/SvJae mice**

| Tissue/tumor | Male | Female | Tissue/tumor | Male | Female |
|---|---|---|---|---|---|
| Adrenal | | | Pancreas | | |
|   Adenoma, cortex | 1/37 (2.7) | 0/48 (0) |   Islet cell adenoma | 0/40 (0) | 1/47 (2.1) |
|   Pheochromocytoma | 4/37 (10.8) | 1/48 (2.1) | Parathyroid | | |
| Brain | 0/39 (0) | 0/47 (0) |   Adenoma | 0/26 (0) | 1/36 (2.8) |
| Epididymis | | | Skin | | |
|   Hemangiosarcoma, | 1/39 (2.6) | |   Hemangioma/sarcoma | 3/40 (7.5) | 0/47 (0) |
|     vas deferens | | |   Papilloma | 0/40 (0) | 1/47 (2.1) |
| Harderian gland | | | Small intestine | | |
|   Adenoma | 20/39 (51.3) | 14/48 (29.2) |   Adenoma | 0/38 (0) | 1/44 (2.3) |
|   Adenocarcinoma | 1/39 (2.6) | 0/48 (0) |   Adenocarcinoma | 1/38 (2.6) | 0/44 (0) |
| Hematopoietic neoplasm | | | Spleen | | |
|   Lymphoma | 1/40 (2.5) | 3/48 (6.3) |   Hemangiosarcoma | 3/39 (7.7) | 0/48 (0) |
|   Histiocytic sarcoma | 0/40 (0) | 2/48 (4.2) | Stomach, nonglandular | | |
| Kidney | | |   Papilloma | 0/39 (0) | 1/47 (2.1) |
|   Tubular adenoma | 1/39 (2.6) | 1/49 (2.2) |   Squamous cell carcinoma | 0/39 (0) | 1/47 (2.1) |
| Liver | | | Testis | | |
|   Adenoma | 6/40 (15) | 3/47 (6.4) |   Teratoma | 1/39 (2.6) | |
|   Hemangioma/sarcoma | 3/40 (7.5) | 1/47 (2.1) | Thyroid | | |
| Lung | | |   Adenoma, follicular cell | 0/40 (0) | 1/48 (2.1) |
|   Adenoma | 16/40 (40) | 12/48 (25) |   C cell carcinoma | 0/40 (0) | 1/48 (2.1) |
|   Carcinoma | 12/40 (30) | 4/48 (8.3) | Uterus | | |
|   Adenoma/carcinoma | 25/40 (62.5) | 15/48 (31.2) |   Hemangioma | | 1/47 (2.1) |
| Mammary | | |   Hemangiosarcoma | | 7/47 (14.9) |
|   Carcinoma | 0/40 (0) | 0/48 (0) |   Stromal polyp | | 4/47 (8.5) |
| Nasal cavity | | |   Stromal sarcoma | | 2/47 (4.3) |
|   Hemangioma | 1/39 (2.6) | 0/47 (0) | Total primary tumors | 78 | 84 |
|   Malignant schwannoma | 1/39 (2.6) | 0/47 (0) | Total animals | 36 | 39 |
| Ovary | | |   with tumors | | |
|   Adenoma | | 6/45 (13.3) | Total animals | 21 | 24 |
|   Granulosa cell tumor | | 5/45 (10.4) |   with multiple tumors | | |
|   Luteoma | | 1/45 (2.2) | Total benign | 54 | 59 |
|   Hemangiosarcoma | | 1/45 (2.2) | Total malignant | 24 | 25 |
|   Theca/sertoli cell tumor | | 1/45 (2.2) | Total malignant | 5 | 7 |
|   Any ovarian tumor | | 12/45 (26.7) |   with metastasis | | |

Note: Figures represent number of mice with lesion/number of mice examined for that tissue (percentage). Forty males and 48 females were maintained until 27 months of age, and all were necropsied.

reported to develop few tumors overall and to be resistant to viral mammary tumor formation (Festing 1996).

Most of our experience has been with a subline presumably originating from the 129/SvTer/+ line; this line was reported by Stevens (1973) to be particularly prone to development of testicular teratomas, but the incidence in our current study populations is much lower than the 30 percent Stevens reported. The animals, which we are referring to as 129/SvTer until the genetics are further analyzed, were produced from breeders kindly provided by Drs. Shioko Kimura, Jeffrey Peters, and Frank Gonzales via Dr. Heiner Westphal's laboratory at the National Institute of Child Health and Development (NICHD), National Institutes of Health (NIH), Bethesda, Maryland. Their origin was Rudolph Janesch's 129/SvTer mice (currently known as 129S4/SvJae mice). The mice produced are largely agouti in color. Mature

mice are fairly small; mature males weigh 30–32 g on average, with females being slightly lighter at 25–30 g. Although the colony was found to be infected with *Helicobacter hepaticus*, the mice were specific pathogen free by conventional pathogen monitoring, and this may have contributed, at least in part, to their relatively long life spans with a mean survival of 105 weeks for both sexes. Our aging study was terminated when surviving mice were 27 months old.

Tumor types and incidences for 40 male and 48 female 129/SvTer (also named 129/SvJae or 129S4/SvJae) mice maintained at the National Cancer Institute-Frederick Cancer Research and Development Center (NCI-FCRDC) for up to 27 months of age are categorized in Table 13.3 and Fig. 13.4. Mice were housed five per cage. As can be seen, the most common neoplasias encountered were Harderian gland adenomas, pulmonary

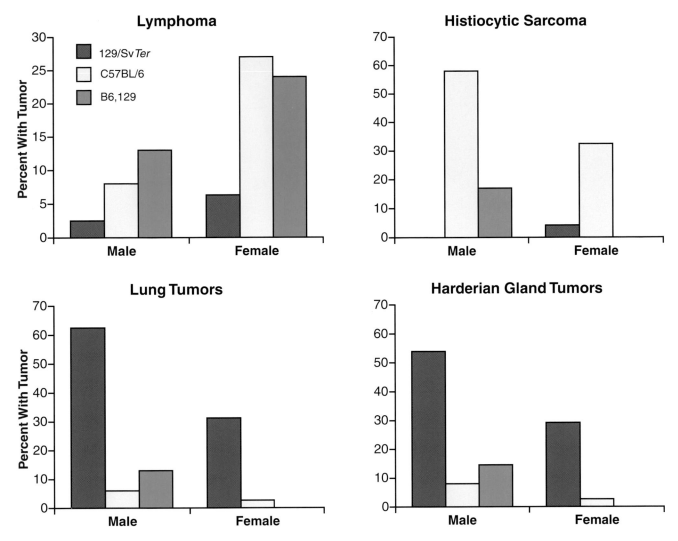

**FIGURE 13.4** Common tumor incidences in C57BL/6, 129, and B6,129 mice (129/Sv*Ter* mice are currently known as 129S4/SvJae mice).

adenomas, carcinomas, and various tumors of the uterus and ovaries (Figs. 13.5–13.8). Hemangiomas and hemangiosarcomas were observed in the uterus, ovary, spleen, liver, and nasal cavity (Figs. 13.7–13.10). In the population studied, few lymphomas or teratomas developed (Fig. 13.11), and no mammary tumors occurred.

Nonneoplastic lesions were commonly found in many tissues (Table 13.4). The most striking degenerative change seen in aging mice occurred in several epithelial tissues. Epithelial cells in the nasal cavity, trachea, lung, glandular stomach, gall bladder, bile ducts, and pancreatic ducts had hyalinized eosinophilic cytoplasmic droplets or inclusions. The incidence was particularly high (>20 percent) in the lung, nasal cavities, and stomach. These lesions have been found in nasal cavities of other strains of mice (Herbert and Leninger 1999; Leninger et al. 1996). Pulmonary macrophages, a

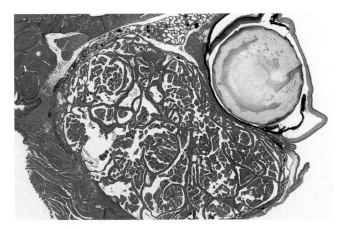

**FIGURE 13.5** Harderian gland papillary adenocarcinoma.

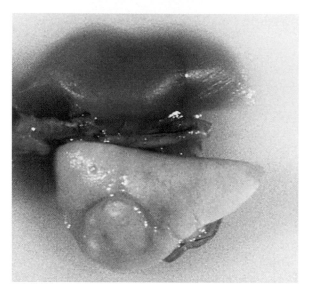

FIGURE 13.6 Grayish lung with acidophilic macrophage pneumonia and one round alveolar Type II cell adenoma.

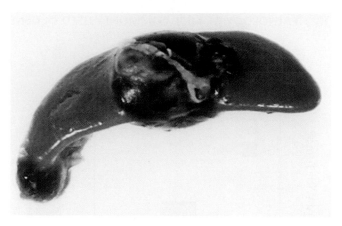

FIGURE 13.9 Spleen with hemorrhagic hemangioma.

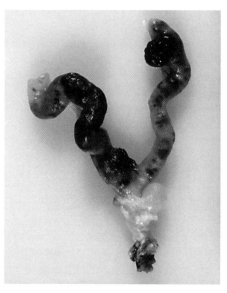

FIGURE 13.7 Hemorrhagic lesions in the uterus. The nodular lesion at the upper right is a hemangioma.

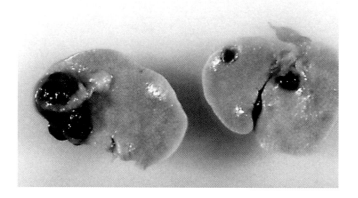

FIGURE 13.10 Multiple hemangiomas in the liver.

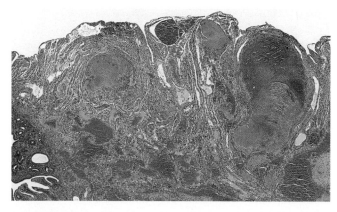

FIGURE 13.8 Hemangioma in the uterine serosa and tunica muscularis with thrombosis in some tumor vessels.

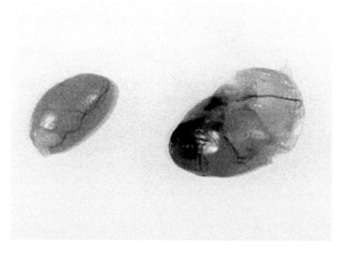

FIGURE 13.11 Testicular enlargement and hemorrhage in 129S4/SvJae mouse with a teratoma.

**TABLE 13.4.  Common nonneoplastic lesions in aging male and female 129S4/SvJae mice**

| Tissue/lesion | Male | Female |
|---|---|---|
| Adrenal | | |
|   Subcapsular cell hyperplasia | 0/37 (0) | 16/48 (33.3) |
|   Hyaline material, zona reticularis | 0/37 (0) | 12/48 (25) |
| Bone | | |
|   Hyperostosis, endosteal | 0/39 (0) | 18/46 (39.1) |
| Bone marrow | | |
|   Hyperplasia, granulocytic | 20/39 (51.3) | 25/46 (54.3) |
|   Myelofibrosis | 0/39 (0) | 18/46 (37) |
| Brain | | |
|   Melanosis, meninges | 9/39 (23.1) | 15/47 (31.9) |
| Epididymis | | |
|   Degeneration | 18/39 (46.2) | |
|   Hypospermia | 18/39 (46.2) | |
|   Inflammation, granulomatous | 12/39 (30.8) | |
| Esophagus | | |
|   Dilatation, lumen | 11/40 (27.5) | 16/48 (33.3) |
|   Foreign material, lumen | 9/40 (22.5) | 13/48 (27.1) |
| Eye | | |
|   Cataract | 5/38 (13.2) | 6/47 (12.8) |
| Gall Bladder | | |
|   Eosinophilic cytoplasmic inclusion bodies, epithelium | 1/38 (2.6) | 5/45 (11.1) |
|   Inflammation (acute, subacute, chronic active) | 7/38 (18.4) | 15/45 (33.3) |
| Harderian gland | | |
|   Hyperplasia, epithelial | 12/39 (30.8) | 6/48 (12.5) |
|   Acinar ectasia | 17/39 (43.6) | 21/48 (43.8) |
|   Lymphocytic infiltrate | 6/39 (15.4) | 26/48 (54.2) |
| Heart | | |
|   Chronic cardiomyopathy | 30/40 (75) | 19/48 (39.6) |
|   Arteritis | 14/40 (35) | 3/48 (6.3) |
|   Mineralization | 5/40 (12.5) | 16/48 (33.3) |
| Kidney | | |
|   Chronic nephropathy | 37/39 (94.9) | 38/47 (80.9) |
|   Mineralization | 38/39 (97.4) | 36/47 (76.6) |
|   Lymphocytic infiltrate | 21/39 (53.8) | 13/47 (27.7) |
|   Cortical tubule vacuolation | 11/39 (28.2) | 2/47 (4.3) |
| Liver | | |
|   Vacuolation, hepatocellular | 7/40 (17.5) | 15/47 (31.9) |
|   Angiectasis | 4/40 (10) | 6/47 (12.8) |
|   Bile duct(ule), inflammation, chronic | 7/40 (17.5) | 18/47 (38.3) |
|   Bile duct(ule), eosinophilic cytoplasmic inclusion bodies, epithelium | 2/40 (5) | 6/47 (12.8) |
|   Bile duct, mucinous metaplasia | 0/40 (0) | 4/47 (8.5) |
|   Inflammation, subacute | 13/40 (32.5) | 17/47 (36.2) |
|   Extramedullary hematopoiesis | 1/40 (2.5) | 26/47 (55.3) |
| Lung | | |
|   Acidophilic macrophage pneumonia | 27/40 (67.5) | 42/48 (87.5) |
|   Eosinophilic crystals | 21/40 (52.5) | 42/48 (87.5) |
|   Bronchi(ole) epithelium, eosinophilic cytoplasmic inclusion bodies | 5/40 (12.5) | 9/48 (18.8) |
|   Mineralization | 8/40 (20) | 12/48 (25) |
| Mammary gland | | |
|   Cystic dilatation, duct | | 14/48 (29.2) |
| Nasal tissues | | |
|   Eosinophilic cytoplasmic inclusion bodies, respiratory epithelium | 12/39 (30.8) | 36/47 (76.6) |
|   Eosinophilic cytoplasmic inclusion bodies, olfactory epithelium | 2/39 (5.1) | 9/47 (19.1) |
|   Inflammation (acute/subacute) | 8/39 (20.5) | 8/47 (17) |
| Ovary | | |
|   Atrophy | | 36/45 (80) |
|   Hyaline material | | 25/45 (55.6) |
|   Pigment | | 23/45 (51.5) |
|   Cyst | | 19/45 (42.2) |
|   Hemorrhagic follicle | | 4/45 (8.9) |
|   Hematocyst | | 7/45 (15.6) |
|   Angiectasis | | 2/45 (4.4) |

*(continued)*

**TABLE 13.4.  Continued**

| Tissue/lesion | Male | Female |
|---|---|---|
| Ovary (continued) | | |
|   Hyperplasia, tubular | | 13/45 (28.9) |
|   Hyperplasia, stromal | | 11/45 (24.4) |
|   Mineralization | | 4/45 (8.9) |
|   Abscess | | 1/45 (2.2) |
|   Lymphocytic infiltrate, periovarian fat | | 4/45 (8.9) |
| Pancreas | | |
|   Islet cell, hyperplasia | 18/39 (46.2) | 13/47 (27.7) |
| Parathyroid | | |
|   Melanin | 2/26 (7.7) | 12/36 (33.3) |
| Pituitary | | |
|   Hyperplasia, diffuse, pars intermedia | 17/34 (50) | 29/41 (70.7) |
|   Hyperplasia, focal, pars distalis | 1/34 (2.9) | 2/41 (4.9) |
| Prostate | | |
|   Hyperplasia, epithelial atypical, dorsolateral | 11/38 (28.9) | |
| Salivary gland | | |
|   Lymphocytic infiltrate | 17/40 (42.5) | 27/48 (56.3) |
| Spleen | | |
|   Hyperplasia, marginal zone | 6/39 (15.4) | 6/48 (12.5) |
|   Increased extramedullary hematopoiesis | 12/39 (30.8) | 32/48 (66.7) |
|   Arteritis | 19/39 (48.7) | 1/48 (2.1) |
| Stomach, glandular | | |
|   Hyperplasia, epithelial | 12/39 (30.8) | 22/46 (47.8) |
|   Eosinophilic cytoplasmic inclusion bodies, epithelium | 8/39 (20.5) | 21/46 (45.7) |
|   Eosinophilic crystals | 3/39 (7.7) | 7/46 (15.2) |
|   Dilated/cystic glands | 19/39 (48.7) | 12/46 (26) |
|   Gland, subserosal | 2/39 (5.1) | 2/46 (4.3) |
|   Gland, submucosal | 6/39 (15.4) | 1/46 (2.2) |
|   Gland, muscularis | 1/39 (2.6) | 0/46 (0) |
|   Inflammation | 11/39 (28.5) | 17/46 (40) |
| Stomach, nonglandular | | |
|   Hyperplasia | 13/39 (33.3) | 21/47 (44.7) |
|   Hyperkeratosis | 9/39 (23.1) | 23/47 (48.9) |
| Teeth | | |
|   Dental dysplasia, incisor | 19/39 (48.7) | 9/47 (19.1) |
| Testis | | |
|   Degeneration, tubular | 25/39 (64.1) | 8/47 (17) |
|   Mineralization | 22/39 (56.4) | |
| Thymus | | |
|   Atrophy, cortex | 21/34 (61.8) | 38/46 (82.6) |
|   Atrophy | 13/34 (38.2) | 3/46 (6.5) |
|   Hyperplasia, medulla | 2/34 (5.9) | 14/46 (30.4) |
| Thyroid | | |
|   Follicular dilatation | 9/40 (22.5) | 20/48 (41.7) |
|   C cell hyperplasia | 5/40 (12.5) | 8/48 (16.7) |
|   Arteritis | 3/40 (7.5) | 1/48 (2.1) |
|   Lymphocytic infiltrate | 5/40 (13.5) | 14/48 (29.2) |
| Trachea | | |
|   Concretion, gland | 22/37 (59.5) | 19/47 (40.4) |
|   Eosinophilic cytoplasmic inclusion bodies, epithelium | 7/37 (18.9) | 12/47 (25.5) |
|   Eosinophilic crystals, gland | 1/37 (2.7) | 9/47 (19.1) |
|   Lymphocytic infiltrate | 5/37 (13.5) | 14/47 (29.8) |
| Urinary bladder | | |
|   Lymphocytic infiltrate | 3/37 (8.1) | 29/46 (63) |
|   Arteritis | 12/37 (32.4) | 3/46 (6.5) |
| Uterus | | |
|   Cystic endometrial hyperplasia | | 28/47 (59.6) |
|   Angiectasis/angiopathy | | 22/47 (46.8) |
| Vertebra | | |
|   Hyperostosis, endosteal | 0/40 (0) | 15/48 (31.3) |
|   Myelofibrosis | 3/40 (7.5) | 12/48 (25) |

Note: Figures represent number of mice with lesion/number of mice examined (percentage). Forty males and 48 females were maintained until 27 months of age, and all were necropsied.

component of acidophilic macrophage pneumonia in our 129S4/SvJae mice, frequently contained intracellular crystals and extracellular crystals (Figs. 13.12-13.14). The macrophage pneumonia (Figs. 13.6, 13.12, 13.13) was frequently severe enough to produce clinical illness and was fatal in some cases. The pulmonary macrophages were found to contain iron, and in this respect, the lesions produced resemble those reported in the motheaten mouse (Green and Shultz 1975; Thrall et al. 1997; Ward 1978) and other mice and are sometimes associated with lung tumors (Ernst et al. 1996). In motheaten mice, the macrophage lesion is apparently induced by a deficiency of SHP-1, a protein tyrosine phosphatase (Khaled et al. 1998). Gall bladders with eosinophilic inclusions were often enlarged with thickened opaque walls (Figs. 13.15, 13.16). Lesions in the bile ducts were associated with mucoid metaplasia and fibrosis (Figs. 13.17, 13.18).

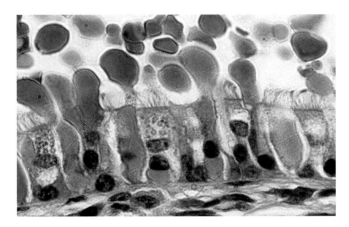

FIGURE 13.14   Respiratory nasal epithelium showing eosinophilic cytoplasm and extracellular protein droplets.

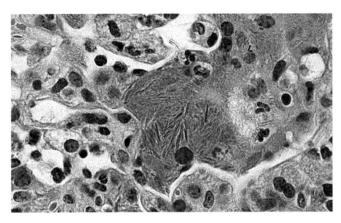

FIGURE 13.12   Prominent cytoplasmic needlelike crystals can be seen in acidophilic pulmonary macrophages in macrophage pneumonia of a 129S4/SvJae mouse.

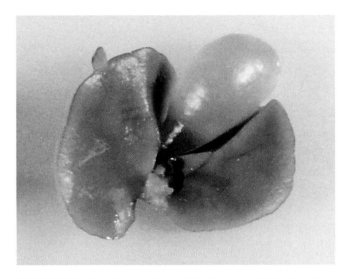

FIGURE 13.15   Enlarged and thickened gall bladder in a 129S4/SvJae mouse. Chronic inflammation, hyperplasia, and eosinophilic inclusions are often present.

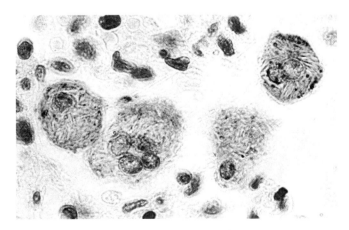

FIGURE 13.13   Acidophilic macrophage pneumonia showing iron and crystals in the pulmonary macrophages. Iron stain.

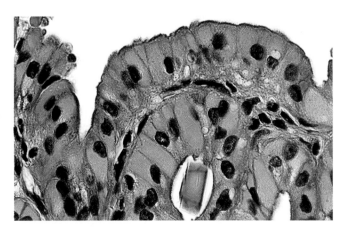

FIGURE 13.16   Eosinophilic hyaline cytoplasm and one large extracellular crystal in a gall bladder.

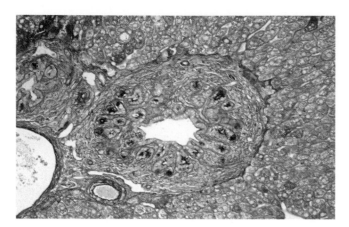

**FIGURE 13.17** Mucus in bile duct epithelium in chronic cholangitis. Alcian blue.

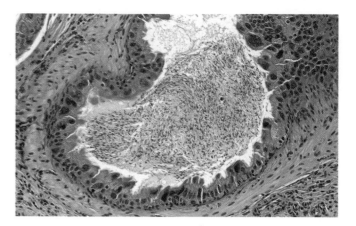

**FIGURE 13.19** Cytomegaly and karyomegaly of epididymal epithelium.

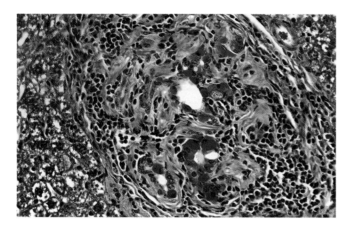

**FIGURE 13.18** Masson's trichrome stain showing much collagen in chronic cholangitis.

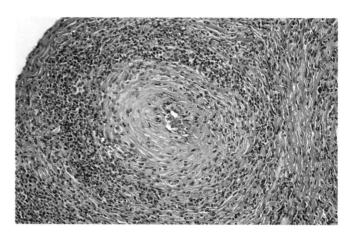

**FIGURE 13.20** Arteritis of lumbar vessel in 129S4/SvJae mouse.

A high frequency of inflammatory lesions, especially lymphocytic foci, were detected in a wide variety of tissues, including the Harderian glands, nasal cavity, salivary glands, trachea, gall bladder, portal areas of the liver, glandular stomach, thyroid, kidney, and urinary bladder. Many male mice had karyomegaly of the epididymal epithelium (Fig. 13.19).

The 129S4/SvJae line also develops aging lesions common to other strains of mice (Table 13.4), including degenerative adrenal lesions, fibrous bone lesions (especially in females), melanosis of meninges and spleen, Harderian gland ectasia, cardiomyopathy, nephropathy, ovarian atrophy, pancreatic islet cell and pituitary hyperplasias, dental dysplasia (Losco 1995), testicular degeneration, uterine angiectasis, and widespread arteritis (Figs. 13.20, 13.21).

Although many of the above lesions were incidental findings, some individual lesions, as well as combinations of lesions, created clinical conditions that justified euthanasia (Table 13.5). The contributing causes of ter-

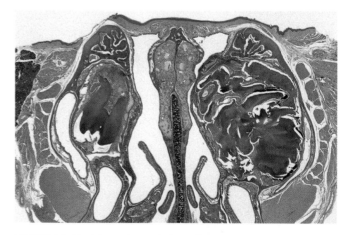

**FIGURE 13.21** Bilateral dental dysplasia.

minal illness and death in the 129S4/SvJae mouse were estimated by gross and histopathological analyses (Table 13.5) based on mortality estimates and severity criteria (Kodell et al. 1995; Hursting et al. 1997). The most common proximal causes of death appeared to be

**TABLE 13.5.  Contributing causes of death of male and female 129S4/SvJae mice**

| Diagnosis | Male | Female |
|---|---|---|
| Pulmonary alveolar carcinoma | 6/40 (15) | 2/48 (4.2) |
| Impaction of esophagus/megaesophagus | 3/40 (7.5) | 7/48 (14.6) |
| Acidophilic macrophage pneumonia | 4/40 (10) | 5/48 (10.4) |
| Abscess, preputial gland/clitoral gland | 4/40 (10) | 0/48 (0) |
| Uterine hemangiosarcoma/hemangioma | | 4/48 (8.3) |
| Uterine hematoma/thrombus | | 4/48 (8.3) |
| Harderian gland adenoma | 3/40 (7.5) | 0/48 (0) |
| Arteritis | 3/40 (7.5) | 0/48 (0) |
| Other uterine neoplasms | | 3/48 (6.3) |
| Mouse urinary syndrome | 2/40 (5) | |
| Other neoplasms | 4/40 (10) | 8/48 (16.7) |
| Indeterminate causes | 4/40 (10) | 4/48 (8.3) |
| Terminal sacrifice, no life-threatening lesions | 3/40 (7.5) | 3/48 (6.3) |

Note: Figures represent number of mice with lesion/number of mice examined (percentage). Forty males and 48 females were maintained until 27 months of age, and all were necropsied.

lung tumors, complications from megaesophagus, and acidophilic macrophage pneumonia. Less frequent mortal lesions included vascular and Harderian gland tumors.

# C57BL/6 BACKCROSS (B6,129)

As stated in the introduction of this chapter, backcrossing of mutant chimeras to one or both of the "parental" strains serves to fix the mutant phenotype on a specific background such that the effects of the targeted mutation can be distinguished from the natural strain phenotype. In addition to choosing the most appropriate ES cell line, backcrossing can be a problem for individuals not well versed in mouse genetics. In the vast majority of cases, the chimeric founder is backcrossed to the B6 line to isolate the ES cell contribution, as most ES cell lines are derived from a 129 subline. However, the investigator cannot consider the resulting hybrid populations to be genetically either B6 or 129. In the case of spontaneous mutations with conventional mouse lines, brother × sister mating subsequent to a number of backcrosses to the parental strain creates a coisogenic line, and the resulting phenotype could be significantly different from either B6 or 129.

The exact genetic contribution of B6 and 129 to the offspring of their chimeras depends on factors that are not completely understood and involve far more than the targeted alteration of one gene (Silver 1995). Donehower et al. (1995) estimated their backcrosses to B6 at least two to four generations to be ~75 percent B6 and ~25 percent 129, but without allelic analysis and a foolproof breeding regime, this should not be taken as a rule. If the situation is reversed, such that it is desired to backcross to 129, it not unreasonable to expect major phenotypic differences, given the emerging information on imprinting. The investigator has only to search the literature to find numerous instances where targeted mutations behave very disparately based on the background genotypes (see Chap. 10).

To our knowledge, the genetics of the more common B6,129 backcross has not been consistently determined to any reliable degree. It might prove to be a very frustrating task due to the numbers of laboratories using the animal and the variability in breeding and record-keeping practices. However, since the number of B6,129 mice increases with each targeted mutation study done, the International Committee on Standardized Genetic Nomenclature for Mice [*http://jaxmice.jax.org/html/nomenclature/nomen_memo.shtml*] has approved the terminology as B6,129.

The advantages of using this backcross versus continual backcrossing in targeted mutant experiments is discussed in detail by Doetschman (1999). In reviewing published data on the pathology of the B6,129 mouse, however, it became apparent that there is a paucity of information about this cross. B6,129s are large mice: males weigh 40–45 g and females 35–40 g at maturity (Hursting et al. 1997). The survival of our studied population was better than the mean of 15.6 months reported by Hursting et al. (1997). In our current aging study of B6,129 mice, more than 80 percent of males and females have survived past 18 months of age. While most mice were either black or agouti, an occasional albino and dilute agouti or brown variant was produced. Mouse litter sizes were moderate to small.

In their relatively limited and low-tumor spectrum, these mice resembled the C57BL/6 more so than strain 129 (Tables 13.6–13.8)(Donehower et al. 1995; Hursting

**TABLE 13.6. Tumors in B6,129 (C57BL/6 × 129) mice**

| Tumor | Donehower et al. 1995[a] (M + F/20+ mo)[b] | McClatchey et al. 1998 (M/21–24 mo)[b] | McClatchey et al. 1998 (F/21–24 mo)[b] | Hursting et al. 1997 (M/24+ mo)[b] | Ward et al. 1999[a] (M/19–31 mo)[b] | Ward et al. 1999[a] (F/19–31 mo)[b] |
|---|---|---|---|---|---|---|
| Lymphoma | 5/11 (56) | 0/11 | 7/12 (58) | 4/30 (13) | 6/41 (15) | 5/21 (24) |
| Histiocytic sarcoma | NR | NR | NR | 5/30 (17) | 0 | 0 |
| Sarcoma | 1/11 (9) | 2/11 (18) | 0/12 (0) | 2/30 7) | 0 | 0 |
| Spleen hemangioma | NR | NR | NR | 0/30 | 2/41 (5) | 1/21 (5) |
| Pulmonary | | | | | | |
|   Adenoma | NR | NR | NR | 1/29 (3) | 5/41 (12) | 0/21 (0) |
|   Carcinoma | 1/11 (9) | 5/11 (46) | 5/12 (42) | 3/29 (10) | 1/41 (2) | 0/21 (0) |
| Hepatic | | | | | | |
|   Adenoma | NR | 2/11 (18) | 1/12 (8) | 6/30 (20) | 3/41 (7) | 1/21 (5) |
|   Carcinoma | NR | 0/11 (0) | 1/12 (8) | 6/30 (20) | 0/41 (0) | 0/21 (0) |
|   Hepatoblastoma | NR | NR | NR | 5/30 (17) | 0/41 (0) | 0/21 (0) |
|   Hemangioma/sarcoma | NR | NR | NR | 4/30 (13) | 3/41 (7) | 2/21 (10) |
| Spleen hemangioma | NR | NR | NR | 0/30 (0) | 2/41 (5) | 1/21 (5) |
| Mammary carcinoma | NR | NR | NR | 0/30(0) | 0/41 (0) | 1/21 (5) |
| Pituitary adenoma | NR | NR | NR | 0/30 (0) | 0/41 (0) | 2/21 (10) |
| Harderian gland | NR | NR | NR | NR | 6/41 (14.6) | 0/21 (0) |
| Brain | NR | NR | NR | 2/30 (7) | 0 | 0 |

Note: Figures represent number of mice with lesion/number of mice examined (percentage). NR = not reported or due to incomplete pathology protocols; it is not known if the mice actually developed these tumors.
[a]Groups described in these sources may not have included mice that died during aging.
[b]Sex/age. Age = allowed to live until this age or mean survival time.

**TABLE 13.7. Common nonneoplastic lesions in aging B6,129 (C57BL/6 × 129) mice**

| Tissue/lesion | Haines and Perkins[a] (M)[c] | Ward[b] (M)[c] | Ward[b] (F)[c] |
|---|---|---|---|
| Lung | | | |
|   Lymphocyte cuffs | 9/30 (31) | 5/41 | 4/21 |
|   Macrophage pneumonia | 1/30 (3) | 0/41 | 0/21 |
| Spleen, marginal zone hyperplasia | | 4/41 | 1/41 |
| Spleen | | | |
|   Hematopoiesis, increased | 19/30 (66) | | 9/21 |
| Stomach, glandular | | | |
|   Eosinophilic plaque | 1/30 (4) | | 0/21 |
| Liver | | | |
|   Hematopoiesis | 16/30 (53) | | |
| Gall bladder | | | |
|   Inflammation | 2/29 (10) | | |
| Pancreas | | | |
|   Islet cell hyperplasia | 7/30 (23) | | |
| Adrenal cortex | | | |
|   Hyperplasia | 8/30 (30) | | |
| Testis | | | |
|   Atrophy | 3/29 (10) | | |
| Epididymis | | | |
|   Karyomegaly | 8/26 (31) | | |
| Prostate | | | |
|   Inflammation | 5/25 (20) | | |
|   Arteritis | 1/25 (4) | | |
| Kidney | | | |
|   Glomerulonephritis | 9/27 (33) | | 11/21 |
|   Nephropathy | 6/27 (22) | | 1/21 |

Note: Figures represent the number of mice with lesion/number of mice examined (percentage). Mice were up to 24-34 months of age.
[a]D.C. Haines and S.N. Perkins, unpublished (from study in Hursting et al. 1997).
[b]J.M. Ward, unpublished.
[c]Sex.

**TABLE 13.8.  Contributing causes of death in male B6,129 (C57BL/6 × 129) mice**

| | |
|---|---|
| Infection | 7/30 (23) |
| Undetermined | 5/30 (17) |
| Histiocytic sarcoma | 4/30 (13) |
| Hemangiosarcoma | 3/30 (10) |
| Hepatoblastoma | 3/30 (10) |
| Other liver tumors | 2/30 (6) |
| Lymphoma | 1/30 (3) |
| Osteosarcoma | 1/30 (3) |
| Astrocytoma | 1/30 (3) |
| Lung carcinoma | 1/30 (3) |

Source: D.C. Haines and S.N. Perkins, unpublished (from study in Hursting et al. 1997).

Note: Figures represent number of mice with lesion/number of mice examined (percentage).

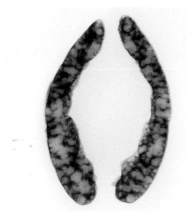

**FIGURE 13.23**  B6,129 mouse with follicular center cell lymphoma showing large white pulp areas in the spleen.

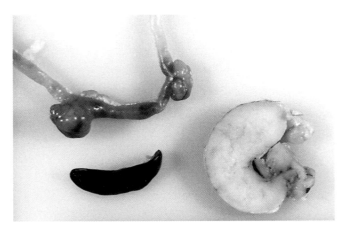

**FIGURE 13.22**  Follicular center cell (B cell) lymphoma showing large Peyer's patches in small intestine, enlarged mesenteric lymph node, and slightly enlarged spleen. B6,129 mouse.

et al. 1997; McClatchey et al. 1998; Perkins et al. 1998; J.M. Ward et al. unpublished). Lymphomas were a common finding through various studies, but histiocytic sarcoma was rare, in contrast to the B6 mouse. The typical B cell lymphomas usually arose in the spleen, mesenteric nodes, or intestinal Peyer's patches (Figs. 13.22, 13.23) and expressed high levels of CD45R, a B lymphocyte marker (Fig. 13.24). (See Chap. 24 for more information.) When reviewing the histology of one earlier aging study (Hursting et al. 1997), however, we recently identified low incidences (<5 percent) of splenic marginal zone lymphoma (MZL) in B6,129 mice. Marginal zone lymphoma is a newly described lymphoma commonly seen in *p53*-null mice on the B6,129 background (Ward et al. 1999). In our own aging study of B6,129 mice, we have since found splenic marginal zone hyperplasia, which may be a possible preneoplastic precursor to MZL, in

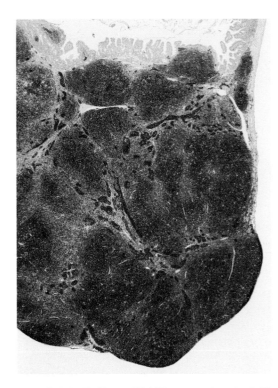

**FIGURE 13.24**  Diffuse CD45R expression in follicular lymphoma arising in Peyer's patch of small intestine in a B6,129 mouse. ABC immunohistochemistry, hematoxylin.

approximately 10 percent (4/41) of male and 2 percent (1/41) of female B6,129 mice in one study (Figs. 13.25, 13.26).

Other less common neoplasias found in B6,129 mice included liver tumors of various phenotypes and pituitary tumors (Table 13.6). The pituitary tumors

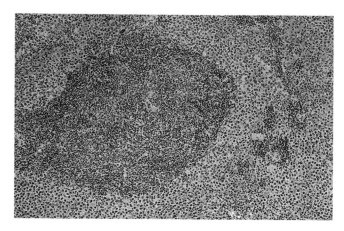

**FIGURE 13.25** Marginal zone lymphoma in a B6,129 mouse. Note expanded marginal zone composed of pale cells.

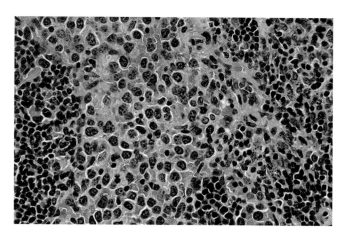

**FIGURE 13.26** Marginal zone lymphoma showing large monocytoid cells with pale eosinophilic cytoplasm.

expressed adrenocorticotropic hormone (ACTH) and, thus, were likely to have arisen from the pars intermedia (Figs. 13.27, 13.28).

Nonneoplastic lesions in the B6,129 line have not been extensively studied (Table 13.7). Similar to the B6 mouse, glomerulonephritis is common in the hybrid, in up to 33 percent of the examined animals in limited reports. Gastric plaques, common in 129 mice and a line of targeted mutant mice (B6,129/Sv-*Cyp1A2*[tm1Gonz]) (see Chap. 19), are rare in B6,129 mice (Figs. 13.29, 13.30). The significance of the increased splenic and hepatic hematopoiesis seen in at least one study (Table 13.7, D.C. Haines and S.N. Perkins, unpublished) remains to be explained. Accompanying this common aging lesion, we find splenic plasmacytosis (Fig. 13.31, 13.32).

Contributing causes of death from one study are compiled in Table 13.8. While tumors accounted for

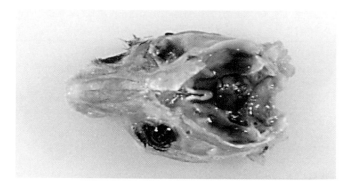

**FIGURE 13.27** Pituitary adenoma appears as a dark mass at the base of the skull.

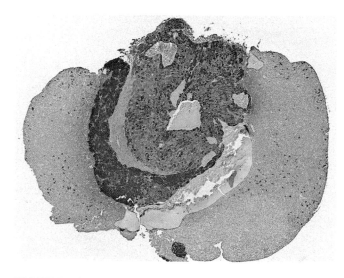

**FIGURE 13.28** ACTH in pituitary adenoma (pale brown mass in upper center of figure) arising from the pars intermedia. Note ACTH also within many cells in the normal pars intermedia (brown band at left side) and scattered cells in the pars distalis. ABC immunohistochemistry, hematoxylin.

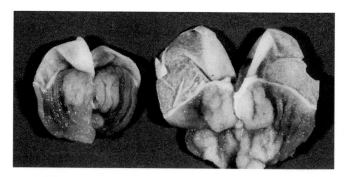

**FIGURE 13.29** Glandular stomach plaques in two B6,129 mice. Note some lesions at junction of forestomach and others in pylorus.

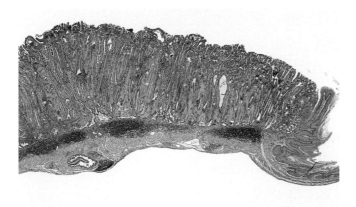

**FIGURE 13.30** Glandular stomach plaque showing diffuse epithelial hyperplasia, accompanied by chronic inflammation and glandular structures in the muscularis (lower left side of tissue) (epithelial herniation/diverticula).

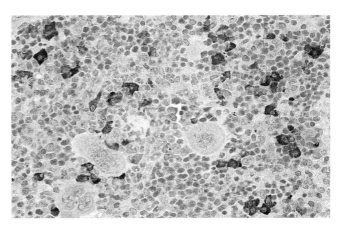

**FIGURE 13.32** Plasma cells among myeloid hyperplasia in red pulp of spleen. ABC immunohistochemistry for human κ light chains, hematoxylin.

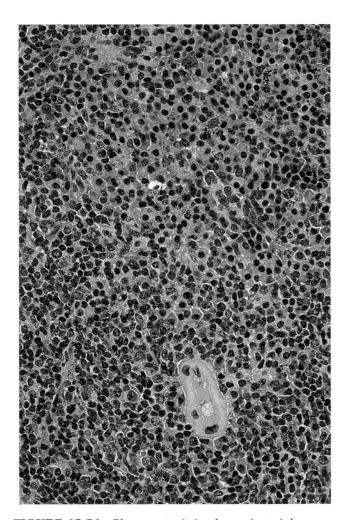

**FIGURE 13.31** Plasmacytosis in the periarteriolar lymphoid sheath (PALS) and B cell zone (upper portion of figure) in aged B6,129 mouse.

many deaths, the largest numbers of animals succumbed to infections (inflammatory lesions) of undetermined etiologies or to death due to other undetermined causes.

## FVB/N

The FVB strain is derived from the outbred NIH general purpose Swiss mouse (N:GP) established there in 1935. It was inbred further from a histamine-sensitive HFSF/N subline for homozygosity at the *Fv1^b* allele, which conferred susceptibility to the B-tropic variant of the Friend leukemia virus (Festing 1996). Today, it is widely used in the production of transgenic mice because of the characteristics listed in the introduction to the chapter (Taketo et al. 1991). Despite its extensive use in this subspecialty, the strain actually has not been well characterized as a laboratory animal, which is a little surprising given the fact that it is used to produce so many transgenic offspring whose mutational effects must be separated from endogenous traits. Hennings et al. (1993) have documented the sensitivity of FVB mice to chemically induced skin carcinogenesis.

FVBs are medium-to-large-sized albinos (adult males frequently reach 32–40 g, females 28–33 g, but both sexes have a tendency to obesity on ad libitum feeding). They resemble the SENCAR or CD-1 strain in appearance and temperament unless they are afflicted with an idiosyncratic neurobehavioral disorder, which is briefly described later in this section. The median life span appears to be greater than 24 months (D.E. Devor-Henneman, personal observations; Mahler et al. 1996). They are normally easy breeders and good parents,

**TABLE 13.9.  Tumors in FVB/N mice**

| Tumor | 14 mo of age | | 24 mo of age | |
|---|---|---|---|---|
| | Males | Females | Males | Females |
| Lung AB adenoma | 3/45 (7) | 9/98 (9) | 4/29 (14) | 11/71 (15) |
| Lung AB carcinoma | 3/45 (7) | 5/98 (5) | 4/29 (14) | 13/71 (18) |
| Lung AB Ad or Ca | 0 | 0 | 4/29 (14) | 2/71 (3) |
| Total Lung AB tumors | 6/45 (13) | 14/98 (14) | 12/29 (41) | 26/71 (37) |
| Hepatocellular adenoma | 0 | 0 | 2/29 (7) | 0 |
| Hepatocellular carcinoma | 0 | 0 | 1/29 (3) | 0 |
| Hepatocellular Ad or Ca | 0 | 0 | 3/29 (10) | 0 |
| Total hepatocellular tumors | 0 | 0 | 6/29 (21) | 0 |
| Malignant lymphoma | 0 | 0 | 0 | 4/71 (6) |
| Histiocytic sarcoma | 0 | 1/98 (1) | 0 | 4/71 (6) |
| Ovarian tumors (combined) | | 2/98 (2) | | 5/71 (7) |
| Pituitary, pars distalis, adenoma | 0 | 5/98 (5) | 0 | 10/71 (14) |
| Adrenal pheochromocytoma | 0 | 0 | 1/29 (4) | 4/71 (6) |
| Subcutis neural crest tumor | 0 | 1/98 (1) | 3/29 (10) | 2/71 (3) |
| Harderian gland adenoma | 0 | 0 | 2/29 (7) | 4/71 (6) |

Source: Adapted from Mahler et al. 1996.

Note: Figures represent number of mice with lesion/number of mice examined (percentage). The 24-month study used FVB/NTac mice, and the 14-month study used FVB/NHsd mice. Tumors occur with greater than 5 percent incidence. AB = alveolar/bronchiolar; Ad = adenoma; Ca = carcinoma.

commonly producing an average of four to six large litters of 8–12 or more pups with excellent survival during their reproductive prime (D.E. Devor-Henneman, personal observations; Silver 1995).

Few papers report spontaneous tumors or lesions in FVB/N mice. Table 13.9 depicts the tumor type and incidence by gender at 14 and 24 months of age from a study by Mahler et al. (1996). The most frequent neoplasm encountered at both time points proved to be pulmonary (alveolar/bronchiolar, alveolar Type II cell) adenomas and carcinomas. Tumor biology and morphology were typical of those found in other mouse strains. The FVB developed several other tumors commonly found in mice in general, including hepatocellular neoplasms, lymphomas and histiocytic sarcomas, prolactin-secreting adenomas of the pituitary pars distalis, and Harderian gland adenomas. A variety of ovarian tumors, including teratoma, granulosa cell tumor, cystadenoma, and Sertoli cell tumors, were observed in the 24-month-old females, and the relatively rare adrenal pheochromocytoma was found in 5 percent of both sexes at 24 months. One unusual tumor characterized in the strain was a subcutis neoplasm, made up of spindle cells arranged in a neural pattern, that showed a site predilection for the pinna and tail. The tumor is diagnosed of neural crest–origin (Mahler et al. 1996), and its occurrence contrasts with the more random distribution of subcutis tumors of various histologic types in other mouse strains.

Nonneoplastic degenerative changes seen in the FVB/N mouse include ovarian atrophy and seminiferous tubule degeneration, inflammatory mononuclear infiltrates in various tissues, and chronic nephropathy (Mahler et al. 1996; D.E. Devor-Henneman and J.M. Ward, unpublished). Peculiar degenerative changes occurring in the adrenal glands demonstrate a sexual dichotomy in phenotype. The adrenal of 24-month-old females showed varying degrees of corticomedullary foamy lipofuscin-laden cells; subcapsular cell hyperplasia was also a concurrent finding in most of these females. The adrenals of age-matched males, in contrast, were small with irregular capsular surfaces caused by cortical atrophy and nodules of compensatory hypertrophy and hyperplasia. Another unusual nonneoplastic lesion of older female mice consisted of focal accumulations of atypical histiocytes in the endometrium, a possible precursor lesion to uterine histiocytic sarcoma. In addition, the presence of the retinal degeneration gene, *rd1*, which predisposes to early apoptotic death of rod and cone photoreceptor cells, has been reported to be widespread in FVB mice (Smith and Sundberg 1996) and probably accounts for the retinal degeneration seen in the strain (Figs. 13.33, 13.34).

Recently, a neuropathological condition has been reported by several investigators (Hsiao et al. 1995; Goelz et al. 1998) in the FVB/NCr subline and in lines derived from NCr stock, encompassing sudden death and various CNS lesions. It appears that this might have

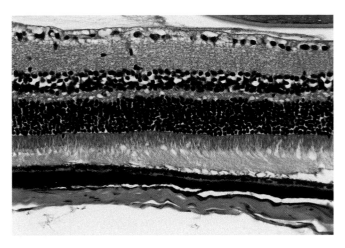

**FIGURE 13.33** Eye of normal 15-month-old B6,129 mouse showing pigmented retina and all normal layers including the outer nuclear layer.

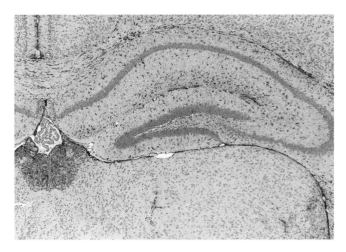

**FIGURE 13.35** Normal glial fibrillary acidic protein (GFAP) immunoreactivity of astrocytes in the hippocampus of a clinically normal FVB/NCr mouse. Note the choroid plexus in the third ventricle on the left.

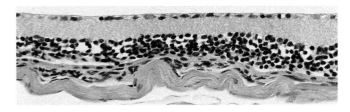

**FIGURE 13.34** Eye of 15-month-old FVB/NCr mouse showing loss of outer nuclear layer of the retina. Retina is nonpigmented in this albino mouse.

been a spontaneous mutation occurring sometime in the early 1990s in the stock maintained at the Animal Production Area at the NCI's Frederick Cancer Research and Development Center. The disease has been further defined to include specific behavioral and tissue lesions (D.E. Devor-Henneman et al., manuscript in preparation). Data from our colonies indicate that, while males are hardly immune, this condition tends to occur more frequently in females and can affect between 20 and 57 percent of a given population. It may become concentrated in "families," although this has not yet been determined. There are behavioral changes, including sudden inappropriate aggression toward never-separated littermates, breeding partners, and pups; declines in fertility; withdrawal from social interaction (hence our "space cadet" description of the condition); and overreaction to stimuli. Seizures, with accompanying laminar necrosis of cerebral cortical and hippocampal neurons and poliomalacia, are the probable cause of sudden death in otherwise healthy animals. Not all seizures, however, are fatal, and many more occur than are actu-

ally recorded. We have observed both violent convulsive episodes and relatively mild seizures involving chewing and salivation with localized muscle spasms. In both cases, mice can survive, and many undergo multiple convulsions during their life spans, which can be within the normal range. There does not appear to be a specific external trigger for these seizures; in this respect, they seem very similar to human epilepsy syndromes.

In contrast to the report by Goelz et al. (1998), we consistently find that there are gross changes in some organs of FVB/NCr mice that are associated with the neurologic syndrome. These lesions include distended gall and urinary bladders, enlarged adrenals, and increased brain weights. In addition to the behavioral changes mentioned, an early indication of the syndrome is increased urination and urinary soiling, which is likely accompanied by increased water consumption, since the animals do not appear to be dehydrated. Copious amounts of normal to dilute urine are voided at death, and the bladders are typically large and flaccid. We confirm the microscopic observations of the brain reported by Goelz et al. (1998). The increase in brain size could be due to gliosis resulting from either primary biochemical defects and resultant seizures or from the acute and chronic neuronal damage incurred by the seizuring itself and subsequent brain repair by astrocytes (Figs. 13.35, 13.36). We cannot rule out a possible neuroendocrine facet, as well, given the polyuria, adrenal hypertrophy, and hyperreactivity to stimuli and, additionally, unusually high serum corticosterone levels, all of which are consistent with a chronic stress response. To support our hypothesis, we found increased pigmentation of neurons

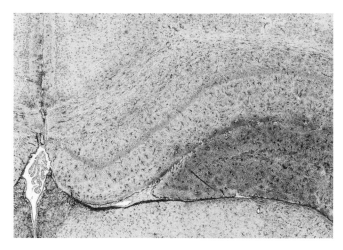

**FIGURE 13.36** Increased glial fibrillary acidic protein (GFAP) immunoreactivity of hypertrophic astrocytes in hippocampus of 60-week-old FVB/NCr mouse with "space cadet syndrome." Note the choroid plexus in the third ventricle on the left.

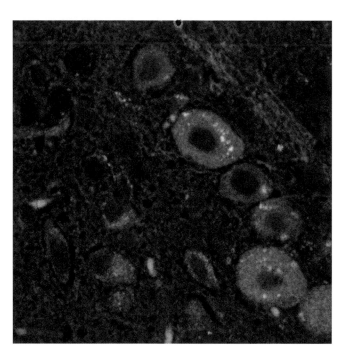

**FIGURE 13.37** Autofluorescent pigment in neurons of the locus coeruleus (small cells) and mesencephalic tract of the trigeminal nerve (large neurons) in a 59-week-old male FVB/NCr mouse with the "space cadet syndrome."

in the mesencephalic tract of the trigeminal nerve and locus coeruleus (Fig. 13.37). One hypothesis that is currently being investigated is that there is an abnormality in the hypothalamic-pituitary-adrenal axis such that, in "space cadets," the modulatory feedback loop is inefficient.

# REFERENCES

Bendele, A.M. and Carlton, W.W. 1998. Urologic syndrome, mouse. In: Urinary System, ILSI Monographs on Pathology of Laboratory Animals, ed. Jones, T.C., Mohr, U., Hunt, R.D. Berlin: Springer-Verlag, pp. 369–375.

Blackwell, B.N., Bucci, T.J., Hart, R.W., et al. 1995. Longevity, body weight, and neoplasia in ad libitum-fed and diet-restricted C57BL6 mice fed NIH-31 open formula diet. Toxicol. Pathol. 23:570–582.

Bronson, R.T., Lipman, R.D., and Harrison, D.E. 1993. Age-related gliosis in the white matter of mice. Brain Res. 609:124–128.

Doetschman, T. 1999. Interpretation of phenotype in genetically-engineered mice. Lab. Anim. Sci. 49:137–143.

Donehower, L.A., Harvey, M., Vogel, H., et al. 1995. Effects of genetic background on tumorigenesis in *p53*-deficient mice. Mol. Carcinog. 14:16–22.

Ernst, H., Dungworth, D.L., Kamino, K., et al. 1996. Nonneoplastic lesions in the lungs. In: Pathobiology of the Aging Mouse, vol. 1, ed. Mohr, U., Dungworth, D.L., Capen, C.C., et al. Washington, DC: ILSI Press, pp. 281–300.

Festing, M.F.W. 1996. Origins and characteristics of inbred strains of mice. In: Genetic Variants and Strains of the Laboratory Mouse, 3rd ed., ed. Lyons, M.F., Rasten, S., and Brown, S.D.M. New York: Oxford University Press, pp. 1537–1576.

Frith, C.H. and Ward, J.M. 1988. Color Atlas of Neoplastic and Non-neoplastic Lesions in Aging Mice. Amsterdam: Elsevier, p. 109.

Frith, C.H., Highman, B., Burger, G., et al. 1983. Spontaneous lesions in virgin and retired breeder BALB/c and C57BL/6 mice. Lab. Anim. Sci. 33:273–286.

Frith, C.H., Ward, J.M., Frederickson, T., et al. 1996. Neoplastic lesions of the hematopoietic system. In: Pathobiology of the Aging Mouse, vol. 1, ed. Mohr, U., Dungworth, D.L. Capen, C.C., et al. Washington, DC: ILSI Press, pp. 2219–2235.

Goelz, M.F., Mahler, J., Harry, J., et al. 1998. Neuropathologic findings associated with seizures in FVB mice. Lab. Anim. Sci. 48:34–37.

Green, M.C. and Shultz, L.D. 1975. Motheaten, an immunodeficient mutant of the mouse. I. Genetics and pathology. *J. Hered.* 66:250–258.

Hard, G.C. and Snowden, R.T. 1991. Hyaline droplet accumulation in rodent kidney proximal tubules: an association with histiocytic sarcoma. *Toxicol. Pathol.* 19:88–97.

Hennings, H., Glick, A.B., Lowry, D.T., et al. 1993. FVB/N mice: an inbred strain sensitive to the chemical induction of squamous cell carcinomas in the skin. Carcinogenesis 14:2353–2358.

Herbert, R.A. and Leninger, J.R. 1999. Nose, larynx, and trachea. In Pathology of the Mouse: Reference and Atlas, ed. Maronpot, R.R., Boorman G.A., and Gaul B.W. Vienna, IL: Cache River Press, pp. 259–292.

Hsiao, K.K., Borchelt, D.R., Olson, K., et al. 1995. Age-related CNS disorder and early death in transgenic FVB/N mice overexpressing Alzheimer amyloid precursor proteins. Neuron 15:1213–1218.

Hursting, S.D., Perkins, S.N., Brown, C.C., et al. 1997. Calorie restriction induces a p53-independent delay of spontaneous carcinogenesis in p53-deficient and wild-type mice. Cancer Res. 57:2843–2846.

Khaled, A.R., Butfiloski, E.J., Sobel, E.S., et al. 1998. Functional consequences of the SHP-1 defect in moth-eaten viable mice: role of NF-kappa B. *Cell Immunol.* 185:49–58.

Kodell, R.L., Blackwell, B.N., Bucci, T.J., et al. 1995. Cause-of-death assignment at the National Center for Toxicological Research. Toxicol. Pathol. 23:241–247.

Leninger, J.R., Herbert, R.A., and Morgan, K.T. 1996. Aging changes in the upper respiratory tract. In: Pathobiology of the Aging Mouse, vol. 1, ed. Mohr, U., Dungworth, D.L., Capen, C.C., et al. Washington, DC: ILSI Press, pp. 247–260.

Losco, P.E. 1995. Dental dysplasia in rats and mice. Toxicol. Pathol.23:677–688.

Lyon, M.F., Rastan, S., and Brown, S.D.M. 1996. Genetic Variants and Strains of the Laboratory Mouse, 3rd ed. vols. 1 and 2. Oxford: Oxford University Press, p. 1807.

Mahler, J.F., Stokes, W., Mann, P.C., et al. 1996. Spontaneous lesions in aging FVB/N mice. Toxicol. Pathol. 24:710–716.

Maronpot, R.R., Boorman, G.A., and Gaul, B.W. 1999. Pathology of the Mouse: Reference and Atlas. Vienna, IL: Cache River Press, p. 699.

McClatchey, A.I., Saotome, I., Mercer, K., et al. 1998. Mice heterozygous for a mutation at the Nf2 tumor suppressor locus develop a range of highly metastatic tumors. Genes Dev. 12:1121–1133.

Mohr, U., Dungworth, D.L., Capen, C.C., et al. 1996. Pathobiology of the Aging Mouse, vols. 1 and 2. Washington, DC: ILSI Press, 505 pages and 527 pages.

Perkins, S.N., Hursting, S.D., Phang, J.M., et al. 1998. Calorie restriction reduces ulcerative dermatitis and infection-related mortality in p53-deficient and wild-type mice. J. Invest. Dermatol. 111:292–296.

Pinkerton, K.E., Cowin, L.L., Witschi, H. 1996. Development, growth and aging of the lungs. In: Pathobiology of the Aging Mouse, vol. 2, ed. Mohr, U., Dungworth, D.L., Capen, C.C., et al. Washington, DC: ILSI Press, pp. 261–272.

Porter, D.D., Porter, H.G., and Cox, N.A. 1973. Immune complex glomerulonephritis in one-year old C57BL/6 mice induced by endogenous murine leukemia virus and erythrocyte antigens. J. Immunol. 111:1626–1633.

Sheldon, W.G., Bucci, T.J., Blackwell, B., et al. 1996. Effect of ad libitum feeding and 40% feed restriction on body weight, longevity, and neoplasms in B6C3F1, C57BL6, and B6D2F1 mice. In: Pathobiology of the Aging Mouse, vol. 2, ed. Mohr, U., Dungworth, D.L., Capen, C.C., et al. Washington, DC: ILSI Press, pp. 21–26.

Silver, L.M. 1995. Mouse Genetics. New York: Oxford University Press, p. 362.

Simpson, E.M., Linder, C.C., Sargent, E.E., et al. 1997. Genetic variation among 129 substrains and its importance for targeted mutagenesis in mice. Nat. Genet. 16:19–27.

Smith, G.S., Walford, R.L., and Mickey, M.R. 1973. Lifespan and incidence of cancer and other diseases in selected long-lived inbred mice and their F1 hybrids. J. Natl. Cancer Inst. 50:1195–1213.

Smith, R.S. and Sundberg, J.P. 1996. Opthalmic abnormalities in inbred mice. In: Pathobiology of the Aging Mouse, vol. 2, ed. Mohr, U., Dungworth, D.L., Capen, C.C., et al. Washington, DC: ILSI Press, pp. 117–123.

Smith, R.S., Roderick, T.H., and Sundberg, J.P. 1994. Microphthalmia and associated abnormalities in inbred black mice. Lab. Anim. Sci. 44:551–560.

Stevens, L.C. 1973. A new inbred subline of mice (129/terSv) with a high incidence of spontaneous congenital testicular teratomas. J. Natl. Cancer Inst. 50:235–242.

Sundberg, J.P., Sundberg, B.A., and King, L.E., Jr. 1996. Cutaneous changes in commonly used inbred mouse strains and mutant stocks. In: Pathobiology of the Aging Mouse, vol. 2, ed. Mohr, U., Dungworth, D.L., Capen, C.C., et al. Washington, DC: ILSI Press, pp. 325–337.

Taketo, M., Schroeder, A.C., Mobraaten, L.E., et al. 1991. FVB/N: an inbred mouse strain preferable for transgenic analyses. Proc. Natl. Acad. Sci. USA 88:2065–2069.

Thrall, R.S., Vogel, S.N., Evans, R., et al. 1997. Role of tumor necrosis factor-alpha in the spontaneous development of pulmonary fibrosis in viable motheaten mutant mice. *Am. J. Pathol.* 151:1303–1310.

Threadgill, D.W., Yee, D., Matin, A., et al. 1997. Genealogy of the 129 inbred strains: 129/SvJ is a contaminated inbred strain. *Mamm. Genome* 8:390–393.

Turusov, V. and Mohr, U., eds. 1994. Pathology of Tumours in Laboratory Animals, vol. 2, Tumours of the Mouse. Lyon: IARC Scientific Publications No. 111, p. 776.

Volk, M.J., Pugh, T.D., Kim, M.J., et al. 1994. Dietary restriction from middle age attenuates age-associated lymphoma development and interleukin 6 dysregulation in C57BL/6 mice. Cancer Res. 54:3054–3061.

Ward, J.M. 1978. Pulmonary pathology of the motheaten mouse. Vet. Pathol. 15:170–178.

Ward, J.M., Weisburger, J.H., Yamamoto, R.S., et al. 1975. Long-term effects of benzene in C57BL/6N mice. Arch. Environ. Health 30:22–25.

Ward, J.M., Taddesse-Heath, L., Perkins, S.N., et al. 1999. Splenic marginal zone B-cell and thymic T-cell lymphomas in p53-deficient mice. Lab. Invest. 79:3–14.

Zurcher, C., van Zweiten, M.J., and Solleveld, H.A. 1982. Aging research. In: The Mouse in Biomedical Research, vol. 4, Experimental Biology and Oncology, American College of Laboratory Animals Medicine Series, ed. Foster, H.L., Small, D.J., Fox, J.G. New York: Academic Press, pp. 11–35.

# IV

# Special Pathology

# 14

# Skin and Its Appendages: Normal Anatomy and Pathology of Spontaneous, Transgenic, and Targeted Mouse Mutations

John P. Sundberg and Lloyd E. King, Jr.

The skin is the largest of the intermediate-sized organs (Goldsmith 1990). Phenotypic deviants (mutant mice) with abnormalities of this organ system are easy to spot, and therefore for over a century large numbers of spontaneous mouse mutations with abnormalities of the skin and adnexa have been accumulated and studied and the gene loci mapped (Fig. 14.1). Many are still available today (Trigg 1972; Sundberg and Shultz 1991; Sundberg 1994h; Sundberg and King 1996b; [*http://www.informatics.jax.org/searches/marker_form. shtml*]). These make up an important resource, the value of which has become increasingly acknowledged by the fact that many gene-targeting studies (creations of partial or complete functional nulls or knockouts) develop phenotypes identical to the spontaneous mouse mutations (Shastry 1998). Gene-targeting technology answers the question of which gene is mutated, information not available for many of the previously identified and well-characterized spontaneous mutant mice (Sundberg 1994h). However, collective knowledge on the biological and pathological aspects of the spontaneous mutant mice provides guidelines or specific

answers on the function of the gene under investigation. For example, the null mutation of fibroblast growth factor 5 (*Fgf5*) turned out not to be an embryonic or neonatal lethal, as the investigators anticipated, but just grew hair that was abnormally long. *Fgf5* mapped near the angora mouse mutation, a spontaneous mutant mouse that has been available for decades and is characterized by prolongation of the hair growth cycle resulting in long hair (Sundberg et al. 1997c). The induced null mutation of *Fgf5* turned out, in breeding studies, to be allelic with angora (Hebert et al. 1994). The massive effort to generate and characterize mutant mice has and will continue to define the molecular and physiological mechanisms of both diseases and normal development (Yamanishi 1998; Ishida-Yamamoto et al. 1998).

Numerous spontaneous mutations are available in which the phenotypes are identical or very similar even though the mutant gene locus maps onto different chromosomes. These are called phenotypic mimics. Defining one phenotypic mimic often permits evaluation of other mimics, with the potential to define the specifically affected biochemical cascade. For example, an induced null mutation of transforming growth factor α (*Tgfα*) resulted in mice with wavy hair. This mutation turned out to be allelic with waved1, a spontaneous mutation that mapped near *Tgfα* (Luetteke et al. 1993; Mann et al. 1993). Another spontaneous mutation that was very similar to waved1 was called waved2. This mutation

This work was supported by grants from the National Alopecia Areata Foundation (JPS, LEK), Council for Nail Research (JPS), National Institutes of Health (CA34196, AR43801, RR00173, JPS; DK26518, LEK), and funds from the Jackson Laboratory (JPS) and the Department of Veterans Affairs (LEK).

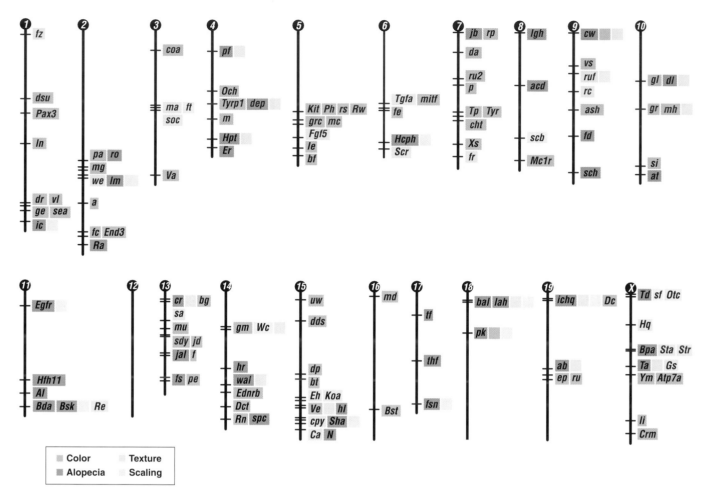

**FIGURE 14.1** Mouse chromosome map. Phenotypes due to pigmentation abnormalities (orange), hair loss (pink), texture of hair fibers (green), or hyperproliferation and scaling (blue) are the result of mutations in genes that are scattered throughout the mouse genome.

mapped near the receptor for *Tgfα*, epidermal growth factor receptor (*Egfr*). Waved2 was subsequently determined to be a mutation of the *Egfr* gene (Luetteke et al. 1994).

While some mutations have no obvious effects (Colucci-Guyon et al. 1994), for others, phenotypes can vary dramatically because of the type of mutation within a gene, the mutation's location within a gene, or the genetic background of the strain the mutation occurs in or is transferred onto. Although some mutations have predictable effects, such as the spontaneous and induced mutations in the desmoglein-3 gene that cause the same pemphigus vulgaris-like disease regardless of background strain or exon mutated (Montagutelli et al. 1997; Koch et al. 1997), many more have great variability. Mutations of *Egfr* have great variability based on the background strain the mutation is maintained on even when the mutated gene is the same, such as between congenic strains (Miettinen et al. 1995;

Threadgill et al. 1995; Sibilia and Wagner 1995). These types of mutations are useful for mapping modifier genes provided by each inbred strain, thereby helping to define genetic influences of phenotypic variability in humans affected with similar types of genodermatoses. Targeted mutagenesis studies utilize C57BL/6 and 129 strains, of which there are many substrains, creating a further complication for those investigators comparing lesions associated with similar mutations that have been created in different laboratories (Simpson et al. 1997).

This chapter provides examples of spontaneous and induced mutant mice with abnormalities of the skin and its appendages to illustrate the general types of abnormalities that occur in this organ system. A categorical approach to defining mutant mouse phenotypes is useful for comparative studies with homologous diseases in humans and domestic animals when one is trying to determine if the mutant mouse is a potential animal model for a particular disease. More importantly, as

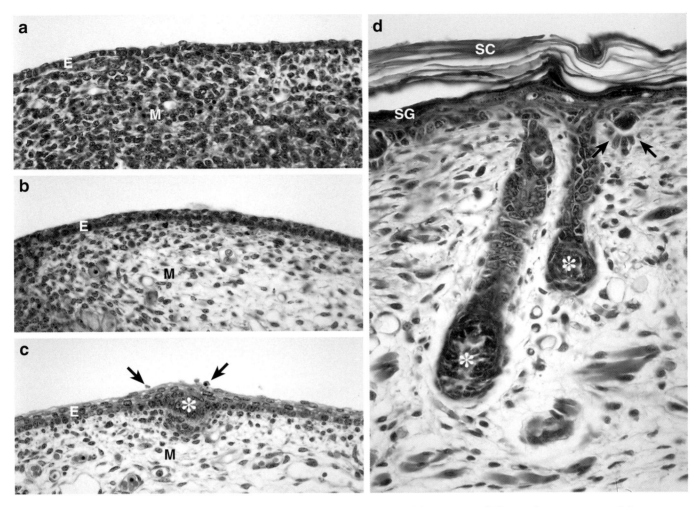

**FIGURE 14.2**  Mouse skin develops from a single layer of epidermis (*E*) into a multilayered structure overlying primitive mesenchyme (*M*) and forms a hair follicle (*). Focal accumulations of epidermal cells and the evolving dermal papilla (*between arrows*) progressively grow down through the dermis into the subcutaneous fat to form the first fully differentiated hair follicles and hair bulb. The follicles produce different fibers and develop at different points in time so various phases of development can be found in the skin near term (**d**). (**a**) embryonic day 12 (E12); (**b**) E14; (**c**) E16; (**d**) E18; *SC*, stratum corneum; *SG*, stratum granulosum.

described above, this approach helps identify phenotypic mimics that are key to defining complex metabolic pathways controled by many seemingly unrelated genes.

General categories of cutaneous disease include (1) hair color (pigmentation) mutations, (2) eccrine gland defects, (3) sebaceous gland defects, (4) primary scarring disorders of the skin, (5) hair shaft growth and structural defects, (6) noninflammatory (ichthyosiform and keratodermas) skin diseases, (7) inflammatory (psoriasiform and proliferative) skin diseases, (8) papillomatous skin diseases, (9) bullous and acantholytic skin diseases, and (10) structural and growth defects in nails. These categories can be increased or subdivided; however, this approach is useful for initial characterization studies and as an approach to identifying potential allelic mutations.

# NORMAL ANATOMY AND EMBRYOLOGY OF MOUSE SKIN AND HAIR

The embryology, anatomy, and physiology of normal mammalian skin, hair, and nails are deceptively complex, as compared with such organs as the liver and lungs, and cannot adequately be described in this chapter. The reader is referred to comprehensive reviews elsewhere (Mann 1962; Holbrook 1991; Holbrook and Smith 1993; Sundberg et al. 1996a; Paus et al. 1999). In brief, as shown in Figure 14.2, the follicle develops from a simple two to three cellular layer structure in early embryogenesis into a complex, multilayered hair follicle and sebaceous gland (Gruneberg 1943; Hardy 1949; Falconer et al. 1951;

Mann 1962; Slee 1962). In addition, follicle density increases during embyronic life (Claxton 1966). The epithelial/mesenchymal interactions that induce hair bulges, hair follicle elongation, and ultimately a hair fiber are just now being described in more precise detail (Paus et al. 1999; Chiang et al. 1999). Melanization first occurs in stage 6 of hair follicle formation in the mouse embryo, at a time when the first hair shaft is formed. In mouse skin all of the pigment is present in the hair fiber, and little or no melanin is present in the interfollicular epidermis, unlike human epidermis. A simple scheme to determine the stage of hair follicle formation by using commonly available histochemical stains and light microscopy is currently available (Paus et al. 1999; Chase et al. 1951).

At birth the truncal epidermis is quite thick but rapidly thins within the first 2 weeks of life (Fig. 14.3; Sundberg et al. 1993, 1997b, 1997c). Hair follicles in the mouse skin produce a variety of fiber types, and each develops at different embryological time points (Fig. 14.3a; Dry 1926; Trigg 1972; Fraser 1951; Yamakado and Yohro 1979). Development of hairs continues to full anagen by 1 week of age (Fig. 14.3b). By the end of the second week of age, follicles enter catagen, and the deep portions of the follicles located in the hypodermal fat layer undergo apoptosis (Fig. 14.3c). This is a very short transition phase, 1–2 days in length, to the resting, or telogen, phase (Fig. 14.3d). The dermis and epidermis normally remain stable in thickness throughout life, but the hair follicle length and hypodermal fat layer increase in size in a regular cyclic basis throughout life (Chase et al. 1953; Chase 1954, 1955; Straile et al. 1961). The mouse hair cycles in a wave beginning cranially and progressing in a somewhat irregular pattern caudally (Chase and Eaton 1959). This is in contrast to the mosaic pattern of hair cycling observed in humans and many domestic animals. When comparing mutant and control mouse skin, it is of paramount importance to match hair cycle stage to avoid the common misinterpretation that any difference seen is due to the mutation being investigated and not the hair cycle. Examples where this was not done are easily found in the literature (Peschon et al. 1998).

Various hair fiber types are found all over the body of the mouse, as is also the case in humans and most other mammals. The most commonly studied hairs, those of the trunk (body or pelage hairs), consist of four anatomically distinct types (Table 14.1; Figs. 14.4, 14.5; Dry 1926; Sundberg and Hogan 1994). Hairs and their follicles are distinct around the ears, vibrissae on the muzzle and around the eyes, cilia on eyelids, and perianal hairs (Sundberg et al. 1996a).

The normal hair follicle is a very complicated structure because it develops into an elongated production unit to form the hair fiber and then undergoes apoptosis to form a tiny resting structure until signals, as yet

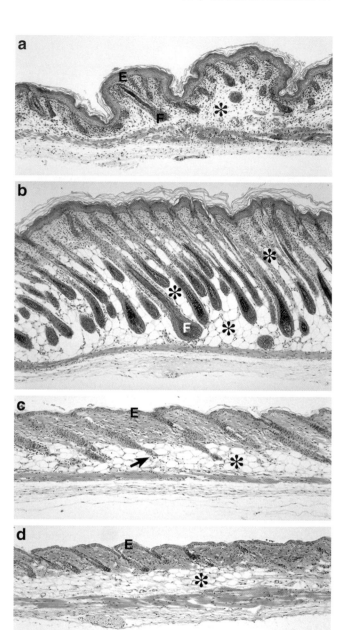

**FIGURE 14.3** The normal mouse epidermis (*E*) is very thick at birth (**a**), and hair follicles (*F*) are completing development. By 1 week of age, follicles are fully formed and in the actively growing, anagen stage (**b**). Around 2 weeks of age the lower third of the anagen follicles undergo apoptosis (*arrow*) and regress in the catagen stage (**c**). The resting phase of normal hair follicles, telogen, is characterized by very small follicles (**d**). Notice the progressive thinning of the epidermis through the first 2 weeks of life and variation of the hypodermal fat layer (*) thickness with stage of the hair cycle.

**TABLE 14.1.  Hair types and subtypes
in the laboratory mouse**

Pelage or truncal hair: guard, awl, auchene, and zigzag
Vibrissae: primary (mystacial vibrissae), secondary
   (supraorbital, postorbital, interramal, ulnar-carpal),
   and supernumerary
Cilia (eyelashes)
Tail hair
Ear hair
Hair around feet
Genital/perianal hair
Nipple hair

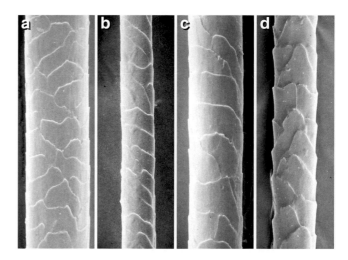

**FIGURE 14.5**  The cuticular scale and midshaft
diameter of the four hair types varies dramatically for
the guard (**a**), auchene (**b**), awl (**c**), and zigzag (**d**) hairs.

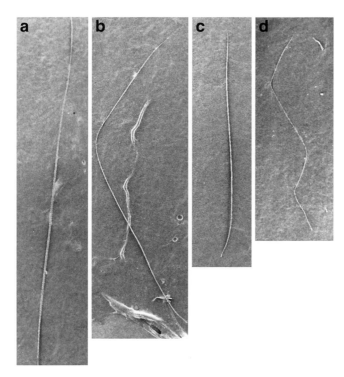

**FIGURE 14.4**  The four major hair fiber types
produced by the truncal or pelage hairs include guard
(**a**), auchene (**b**), awl (**c**), and zigzag (**d**).

unknown, start the growth phase all over again. Details
of an anagen-stage follicle that is actively producing a
hair fiber are shown in Figure 14.6. The deepest part of
the follicle is bulbous in appearance and is known as the
hair bulb. It consists of layers of epithelial cells that surround a core of specialized fibroblasts known historically as the dermal papilla (Jamieson, 1888). This term,
*dermal papilla,* is commonly used by researchers working on hair follicle biology; however, some dermatolo-
gists consider this term to relate to the upper part of the
dermis where it lies between rete ridges in human skin.
For this reason some prefer the term *follicular papilla*
(Williams et al. 1994). Since mice do not have rete

ridges, this is not an issue. The epithelial layers of the
hair bulb differentiate to form a number of layers. The
outer junction of the follicle with the dermis is the basement membrane that is often called the glassy membrane since it becomes very hyalinized and prominent
during catagen. The epithelial layers adjacent to this
basement membrane are called the outer root sheath.
These structures can be identified using keratins 5 and
14 as markers for basal keratinocytes (Sundberg et al.
1994e). The inner layer of the outer root sheath is called
the companion layer, and its cells are normally the only
ones that express keratin 6 (Fig. 14.6). Keratin 6–positive
companion layer cells are a useful histologic marker to
define the extent of the outer and inner root sheaths
(Sundberg et al. 1994e). Mouse keratin-specific antibodies can be very useful for defining affected cell
layers in some mutant mice (Montagutelli et al. 1997;
Sundberg et al. 1994d; HogenEsch et al. 1999). The
inner root sheath can be differentiated into two layers
based on anatomical features with names descriptive of
cytoplasmic granules: pale epithelial, or Henle's (outer)
layer, and granular epithelial, or Huxley's (inner) layer,
respectively (Calhoun and Stinson 1981; Bloom and
Fawcett 1968). These inner root sheath layers are
covered by a thin layer of cells, the cuticle of the inner
root sheath, that interlocks with the cuticle of the hair
shaft. The hair shaft consists of epithelial cells that
form a cortex and medulla of the hair shaft or fiber. The
hair fiber is formed from a triangular cluster of keratinocytes located directly above the dermal papilla
called the matrix region (Parakkal 1969; Sperling 1991;
Sundberg et al. 1996a). The size, shape, tinctorial characteristics, cytoplasmic granules, and other features
change as the hair shaft is formed and approaches the

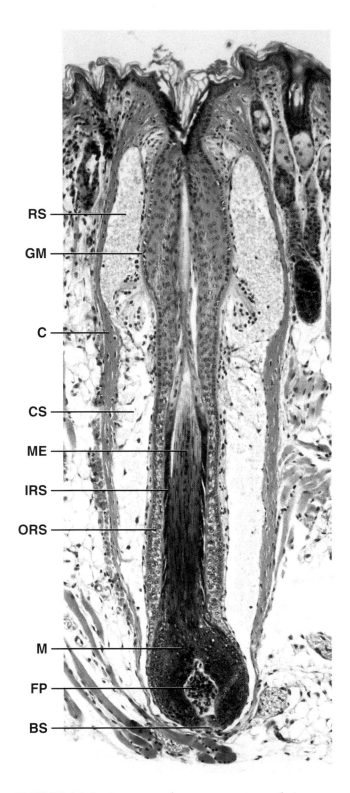

**FIGURE 14.6** Anatomy of an anagen-stage vibrissa follicle includes *RS*, ring sinus; *GM*, glassy membrane; *C*, capsule; *CS*, cavernous sinus; *ME*, medulla; *IRS*, inner root sheath; *ORS*, outer root sheath; *M*, matrix; *FP*, follicular papilla; and *BS*, basal stalk. (Williams et al. 1994; Oliver 1966)

epidermis. These changes make interpretation of tangential sections difficult (Headington 1984; Bergfeld 1990). Examination of hair follicles and fibers using dark-field illumination can emphasize the differences both between the layers and as the layers differentiate (Fig. 14.20b).

The details of the evolution of a cutaneous barrier in truncal mouse skin are less well understood than in humans even though extensive studies have been performed on fatty acid–deficient and other mouse models with increased transepidermal water loss (Roop 1995; Imakado et al. 1995; Yosipovitch et al. 1998; Sundberg et al. in press—b). Such studies are hampered by the lack of information about the biochemical and molecular bases of epidermal maturation in mice and the formation of thick and thin (epidermis) skin at different anatomic sites. For example, the truncal skin of the mouse is thick at birth and thins dramatically by 2 weeks of age and remains that way throughout life (Fig. 14.3). In contrast, the epidermis of the tail skin and foot pads remains very thick throughout life (Fig. 14.9).

General mechanisms of normal nail and appendage formation have been described in reviews of mouse, human, and domestic animals (Calhoun and Stinson 1981; Fleckman and Sundberg submitted). The formation of normal functioning nails in mice has not been extensively investigated due to their small size (Fleckman et al. submitted). The normal features of nails and glands of the skin are described in the appropriate sections below.

# BIOLOGICAL CHARACTERIZATION OF A NEW MUTATION

Mice, like other mammals, undergo major changes in their lives that may affect the phenotype of a mutation. These life changes can provide points to focus systemic investigations, while knowledge of aging changes of the organ system being studied defines a second set of observation points. Major life changes include birth (0–1 day, depending upon how this is calculated), weaning (3–4 weeks), sexual maturity (6–8 weeks), sexual quiescence (6–8 months), and geriatric stages (2 years +). The age range provided reflects strain-specific differences (Green and Witham 1991). The cost of maintaining mice to geriatric age is often prohibitive, and many mice with genetic mutations never live that long, so this age group is rarely studied.

Skin and its appendages undergo very dramatic changes during the first 3 weeks of life, as described above. All of these features can be evaluated if skin is collected at 2- or 3-day intervals during the first 3 weeks of life.

Numbers of mice can easily become quite large. If inbred mice are being studied and are maintained in a clean, environmentally controlled, pathogen-free facility, as few as two mutants and two controls can be used of each sex (eight total per time point). Complete sets of organs should be collected to study major life changes (see below), while skin and appendage evaluation can be limited to collection of selected skin. Use of the same individual for multiple biopsies can reduce the numbers of animals used but with a skin mutant may cause a problem if the phenotype has a positive Köbner reaction, as is the case with some of the scaly skin mutations (Sundberg, et al. 1990a; Nanney et al. 1996).

Injection of mice with bromodeoxyuridine or tritiated thymidine prior to euthanasia provides the opportunity to do later kinetic studies. Necropsy methods vary, but procedures for mice and other rodents have been detailed elsewhere (Smith et al. 1999). Mice can be euthanized by numerous methods depending upon institutional regulations. Carbon dioxide asphyxiation in a chamber is an American Veterinary Medical Association–approved method for adults. Asphyxiation followed by decapitation is necessary for pups less than 12 days of age since they rarely die by the gas alone. Other methods are available and approved (Relyea et al. 1999). Skin is collected from the dorsal and ventral trunk, eyelids, ear, muzzle, tail, and foot pads. Although dorsal and ventral skin can not be easily differentiated histologically when normal, the other skin sites can. For this reason, we place dorsal skin with tail and ear skin in one casset. Ventral skin is processed in a casset with muzzle and eyelid skin. Foot pad skin with eccrine glands is processed separately since it has a very different consistency, sometimes including bone. Both vertical and horizontal sections can be prepared for dorsal and ventral skin (Headington 1984; Whiting et al. 1990). More general necropsy procedures for collection of all organs are described elsewhere (Feldman and Seely 1988; Sundberg et al. 1998; Relyea et al. 1999). All tissues should be handled delicately to avoid crushing artifact that will be obvious during microscopic evaluation and interfere with interpretation.

Skin should be laid out flat, epidermal (haired) surface up, on an unlined index-type card or aluminum foil. The hair can be left on or removed, depending upon the ability of your histology laboratory and goals of the study. We have shaved and depilated mice with no change in histologic features or epitope expression patterns for keratins compared with haired skin samples. The skin should be oriented on the card or foil in a head-to-tail (cranial-caudal) fashion and labeled (in pencil) as such along with where the skin came from.

When the tissue is trimmed, it should be cut in the cranial-caudal orientation (lengthwise) to follow the lay of the hair, which reflects the angle of the follicle within the skin. This will maximize the chances of obtaining most or all of the follicle in a section. Tissues can also be oriented using a dissection microscope one block at a time to obtain this type of result. Since the dermis will adhere to the card or foil and not fall off when fresh, tissues can be placed in the same bottle of fixative regardless of the anatomic site as long as each is labeled. Most pen ink will wash off the cards in the fixatives, so pencil is necessary to maintain a legible label.

Tissue fixation is as critical as tissue collection. A large number of fixatives are available, each with their own advantages and disadvantages. We have found formalin-based fixatives, especially acid-alcohol-formalin (5 ml glacial acetic acid, 100 ml of 70 percent ethanol, 10 ml formaldehyde solution), to yield fine detail in well-preserved specimens while also maintaining many epitopes for immohistochemical studies. All organs should be routinely fixed by immersion. Serial sections of skin can be stained with Masson's trichrome (for scarring), Verhoeffvan Gieson (for elastic fibers), periodic acid-Schiff (PAS; for fungi, glycogen, glycoproteins, and glycolipids), and von Kossa (for mineralization) stains, among others.

Skin can also be frozen for use in various biochemical, molecular, or immunofluorescence studies. Frozen sections lack detail but maintain epitopes for immunohistochemical studies or lipids that can be detected with oil red O, Sudan black, osmium, and other stains. We routinely take a 1.5 × 2.0 cm section of skin that is removed from the dorsal surface of the mouse at a standardized location, usually at the withers (tissue overlying the shoulders). This skin is trimmed to approximately 0.3 × 1.5 cm to form strips that run lengthwise from the head to the tail to properly orient hair follicles. The strips of skin are placed on a piece of aluminum foil, and a bead of OCT solution (Miles Inc., Elkhart, IN) is run along one edge. The foil is then dipped into liquid nitrogen to instantly freeze the samples. Once frozen, samples are quickly removed from the foil and placed on edge in a clear plastic mold (HistoPrep disposable base molds, Fisher Scientific, Pittsburgh, PA) and filled with OCT solution. The mold is then placed back into the liquid nitrogen and allowed to freeze. Frozen molds are wrapped in foil and stored at −80°C until needed. Both the molds and the foil are labeled with the accession number used for the animal being necropsied.

In situ hybridization techniques can utilize tissues collected in fixatives routinely used for histopathology. However, use of these types of fixatives often is associated with high background signals. One approach that has yielded high-quality results is the following. Strips of skin are collected in the same manner as for freezing (described above). The skin is placed on nylon mesh, placed in 4 percent paraformaldehyde, and fixed overnight at 4°C. The following day the paraformaldehyde is replaced with 30 percent sucrose in phosphate-buffered saline (pH 7.6), where it remains until the following day at 4°C. On day 3 tissues are removed, trimmed, and embedded in OCT solution as described above. These tissues can now be sectioned for in situ hybridization studies or shipped to collaborators on dry ice (Keeney 1999; Limberg and Bascom 1999).

For molecular studies (gene mapping), spleen, liver, and kidneys are routinely removed at necropsy, snap frozen in liquid nitrogen in screw-capped plastic vials (NUNC tubes, Nalgen Nunc International, Denmark), and stored at −80°C for subsequent DNA extraction.

Transmission electron microscopy can be a useful adjunct to standard histological studies. However, the relatively high cost of processing and viewing specimens warrants its judicious use. Skin is fixed for 18 hours in 2.5 percent glutaraldehyde in 0.1M cacodylate buffer, pH 7.4, and postfixed for 18 hours in aqueous 1 percent osmium or rhuthenium tetroxide. Tissues are stained en bloc with 2 percent uranyl acetate in 10 percent ethanol and further dehydrated in a graded ethanol series. Samples embedded in Spurrs-Mollenhauer resin are polymerized at 65°C for 48 hours. Ultrathin sections are collected, stained with uranyl acetate and lead citrate, and examined in a transmission electron microscope (Bechtold 1999).

Scanning electron microscopy can be done on nails, skin punches, and plucked hairs. At the time of necropsy, 1.5–2.0 cm square samples of mouse skin can be removed from mutant and control mice avoiding the subcutaneous fat layer. The samples are placed, connective tissue side down, on dry nylon mesh and immersed in cold 2.5 percent glutaraldehyde in 0.1M cacodylate buffer. In addition, during necropsy the left front and rear feet can be amputated at the carpus/tarsus and prepared in a similar manner. After overnight fixation at 4°C, samples are washed twice with 0.1M cacodylate buffer and postfixed in 0.5 percent osmium tetroxide in 0.1M cacodylate buffer. Some of the skin samples can be first fractured in liquid nitrogen and then processed. Samples are subsequently dehydrated in a series of graded ethanols to 100 percent. After three changes in 100 percent ethanol, the samples are critical point dried, attached to aluminum stubs with silver adhesive, and sputter coated with 15 nm of gold. Samples are examined in a scanning electron microscope operated at 10 kV. Plucked hairs from mice are directly mounted onto aluminum stubs with double-stick tape. Hair samples are sputter coated with gold and examined as described above (Bechtold 1999).

# CATEGORIES OF DISEASES OF THE SKIN AND ADNEXA

## Hair Color (Pigmentation) Mutations

Large numbers of mouse mutations exhibit phenotypes of various coat colors. Some are color dilutions, like beige, a homologue for Chédiak-Higashi syndrome in humans (Windhorst and Padgett 1973; Sundberg 1994d), or unique colors, like yellow, a mutation that has been useful in working out pigmentation and obesity biochemistry (J. Naggert, personal commmunication). Mutations of these types are numerous, are beautiful to look at, and have been studied extensively for decades to provide, collectively, panels of tools to dissect out the regulatory pathways of melanogenesis (Bailin et al. 1996; Xu et al. 1998; Lamoreux et al. 1995; Orlow et al. 1993; Rosemblat et al. 1994, 1998; Sakai et al. 1997; Wilson et al. 1995). Readers are referred to several detailed reviews (Sundberg 1994i; Barsh 1996; Orlow 1996).

Melanomas in mice are extremely rare, possibly because pigmentation is limited to anagen bulbs and hair fibers but not the interfollicular epidermis, as in many other mammals. Mice are also housed in areas with limited exposure to ultraviolet irradiation. Mutant mice, like adrenocortical dysplasia (acd) (Fig. 14.7) mice, have interfollicular epidermal pigmentation (Sundberg et al. 1994f) and may provide useful tools for studying melanomas if exposed to ultraviolet light. Some mice do develop malignant melanomas on skin with little hair, such as the tail (Fig. 14.8; J.P. Sundberg, personal observation). Transgenic mice have been created that develop melanomas spontaneously in the absence of any known chemical carcinogen or ultraviolet light and are providing useful models to identify the genes involved in this process (Zhu et al. 1998).

Mutant mice with abnormal coat colors make up one of the most numerous groups of skin and hair phenotypes available in repositories (Green 1989; Peters and Cocking 1994). These mutant mice have been described collectively in detail (Silvers 1979) and are beyond the scope of this overview. Several mutations with pigmentation abnormalities are included here because they are being studied for structural defects of the hair shaft or skin. Mutations, such as adrenocortical dysplasia (acd), have severe follicular defects associated with hyperpigmentation (Beamer et al. 1994; Sundberg et al. 1994f). Beige (lysosomal trafficking regulator, Lyst$^{bg}$) and mottled (ATPase, Cu$^{++}$ transporting α polypeptide, Atp7a$^{Mo}$)

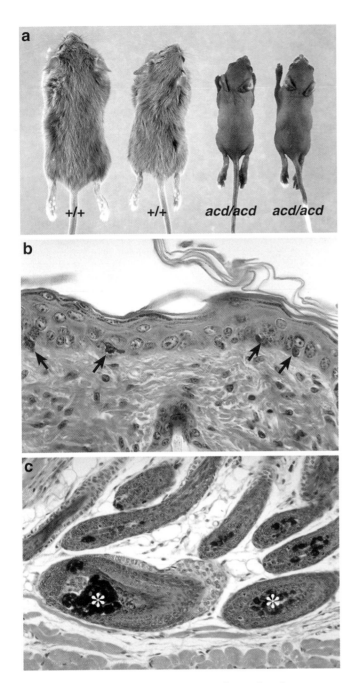

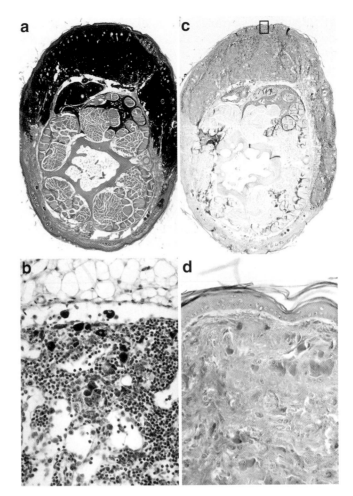

**FIGURE 14.8** Malignant melanomas rarely occur in mice. An example of a malignant melanoma found in the tail of a 3-month-old male T(12:17)4Rk mouse (**a**) reveals the focal invasion of neoplastic cells. The melanoma cells in this mouse metastasized to the regional lymph nodes (**b**). The malignant melanoma was bleached to remove melanin and show cellular detail (**c, d**).

**FIGURE 14.7** Some mutant mice have deeply pigmented skin such as alopecic adrenocortical dysplasia mice (*acd/acd*, **a**) as compared with their littermate controls (+/+, **a**). The dark skin is due to the presence of interfollicular epidermal melanin (*arrow*, **b**) and pigment overproduction within anagen bulbs (*, **c**). In normal mice, melanin is only found in anagen bulbs and hair fibers, not in interfollicular epidermis as seen in humans.

have primary coat color defects but represent well-established groups of mutations that are analogous to the human diseases Chédiak-Higashi syndrome (Oliver and Essner 1973) and Menke's kinky hair disease (Sundberg 1994i), respectively. Multiple remutations at these loci result in mice with various modifications of the phenotype, providing good examples of how a single disease with variations in presentation can be the result of different mutations in the same gene.

## Eccrine Gland Defects

Eccrine glands, or sweat glands, are only located within the dermis of foot pads in rodents. These glands consist of cuboidal cells arranged in small islands with a tortuous, long duct leading to the epidermal surface. Eccrine gland secretions and excretions soften and lubricate the skin and regulate body temperature (Munger and Brusilow 1971; Briggs 1987; Sundberg et al. 1996a). Some mouse mutations lacking meibomian glands also lack eccrine glands (i.e., crinkled, *cr*; downless, *dl*; sleek, *dl^{Slk}*; and tabby, *Ta*) (Fig. 14.9; Sundberg 1994h). These mice provide a group of phenotypic mimics of the human disease anhydrotic ectodermal dysplasia. The tabby mutation has been defined on the mouse X chromosome (Montreal et al. 1998; Bayes et al. 1998; Ferguson et al. 1997; Srivastava et al. 1997). The other loci, crinkled and downless, are on other mouse chromosomes representing additional mutated genes resulting in phenotypic mimics (also called phenocopies) of the disease (Fig. 14.1; Crocker and Cattanach 1979; Sofaer 1969). Identification of the mutated genes and their function will help define the biochemical pathways

involved in this disease and also the normal physiology of eccrine glands.

## Sebaceous Gland Defects

Five types of sebaceous glands or modified sebaceous glands are found in the mouse skin. These include (1) sebaceous glands of the hair follicles (pilosebaceous unit; Figs. 14.3 , 14.9i), (2) meibomian glands adjacent to the cilia in the eyelids (Fig. 14.9h), (3) preputial (males) or clitoral (females) glands adjacent to the prepuce or vulva, respectively, (4) ceruminous glands within the external ear canal, and (5) perianal glands. The sebaceous glands produce a lipid film that functions to soften the skin and provide a chemical barrier (Briggs 1987; Strauss et al. 1991).

All of these sebaceous glands have similar morphologic features but vary in size and where their ducts empty. Reserve cells, the transient amplifying cells that

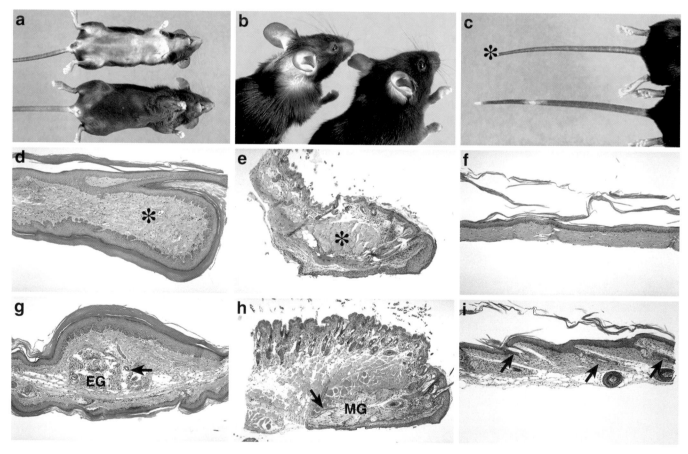

**FIGURE 14.9** Phenotypic mimics such as tabby (*Ta*), crinkled (*cr*), and downless (*dl*, **a–c**), all homologous for human anhydrotic ectodermal dysplasia, have local areas of alopecia due to lack of specific hair types, no eccrine glands in their foot pads (*\**, **d**), no meibomian glands in their eyelids (*\**, **e**), and no tail pilosebaceous units (**f**), resulting in tails with a smooth surface. Eccrine glands (*EG*, **g**), meibomian glands (*MG*, **h**), and tail pilosebaceous units (*arrows*, **i**) from normal littermates are shown for comparison.

differentiate into sebocytes, form a crescent of flattened, hyperchromatic cells around the gland. These cells presumably differentiate from the bulge region (stem cells), located immediately below the sebaceous gland on hair shafts. The reserve cells differentiate into polygonal cells with abundant, finely vacuolated cytoplasm, the sebocytes. The differentiated cells are excreted in toto and rupture to release their oily contents.

Sebaceous glands of the hair follicles empty, via a short duct, directly into the piliary canal. Meibomian glands, located adjacent to cilia in the eyelids, have separate ducts from follicles that empty directly onto the mucocutaneous junction of the eyelid. Preputial and clitoral glands are large glands that have stratified squamous epithelial-lined ducts within the glands that often enlarge and efface the glands as mice age (J.P. Sundberg, unpublished observations). Ceruminous glands empty directly into the ear canal. Perianal glands are large sebaceous glands that empty directly into the piliary canal of the large perianal hair follicles. Several single-gene mouse mutations exist in which some of the sebaceous glands develop normally while others do not develop at all (crinkled, downless, sleek, and tabby; Sundberg 1994h), suggesting that although the five groups of glands listed here have morphologic similarities, there may be major developmental and biochemical differences between them. Mice carrying a spontaneous mutation in the *Hoxd13* gene lack preputial glands but not other types of sebaceous glands (Johnson et al. 1998). Other mutant mice have marked hypoplasia of most sebaceous glands, like asebia (*ab, ab^J, ab^2J*), a group of spontaneous null alleles of the Stearoyl-CoA Desaturase-1 gene (Fig. 14.10; Sundberg 1994a; Zheng et al. 1999; Sundberg et al. in press—b; Eilersten et al. 2000). These mice have illustrated the role of their excretory products in controlling the barrier around emerging hair fibers. Asebia mice develop very long anagen and catagen follicles because hairs can not easily emerge. Some rupture through the follicular bulb, causing a foreign body response. Secondary scarring alopecia may develop (see below; Stenn et al. 1999; Sundberg et al. in press—b). Null mutations of the parathyroid hormone–related peptide (*PTHrP*) rescued with various transgenes may have hypoplastic or hyperplastic sebaceous glands (Foley et al. 1998). Dominant-negative retinoic acid receptor mutant mice have a loss of cutaneous barrier function attributed to absence of the lipid multilamellar structures in the stratum corneum of the epidermis although no mention of the sebaceous glands or their function are made in Imakado et al. 1995.

The size of the sebaceous glands of the pilosebaceous unit varies with the stage of the mouse hair cycle. These glands are generally larger during telogen and smaller

during middle and late anagen (Chase et al. 1953; Chase 1954). To avoid misinterpretation, it is imperative to compare mutant and control age- and sex-matched mice at the same hair cycle stage.

## Primary Scarring Disorders of the Skin

Fibroblasts are spindle-shaped cells located throughout the dermis that produce collagen, fibronectin, and elastin. These cells also produce and release a variety of cytokines required for keratinocyte maintenance and differentiation (Green et al. 1979; Bell et al. 1983; Pittelkow 1994; Shipley et al. 1989).

The subcutaneous fascia, or stratum fibrosus (English and Munger 1994), is the layer of connective tissue located immediately below the panniculus carnosus muscle. This layer does not often remain attached when skin is removed at the time of necropsy, so it may be overlooked. This layer can become markedly thickened in some mouse mutations, such as tight skin (*Tsk*) (Green et al. 1976; Sundberg 1994j) and its phenotypic mimic, tight skin2 (*Tsk2*) Christner et al. 1995; Li et al. 1993; Christner et al. 1996). These mutant mice have been used as models for progressive systemic sclerosis (scleroderma). Aging *cpdm/cpdm* mice, a mutation with a progressive psoriasiform dermatitis, develop a severe diffuse scarring alopecia that is not a feature of *fsn/fsn*

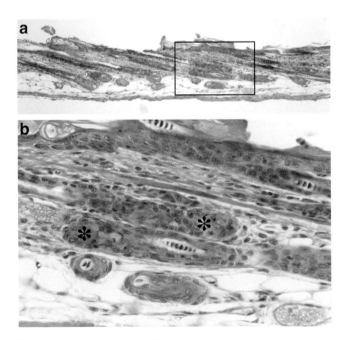

**FIGURE 14.10** Asebia2J mice (*ab^2J/ab^2J*) have hypoplastic sebaceous glands (*) that are associated with defects in hair fiber eruption. **b** is an enlargement of the boxed area in **a**.

mice, another mutation with psoriasiform dermatitis (Sundberg et al. 1995). This scarring phenotype can become common and very severe when the *cpdm/cpdm* mutation is on a hybrid background from a C57BL/Kaal × CAST/EiJ cross (Sundberg, personal observations). Other mouse mutations with severe and generalized alopecia throughout life may develop a scarring alopecia with loss of hair follicles, particularly when maintained on certain genetic backgrounds. For example, the nude (*Hfh11^{nu}/Hfh11^{nu}*) mouse can have a scarring alopecia with loss of follicles in mice over 1 year of age on the Nu/J inbred background (Sundberg and King 1996a). Abnormalities of the inner root sheath, as seen in the bare skin mutation (*Bsk*) (Fig. 14.11), or hypoplasia of the sebaceous glands in the asebia mutation

(*ab*), can result in an age-dependent loss of the hair follicle and scarring of the region where the follicle was located (Stenn et al. 1999; Sundberg et al. in press—b; Sundberg and King 1996b; Sundberg 1994c).

The C57BL/6 and its related strains, regardless of distributor, are prone to development of alopecia around the time of weaning that usually begins on the dorsal skin (Fig. 14.12). Early lesions consist of focal follicular dystrophy with production of an abnormal hair fiber. Dystrophic fibers can rupture and cause a local foreign body reaction. A subpopulation of these mice will develop various degrees of ulcerative dermatitis. When observed in isolation, the mice have actively engaged in self-mutilation behavior. This observation has led to the suggestion that these mice may serve as a model for Tourette's disorder or obsessive compulsive disorder (Sundberg et al. 1994b). Histologically, these lesions appear as ulcers at various stages of healing. There is usually marked pseudoepitheliomatous hyperplasia along the borders of the ulcers (Fig. 14.13). These ulcers heal by diffuse scarring, and hair does not regrow. Reports have suggested that this may be secondary to an autoimmune vasculitis (Andrews et al. 1994). Polyarteritis nodosa is a common background lesion in C57BL/6J mice but is rarely associated with skin lesions (J.P. Sundberg, unpublished observations). It is likely that the immune complex deposition reported is secondary to the extensive inflammation and constant traumatization of the wounds by affected mice. The severity and frequency of disease within a colony is dependent upon many epigenetic events, including, for example, diet, weaning times, and humidity. Experimentally, dietary restriction has been effective in reducing the incidence of disease in both wild-type and p53-null mice (Witt 1989; Perkins et al. 1998). Extensive clinical investigations are summarized on the Jackson Laboratory web site, which is updated periodically [*http://www.jax.org*].

It is likely that the list of mouse mutations with scarring alopecia or dermatitis will expand if other mouse mutations with structural defects of hair shafts are carefully evaluated at ages 18 months and older.

Experimentally induced wound healing has been used to stress mutant mouse skin to try to identify a function of a transgene or null mutation. The effects can be either exacerbation of the wound process or normal wound healing (Connolly et al. 1997; Kaiser et al. 1998).

## Hair Follicle Cycling and Structural Defects of Fibers

### HAIR CYCLE

The mouse loses and replaces hair in a regular cycle. The hair is shed in a wave from the head to the tail (Chase and Eaton 1959; Straile et al. 1961) rather than in a mosaic pattern as seen with humans and many

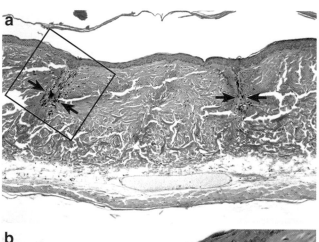

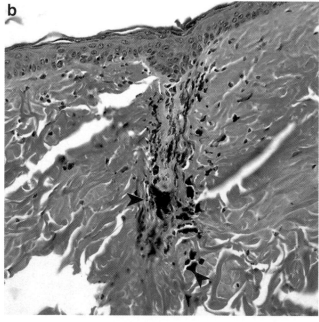

**FIGURE 14.11** A scarring alopecia is present in bareskin (*Bsk/+*) mice with fibrous tracts in the dermis (*arrows*, **a**) and pigmentary incontinence (*arrowheads*, **b**).

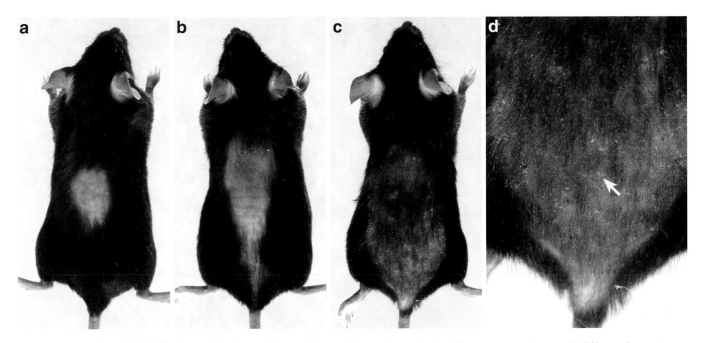

**FIGURE 14.12**   C57BL/6J dermatitis is an idiopathic condition characterized by a progressive and diffuse alopecia with scaling in the early phases (**a–c**). Magnification of mouse in **c** illustrates the fine scaling (*arrow*, **d**).

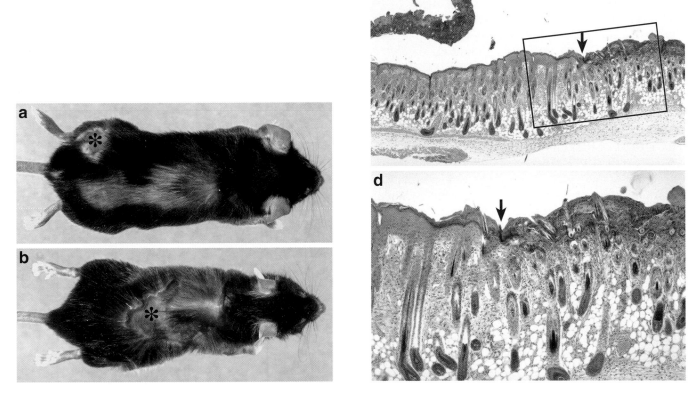

**FIGURE 14.13**   C57BL/6J mice also develop alopecia that may progress to ulceration (*, **a** and **b**) with subsequent scarring. The epidermis adjacent to an ulcer (*left of arrow*, **c** and **d**) undergoes pseudoepitheliomatous hyperplasia and heals by severe, diffuse dermal scarring.

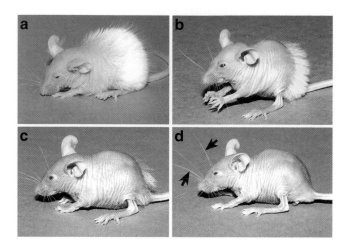

**FIGURE 14.14**   Hair cycle defects are exemplified by the progressive loss of hair at 2–3 weeks of age by mice with mutations at the hairless locus. This hairless mouse (HRS/J—*hr/hr*) lost all truncal hair during its third week of life (**a–d:** successive daily changes in the same mouse). Vibrissae (*arrow*) will eventually be lost as well.

domestic species (Chase 1955; Muller et al. 1983). This is most evident in mouse mutations at the hairless locus (*hr*) in which affected mice lose hair progressively from the head to the tail at the end of the first hair cycle because the second hair cycle is defective (Figs. 14.14, 14.15; Sundberg et al. 1991; Panteleyev et al. 1998b, 1998c). A number of spontaneous mutations have occurred at the hairless locus (Ahmad et al. 1998b, 1998c; Panteleyev et al. 1998a; Sundberg and Boggess 1998; Blandova et al. 1984; Garber 1952; Stelzner 1983). At least one mutation is due to the integration of a transgene (*hr*^TgN5053Mm^; Jones et al. 1993). Ornithine decarboxylase transgenic lines all are dominant phenotypic mimics of the rhino variation at the hairless locus (Megosh et al. 1995; Soler et al. 1995). As the human and other mammalian homologues of the hairless mutations are unraveled (Ahmad et al. 1998a, submitted; Christiano et al. 1998), identification of phenotypic mimics that involve additional genes becomes more useful.

   The mechanisms controlling the hair cycle have been and remain poorly understood. Targeted mutagenesis has opened many doors for investigating regulation of the hair cycle. Many genes are being identified that appear to be involved in hair follicle cycling and growth regulation (Suzuki et al. 1998; Botchkarev et al. 1998a, 1998b; Linder et al. 1997; Maurer et al. 1997; Paus et al. 1997, 1998; Schilli et al. 1997; Combates et al. 1997; Cotsarelis 1997; Matzuk et al. 1995; Guo et al. 1993, 1996; Chiang et al. 1999; Blessing et al. 1993). The first mutation that had an impact on the field of hair growth regulation involved creation of a fibroblast growth

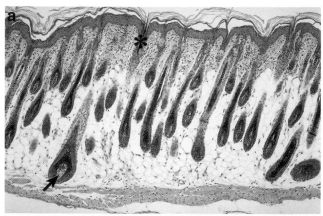

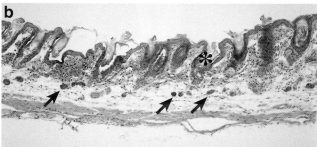

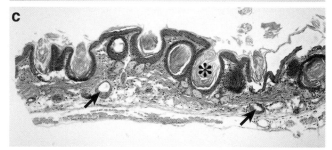

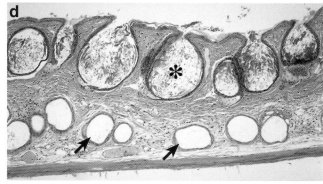

**FIGURE 14.15**   Hair cycle defects are also present in rhino, a mutation allelic with hairless. Rhino mice have normal hair follicle development at birth through the first hair cycle (**a**). In the second and subsequent hair cycles, the migration of the early anagen follicle fails to interact with the dermal papilla (*arrows*), resulting in an isolated dermal papilla and progressive dilation of the upper portion of the hair follicle (**b,** 3 weeks of age; **c,** 6 weeks of age). The follicular infundibulum (*) becomes plugged with cornified material and the residual dermal papilla becomes cystic and progressively enlarges (*, utricles, **d,** 6 months of age).

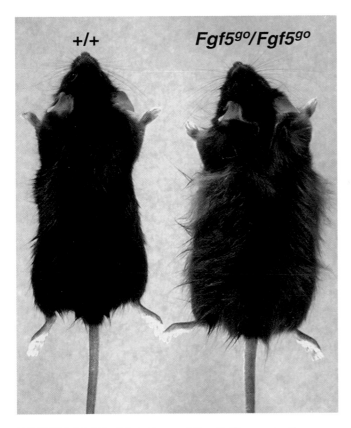

**FIGURE 14.16** Mutations of the *Fgf5* gene in the angora mouse (*Fgf5^go^/Fgf5^go^*) develop abnormally long hair compared with normal littermates (+/+) due to prolongation of the growth phase of the hair cycle.

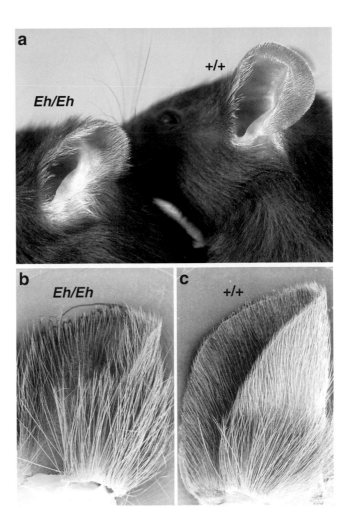

**FIGURE 14.17** The hairy ears mutation (*Eh*) results in small pinna with slightly longer hairs compared with normal littermate (+/+) (**a**). The *Eh* phenotype is best seen with scanning electron microscopy (**b, c**).

factor 5–null (*Fgf5*-null) mutation (Hebert et al. 1994). This null mutation of *Fgf5* turned out to be allelic with angora (Fig. 14.16), a mutant mouse that has a 3-day prolongation of the hair growth cycle resulting in long hair (Sundberg et al. 1997c). Other studies have implicated additional members of the FGF (fibroblast growth factor) family of cytokines (Rosenquist and Martin 1996; DuCros 1993; Danilenko et al. 1995). A new spontaneous mutation, juvenile alopecia (*jal*), may be due to a mutation in one of the fibroblast growth factor receptor genes (Sundberg et al. submitted). Other types of mutant mice with localized long hair that have yet to be defined include hairy ears (*Eh*) (Fig. 14.17; Davisson et al. 1990) and its phenotypic mimic, koala (*Koa*) (Ball and Peters 1989). Many other genes are being identified that modulate the hair cycle, but it is beyond the scope of this chapter to review them all.

## HAIR TEXTURE ABNORMALITIES

Mice may be essentially normal and have normal hair coats and cycles, but the texture of the hairs may be abnormal. The best-characterized hair texture mutations are the spontaneous mutations known as waved1

(*Tgfα^wa1^*) and waved2 (*Egfr^wa2^*) that are allelic with mutations at the *Tgfα* and *Egfr* loci as described above (Fig. 14.18; Mann et al. 1993; Luetteke et al. 1993, 1994). From the updated nomenclature, it is obvious what the mutated gene is for each allelic mutation. Null and dominant negative mutations of *Egfr* have proven to have more severe phenotypes (Miettinen et al. 1995; Threadgill et al. 1995; Sibilia and Wagner 1995; Murillas et al. 1995). New spontaneous mutations, tentatively called waved3 and waved4, may identify other genes involved in these biochemical cascades (J.P. Sundberg, unpublished data). Other hair types may also be waved or curly, such as curly whiskers (*cw*) (Sundberg 1994e).

## STRUCTURAL DEFECTS OF HAIR SHAFTS

Phenotypic deviants with alopecia, coat color changes, or oddly shaped hair represent the most obvious clinical features used for identifying potential new mutations.

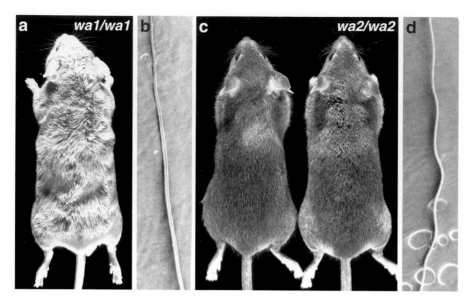

**FIGURE 14.18** Waved1 (*wa1*) (**a**, **b**) and its phenotypic mimic, waved2 (*wa2*) (**c**, **d**), are examples of mutant mice with hair texture defects. Scanning electron micrographs of hairs are shown (**b**, **d**).

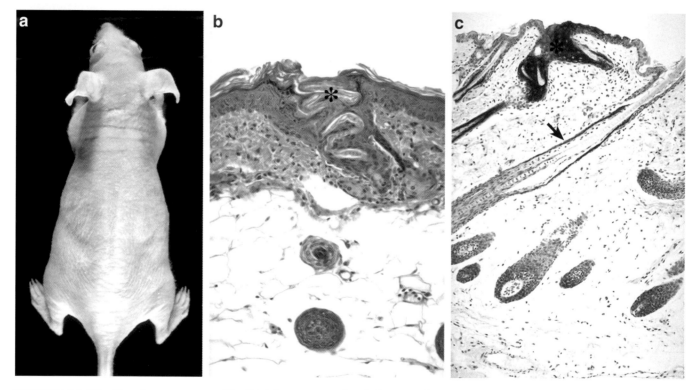

**FIGURE 14.19** The shaven mouse (*Sha/Sha*) is an example of alopecia due to structural defects in hair fibers (**a**). The twisting of hair fibers within the follicle (**b**) is associated with the alopecia in *Sha/Sha* mice. Not all hair fibers are twisted in young *Sha/Sha* mice. When hair fiber twisting occurs within the follicles, it results in outer root sheath hyperplasia associated with keratin 6 overexpression (*, **c**). Expression of keratin 6 in normal follicles is limited to the inner layer of the outer root sheath (*arrow*, **c**).

Therefore, these types of mouse mutations are disproportionately represented in colonies that maintain spontaneous mutations. As a result, a large variety of such mutations arising from changes in many different chromosomes are known and maintained. The majority of these mutations are due to structural defects of the hair shaft that result in weakness and breakage. These structural defects may be very subtle in histologic sections for forms of trichothiodystrophy such as ichthyosis (*ic*) (Itin et al. 1990) and xeroderma pigmentosa nulls (Berg et al. 1998) to nude (*Hfh11^{nu}*), shaven (*Sha*) (Fig. 14.19), or naked (*N*) in which shafts twist and deform within the

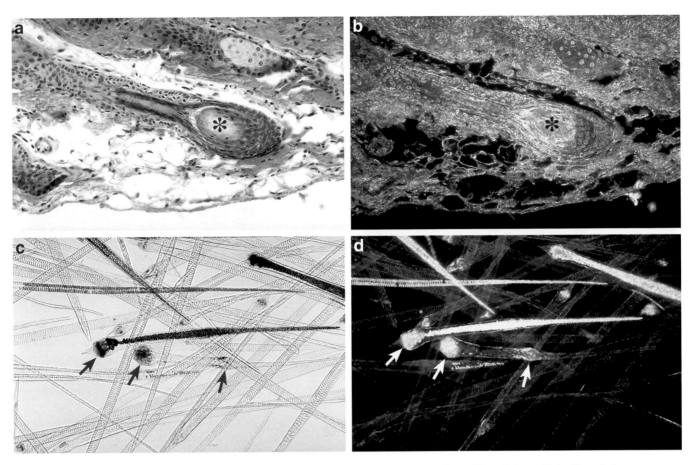

**FIGURE 14.20** Lanceolate hair (*lah/lah*) is another example of a structural hair fiber defect. Hair fiber defects occur periodically throughout anagen. Structural defects in hair fibers (*) may result in focal weak points that break when the hair emerges from the follicle, as is seen in *lah/lah* mice (**a,** light microscopy; **b,** same field by dark-field microscopy). The affected hairs have focal swellings at break points resembling a lance head, and occasionally multiple nodules can be observed (*arrows,* **c,** light microscopy; *arrows,* **d,** same field, dark-field).

follicle or as the shaft emerges (Sundberg 1994h; Hogan et al. 1995). Little is known about the specific biochemical defects that produce the structural defects in the follicles of these mutations. However, a number of targeted mutagenesis studies, in which the inactivated genes are known, are under investigation to define the role of these genes in structural integrity of hair fibers in the mouse and presumably in man (J.P. Sundberg, unpublished data). Others, such as the spontaneous mutations that occur in the lanceolate hair locus (*lah*), are located within a cluster of genes coding for adhesion molecules (Fig. 14.20; Montagutelli et al. 1996; Sundberg et al. 2000). The interaction between the hair keratins and these adhesion molecules are abnormal, resulting in periodic deformities in hair fibers (Sundberg et al. 2000). When these fibers emerge above the surface of the skin, they are rapidly broken off, resulting in the clinical appearance of alopecia.

## MISSING HAIR TYPES

Mice have a variety of distinct hair types depending upon their anatomic location (Table 14.1). Superficially, the obvious types are vibrissae (long, thick, tactile hairs on the head that are often incorrectly referred to as whiskers) and truncal or pelage hairs (those that cover most of the body). The pelage hairs, and probably other types, have at least four well-defined subtypes (Table 14.1; Dry 1926; Sundberg 1994h). It is therefore not surprising that mouse mutations may affect only one hair fiber/follicle type. Examples in which specific fiber types appear to be missing include long hair (Sweet et al. 1989), downless, crinkled, sleek, tabby (Fig. 14.9; Crocker and Cattanach 1979; Falconer et al. 1951; Sofaer 1969; Vielkind and Hardy 1996), hair patches (Shultz et al. 1991), and opossum (Mann 1963). Others may have reduced numbers of follicles (Sellheyer et al. 1993).

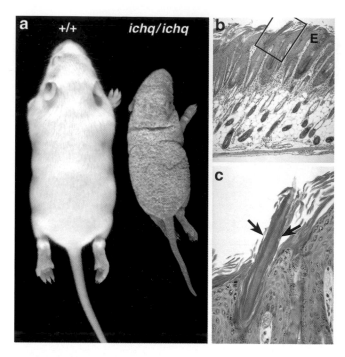

**FIGURE 14.21** The harlequin ichthyosis mutation (*ichq/ichq*) results in mice that develop a thick, scaly skin with essentially no inflammation (**a**). The epidermis (*E*) is markedly thickened (**b**) with densely packed cornified cell sheaths (*arrows*) forming around emerging hair fibers (**c**).

# Noninflammatory (Ichthyosiform and Keratodermas) Skin Diseases

The majority of mouse mutations with skin and hair defects have limited histological evidence of dermal inflammatory cell infiltrates. The exception is rare and widely scattered hair follicles perforated by structurally abnormal hair shafts that result in secondary, local, dermal inflammation. It is in this context that the term noninflammatory skin disease is used. Several mouse mutations have epidermal thickening (acanthosis and orthokeratosis) without marked dermal inflammation, making them likely candidates for some of the ichthyosiform dermatidites (Sundberg et al. 1995). These include ichthyosis (*ic*) (Carter and Phillips 1950; Itin et al. 1990; Sundberg and Pittelkow 1994), harlequin ichthyosis (*ichq*) (Fig. 14.21; Sundberg et al. 1997a), and flaky tail (*ft*) (Lane 1972; Rothnagel et al. 1994; Sundberg 1994f) as well as a number of new mutations currently being investigated.

Trichothiodystrophy is a relatively rare human disease that results in a marked decrease in the ultrahigh–sulfur-containing amino acids in the hair. Hairs become brittle and break off. Other, more serious cutaneous problems are found in the related disease xeroderma pigmentosa (Cleaver 1998). The spontaneous ichthyosis

mutant mouse was first reported in 1950 (Carter and Phillips 1950; Sundberg and Pittelkow 1994) and has been shown to have many similarities to human trichothiodystrophy (Itin et al. 1990).

Harlequin ichthyosis is a rare neonatal lethal human disease of which there are three distinct subtypes (Dale et al. 1990). This human disease is difficult to study because of the small numbers of patients and families available. Use of a high-resolution map to identify a spontaneous mutation in BALB/cJ mice (Fig. 14.21) that closely resembled type II human harlequin ichthyosis (Sundberg et al. 1997a) has led to the identification of candidate genes (B. Dale and J.P. Sundberg, unpublished data).

Flaky tail is another example of a spontaneous mutation that has been available for many decades that has an ichthyosiform phenotype early in life but clears as the mouse ages (Lane 1972). The mutation maps to mouse Chromosome 3 near the loricrin gene (Rothnagel et al. 1994). Loricrin is mutated in the human disease known as Vohwinkel's syndrome, a disease clinically similar to the mouse flaky tail mutation (Maestrini et al. 1996; Korge et al. 1997). Studies are in progress to define this mouse mutation and compare it with Vohwinkel's syndrome and other human ichthyosiform dermatitides.

Ichthyosiform dermatitis, nonspecific epidermal hyperplasia without dermal inflammation, is the phenotype of a number of transgenic and targeted mutagenesis developments and has to be viewed carefully until characterized and compared with various human and domestic animal diseases (Tarutani et al. 1997; Allen et al. 1996; Matsuki et al. 1998; Bickenbach et al. 1996; Fuchs et al. 1992; Andersen et al. 1997; Porter et al. 1998; Emami et al. 1994; Turksen et al. 1992; Werner et al. 1993; Sellheyer et al. 1993; Matzuk et al. 1995).

A few induced mutations have phenotypes essentially opposite that of ichthyosiform dermatitis. There is no inflammation, and the epidermis is unusually thin (Saltou et al. 1995; Hanada et al. 1998). These mutations may be useful for understanding the negative regulatory mechanisms of the epidermis.

# Inflammatory (Psoriasiform and Proliferative) Skin Diseases

Small numbers of lymphocytes and macrophages can be identified in normal skin. These cells function as part of the normal immune surveillance system but also produce a variety of cytokines important to the function of the skin. Large influxes of neutrophils into the dermis can result in intraepidermal abscesses and ulceration, as is the case with the motheaten and viable motheaten mutations (Green and Shultz 1975; Shultz et al. 1993; Shultz and Sundberg 1994). Single-gene mutations can

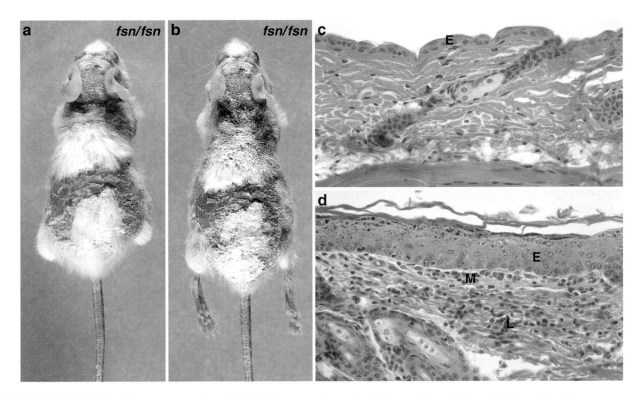

**FIGURE 14.22**   Flaky skin mutant mice (*fsn/fsn*) become alopecic with age (**a**) and have thick scales (**b**, same mouse shaved). Normal littermate control (+/+) skin (**c**) has a thin epidermis (*E*) with no dermal inflammation. Flaky skin mice (**d**) have a markedly thickened epidermis (*E*), mast cells (*M*) marginating under the basement membrane, and large numbers of lymphocytes (*L*) infiltrating into the dermis.

be used to identify the roles of some types of inflammatory cells in the skin when there are no other insults involved. For example, infiltration of some neutrophils but large numbers of lymphocytes can result in marked, abnormal proliferation of epidermal keratinocytes, as is the case with the flaky skin mutation (Figs. 14.22, 14.23; Morita et al. 1995; Pelsue et al. 1998; Sundberg et al. 1994a, 1997b). The chronic proliferative dermatitis mouse mutation looks histologically very similar to psoriasis; however, many of the infiltrating dermal cells are eosinophils (Fig. 14.24; HogenEsch et al. 1993, 1994, 1999). A number of induced mutations resemble psoriasis to various degrees, and current work will determine their usefulness as models (Blessing et al. 1996; Klement et al. 1996; Bullard et al. 1996; Uehira et al. 1998; Carroll et al. 1997). Transgenic mice that overexpress vascular endothelial growth factor in the skin have been used to study the dermal neovascularization associated with psoriasis without other dermatological features (Detmar et al. 1998).

Infiltration of lymphocytes in and around hair follicles can result in disruption of normal follicular function, resulting in the production of a defective hair shaft without significant hyperplasia of the epidermis, as is the case with alopecia areata in aging C3H/HeJ mice (Fig. 14.25; Sundberg et al. 1994c). This is not psoriasiform dermatitis since any epidermal hyperplasia is mild and secondary to the alopecia, not induced by the inflammation.

Mast cells are normally found widely scattered throughout the dermis of mouse skin. These cells have numerous basophilic granules of uniform size. The granules are metachromatic when stained with toluidine blue and stain nonspecifically with some immunohistochemical techniques (Bergstresser et al. 1984; Bolon and Calderwood-Mays 1988). The cytoplasmic granules are round to oval and are electron dense. Mast cells secrete a variety of vasoactive amines including serotonin, histamine, and heparin during inflammatory processes (Morrison et al. 1974; Sullivan et al. 1975; Theoharides and Douglas 1978; Greenberg and Burnstock 1983; Tharp 1991). A variety of mouse mutations affect the normal function and numbers of mast cells in the skin and other organs. The beige mutation (*Lyst^{bg}*) results in failure of cells containing cytoplasmic granules to degranulate normally as a result of a cytoskeletal defect (Sundberg 1994d). Mast cell numbers are decreased in dominant spotting (*W/W^v*) (Tharp 1997) or increased in the asebia (*ab*) (Brown and Hardy 1989) and flaky skin (*fsn*) mutations (Sundberg et al. 1997b; Pelsue et al. 1998). A reduced number of degranulated mast cells has been associated with dermal sclerosis in the tight skin (*Tsk*) mouse mutation (Walker et al. 1985, 1987, 1989).

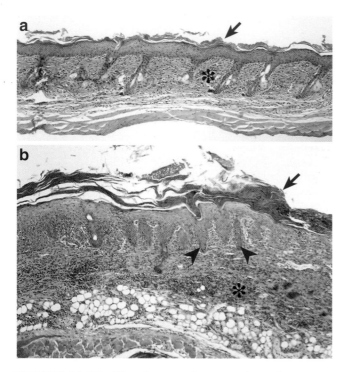

**FIGURE 14.23** The phenotypic expression of a mutation is dependent upon the inbred background and may be modified when a mutation is transferred to develop a congenic line or a double mutation. Changes in phenotype may be detected grossly by dramatic changes in hair color and texture or more subtly by changes in histologic features. Phenotypic changes due to different genetic backgrounds are easily detected in *fsn/fsn* mice when the phenotype on the CBy.A (**a**) is compared with an IL-4-null targeted mutation on a 129 background (**b**). Notice the psoriasiform hyperplasia (*arrowheads*), variation in scale formation (*arrows*), and dermal inflammation (*).

Hyperproliferation of the epidermis associated with dermal inflammation can be associated with ectoparasites (mange mites) or bacterial infections. These are common problems in mice not maintained in specific pathogen-free environments that are tightly controlled and monitored. The mites can be found if mice are examined carefully at both the gross and histologic levels (Weisbroth 1982). *Corynebacterium pseudodiphtheriticum* has been associated with a proliferative dermatitis in athymic (nude, *Hfh11^{nu}*) mice. Once a colony is infected, the disease can become endemic (Clifford et al. 1995).

## Papillomatous Skin Diseases

### EPIDERMAL RESPONSE TO INJURY

Response to injury of mouse epidermis (i.e., trauma or topical application of irritants), although similar to that of other mammals, has several species-specific features. Mouse skin does not respond to injury by producing rete

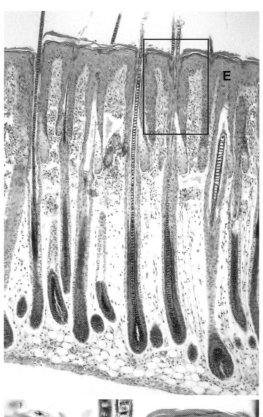

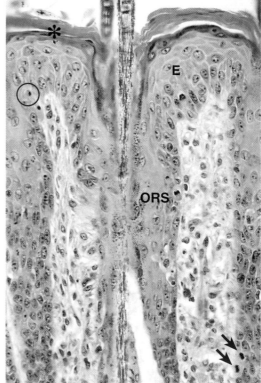

**FIGURE 14.24** Psoriasiform dermatitis is a feature of the chronic proliferative dermatitis (*cpdm/cpdm*) mutation in which there are numerous mitotic figures, thickening of the epidermis (*E*) and outer root sheaths (*ORS*), focal parakeratosis (*), scattered apoptotic cells (*circle*), and dermal inflammation.

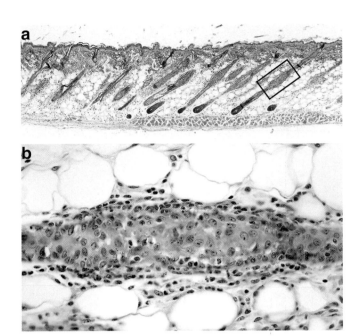

**FIGURE 14.25** Alopecia areata–like disease in A/J mice consists of disruption of anagen-stage follicles by a mixed, mostly lymphocytic, infiltrate in and around the middle of the follicle. The boxed area in (**a**) is magnified in (**b**) to show the infiltration in and around the follicle.

ridges. This lack of response may be a result of the high hair follicle density in this species. In addition, pseudoepitheliomatous hyperplasia adjacent to ulcers in mouse skin can become prominent enough to be misinterpreted as a papilloma (pseudopapilloma) at both gross and microscopic levels. Changes in keratin gene expression, as revealed by alterations in immunohistochemical staining patterns, cannot be used to differentiate these events. These biochemical features are discussed in greater detail elsewhere (Conti et al. 1996; Aldaz et al. 1988; Roop et al. 1988; Sundberg et al. 1994e).

Various degrees of acanthosis (thickening of the viable cell layers) and orthokeratosis (thickening of the stratum corneum without nuclear retention) may be focal (healing ulcer) or diffuse (irritant application). Chronic applications of irritants such as phorbol esters may produce foci of parakeratosis (retention of the keratinocyte nuclei into the stratum corneum). Terminal differentiation markers (loricrin, filaggrin, K1, and K10) are not identifiable in foci of parakeratosis (Conti et al. 1996; Sundberg et al. 1994e).

### TRANSGENICS AND TARGETED MUTAGENESIS NULLS FOR UNDERSTANDING CARCINOGENESIS

The study of two-stage carcinogenesis has utilized laboratory mice for decades. Selective breeding resulted in the development of mice sensitive to carcinogens (SENCAR mice), initially as an outbred strain. A number of inbred strains have now been developed including the super SENCAR, and SENCAR lines A, B, and C (Gimenez-Conti et al. 1992; Hennings et al. 1997; Slaga et al. 1996; Stern and Conti 1996; Stern et al. 1995, 1998). Identification of a single base pair mutation in the *Hras1* gene at codon 61 has led to the development of numerous transgenic lines using keratin promoters in the epidermis. Some of these transgenic lines are heavily used in carcinogenesis screening currently (Blanchard et al. 1998; Cannon et al. 1997; Hansen et al.1995; Hansen and Tennant 1994; Spalding et al. 1993; Thompson et al. 1998). As the processes of cutaneous chemical- and light-induced carcinogenesis are better understood, mutations in critical genes are being created to validate these observations. Some will increase while others decrease inducibility and types of tumors (Berg et al. 1998; Kiguchi et al. 1997).

### PAPILLOMAVIRUSES

Papillomaviruses naturally induce papillomas and squamous cell carcinomas in most mammalian species and birds (Sundberg et al. 1996b). Rodents are no exception. Wild mice have been reported to be infected with species-specific papillomaviruses (O'Banion et al. 1988; Sundberg et al. 1988), but none have been convincingly identified in laboratory mice (Sundberg et al. 1990b, 1997d). Regardless, a number of transgenic mice have been produced using the purported oncogenes of various human papillomaviruses driven by epidermal keratin promoters. Not all induce tumors of the skin, such as papillomas and squamous cell carcinomas, making this approach questionable (Doan et al. 1998; Frazer et al. 1995; Gulliver et al. 1997; Kondoh et al. 1995; Michelin et al. 1997; Arbeit 1996; Arbeit et al. 1996; Coussens et al. 1996; Herber et al. 1996).

## Bullous and Acantholytic Skin Diseases

The bullous or blistering skin diseases of mammals involve two groups of proteins, those involved in adhesion between cells (primarily desmosome and hemidesmosomal proteins) and those that make up the cytoskeletal system (primarily the keratin proteins). The first spontaneous mutation in the mouse that resulted in blister formation involved balding (*bal*) and subsequently two allelic mutations, balding-2J and balding-Pas (Montagutelli et al. 1997; Davisson et al. 1994; Sundberg 1994b). Concurrently, targeting mutagenesis studies for the desmoglein-3 gene created a fourth allelic mutation and verified that all four were due to mutations within the same gene with the same resulting phenotype (Figs. 14.26, 14.27; Koch et al. 1997).

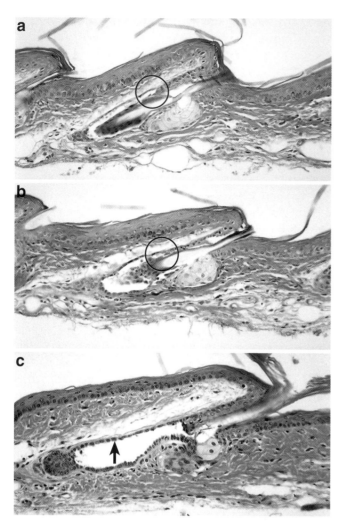

**FIGURE 14.26** Structural defects in hair fibers and follicles due to mutations in cellular adhesion molecules may produce blistering and alopecia. In mice with a null mutation of the desmoglein-3 gene, a member of the cadherin family of adhesion molecules, blisters due to acantholysis in the hair follicle cause hair loss. Progressive loss (**a–c**) of hair follicle structures in tail skin results from separation of the inner and outer root sheaths (circled areas), leaving a "tombstone" pattern (*arrow*) of remaining outer root sheath cells.

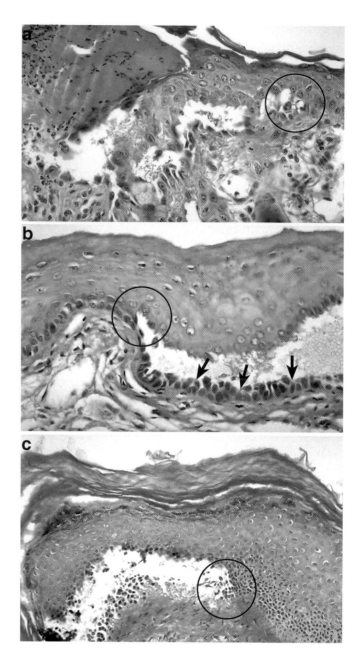

**FIGURE 14.27** The desmoglein-3–null mutant mice may also have blister formation in the interfollicular epidermis and at sites of constant friction, such as the eyelid margin (**a**), ventral tongue (**b**), and foot pads (**c**). Circled areas illustrate site of separation. Arrows highlight "tombstone" pattern of basal cells.

Desmoglein-3 is part of the adhesion molecule matrix that holds the basal cells to the rest of the epidermis or holds the root sheaths of the hair follicle together. With loss of adhesive function, these stuctures develop vesicles and blisters or entire loss of the follicle, respectively, leaving the classic "tombstonelike" appearance of the basal cells. Induced mutations in other structural genes have resulted in creations of additional blistering phenotypes. Overexpression of the desmoglein-3 gene resulted in disruption of desmosomes, where epidermis

was normally thick, but histologic changes included epidermal thickening with a marked increase in the strata spinosum and corneum (Allen et al. 1996). Pemphigus vulgaris is commonly considered to be an autoimmune disease due to production of autoantibodies against desmoglein-3. Recent studies indicate the disease can be subtyped by the types of autoantibodies produced to this and other desmogleins (Amagai et al. 1999).

Induced mutations have reproduced many of the blistering genodermatoses found in mammals. The targeted genes have included the adhesion molecules such as integrins (Dowling et al. 1996; van derNeut et al. 1996; Georges-Labouesse et al. 1996) and plectins (Andra et al. 1997) or various keratins (Vassar et al. 1991; Fuchs and Coulombe 1992; Lloyd et al. 1995; Chan et al. 1994; Guo et al. 1995; Paller 1996).

## Structural and Growth Defects in Nails

A nail covers the distal phalanx of each digit, providing both protection and a gripping device. The gross structure appears to be very different in the mouse compared with that in humans; however, the only real difference is that the nail plate in mice tends to be laterally compressed, forming a semiconical structure (resulting in a clawlike structure) rather than a flat plate. Sagittal sections reveal that, other than size, the anatomical structures forming the nail plate and maintaining its adhesion to the nail bed are essentially the same between the two species (Fleckman and Sundberg submitted). These structures are illustrated in Figure 14.28.

Defects of nails are common problems that occur in some human skin and hair diseases such as alopecia areata (Staughton 1988) and psoriasis (Scher 1991). Unless mouse nails have prominent abnormalities, subtle defects in nails are usually overlooked due to their small size. Spontaneous mutant mice such as hairless (*hr*) (Fig. 14.29) and ichthyosis (*ic*) have severely overgrown and curved nails (Sundberg et al. 1989; Sundberg and Pittelkow 1994; Sundberg 1994g; Fleckman et al. submitted). Similar gross changes are found in transgenic (Soler et al. 1995) and targeted mouse mutations (Jiang et al. 1998; Fleckman et al. submitted). Complete destruction of the nail plate and bed may occur as a sequelae to loss of sensation, as is the case with the nerve growth factor receptor null mutation (Fig. 14.30; Lee et al. 1992). These mice traumatize their nails when feeding on wire mesh or grooved metal feed hoppers embedded in the cage lids. As the mice age, the lesions result in complete loss of nails, with ulcerations and secondary infections of the remaining soft tissues. More subtle lesions, such as longitudinal striations on the nails of flaky skin (*fsn*) mice, may only be identified by scanning electron microscopy (Morita et al. 1995). Detailed evaluation of mouse nails should be included in routine characterization studies of new mutations, especially when nail defects are a feature of potentially analogous human diseases.

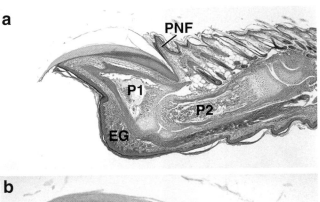

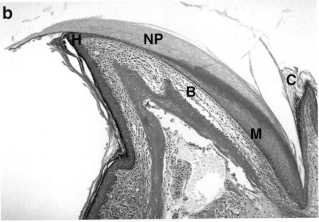

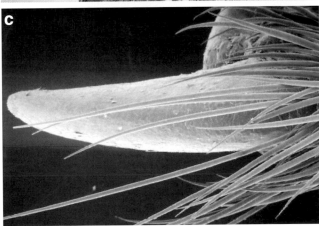

**FIGURE 14.28** The normal nail of a mouse is anatomically very similar in longitudinal section with the human nail. Low magnification of a sagittal section illustrates the bones, skin, and nail (**a**). Higher magnification (**b**) details the normal nail structures. Scanning electron microscopy (**c**) details the nail surface. *P1*, first phalanx; *P2*, second phalanx; *EG*, eccrine gland; *PNF*, proximal nail fold; *C*, cuticle; *NP*, nail plate, *M*, matrix; *B*, nail bed; *H*, hyponechium. (Baden 1987)

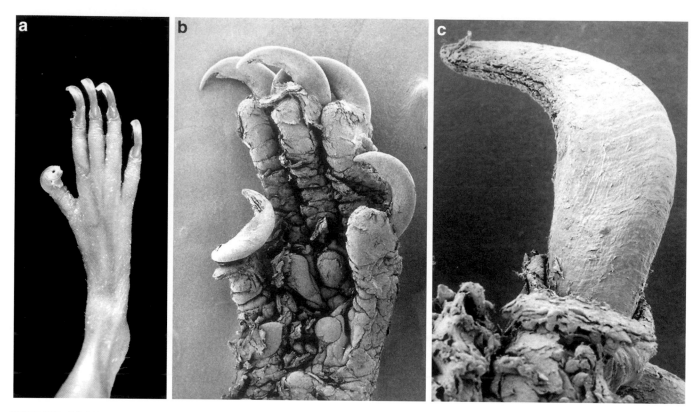

**FIGURE 14.29**  Structural abnormalities of mouse nails are often overlooked due to their small size. Rhino mutant mice (**a–c**), allelic mutations at the hairless locus, have nail plate overgrowth as a common phenotype. The nail abnormalities seen in the rhino and hairless mouse mimic those seen in ornithine decarboxylase transgenic mice.

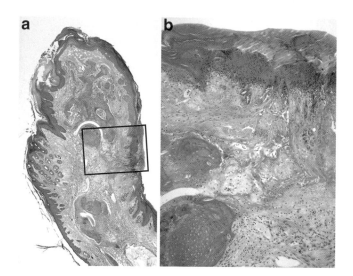

**FIGURE 14.30**  Defects in the sensory innervation of cutaneous structures, including joints, may result in subtle (nails) or gross (loss of a portion of an extremity) changes. In nerve growth factor receptor (*p75*) null mutant mice (Ngfr$^{tm1Jae}$), the loss of sensation results in trauma to the nail and distal phalanx with eventual loss of the entire nail structure with ulceration (**a, b**).

# REFERENCES

Ahmad, W., Haque, M.F., Brancolini, V., et al. 1998a. Alopecia universalis associated with a mutation in the human hairless gene. Science 279:720–724.

Ahmad, W., Panteleyev, A., Sundberg, J.P., et al. 1998b. Molecular basis for the rhino-8J mouse mutation: a nonsense mutation in the mouse hairless gene. Genomics 53:383–386.

Ahmad, W.A., Panteleyev, A.A., Henson-Apollonio, V., et al. 1998c. Molecular basis of a novel rhino (*hr$^{rh-CF4}$*) phenotype: a nonsense mutation in the mouse hairless gene. Exp. Dermatol. 7:298–301.

Ahmad, W., Ratteree M.S., Panteleyev, A.A., et al. Submitted. Evolution of the hairless phenotype in a Rhesus monkey. Proc. Natl. Acad. Sci. USA.

Aldaz, C.M., Conti, C.J., Larcher, F., et al. 1988. Sequential development of aneuploidy, keratin modifications, and gamma-glutamyltransferase in mouse skin papillomas. Cancer Res. 48:3253–3257.

Allen, E., Yu, Q.-C., Fuchs, E. 1996. Mice expressing a mutant desmosomal cadherin exhibit abnormalities in desmosomes, proliferation, and epidermal differentiation. J. Cell. Biol. 133:1367–1382.

Amagai, M., Tsunoda, K., Zillikens, D., et al. 1999. The clinical phenotype of pemphigus is defined by the anti-desmoglein autoantibody profile. J. Am. Acad. Dermatol. 40:167–170.

Andersen, B., Weinberg, W.C., Rennekampff, O., et al. 1997. Functions of the POU domain genes *Skn-1a/i* and *Tst-1/Oct-6/SCIP* in epidermal differentiation. Genes Dev. 11:1873–1884.

Andra, K., Lassmann, H., Bittner, R., et al. 1997. Targeted inactivation of plectin reveals essential function in maintaining the integrity of skin, muscle, and heart cytoarchitecture. Genes Dev. 11:3143–3156.

Andrews, A.G., Dysko, R.C., Spilman, S.C., et al. 1994. Immune complex vasculitis with secondary ulcerative dermatitis in aged C57BL/6NNia mice. Vet. Pathol. 31:293–300.

Arbeit, J.M. 1996. Transgenic models of epidermal neoplasia and multistage carcinogenesis. Cancer Surv. 26:7–34.

Arbeit, J.M., Howley, P.M., Hanahan, D. 1996. Chronic estrogen-induced cervical and vaginal squamous carcinogenesis in human papillomavirus type 16 transgenic mice. Proc. Natl. Acad. Sci. USA 93:2930–2935.

Baden, H.P. 1987. Diseases of the Hair and Nails. Chicago: Year Book Medical Publishers.

Bailin, T., Lee, S.-T., Spritz, R.A. 1996. Genomic organization and sequence of D12S53E (*Pmel 17*), the human homologue of the mouse silver (*si*) locus. J. Invest. Dermatol. 106:24–27.

Ball, S.T., Peters, J. 1989. Koala, a dominant mutation. Mouse News Lett. 83:163.

Barsh, G.S. 1996. The genetics of pigmentation: from fancy genes to complex traits. Trends Genet. 12:299–305.

Bayes, M., Hartung, A.J., Ezer, S., et al. 1998. The anhidrotic ectodermal dysplasia gene (EDA) undergoes alternative splicing and encodes ectodyplasin-A with deletion mutations in collagenous repeats. Hum. Mol. Genet. 7:1661–1669.

Beamer, W.G., Sweet, H.O., Bronson, R.T., et al. 1994. Adrenocortical dysplasia: a mouse model system for adrenocortical insufficiency. J. Endocrinol. 141:33–43.

Bechtold, L.S. 1999. Ultrastructural evaluation of mouse mutations. In: Sundberg, J.P., Boggess, D. (eds.), Systematic Approach to Evaluation of Mouse Mutations. Boca Raton, FL: CRC Press, pp. 121–129.

Bell, E., Sher, S., Hull, B., et al. 1983. The reconstruction of living skin. J. Invest. Dermatol. 81:2S–10S.

Berg, R.J.W., Ruven, H.J.T., Sands, A.T., et al. 1998. Defective global genome repair in XPC mice is associated with skin cancer susceptibility but not with sensitivity to UVB induced erythema and edema. J. Invest. Dermatol. 110:405–409.

Bergfeld, W.F. 1990. Noninflammatory reactions of the pilosebaceous unit and disorders of the hair shaft. In: Farmer, E.R., Hood, A.F. (eds.), Pathology of the Skin. Norwalk, CT: Appleton and Lange, pp. 941–951.

Bergstresser, P.R., Tigelaar, R.E., Tharp, M.D. 1984. Conjugated avidin identifies cutaneous rodent and human mast cells. J. Invest. Dermatol. 83:214–218.

Bickenbach, J.R., Longley, M.A., Bundman, D.S., et al. 1996. A transgenic mouse model that recapitulates the clinical features of both neonatal and adult forms of the skin disease epidermolytic hyperkeratosis. Differentiation 51:129–139.

Blanchard, K.T., Ball, D.J., Holden, H.E., et al. 1998. Dermal carcinogenicity in transgenic mice: relative responsiveness of male and female hemizygous and homozygous Tg.AC mice to 12-O-tetradecanoylphorbol 13-acetate (TPA) and benzene. Toxicol. Pathol. 26:541–547.

Blandova, Z.K., Beletskaya, L.V., Belyaev, D.L., et al. 1984. Genetic analysis and investigation of immunopathology in nude B10-*hr^{rhY}* mice. Immunology 3:25–28.

Blessing, M., Nanney, L.B., King, L.E., et al. 1993. Transgenic mice as a model to study the role of TGF-β-related molecules in hair follicles. Genes Dev. 7:204–215.

Blessing, M., Schirmacher, P., Kaiser, S. 1996. Overexpression of bone morphogenetic protein-6 (BMP-6) in the epidermis of transgenic mice: inhibition or stimulation of proliferation depending on the pattern of transgene expression and formation of psoriatic lesions. J. Cell Biol. 135:227–239.

Bloom, W., Fawcett, D.W. 1968. Textbook of Histology. Philadelphia: WB Saunders.

Bolon, B., Calderwood-Mays, M.B. 1988. Conjugated avidin-peroxidase as a stain for mast cell tumors. Vet. Pathol. 25:523–525.

Botchkarev, V.A., Botchkarev, N.V., Albers, K.M., et al. 1998a. Neurotrophin-3 involvement in the regulation of hair follicle morphogenesis. J. Invest. Dermatol. 111:279–285.

Botchkarev, V.A., Welker, P., Albers, K.M., et al. 1998b. A new role for neurotrophin-3. Involvement in the regulation of hair follicle regression (catagen). Am. J. Pathol. 153:785–799.

Briggs, O.M. 1987. Practical small animal dermatology. I. Structure and function of the skin. J. S. Afr. Vet. Assoc. 4:229–231.

Brown, W.R., Hardy, M.H. 1989. Mast cells in asebia mouse skin. J. Invest. Dermatol. 93:708.

Bullard, D.C., Scharffetter-Kochanek, K., McArthur, M.J., et al. 1996. A polygenic mouse model of psoriasiform skin disease in CD18-deficient mice. Proc. Natl. Acad. Sci. USA 93:2116–2121.

Calhoun, M.L., Stinson, A.W. 1981. Integument. In Dellmann, H.D., Brown, E.M. (eds.), Textbook of Veterinary Histology. Philadelphia: Lea and Febiger, pp. 378–411.

Cannon, R.E., Spalding, J.W., Trempus, C.S., et al. 1997. Kinetics of wound-induced *v-Ha-ras* transgene expression and papilloma development in transgenic Tg.AC mice. Mol. Carcinogen. 20:108–114.

Carroll, J.M., Crompton, T., Seery, J.P., et al. 1997. Transgenic mice expressing IFN-γ in the epidermis have eczema, hair hypopigmentation, and hair loss. J. Invest. Dermatol. 108:412–422.

Carter, T.C., Phillips, R.S. 1950. Ichthyosis, a new recessive mutation in the house mouse. J. Hered. 41:297–300.

Chan, Y.-M., Anton-Lamprecht, I., Yu, Q.-C., et al. 1994. A human keratin 14 "knockout": the absence of K14 leads to severe epidermolysis bullosa simplex and a function for an intermediate filament protein. Genes Dev. 8:2574–2587.

Chase, H.B. 1954. Growth of the hair. Physiol. Rev. 34:113–126.

Chase, H.B. 1955. The physiology and histochemistry of hair growth. J. Soc. Cosmetic. Chem. 6:9–14.

Chase, H.B., Eaton, G.J. 1959. The growth of hair follicles in waves. Ann. N.Y. Acad. Sci. 83:365–368.

Chase, H.B., Rauch, H., Smith, V.W. 1951. Critical stages of hair development and pigmentation in the mouse. Physiol. Zool. 24:1–10.

Chase, H.B., Montagna, W., Malone, J.D. 1953. Changes in the skin in relation to the hair growth cycle. Anat. Rec. 116:75–82.

Chiang, C., Swan, R.Z., Grachtchouk, M., et al. 1999. Essential role for sonic hedgehog during hair follicle morphogenesis. Dev. Biol. 205:1–9.

Christiano, A.M., Irvine, A., McGrath, J.A., et al. 1998. Molecular pathology of papular atrichia: hairless gene mutations in humans and rhino mice. In Third International Alopecia Areata Workshop. Washington, DC.

Christner, P.J., Peters, J., Hawkins, D., et al. 1995. The tight skin 2 mouse. An animal model of scleroderma displaying cutaneous fibrosis and mononuclear cell infiltration. Arthritis Rheum. 38:1791–1798.

Christner, P.J., Siracusa, L.D., Hawkins, D.F., et al. 1996. A high resolution linkage map of the tight skin 2 (*Tsk2*) locus: a mouse model for scleroderma (SSc) and other cutaneous fibrotic diseases. Mamm. Genome 7:610–612.

Claxton, J.H. 1966. The hair follicle group in mice. Anat. Rec. 154:195–208.

Cleaver, J.E. 1998. Hair today, gone tomorrow: transgenic mice with human repair deficient hair disease. Cell 93:1099–1102.

Clifford, C., Walton, B., Reed, T., et al. 1995. Hyperkeratosis in athymic nude mice caused by a coryneform bacterium: microbiology, transmission, clinical signs, and pathology. Lab. Anim. Sci. 45:131–139.

Colucci-Guyon, E., Portier, M.-M., Dunia, I., et al. 1994. Mice lacking vimentin develop and reproduce without an obvious phenotype. Cell 79:679–694.

Combates, N.J., Chuong, C.-M., Stenn, K.S., et al. 1997. Expression of two Ig family adhesion molecules in the murine hair cycle: DCC in the bulge epithelia and NCAM in the follicular papilla. J. Invest. Dermatol. 109:672–678.

Connolly, A.J., Suh, D.Y., Hunt, T.K., et al. 1997. Mice lacking the thrombin receptor, PAR1, have normal skin wound healing. Am. J. Pathol. 151:1199–1204.

Conti, C., Binder, R., Sundberg, J.P. 1996. Histological, biochemical, and molecular evolution of skin lesions using a two-stage chemical carcinogenesis protocol. In Mohr, U., Dungworth, D.L., Capen, C.C., et al. (eds.), Pathobiology of the Aging Mouse, vol. 2. ILSI Press: Washington, DC.

Cotsarelis, G. 1997. The hair follicle: dying for attention. Am. J. Pathol. 151:1505–1509.

Coussens, L.M., Hanahan, D., Arbeit, J.M. 1996. Genetic predisposition and parameters of malignant progression in K14-HPV16 transgenic mice. Am. J. Pathol. 149:1899–1917.

Crocker, M., Cattanach, B.M. 1979. The genetics of Sleek: a possible regulatory mutation of the tabby-crinkled-downless syndrome. Genet. Res. 34:231–238.

Dale, B.A., Holbrook, K.A., Fleckman, P., et al. 1990. Heterogeneity in harlequin ichthyosis, an inborn error of epidermal keratinization: Variable morphology and structural protein expression and a defect in lamellar granules. J. Invest. Dermatol. 94:6–18.

Danilenko, D.M., Ring, B.D., Yanagihara, D., et al. 1995. Keratinocyte growth factor is an important endogenous mediator of hair follicle growth, development, and differentiation. Normalization of the *nu/nu* follicular differentiation defect and amelioration of chemotherapy-induced alopecia. Am. J. Pathol. 147:145–154.

Davisson, M.T., Roderick, T.H., Akeson, E.C., et al. 1990. The hairy ears (*Eh*) mutation is closely associated with a chromosomal rearrangement in mouse chromosome 15. Genet. Res. 56:167–178.

Davisson, M.T., Cook, S.A., Johnson, K.R., et al. 1994. Balding: a new mutation on mouse Chromosome 18 causing hair loss and immunological defects. J. Hered. 85:134–136.

Detmar, M., Brown, L.F., Schon, M.P., et al. 1998. Increasing microvascular density and enhanced leukocyte rolling and adhesion in the skin of VEGF transgenic mice. J. Invest. Dermatol. 111:1–6.

Doan, T., Chambers, M., Street, M., et al. 1998. Mice expressing the E7 oncogene of HPV16 in epithelium show central tolerance, and evidence of peripheral anergising tolerance, to E7-encoded cytotoxic T lymphocyte epitopes. Virology 244:352–364.

Dowling, J., Yu, Q.-C., Fuchs, E. 1996. B4 integrin is required for hemidesmosome formation, cell adhesion and cell survival. J. Cell. Biol. 134:559–572.

Dry, F.W. 1926. The coat of the mouse (*Mus musculus*). J. Genet. 16:287–340.

DuCros, D.L. 1993. Fibroblast growth factor influences the development and cycling of murine hair follicles. Dev. Biol. 156:444–453.

Eilersten, K.J., Tran, T., Sundberg, J.P., et al. 2000. High resolution genetic and physical mapping of the mouse asebia locus: a key gene locus for sebaceous gland differentiation. J. Exp. Anim. Sci. 40:165–170.

Emami, S., Hanley, K.P., Esterly, N.B., et al. 1994. X-linked dominant ichthyosis with peroxisomal deficiency: an ultrastructural and ultracytochemical study of the Conradi-Hunermann syndrome and its murine homologue, the bare patches mouse. Arch. Dermatol. 130:325–336.

English, K.B., Munger, B.L. 1994. Normal development of the skin and subcutis of the albino rat. In Mohr, U., Dungworth, D.L., Capen, C.C. (eds.), Pathobiology of the Aging Rat. Washington, DC: ILSI Press, pp. 363–389.

Falconer, D.S., Fraser, A.S., King, J.W.B. 1951. The genetics and development of "crinkled": a new mutant in the house mouse. J. Genet. 50:324–344.

Feldman, D.B., Seely, J.C. 1988. Necropsy Guide to Rodents and the Rabbit. Boca Raton, FL: CRC Press.

Ferguson, B.M., Brockorff, N., Formstone, E., et al. 1997. Cloning of Tabby, the murine homolog of the human EDA gene: evidence for a membrane-associated protein with a short collagenous domain. Hum. Mol. Genet. 6:1589–1594.

Fleckman, P., Sundberg, J.P. Submitted. Anatomy of mouse and human nails. Exp. Dermatol.

Fleckman, P., Raymond, J.T., Hogan, M.E., et al. Submitted. Nail defects in mutant mice. Exp. Dermatol.

Foley, J., Longely, J., Wysolmerski, J.J., et al. 1998. PTHrP regulates epidermal differentiation in adult mice. J. Invest. Dermatol. 111:1122–1128.

Fraser, A.S. 1951. Growth of the mouse coat. J. Exp. Zool. 117:15–29.

Frazer, I.H., Leippe, D.M., Dunn, L.A., et al. 1995. Immunologic responses in human papillomavirus 16 E6/E7-transgenic mice to E7 protein correlate with the presence of skin disease. Cancer Res. 55:2635–2639.

Fuchs, E., Coulombe, P.A. 1992. Of mice and men: genetic skin diseases of keratin. Cell 69:899–902.

Fuchs, E., Esteves, R.A., Coulombe, P.A. 1992. Transgenic mice expressing a mutant keratin 10 gene reveal the likely genetic basis for epidermolytic hyperkeratosis. Proc. Natl. Acad. Sci. USA 89:6906–6910.

Garber, E.D. 1952. Bald, a second allele of hairless in the house mouse. J. Hered. 43:45–46.

Georges-Labouesse, E., Messaddeq, N., Yehia, G., et al. 1996. Absence of integrin α6 leads to epidermolysis bullosa and neonatal death in mice. Nat. Genet. 13:370–373.

Gimenez-Conti, I.B., Bianchi, A.B., Fischer, S.M., et al. 1992. Dissociation of sensitivities to tumor promotion and progression in outbred and inbred SENCAR mice. Cancer Res. 52:3432–3435.

Goldsmith, L.A. 1990. My organ is bigger than your organ. Arch. Dermatol. 126:301–302.

Green, H., Kehinde, O., Thomas, J. 1979. Growth of cultured human epidermal cells into multiple epithelia suitable for grafting. Proc. Natl. Acad. Sci. USA 76:5665–5668.

Green, M.C. 1989. Catalog of mutant genes and polymorphic loci. In: Lyons, M.F., Searle, A.G. (eds.), Genetic Variants and Strains of the Laboratory Mouse, 2nd ed. Oxford: Oxford University Press, pp. 12–403.

Green, M.C., Shultz, L.D. 1975. Motheaten, an immunodeficient mutant of the mouse. I. Genetics and pathology. J. Hered. 66:250–258.

Green, M.C., Witham, B.A. 1991. Handbook on Genetically Standardized Jax Mice, 4th ed. Bar Harbor: The Jackson Laboratory.

Green, M.C., Sweet, H.O., Bunker, L.E. 1976. Tight-skin, a new mutation of the mouse causing excessive growth of connective tissue and skeleton. Am. J. Pathol. 82:493–512.

Greenberg, G., Burnstock, G. 1983. A novel cell-to-cell interaction between mast cells and other cell types. Exp. Cell. Res. 147:1–13.

Gruneberg, H. 1943. The development of some external features in mouse embryos. J. Hered. 34:88–92.

Gulliver, G.A., Herber, R.L., Liem, A., et al. 1997. Both conserved region 1 (CR1) and CR2 of the human papillomavirus type 16 E7 oncogene are required for induction of epidermal hyperplasia and tumor formation in transgenic mice. J. Virol. 71:5905–5914.

Guo, L., Yu, Q.-C., Fuchs, E. 1993. Targeting expression of keratinocyte growth factor to keratinocytes elicits striking changes in epithelial differentiation in transgenic mice. EMBO J. 12:973–986.

Guo, L., Degenstein, L., Dowling, J., et al. 1995. Gene targeting of BPAG1: abnormalities in mechanical strength and cell migration in stratified epithelia and neurologic degeneration. Cell 81:233–243.

Guo, L., Degenestein, L., Fuchs, E. 1996. Keratinocyte growth factor is required for hair development but not for wound healing. Genes Dev. 10:165–175.

Hanada, K., Sawamura, D., Hashimoto, I., et al. 1998. Epidermal proliferation of the skin in metallothionein-null mice. J. Invest. Dermatol. 110:259-262.

Hansen, L.A., Tennant, R. 1994. Focal transgene expression associated with papilloma development in v-Ha-ras-transgenic TG.AC mice. Mol. Carcinog. 9:143–154.

Hansen, L.A., Spalding, J.W., French, J.E., et al. 1995. A transgenic mouse model (TG.AC) for skin carcinogenesis: inducible transgene expression as a second critical event. Prog. Clin. Biol. Res. 391:223–235.

Hardy, M.H. 1949. The development of mouse hair in vitro with some observations on pigmentation. J. Anat. 83:364–384.

Headington, J.T. 1984. Transverse microscopic anatomy of the human scalp. A basis for a morphologic approach to disorders of the hair cycle. Arch. Dermatol. 120:449–456.

Hebert, J.M., Rosenquist, T., Gotz, J., et al. 1994. Fgf5 as a regulator of the hair growth cycle: evidence from targeted and spontaneous mutations. Cell 78:1017–1025.

Hennings, H., Lowry, D.T., Yuspa, S.H., et al. 1997. New strains of inbred SENCAR mice with increased susceptibility to induction of papillomas and squamous cell carcinomas in skin. Mol. Carcinog. 20:143–150.

Herber, R., Liem, A., Pitot, H., et al. 1996. Squamous epithelial hyperplasia and carcinoma in mice transgenic for the human papillomavirus type 16 E7 oncogene. J. Virol. 70:1873–1881.

Hogan, M.E., King, L.E., Sundberg, J.P. 1995. Defects of pelage hairs in 20 mouse mutations. J. Invest. Dermatol. 104:31s–32s.

HogenEsch, H., Gijbels, M., Offerman, E., et al. 1993. A spontaneous mutation characterized by chronic proliferative dermatitis in C57BL mice. Am. J. Pathol. 143:972–982.

HogenEsch, H., Gijbels, M.J.J., Zurcher, C. 1994. The chronic proliferative dermatitis (cpd) mutation, Chromosome? In: Sundberg, J.P. (ed.), Handbook of Mouse Mutations with Skin and Hair Abnormalities: Animal Models and Biomedical Tools. Boca Raton, FL: CRC Press, pp. 217–220.

HogenEsch, H., Boggess, D., Sundberg, J.P. 1999. Changes in keratin and filaggrin expression in the skin of chronic proliferative dermatitis (cpdm) mutant mice. Pathobiology 67:45–50.

Holbrook, K.A. 1991. Structure and function of the developing human skin. In: Goldsmith, L.A. (ed.), Physiology, Biochemistry, and Molecular Biology of the Skin, 2nd ed. New York: Oxford University Press, pp. 63–110.

Holbrook, K.A., Smith, L.T. 1993. Morphology and connective tissue: structure of the skin and tendon. In: Royce, P.M., Steinmann, B. (eds.), Connective Tissue and Its Heritable Disorders: Molecular, Genetic, and Medical Aspects. New York: Wiley-Liss, pp. 51–71.

Imakado, S., Bickenbach, J.R., Bundman, D.S., et al. 1995. Targeting expression of a dominant-negative retinoic acid receptor mutant in the epidermis of transgenic mice results in loss of barrier function. Genes Dev. 9:317–329.

Ishida-Yamamoto, A., Tanaka, H., Nakane, H., et al. 1998. Inherited disorders of epidermal keratinization. J. Dermatol. Sci. 18:139–154.

Itin, P.H., Sundberg, J.P., Dunstan, R.W., et al. 1990. Ichthyosis mouse-structural and biochemical analysis of the hair defect. J. Invest. Dermatol. 94:537.

Jamieson, W.A. 1888. Diseases of the Skin. Philadelphia: JB Lippincott Company, p. 546.

Jiang, R., Lan, Y., Norton, C.R., et al. 1998. The slug gene is not essential for mesoderm or neural crest development in mice. Dev. Biol. 198:277–285.

Johnson, K.R., Sweet, H.O., Donahue, L.R., et al. 1998. A new spontaneous mouse mutation of Hoxd13 with a polyalanine expansion and phenotype similar to human synpolydactyly. Hum. Mol. Genet. 7:1033–1038.

Jones, J.M., Elder, J.T., Simin, K., et al. 1993. Insertional mutation of the hairless locus on mouse chromosome 14. Mamm. Genome 4:639–643.

Kaiser, S., Schirmacher, P., Philipp, A., et al. 1998. Induction of bone morphogenetic protein-6 in skin wounds. Delayed reepithelialization and scar formation in BMP-6 overexpressing transgenic mice. J. Invest. Dermatol. 111:1145–1152.

Keeney, D.S. 1999. Radiolabeled cRNA in situ hybridization. In: Sundberg, J.P., Boggess, D. (eds.), Systematic Approach to Evaluation of Mouse Mutations. Boca Raton, FL: CRC Press, pp. 145–167.

Kiguchi, K., Beltran, L., Dubowski, A., et al. 1997. Analysis of the ability of 12-O-tetradecanoylphorbol-13-acetate to induce epidermal hyperplasia, transforming growth factor-α, and skin tumor promotion in wa-1 mice. J. Invest. Dermatol. 108:784–791.

Klement, J.F., Rice, N.R., Car, B.D., et al. 1996. IkBα deficiency results in a sustained NF-kβ response and severe widespread dermatitis in mice. Mol. Cell. Biol. 16:2341–2349.

Koch, P.J., Mahoney, M.G., Ishikawa, H., et al. 1997. Targeted disruption of the pemphigus vulgaris antigen (desmoglein 3) gene in mice causes loss of keratinocyte cell adhesion with a phenotype similar to pemphigus vulgaris. J. Cell. Biol. 137:1091–1102.

Kondoh, G., Li, Q., Pan, J., et al. 1995. Transgenic models for papillomavirus-associated multistep carcinogenesis. Intervirology 38:181–186.

Korge, B.P., Ishida-Yamamoto, A., Punter, C., et al. 1997. Loricrin mutation in Vohwinkel's keratoderma is unique to the variant with ichthyosis. J. Invest. Dermatol. 109:604–610.

Lamoreux, M.L., Zhou, B.K., Rosemblat, S., et al. 1995. The pinkeyed-dilution protein and the eumelanin/pheomelanin switch: in support of a unifying hypothesis. Pigment Cell Res. 8:263–270.

Lane, P. 1972. Two new mutations in linkage group XVI of the house mouse. Flaky tail and varitint-waddler-J. J. Hered. 63:135–140.

Lee, K.-F., Li, E., Huber, J., et al. 1992. Targeted mutation of the gene encoding the low affinity NGF receptor p75 leads to deficits in the peripheral sensory nervous system. Cell 69:737–749.

Li, X., Pereira, L., Zhang, H., et al. 1993. Fibrillin genes map to regions of conserved mouse/human synteny on mouse chromosomes 2 and 18. Genomics 18:667–672.

Limberg, B.J., Bascom, C.C. 1999. In situ hybridization with non-radiolabeled probes. In: Sundberg, J.P., Boggess, D. (eds.), Systematic Approach to Evaluation of Mouse Mutations. Boca Raton, FL: CRC Press, pp. 169–178.

Linder, G., Botchkarev, V.A., Botchkarev, N.V., et al. 1997. Analysis of apoptosis during hair follicle regression. Am. J. Pathol. 151:1601–1617.

Lloyd, C., Yu, Q.-C., Cheng, J., et al. 1995. The basal keratin network of stratified squamous epithelia: defining K15 function in the absence of K14. J. Cell. Biol. 129:1329–1344.

Luetteke, N.C., Qiu, T.H., Peiffer, R.L., et al. 1993. TGF deficiency results in hair follicle and eye abnormalities in targeted and waved-1 mice. Cell 73:263–278.

Luetteke, N.C., Phillips, H.K., Qiu, T.H., et al. 1994. The mouse waved-2 phenotype results from a point mutation in the EGF receptor tyrosine kinase. Genes Dev. 8:399–413.

Maestrini, E., Monaco, A., McGrath, J., et al. 1996. A molecular defect in loricrin, the major component of the cornified cell envelope, underlies Vohwinkel's syndrome. Nat. Genet. 13:70–77.

Mann, G.B., Fowler, K.J., Gabriel, A., et al. 1993. Mice with a null mutation of the TGF gene have abnormal skin architecture, wavy hair, and curly whiskers and often develop corneal inflammation. Cell 73:249–261.

Mann, S.J. 1962. Prenatal formation of hair follicle types. Anat. Rec. 144:135–142.

Mann, S.J. 1963. The phenogenetics of hair mutants in the house mouse: opossum and ragged. Genet. Res. 4:1–11.

Matzuk, M.M., Lu, N., Vogel, H., et al. 1995. Multiple defects and perinatal death in mice deficient in follistatin. Nature 374:360–363.

Matsuki, M., Yamashita, F., Ishida-Yamamoto, A., et al. 1998. Defective stratum corneum and early neonatal death in mice lacking the gene for transglutaminase 1 (keratinocyte transglutaminase). Proc. Natl. Acad. Sci. USA 95:1044–1049.

Maurer, M., Handjiski, B., Paus, R. 1997. Hair growth modulation by topical immunophilin ligands. Am. J. Pathol. 150:1433–1441.

Megosh, L., Gilmour, S.K., Rosson, D., et al. 1995. Increased frequency of spontaneous skin tumors in transgenic mice which overexpress ornithine decarboxylase. Cancer Res. 55:4205–4209.

Michelin, D., Gissmann, L., Street, D., et al. 1997. Regulation of human papillomavirus type 18 *in vivo*: effects of estrogen and progesterone in transgenic mice. Gynecol. Oncol. 66:202–208.

Miettinen, P.J., Berger, J.E., Meneses, J., et al. 1995. Epidermal immaturity and multiorgan failure in mice lacking epidermal growth factor receptor. Nature 376:337–341.

Montagutelli, X., Hogan, M.E., Aubin, G., et al. 1996. Lanceolate hair (*lah*): a recessive mouse mutation with alopecia and abnormal hair. J. Invest. Dermatol. 107:20–25.

Montagutelli, X., Lalouette, A., Boulouis, H.J., et al. 1997. Vesicle formation and follicular root sheath separation in mice homozygous for deleterious alleles at the mouse balding (*bal*) locus. J. Invest. Dermatol. 109:324–328.

Montreal, A.W., Zonana, J., Ferguson, B. 1998. Identification of a new splice form of the EDA1 gene permits detection of nearly all X-linked hypohidrotic ectodermal dysplasia mutations. Am. J. Hum. Genet. 63:380–389.

Morita, K., Hogan, M.E., Nanney, L.B., et al. 1995. Cutaneous ultrastructural features of the flaky skin (*fsn/fsn*) mouse mutation. J. Dermatol. 22:385–395.

Morrison, D.C., Rosser, J.F., Henson, P.M., et al. 1974. Activation of rat mast cells by low molecular weight stimuli. J. Immunol. 112:573–582.

Muller, G.H., Kirk, R.W., Scott, D.W. 1983. Small Animal Dermatology. 3rd ed. Philadelphia: WB Saunders.

Munger, B.L., Brusilow, S.W. 1971. The histophysiology of rat plantar sweat glands. Anat. Rec. 169:1–22.

Murillas, R., Larcher, F., Conti, C.J., et al. 1995. Expression of a dominant negative mutant of epidermal growth factor receptor in the epidermis of transgenic mice elicits striking alterations in hair follicle development and skin structure. EMBO J. 14:5216–5223.

Nanney, L.B., Sundberg, J.P., King, L.E. 1996. Increased epidermal growth factor receptor in *fsn/fsn* mice. J. Invest. Dermatol. 106:1169–1174.

O'Banion, M.K., Reichmann, M.E., Sundberg, J.P. 1988. Cloning and characterization of a papillomavirus associated with papillomas and carcinomas in the European harvest mouse (*Micromys minutus*). J. Virol. 62:226–233.

Oliver, C., Essner, E. 1973. Distribution of anomalous lysosomes in the beige mouse. A homologue of Chediak-Higashi syndrome. J. Histochem. Cytochem. 21:218–228.

Oliver, R.F. 1966. Whisker growth after removal of the dermal papilla and lengths of follicle in the hooded rat. J. Embryol. Exp. Morphol. 15:331–347.

Orlow, S.J. 1996. Aging of the pigmentary system in normal and pathological states. In: Mohr, U., Dungworth, D.L., Capen, C.C., et al. (eds.), Pathobiology of the Aging Mouse, vol. 2. Washington DC: ILSI Press, pp. 351–357.

Orlow, S.J., Lamoreux, M.L., Pifko-Hirst, S., et al. 1993. Pathogenesis of the platinum (*cp*) mutation, a model for oculocutaneous albinism. J. Invest. Dermatol. 101:137–140.

Paller, A.S. 1996. Lessons from skin blistering: molecular mechanisms and unusual patterns of inheritance? Am. J. Pathol. 148:1727–1731.

Panteleyev, A.A., Ahmad, W., Malashenko, A.M., et al. 1998a. Molecular basis for the rhino Yurlovo (*hr^{rhY}*) phenotype: severe skin abnormalities and female reproductive defects associated with an insertion in the hairless gene. Exp. Dermatol. 7:281–288.

Panteleyev, A.A., Paus, R., Ahmad, W., et al. 1998b. Molecular and functional aspects of the hairless (*hr*) gene in laboratory rodents and humans. Exp. Dermatol. 7:249–267.

Panteleyev, A.A., vanderVeen, C., Rosenbach, T., et al. 1998c. Towards defining the pathogenesis of the hairless phenotype. J. Invest. Dermatol. 110:902–907.

Parakkal, P.F. 1969. The fine structure of anagen hair follicle of the mouse. Adv. Biol. Skin 9:441–469.

Paus, R., Foitzik, K., Welker, P., et al. 1997. Transforming growth factor-B receptor type 1 and type II expression during murine hair follicle development and cycling. J. Invest. Dermatol. 109:518–526.

Paus, R., vanderVeen, C., Eichmuller, S., et al. 1998. Generation and cyclic remodeling of the hair follicle immune system in mice. J. Invest. Dermatol. 111:7–18.

Paus, R., Muller-Rover, S., van der Veen, C., et al. 1999. A comprehensive guide for the recognition and classification of distinct stages of hair follicle morphogenesis. J. Invest. Dermatol. 113:523–532.

Pelsue, S.C., Schweitzer, P.A., Schweitzer, I.B., et al. 1998. Lymphadenopathy, hyper-IgE, autoimmunity, and mast cell accumulation in flaky skin (*fsn*) mice. Eur. J. Immunol. 28:1379–1388.

Perkins, S.N., Hursting, S.D., Phang, J.M., et al. 1998. Calorie restriction reduces ulcerative dermatitis and infection-related mortality in p53-deficient and wild-type mice. J. Invest. Dermatol. 111:292–296.

Peschon, J.J., Slack, J.L., Reddy, P., et al. 1998. An essential role for ectodermal shedding in mammalian development. Science 282:1281–1284.

Peters, J., Cocking, Y. 1994. Mouse gene list. Mouse Genome 92:169–299.

Pittelkow, M.R. 1994. Keratinocyte cultures as models for dermatologic disease. In: Sundberg, J.P. (ed.), Handbook of Mouse Mutations with Skin and Hair Abnormalities: Animal Models and Biomedical Tools. Boca Raton, FL: CRC Press, pp. 117–127.

Porter, R.M., Leitgeb, S., Melton, D.W., et al. 1998. Gene targeting at the mouse cytokeratin 10 locus: severe skin fragility and changes of cytokeratin expression in the epidermis. J. Cell Biol. 132:925–936.

Relyea, M.J., Miller, J., Boggess, D., et al. 1999. Necropsy methods for laboratory mice. Biological characterization of a new mutation. In: Sundberg, J.P., Boggess, D. (eds.), Systematic Approach to Evaluation of Mouse Mutations. Boca Raton, FL: CRC Press.

Roop, D. 1995. Defects in the barrier. Science 267:474–475.

Roop, D.R., Krieg, T.M., Cheng, C.K., et al. 1988. Transcriptional control of high molecular weight keratin gene expression in multistage mouse skin carcinogenesis. Cancer Res. 48:3245–3252.

Rosemblat, S., Durham-Pierre, D., Gardner, J.M., et al. 1994. Identification of a melanosomal membrane protein encoded by the pink-eyed dilution (type II oculocutaneous albinism) gene. Proc. Natl. Acad. Sci. USA 91:12071–12075.

Rosemblat, S., Sviderskaya, E.V., Easty, D.J., et al. 1998. Melanosomal defects in melanocytes from mice lacking expression of the pink-eyed dilution gene: correction by culture in the presence of excess tyrosine. Exp. Cell. Res. 239:344–352.

Rosenquist, T.A., Martin, G.R. 1996. Fibroblast growth factor signalling in the hair growth cycle. Expression of the fibroblast growth factor receptor and ligand genes in the murine hair follicle. Dev. Dyn. 205:379–386.

Rothnagel, J., Longley, M., Bundman, D., et al. 1994. Characterization of the mouse loricrin gene: linkage with profilaggrin and the flaky tail and soft coat mutant loci on chromosome 3. Genomics 23:450–456.

Sakai, C., Ollmann, M., Kobayashi, T., et al. 1997. Modulation of murine melanocyte function *in vitro* by agouti signal protein. EMBO J. 16:3544–3552.

Saltou, M., Sugal, S., Tanaka, T., et al. 1995. Inhibition of skin development by targeted expression of a dominant-negative retinoic acid receptor. Nature 374:159–162.

Scher, R.K. 1991. The nails. In: Roenigk, H.H., Maibach, H.I. (eds.), Psoriasis. New York: Marcel Dekker, pp. 131–134.

Schilli, M.B., Ray, S., Obi-Tabot, E., et al. 1997. Control of hair growth with parathyroid hormone (7-34). J. Invest. Dermatol. 108:928–932.

Sellheyer, K., Bickenbach, J.R., Rothnagel, J.A., et al. 1993. Inhibition of skin development by overexpression of transforming growth factor B1 in the epidermis of transgenic mice. Proc. Natl. Acad. Sci. USA 90:5237–5241.

Shastry, B.S. 1998. Gene disruption in mice: models of development and disease. Mol. Cell. Biochem. 181:163–179.

Shipley, G.D, Keeble, W.W., Hendrickson, J.E., et al. 1989. Growth of normal human keratinocytes and fibroblasts in serum-free medium is stimulated by acidic and basic fibroblast growth factor. J. Cell. Physiol. 138:511–518.

Shultz, L.D., Sundberg, J.P. 1994. The motheaten (*me*) and viable motheaten (*me*ᵛ) mutations, chromosome 6. In: Sundberg, J.P. (ed.), Handbook of Mouse Mutations with Skin and Hair Abnormalities: Animal Models and Biomedical Tools. Boca Raton, FL: CRC Press, pp. 351–358.

Schultz, L.D., Lane, P.W., Coman, D.R., et al. 1991. Hairpatches, a single gene mutation characterized by progressive renal disease and alopecia in the mouse: a potential model for a newly described heritable human disorder. Lab. Invest. 65:588–600.

Shultz, L.D., Schweitzer, P.A., Rajan, T.V., et al. 1993. Mutations at the murine motheaten locus are within the hematopoietic cell protein-tyrosine phosphatase (*Hcph*) gene. Cell 73:1445–1454.

Sibilia, M., Wagner, E.F. 1995. Strain-dependent epithelial defects in mice lacking the EGF receptor. Science 269:234–239.

Silvers, W.K. 1979. The Coat Colors of Mice. New York: Springer-Verlag.

Simpson, E.M., Linder, C.C., Sargent, E.E., et al. 1997. Genetic variation among 129 substrains and its importance for targeted mutagenesis in mice. Nat. Genet. 16:19–27.

Slaga, T.J., Budunova, I.V., Gimenez-Conti, I.B., et al. 1996. The mouse skin carcinogenesis model. J. Invest. Dermatol. Symp. Proc. 1:151–156.

Slee, J. 1962. Developmental morphology of the skin and hair follicles in normal and "ragged" mice. J. Embryol. Exp. Morphol. 10:507–529.

Smith, R.S., Martin, G., Boggess, D. 1999. Kinetics and morphometrics. In: Sundberg, J.P., Boggess, D. (eds.), Systematic Approach to Evaluation of Mouse Mutations. Boca Raton, FL: CRC Press.

Sofaer, J.A. 1969. Aspects of the tabby-crinkled-downless syndrome. II. Observations on the reaction to changes of genetic background. J. Embryol. Exp. Morphol. 22:207–227.

Soler, A.P., Gilliard, G., Megosh, L.C., et al. 1995. Modulation of hair follicle function by alterations of ornithine decarboxylase activity. J. Invest. Dermatol. 106:1108–1113.

Spalding, J.W., Momma, J., Elwell, M.R., et al. 1993. Chemically induced skin carcinogenesis in a transgenic mouse line (TG.AC) carrying a *v-Ha-ras* gene. Carcinogenesis 14:1335–1341.

Sperling, L.C. 1991. Hair anatomy for the clinician. J. Am. Acad. Dermatol. 25:1–17.

Srivastava, A.K., Pispa, J., Hartung, A.J., et al. 1997. The Tabby phenotype is caused by mutation in a mouse homologue of the EDA gene that reveals novel mouse and human exons and encodes a protein (ectodysplasin-A) with collagenous domains. Proc. Natl. Acad. Sci. USA 94:13069–13074.

Staughton, R.C.D. 1988. The Color Atlas of Hair and Scalp Disorders. London: Wolfe Publishing.

Stelzner, K.F. 1983. Four dominant autosomal mutations affecting skin and hair development in the mouse. J. Hered. 74:193–196.

Stenn, K., Sundberg, J.P., Sperling, L.C. 1999. Hair follicle biology, the sebaceous gland, and scarring alopecias. Arch. Dermatol. 135:973–974.

Stern, M.C., Conti, C.J. 1996. Genetic susceptibility to tumor progression in mouse skin carcinogenesis. Prog. Clin. Biol. Res. 395:47–55.

Stern, M.C., Gimenez-Conti, I.B., Conti, C.J. 1995. Genetic susceptibility to papilloma progression in SENCAR mice. Carcinogenesis 16:1947–1953.

Stern, M.C., Gimenez-Conti, I.B., Budunova, I., et al. 1998. Analysis of two inbred strains of mice derived from the SENCAR stock with different susceptibility to skin tumor progression. Carcinogenesis 19:125–132.

Straile, W.E., Chase, H.B., Arsenault, C. 1961. Growth and differentiation of hair follicles between periods of activity and quiescence. J. Exp. Zool. 148:205–216.

Strauss, J.S., Downing, D.T., Ebling, F.J., et al. 1991. Sebaceous glands. In: Goldsmith, L.A. (ed.), Physiology, Biochemistry, and Molecular Biology of the Skin. New York: Oxford University Press, pp. 712–740.

Sullivan, T.J., Parker, K.L., Stenson, W., et al. 1975. Modulation of cyclic AMP in purified rat mast cells. I. Response to pharmacologic, metabolic, and physiologic stimuli. J. Immunol. 114:1473–1479.

Sundberg, J.P. 1994a. The asebia (ab, ab^J) mutations, chromosome 19. In: Sundberg, J.P. (ed.), Handbook of Mouse Mutations with Skin and Hair Abnormalities: Animal Models and Biomedical Tools. Boca Raton, FL: CRC Press, pp. 171–177.

Sundberg, J.P. 1994b. The balding (bal) mutation, chromosome 18. In: Sundberg, J.P. (ed.), Handbook of Mouse Mutations with Skin and Hair Abnormalities: Animal Models and Biomedical Tools. Boca Raton, FL: CRC Press, pp. 187–191.

Sundberg, J.P. 1994c. The bareskin (Bsk) mutation, Chromosome 11. In: Sundberg, J.P. (ed.), Handbook of Mouse Mutations with Skin and Hair Abnormalities: Animal Models and Biomedical Tools. Boca Raton, FL: CRC Press, pp. 197–202.

Sundberg, J.P. 1994d. The beige (bg) mutation, Chromosome 3. In: Sundberg, J.P. (ed.), Handbook of Mouse Mutations with Skin and Hair Abnormalities: Animal Models and Biomedical Tools. Boca Raton, FL: CRC Press, pp. 03–210.

Sundberg, J.P. 1994e. The curly-whisker (cw) mutation, chromosome 9. In: Sundberg, J.P. (ed.), Handbook of Mouse Mutations with Skin and Hair Abnormalities: Animal Models and Biomedical Tools. Boca Raton, FL: CRC Press, pp. 231–234.

Sundberg, J.P. 1994f. The flaky tail (ft) mutation, chromosome 3. In: Sundberg, J.P. (ed.), Handbook of Mouse Mutations with Skin and Hair Abnormalities: Animal Models and Biomedical Tools. Boca Raton, FL: CRC Press, pp. 269–273.

Sundberg, J.P. 1994g. The hairless (hr) and rhino (hr^rh) mutations, chromosome 14. In: Sundberg, J.P. (ed.), Handbook of Mouse Mutations with Skin and Hair Abnormalities: Animal Models and Biomedical Tools. Boca Raton, FL: CRC Press, pp. 291–312.

Sundberg, J.P. (ed.). 1994h. Handbook of Mouse Mutations with Skin and Hair Abnormalities: Animal Models and Biomedical Tools. Boca Raton, FL: CRC Press.

Sundberg, J.P. 1994i. The mottled locus: mottled (Mo), blotchy (Mo^blo), brindled (Mo^br), dappled (Mo^dp), mosaic (Mo^ms), tortoiseshell (Mo^to), and viable brindled (Mo^vbr), chromosome X. In: Sundberg, J.P. (ed.), Handbook of Mouse Mutations with Skin and Hair Abnormalities: Animal Models and Biomedical Tools. Boca Raton, FL: CRC Press, pp. 359–369.

Sundberg, J.P. 1994j. The tight-skin (Tsk) mutation, chromosome 2. In: Sundberg, J.P. (ed.), Handbook of Mouse Mutations with Skin and Hair Abnormalities: Animal Models and Biomedical Tools. Boca Raton, FL: CRC Press, pp. 463–470.

Sundberg, J.P., Boggess, D. 1998. Rhino-9J (hr^rh9J). A new allele at the hairless locus. Vet. Pathol. 35:297–299.

Sundberg, J.P., Hogan, M.E. 1994. Hair types and subtypes in the laboratory mouse. In: Sundberg, J.P. (ed.), Handbook of Mouse Mutations with Skin and Hair Abnormalities: Animal Models and Biomedical Tools. Boca Raton, FL: CRC Press, pp. 57–68.

Sundberg, J.P., King, L.E. 1996a. Mouse models for the study of human hair loss. Dermatol. Clin. 14:619–632.

Sundberg, J.P., King, L.E. 1996b. Mouse mutations as animal models and biomedical tools for dermatological research. J. Invest. Dermatol. 106:368–379.

Sundberg, J.P., Pittelkow, M.R. 1994. The ichthyosis (ic) mutation, Chromosome 1. In: Sundberg, J.P. (ed.), Handbook of Mouse Mutations with Skin and Hair Abnormalities: Animal Models and Biomedical Tools. Boca Raton, FL: CRC Press, pp. 327–335.

Sundberg, J.P., Shultz, L.D. 1991. Inherited mouse mutations: models for the study of alopecia. J. Invest. Dermatol. 96:95S–96S.

Sundberg, J.P., O'Banion, M.K., Shima, A., et al. 1988. Papillomas and carcinomas associated with a papillomavirus in European harvest mice (Micromys minutus). Vet. Pathol. 25:356–361.

Sundberg, J.P., Dunstan, R.W., Compton, J.G. 1989. In: Jones, T.C. (ed.), Hairless Mouse, HRS/J hr/hr. Heidelberg, Germany: Springer-Verlag, pp.192–197.

Sundberg, J.P., Beamer, W.G., Shultz, L.D., et al. 1990a. Inherited mouse mutations as models of human adnexal, cornification, and papulosquamous dermatoses. J. Invest. Dermatol. 95:62S–63S.

Sundberg, J.P., Binder, R.L., Maurer, J.K., et al. 1990b. Absence of papillomavirus in skin tumors induced in SENCAR mice by a two-stage carcinogenesis protocol. Carcinogenesis 11:341–344.

Sundberg, J.P., Roop, D.R., Dunstan, R., et al. 1991. Interaction between dermal papilla and bulge: the rhino mouse mutation as a model system. Ann. N.Y. Acad. Sci. 642:496–499.

Sundberg, J.P., Boggess, D., Sundberg, B.A., et al. 1993. Epidermal dendritic cell populations in the flaky skin mutant mouse. Immunol. Invest. 22:389–401.

Sundberg, J.P., Boggess, D., Shultz, L.D., et al. 1994a. The flaky skin (fsn) mutation, chromosome? In: Sundberg, J.P. (ed.), Handbook of Mouse Mutations with Skin and Hair Abnormalities: Animal Models and Biomedical Tools. Boca Raton, FL: CRC Press, pp. 253–268.

Sundberg, J.P., Brown, K.S., McMahon, W.M. 1994b. Chronic ulcerative dermatitis in black mice. In: Sundberg, J.P. (ed.), Handbook of Mouse Mutations with Skin and Hair Abnormalities: Animal Models and Biomedical Tools. Boca Raton, FL: CRC Press, pp. 485–492.

Sundberg, J.P., Cordy, W.R., King, L.E. 1994c. Alopecia areata in aging C3H/HeJ mice. J. Invest. Dermatol. 102:847–856.

Sundberg, J.P., Dunstan, R.W., Roop, D.R., et al. 1994d. Full thickness skin grafts from flaky skin mice to nude mice: maintenance of the psoriasiform phenotype. J. Invest. Dermatol. 102:781–788.

Sundberg, J.P., Erickson, A.A., Roop, D.R., et al. 1994e. Ornithine decarboxylase expression in cutaneous papillomas in SENCAR mice is associated with altered expression of keratins 1 and 10. Cancer Res. 54:1344–1351.

Sundberg, J.P., Orlow, S.J., Sweet, H.O., et al. 1994f. The adrenocortical dysplasia (*acd*) mutation, Chromosome 8. In: Sundberg, J.P. (ed.), Handbook of Mouse Mutations with Skin and Hair Abnormalities: Animal Models and Biomedical Tools. Boca Raton, FL: CRC Press, pp. 159–164.

Sundberg, J.P., HogenEsch, H., King, L.E. 1995. In: Maibach, H.I. (ed.), Mouse Models for Scaly Skin Diseases. Boca Raton, FL: CRC Press, pp. 61–89.

Sundberg, J.P., Hogan, M.E., King, L.E. 1996a. Normal biology and aging changes in skin and hair. In: Mohr, U., Dungworth, D.L., Capen, C.C., et al. (eds.), Pathobiology of the Aging Mouse, vol. 2. Washington, DC: ILSI Press, pp. 303–323.

Sundberg, J.P., VanRanst, M., Burk, R.D., et al. 1996b. The nonhuman (animal) papillomaviruses: host range, epitope conservation, and molecular diversity. In: Gross, G., vonKrogh, G. (eds.), Human Papillomavirus Infections in Dermatology and Venereology. Boca Raton, FL: CRC Press, pp. 47–68.

Sundberg, J.P., Boggess, D., Hogan, M.E., et al. 1997a. Harlequin ichthyosis. A juvenile lethal mouse mutation with ichthyosiform dermatitis. Am. J. Pathol. 151:293–310.

Sundberg, J.P., France, M., Boggess, D., et al. 1997b. Development and progression of psoriasiform dermatitis and systemic lesions in the flaky skin (*fsn*) mouse mutant. Pathobiology 65:271–286.

Sundberg, J.P., Rourk, M., Boggess, D., et al. 1997c. Angora mouse mutation: altered hair cycle, follicular dystrophy, phenotypic maintenance of skin grafts, and changes in keratin expression. Vet. Pathol. 34:171–179.

Sundberg, J.P., Sundberg, B.A., Beamer, W.G. 1997d. Comparison of chemical carcinogen skin tumor induction efficiency in inbred, mutant, and hybrid strains of mice: morphologic variations of induced tumors and absence of a papillomavirus co-carcinogen. Mol. Carcinog. 20:19–32.

Sundberg, J.P., Montagutelli, X., Boggess, D. 1998. Systematic approach to evaluation of mouse mutations with cutaneous appendage defects. In: Chuong, C.-M. (ed.), Molecular Basis of Epithelial Appendage Morphogenesis. Austin, TX: RG Landes, pp. 421–435.

Sundberg, J., Boggess, D., Bascom, C., et al. 2000. Lanceolate hair-J (*lah^J*): a mouse model for human hair disorders. Exp. Dermatol. 9:201–213.

Sundberg, J.P., Boggess, D., Sundberg, B.A., et al. In press—b. Asebia-2J (*ab^2J*): a mouse mutation with sebaceous gland hypoplasia, alopecia, dermal scarring, and lipid abnormalities: characterization and comparison with asebia-J (*ab^J*). Am. J. Pathol.

Sundberg, J.P., Boggess, D., Sundberg, B.A., et al. Submitted. Juvenile alopecia (*jal*): a new mouse mutation with curly hair, focal alopecia, and cuticle defects on chromosome 13. Exp. Dermatol.

Suzuki, S., Kato, T., Takimoto, H., et al. 1998. Localization of rat FGF-5 protein in skin macrophage-like cells and

FGF-5S protein in hair follicle: possible involvement of two *Fgf-5* gene products in hair growth cycle regulation. J. Invest. Dermatol. 111:963–972.

Sweet, H.O., Davisson, M.T., Akeson, E.C., et al. 1989. Long hair (*lgh*). Mouse News Lett. 83:166–167.

Tarutani, M., Itami, S., Okabe, M., et al. 1997. Tissue-specific knockout of the mouse Pig-a gene reveals important roles of GPI-anchored proteins in skin development. Proc. Natl. Acad. Sci. USA 94:7400–7405.

Tharp, M.D. 1991. The mast cell and its mediators. In: Goldsmith, L.A. (ed.), Physiology, Biochemistry, and Molecular Biology of the Skin, 2nd ed. New York: Oxford University Press, pp. 1099–1120.

Tharp, M.D. 1997. Understanding mast cells and mastocytosis. J. Invest. Dermatol. 108:698–699.

Theoharides, T.C., Douglas, W.W. 1978. Serotonin in mast cells induced by calcium entrapped within phospholipid. Vesicles Sci. 201:1143–1145.

Thompson, K.L., Rosenzweig, B.A., Sistare, F. 1998. An evaluation of the hemizygous transgenic Tg.AC mouse for carcinogenicity testing of pharmaceuticals. II. A genotypic marker that predicts tumorigenic responsiveness. Toxicol. Pathol. 26:548–555.

Threadgill, D.W., Dlugosz, A.A., Hansen, L.A., et al. 1995. Targeted disruption of mouse EGF receptor: effect of genetic background on mutant phenotype. Science 269:230–233.

Trigg, M.J. 1972. Hair growth in mouse mutants affecting coat texture. J. Zool., Lond. 168:165–198.

Turksen, K., Kupper, T., Degenstein, L., et al. 1992. Interleukin 6: insights to its function in skin by overexpression in transgenic mice. Proc. Natl. Acad. Sci. USA 89:5068–5072.

Uehira, M., Matsuda, H., Nakamura, A., et al. 1998. Immunologic abnormalities exhibited in IL-7 transgenic mice with dermatitis. J. Invest. Dermatol. 110:740–745.

van der Neut, R., Krimpenfort, P., Calafat, J., et al. 1996. Epithelial detachment due to absence of hemidesmosomes in integrin β4 null mice. Nat. Genet. 13:366–369.

Vassar, R., Coulombe, P.A., Degenstein, L., et al. 1991. Mutant keratin expression in transgenic mice causes marked abnormalities resembling a human genetic skin disease. Cell 64:365–380.

Vielkind, U., Hardy, M.H. 1996. Changing patterns of cell adhesion molecules during mouse pelage hair follicle development. 2. Follicle morphogenesis in the hair mutants Tabby and downy. Acta. Anat. Basel 157:183–194.

Walker, M.A., Harley, R., Maize, J., et al. 1985. Mast cells and their degranulation in the *Tsk* mouse model of scleroderma. Proc. Soc. Exp. Biol. Med. 180:323–328.

Walker, M.A., Harley, R.A., LeRoy, E.C. 1987. Inhibition of fibrosis in TSK mice by blocking mast cell degranulation. J. Rheumatol. 14:299–301.

Walker, M.A., Harley, R., Delustro, F., et al. 1989. Adoptive transfer of tsk skin fibrosis to +/+ recipients by tsk bone marrow and spleen cells. Proc. Soc. Exp. Biol. Med. 192:196–200.

Weisbroth, S.H. 1982. Arthropods. In: Foster, H.L. (ed.), The Mouse in Biomedical Research. II. Diseases. New York: Academic Press, pp. 388–390.

Werner, S., Weinberg, W., Liao, X., et al. 1993. Targeted expression of a dominant-negative FGF receptor mutant in the epidermis of transgenic mice reveals a role of FGF in keratinocyte organization and differentiation. EMBO J. 12:2635–2643.

Whiting, D.A. 1990. The value of horizontal sections of scalp biopsies. J. Cut. Aging. Cosmet. Dermatol. 1:165–173.

Williams, D., Profeta, K., Stenn, K.S. 1994. Isolation and culture of follicular papillae from murine vibrissae: an introductory approach. Br. J. Dermatol. 130:290–297.

Wilson, B.D., Ollmann, M.M., Kang, L., et al. 1995. Structure and function of ASP, the human homolog of the mouse agouti gene. Hum. Mol. Genet. 4:223–230.

Windhorst, D.B., Padgett, G. 1973. The Chediak-Higashi syndrome and the homologous trait in animals. J. Invest. Dermatol. 60:529–537.

Witt, W.M. 1989. An idiopathic dermatitis in C57BL/6N mice effectively modulated by dietary restriction. Lab. Anim. Sci. 39:470.

Xu, Y., Vijayasaradhi, S., Houghton, A.N. 1998. The cytoplasmic tail of the mouse brown locus product determines intracellular stability and export from the endoplasmic reticulum. J. Invest. Dermatol. 110:324–331.

Yamakado, M., Yohro, T. 1979. Subdivision of mouse vibrissae on an embryological basis, with descriptions of variations in the number and arrangement of sinus hairs and cortical barrels in BALB/c (*nu/+*; nude, *nu/nu*) and hairless (*hr/hr*) strains. Am. J. Anat. 155:153–174.

Yamanishi, K. 1998. Gene-knockout mice with abnormal epidermal and hair follicular development. J. Dermatol. Sci. 18:75–89.

Yosipovitch, G., Xiong, G.L., Haus, E., et al. 1998. Time-dependent variations of the skin barrier function in humans: transepidermal water loss, stratum corneum hydration, skin surface pH, and skin temperature. J. Invest. Dermatol. 110:20–23.

Zheng, Y., Eilertsen, K.J., Ge, L., et al. 1999. *Scd1* is expressed in sebaceous glands and is disrupted in the asebia mouse. Nat. Gen. 23:268–270.

Zhu, H., Reuhl, K., Zhang, X., et al. 1998. Development of heritable melanoma in transgenic mice. J. Invest. Dermatol. 110:247–252.

# 15

# Interpretation of Ocular Pathology in Genetically Engineered and Spontaneous Mutant Mice

Richard S. Smith, Patsy M. Nishina, Sakae Ikeda, Priscilla Jewett, Adriana Zabaleta, and Simon W.M. John

The advantages of using mice to study molecular and genetic aspects of human eye disease are well documented (Leiter et al. 1987; Sundberg and Shultz 1993; Sundberg and King 1996; Smith et al. 1997; John et al. 1998). Genetic homogeneity within a given strain, a high degree of homology with the human genome, physiology similar to that of humans, development of adult phenotypes in a relatively short time, and the ability to control environmental factors are some of the more obvious benefits provided by mice. The advent of successful transgenic and gene-targeting (knockout) technology (hereafter, *genetically engineered mice* [GEM]) has established the mouse as a very important experimental mammal in establishing mechanisms of human disease.

The frequency of disabling eye diseases, such as diabetic retinopathy, cataracts, and retinal degeneration, provides adequate reasons for studying the genetic aspects of ocular pathology. The rapidly increasing knowledge of mouse and human genomes, therefore, makes mice particularly useful for establishing disease mechanisms.

Genetically engineered mice often manifest ocular disease as part of a spectrum of systemic disease. For this reason, it is important to check the eyes of GEM created for studies of diffuse disease to determine if the eyes are affected. Care must be taken in interpretation of findings in order not to confuse strain-specific background lesions with other effects of the gene alteration. Appropriate control mice must be chosen to prevent a background disease with effects that might be confused with those of the targeted mutation.

For the investigator interested in disease not specific to the eye, such as central nervous system or vascular disease, the eye offers several advantages: (1) the cornea is the most accessible naturally avascular tissue in the body—as such it offers an excellent site for studies of factors that induce or inhibit angiogenesis (Folkman and D'Amore 1996), (2) the retina is the only place where healthy or diseased arterioles (Lutty et al. 1994) can be visualized in vivo, *without* surgical intervention, and (3) the optic nerve is the only part of the central nervous system visible without manipulation (Sadun et al. 1994).

Histologists generally agree that the eye is one of the more difficult organs to section. Once sections are prepared, it is necessary to separate artifact from true abnormalities. Also, regional differences in morphology within the eye must be recognized to avoid making erroneous interpretations. The first goal of this chapter is to review the anatomy and embryology of the eye, to outline techniques that enhance quality of histological material, and discuss necessary approaches to ensure accurate analysis of ocular disease. Spontaneous mutations

Supported in part by NCI Cancer Core Center Grant CA 34196 and by NIH grants EY07758 and EY 12093, by a grant from Foundation Fighting Blindness, and by funds from the Howard Hughes Medical Institute. We would like to thank John P. Sundberg, Bo Chang, and Peggy Danneman for critical reading of the manuscript and Jennifer L. Smith for graphics assistance.

and GEM are used to illustrate approaches to the study of eye disease and to demonstrate additional pitfalls in interpreting histopathology. The great volume of literature available and its continual expansion makes a complete review of ocular genetic engineering impossible, but some of the major uses of GEM in eye research are listed in Table 15.1 on page 229.

# ANATOMY AND EMBRYOLOGY

An understanding of the anatomy of the mouse eye is needed for evaluation of histopathologic findings. The outer layer of the eye includes cornea and sclera, which are largely composed of collagen. In the cornea the highly ordered arrangement of collagen fibers contributes to the transparency of this organ. The middle, or uveal, layer is composed of choroid, ciliary body, and iris. This layer is characterized by dense melanin pigmentation (except in albinos) and is highly vascular. The inner, or neural, layer includes the sensory retina, retinal pigment epithelium, and optic nerve. In the mouse, the lens fills about two-thirds of the inner volume of the eye. The space between lens and retina is filled with vitreous. The anterior chamber is bounded by cornea, iris, and the anterior portion of the lens and is filled with the aqueous humor (see Figs. 15.1 and 15.5, discussed below). A complete discussion of ocular anatomy is beyond the scope of this book and is available elsewhere (Hogan et al. 1971). The following brief review covers important structures discussed elsewhere in this chapter.

The corneal surface is covered by five to six layers of stratified squamous epithelial cells that become flattened toward the surface but differ from cutaneous epithelium in that they do not become cornified. Beneath the epithelium is a thin acellular layer of basal lamina and collagen (Bowman's membrane). The bulk of the corneal thickness is supplied by the corneal stroma that consists of multiple, highly organized layers of uniform diameter collagen fibers and scattered keratocytes. Internal to the stroma is a thick layer of basal lamina with periodic deposits of long-spacing collagen (Descemet's membrane). Facing the anterior chamber is the monolayer corneal endothelium, which produces Descemet's membrane and engages in active transport of fluids and electrolytes in the cornea (Fig. 15.1a). The normal cornea is avascular.

The iris is a complex structure consisting of the iris stroma (neural crest/mesodermal derivation) and the bilayered posterior iris pigment epithelium (neuroepithelial origin). The smooth muscle of the iris sphincter and dilator is derived from the anterior layer of iris pigment epithelium. The iris stroma contains dendritic melanocytes, capillaries, collagen, and extracellular matrix (Fig. 15.1b).

The region around the junction between iris and cornea is referred to as the anterior chamber angle and includes the structures of the trabecular meshwork that play a critical role in aqueous humor outflow and control of intraocular pressure. The trabecular meshwork is a complex structure composed of collagen and elastic tissue bands surrounded by endothelial cells. The aqueous humor passes through the meshwork before leaving the eye through the endothelial-lined channel known as Schlemm's canal, which is located just external to the meshwork. Schlemm's canal connects to the systemic circulation by a series of aqueous veins (Fig. 15.1c).

The ciliary body lies directly behind the iris and is covered by single layers of nonpigmented and pigmented epithelium (Fig. 15.1d). These two cell layers and the fibrovascular tissue beneath them make up the ciliary processes that produce aqueous humor and also produce the zonules that suspend the lens. External to these structures in primates is a large triangular bed of smooth muscle. The ciliary muscle is very small in mice and may have little function. Only a few muscle cells are found external to the ciliary processes, sometimes extending as far forward as the posterior termination of Schlemm's canal. The lens fibers are produced by the lens epithelium, which is normally found in only the anterior half of the lens. The lens capsule surrounds the lens epithelium.

The two layers of ciliary epithelium thicken abruptly at the posterior end of the ciliary body, marking the beginning of the peripheral retina. The pigmented ciliary epithelium is continuous with the retinal pigment epithelium, while the nonpigmented ciliary epithelium corresponds embryologically to the multilayered sensory retina. The retinal layers are illustrated in Fig. 15.1e. In the periphery there are fewer retinal ganglion cells, and the nerve fiber layer is extremely thin. Near the optic nerve, the ganglion cell layer is 2–4 cells thick, and the nerve fiber layer is prominent.

The axons of the retinal ganglion cells give rise to the nerve fiber layer, which exits the globe via the optic nerve. As it leaves the globe, the optic nerve is traversed by the collagen meshwork of the lamina cribrosa. Posterior to the lamina, the axons of the optic nerve are myelinated and separated into smaller bundles by the pia. As with other structures of the central nervous system, the optic nerve is surrounded by arachnoid and dura, which is continuous with the meninges of the brain (Fig. 15.1f).

Many of the differences between human and mouse eyes are those of absolute size. Although the basic structure of its trabecular meshwork is identical to that in the human eye, the mouse's eye has smaller numbers of

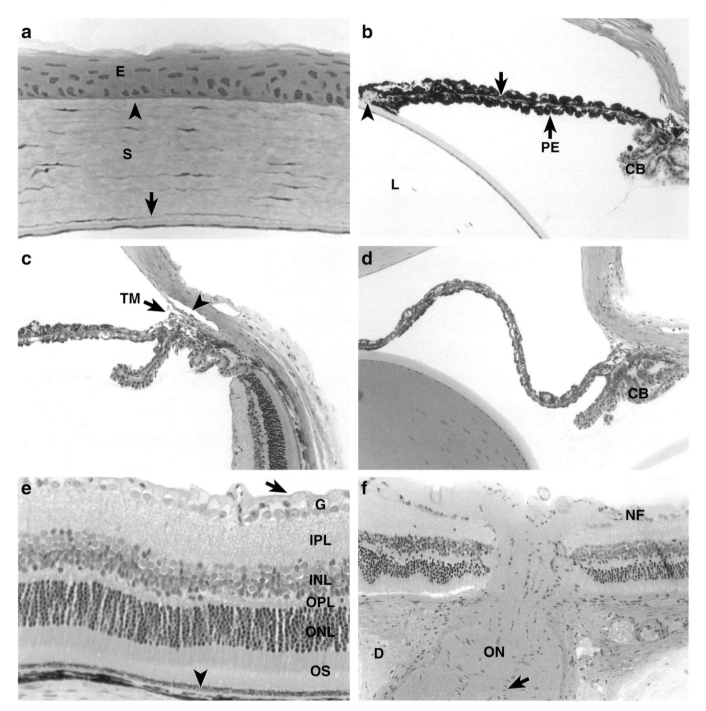

**FIGURE 15.1** (**a**) The cornea consists of the epithelium (*E*), Bowman's membrane (*arrowhead*), the corneal stroma (*S*), Descemet's membrane (*arrow*), and the single layer of corneal endothelium (not labeled). (**b**) The anterior iris stroma is separated from the posterior iris pigment epithelium (*PE*) by the thin dilator muscle (*arrow*). The sphincter muscle (*arrowhead*) is located at the pupillary border. The ciliary body (*CB*) begins directly posterior to the iris root. (**c**) The trabecular meshwork (*TM*) is located at the junction between iris and cornea. Aqueous humor drains through the trabecular meshwork into Schlemm's canal (*arrowhead*). (**d**) The ciliary body (*CB*) is composed of the inner nonpigmented ciliary epithelium and an outer layer of pigmented epithelium. The vascular channels beneath the epithelium and the small amount of smooth muscle are not seen at this magnification. (**e**) The innermost portion of the retina is the nerve fiber layer (*arrow*). It arises from the retinal ganglion cells (*G*). Next is the inner plexiform layer (*IPL*), where the retinal ganglion cells connect with the neurons of the inner nuclear layer (*INL*). The outer plexiform layer (*OPL*) is the site of synapse of the INL neurons with the photoreceptor cells. The nuclei of the photoreceptor layer are found in the outer nuclear layer (*ONL*), while the outer segments (*OS*) of the photoreceptors are the site of phototransduction. External to the retina is the single layer of retinal pigment epithelium (*arrowhead*). (**f**) The thickened nerve fiber layer (*NF*) forms the optic nerve (*ON*), which becomes myelinated and thicker posterior to the lamina cribrosa (not seen at this magnification). The bundles of nerve fibers are separated by pial septae (*arrow*), and the nerve is covered by dura and arachnoid (*D*).

trabecular beams than the human eye as well as a slightly different termination in the area of the anterior ciliary body. The mouse lens occupies a larger portion of the eye than the human lens, while the mouse has proportionately less vitreous. The specialized area of the human retina, known as the macula, is absent in mice, although there are increased numbers of cone photoreceptors near the optic nerve (Hogan et al. 1971). Because of the large number of albino mouse strains, it should be emphasized that, except for the absence of melanosomes, albino and pigmented mice are anatomically similar.

Many mouse structures are not anatomically mature in the weeks immediately after birth. The short gestation period of the mouse results in immature pups, so the onset of neonatal phenotypes is different between mice and humans. Except for the time scale, the stages of ocular embryologic development are similar in mice and humans with a few exceptions. The hyaloid vessels, especially those surrounding the lens, usually persist for 2–3 weeks after birth in mice. The final structure of the trabecular meshwork is not achieved until 6–8 weeks after birth (R.S. Smith and S.W.M. John, unpublished observations). The retina is not mature until the second week of life. A number of useful reviews of the details of mouse embryology are available (Rugh 1968; Pei and Rhodin 1970; Coulombre and Coulombre 1964; Hero et al. 1991; Graw 1996; Fini et al. 1997; Oliver and Gruss 1997; Reme et al. 1983; Dahl et al. 1997).

# TISSUE PROCESSING

## Collection

Removal of the eye, fixation, and sectioning require specialized techniques to avoid inducing artifacts that lead to incorrect conclusions. There are many approaches to handling tissue and no single "right" way to do it. Because ocular tissues are often particularly troublesome to process, the material that follows represents techniques that have proven useful in our laboratory. Investigators must adapt published techniques to the specific ends they wish to reach.

Enucleation must be done gently to avoid damaging the optic nerve and intraocular structures. The thin sclera and small size of the mouse eye makes it vulnerable to trauma. Rough handling can produce intraocular hemorrhage, cause retinal detachment, and crush artifacts of the optic nerve. A curved forceps with fine serrations is the safest instrument to use. This is available from many manufacturers. We prefer a forceps of the style generally labeled as fine dressing forceps, iris forceps, or microdissecting forceps. Immediately after

euthanasia, the forceps are directed posterior to the globe and gently pushed as far back in the orbit as possible. The forceps are then closed and pulled forward. This provides a long piece of optic nerve attached to the globe, as well as portions of extraocular muscle. Grasping the nerve close to the globe can produce myelin artifacts (myelin is pushed into the subretinal space as a result of crushing). In older mice that may have atrophic optic nerves, careful scissors dissection and enucleation without any traction may be needed. For purposes of orientation, the eye of an albino mouse may be marked in the twelve o'clock meridian with a red pencil moistened in alcohol or with an indelible dye. This approach does not work with pigmented mice, in which the best alternative is to make a small slit at a known location that can be identified later by using a dissecting microscope.

Different techniques are required for excision of the optic chiasm and tracts. After removal of the skin and top of the skull, the brain is excised with a small scalpel, leaving a thin layer of brain tissue so that the optic tracts and chiasm are not stretched. After fixation the optic tracts are cut, using Vannas scissors, and the chiasm and the intracranial portion of the optic nerves are removed.

## Fixation

The choice of fixative depends on the potential final use for the tissue: what is satisfactory for routine stains may not be useful for immunohistochemistry. The eye should be placed in fixative immediately after enucleation (Sundberg and Boggess 1999). We have explored a variety of fixatives in an effort to achieve the best sections. Bouin's solution and 10 percent neutral buffered formalin are disappointing for ocular tissue, the former because of loss of cellular definition and eosin overstaining, the latter due to its tendency to harden the lens and make it shatter on sectioning. However, the advantages of Bouin's solution for whole head fixation outweigh the tissue definition issues (see below) because it facilitates sectioning due to decalcification by the picric acid in the fixative. For paraffin sectioning and immunohistochemistry, we use Fekete's acid-alcohol-formalin; tissues may be stored in 70 percent ethanol. A phosphate-buffered glutaraldehyde-paraformaldehyde mixture (Smith and Rudt 1973) produces good results for plastic embedding and is also our fixative of choice for transmission electron microscopy. Tissues are fixed for 24 hours and stored in 0.1M phosphate buffer, pH 7.4. Recently, satisfactory results have also been achieved with a 4 percent paraformaldehyde fixative (Schlamp and Nickells 1996; Schlamp and Williams 1996) that offers the advantage of being useful for plastic embedding and immunohistochemical studies.

Storage of tissue in 0.4 percent paraformaldehyde fixative is possible for at least 1 year without deterioration. (Both the 4 percent and 0.4 percent paraformaldehyde are made in 0.2M phosphate buffer, pH 7.2.)

The combination of closed eyelids and the small size of the perinatal eye makes enucleation difficult in embryos and newborns until 2 weeks of age, so the best tissue sections come from processing the whole head in Bouin's solution for 24–48 hours. After fixation the nose and back of the head are removed, and the remaining tissues washed in running water for at least 4 hours. Using a 2-hour tissue processor program, tissues are dehydrated and embedded in paraplast (65 percent alcohol; 80 percent alcohol × 2; 95 percent alcohol; absolute alcohol × 3; xylene × 3; paraplast × 4). Decalcification is not needed in mice of these ages. Because of the size of the head by 7–14 days of age, it is best to hemisect the skull along the midline and section separately for each eye.

For in situ hybridization, tissues are fixed in 4 percent paraformaldehyde and processed through graded alcohols (65 percent alcohol; 80 percent alcohol × 2; 95 percent alcohol; absolute alcohol × 3; xylene × 3; paraplast × 4) made in diethyl pyrocarbonate (depec) water (Sigma Chemical Company, St. Louis, MO). The length of time chosen depends on the size of the tissue, but 1 hour is satisfactory for whole eyes. The embedding cycle is completed with four changes of paraffin. Blocks are kept at 4°C before sectioning, and depec water is used in the water bath. Sections (4–5 μm) are placed on glass slides and stored at 4°C until used. The slides are rehydrated through depec water alcohols and stained as described elsewhere in this book (Sundberg and Boggess 1999).

## Tissue Processing—Plastic

Eyes are dehydrated for 1 hour in each of several progressive ethanol concentrations (25 percent, 50 percent, 70 percent, two changes of 95 percent). All dehydration and infiltration steps are done on a shaker set at slow speed. Infiltration is done with degassed Leica historesin at 4°C (day 1: prepare 1:1 solution of historesin and 95 percent ethanol and infiltrate 24 hours; day 2: replace with 100 percent historesin for 24 hours; day 3: replace with fresh 100 percent historesin and infiltrate for 4 days; day 7: replace with fresh 100 percent historesin for 4 days and then embed).

Fresh embedding medium with hardener added according to the kit instructions is used to fill the mold tray to 3–4 mm from the top. The eyes are immersed in embedding medium and oriented under a dissecting microscope. A plane through the cornea and optic nerve must be positioned as parallel as possible with the bottom of the tray. If orienting marks have been placed on the eye, they should be positioned to produce the appropriate plane of section. A total of 16 ml of embedding medium is sufficient to embed 12 eyes in small trays, and the rate of polymerization allows all 12 eyes to be properly oriented. Polymerization should continue overnight before removal of the trays.

## PLASTIC SECTIONING

In humid weather, the plastic blocks are left in a dessicator for 24 hours prior to sectioning to provide better sectioning quality. If blocks are sticky or sections stretch or wrinkle, it may be useful to place the blocks in an incubator set at 45–65°C for 1 hour followed by cooling in the dessicator. The plastic block should be oriented in the microtome with the optic nerve at the bottom and the cornea at the top. Rough cuts are made at a maximum thickness of 3 μm (to avoid damage to the block), and sections are collected at 1.5 μm. When sectioning mouse eyes, the lens always presents the biggest problem because of its hardness and tendency to shatter. Section quality with a brittle lens is sometimes helped by temporarily cutting sections at 0.5-1 μm. In our hands, tungsten carbide knives produce better sections than glass knives. The selection of clearance angle depends on the microtome, personal preference, and the type of knife used. For eye sectioning, a clearance angle of 4 degrees is recommended with glass knives and 12–14 degrees with tungsten carbide knives. When sectioning the entire optic nerve (approximately 16 slides with eight sections per slide), if glass knives are being used, freshly made glass knives produce the best results.

Thin-tipped forceps are used to collect sections from the knife. The forceps tip must be very clean and dry, or sections will adhere to the forceps. To avoid wrinkles, sections are flattened as much as possible before placing them in the water bath. Distilled water in the water bath is filtered (22 μm filter) to remove dust and also appears to decrease surface tension of the water. The water bath temperature is set at 28°C. Sections are picked up from the water bath and placed on precleaned slides with the help of thin-tipped brushes. Fresh slides are dried first on a hot plate at 55°C and then overnight in an incubator at 45–65°C. Slides are kept in a dessicator until ready for staining.

## Tissue Processing—Paraffin

Eyes are dehydrated for 1 hour in each of a series of alcohol concentrations (65 percent, 80 percent × 2, 95 percent, 100 percent × 3). The eyes then pass through three 1-hour changes of xylene, followed by four changes of paraffin at 60°C under 15 mm Hg of vacuum. At the time of embedding, the eyes are oriented as described for plastic embedding in "Tissue Processing—Plastic" (above).

## PARAFFIN SECTIONING

Plastic sections are always superior to paraffin for morphology, but with patience, good quality paraffin sections can be produced that are satisfactory for many purposes. Paraffin sections also permit use of techniques such as immunohistochemistry that are very difficult with plastic. After initial rough cutting to the lens, prior to sectioning, 3–4 drops of 10 percent ammonium hydroxide are applied to the surface of the block, which is placed face down on an ice cube for 15–30 minutes before sectioning (*caution:* ammonium hydroxide cannot be used with in situ techniques). This maneuver softens the lens and decreases the risk of shattering. If a very brittle lens is encountered, the block is soaked overnight at 4°C in a cloth saturated with 10 percent ammonium hydroxide. These procedures should be done with adequate ventilation. The block is placed in the microtome chuck with the cornea and optic nerve at the *sides* of the block. Note that this is different than when sectioning plastic blocks. The lens has a strong tendency to become detached from the slide. Addition of a single drop of Elmer's® glue (Borden, Inc., Columbus, OH) or polylysine to the water bath helps to minimize this problem. Rough handling during the staining procedure can also cause lens detachment from the slide.

# INTERPRETING EYE SECTIONS

Since the eye is an asymmetric structure with regional variations in anatomy, careful attention to plane of section is *critical* for correct interpretation. At the junction between cornea and sclera, the surface epithelium of the conjunctiva becomes thicker and folded, as opposed to the uniform 5- to 7-cell-thick corneal epithelium. The cornea is avascular, while the sclera is vascular. The highly ordered arrangement of collagen in the corneal stroma becomes irregular in the sclera (Fig. 15.2).

At the junction (referred to as the pars plana) between ciliary body and retina, there is a transition, within about 50 μm, from a single layer of epithelium to the full thickness multilayer retina (Fig. 15.3). The peripheral retina contains fewer ganglion cells than the posterior retina, and it is usually not possible to identify the nerve fiber layer. In the posterior retina, the ganglion cell layer is usually 2–3 cells thick, and the nerve fiber layer is prominent, especially near the entrance of the optic nerve (Fig. 15.4). The mouse lacks a macula (the area of acute vision found in primates), but there is a region of increased density of cones temporal to the optic nerve, whereas rods predominate elsewhere.

These regional anatomic differences become important when localization of specific structures is necessary, when comparative cell counts are done to compare

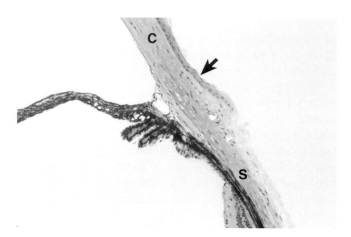

**FIGURE 15.2** The limbus (*arrow*) is the junction between the cornea (*C*) and sclera (*S*). The presence of blood vessels and an irregular arrangement of collagen is characteristic of the sclera.

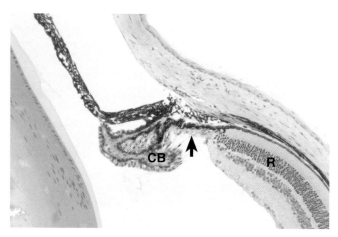

**FIGURE 15.3** The junction between the ciliary body (*CB*) and retina (*R*) is known as the pars plana (*arrow*). The single layer of pigmented epithelium in this region is continuous with the retinal pigment epithelium and the pigmented ciliary epithelium. The nonpigmented layer thickens rapidly to form the neural retina.

mutant versus control (West et al. 1997), and when precise morphometric analysis is required to quantitate the effects of a mutant gene. If sections are cut in plastic at 1.5 μm or in paraffin at 5–6 μm, it is apparent that serial sectioning of the eye is an expensive and time-consuming process. Since the most important information is usually found in a central sagittal cut that contains central cornea, pupil, lens, and optic nerve, our laboratory has developed a modification of step-sectioning that is efficient and effective. The technician cuts the tissue block a short way into the lens (Fig. 15.5a and 15.6). A series of three to four slides, each containing 8–12 sections, is taken and labeled A. More sections are cut and discarded until a point is

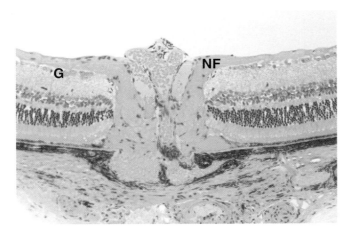

**FIGURE 15.4** Near the optic nerve, the ganglion cell layer (*G*) is usually 2–3 cells thick, and the nerve fiber layer (*NF*) is more prominent than in the peripheral retina.

reached midway between the A level and the central lens. The next set of three to four slides is labeled B1, B2, and so on, and sectioning then moves to the most critical central cut (C level). Sectioning may stop at this level or continue to the D and E levels (at locations similar to A and B, but on the opposite side of the eye). If the eye was correctly oriented at the time of embedding, the C-level sections should include central cornea, central lens, pupil, and optic nerve. However, if the globe became tipped during embedding, this approach at least ensures that the optic nerve will not be missed. The number of sections taken at each level can be adjusted as needed, and often only the C-level sections are needed. This approach is most appropriate for a normal eye or one with evenly distributed abnormalities. Adjustments must be made if focal disease is present. For example, if the pupil is displaced because of synechias, the technician must be made aware of this before sectioning begins.

The modified step-section technique must be coupled with careful analysis of an individual section to make certain that orientation of the eye in the block does not produce confusion. Fig. 15.5b illustrates the potential problem when an obliquely sectioned eye is analyzed: although the section includes the pupil, the optic nerve is not present. Knowledge of ocular anatomy will provide orientation clues in the examples that follow. In Fig. 15.6a, the plane of section is both oblique and peripheral. The cornea and retina appear thickened (oblique), and ciliary processes are seen, accompanying a lens of small diameter (peripheral). Although iris is present in Fig. 15.6b, there is no pupil or optic nerve, and the lens is smaller than expected. This corresponds to the A level of section. The lens is approaching full diameter in Fig. 15.6c, but pupil and optic nerve are still

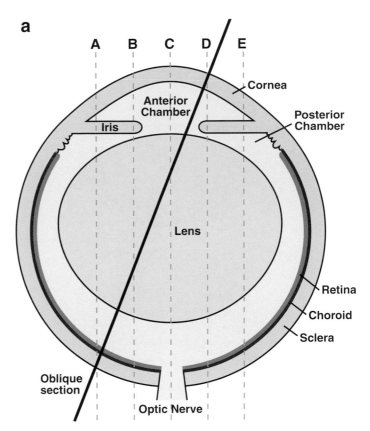

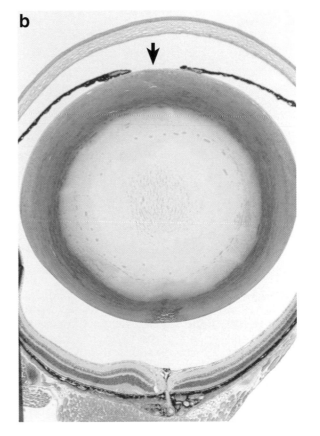

**FIGURE 15.5** (**a**) The levels for step-sectioning are indicated by dotted lines and the letters *A–E*. (**b**) In an eye cut in a slightly oblique plane, the pupil (*arrow*) is present, but the optic nerve is missing.

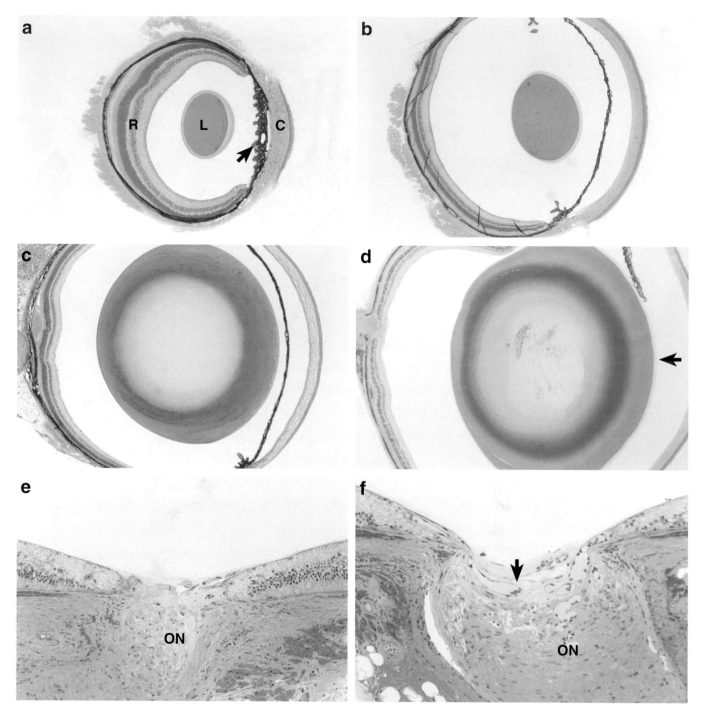

**FIGURE 15.6**   (**a**) The plane of section is oblique, as indicated by the artifactual thickening of the cornea (*C*) and retina (*R*). The apparent small size of the lens (*L*) and the presence of ciliary processes (*arrow*) reveal that the section is through the edge of the eye. (**b**) The iris is present in this section, but the lens is small, and the pupil and optic nerve are absent. This section is at the "A level." A few artifactual wrinkles are present in the retina. (**c**) With a lens of nearly normal diameter, this section is near the "B level." (**d**) A "C-level" section, demonstrating central cornea, pupil (*arrow*), and optic nerve. (**e**) The optic nerve (*ON*) appears normal in this DBA/2J mouse with advanced glaucoma. (**f**) A deeper cut of the same eye shown in **e** reveals deep cupping (*arrow*) of the optic nerve (*ON*), diagnostic of advanced glaucoma.

missing (B level). Central cornea, pupil, central lens, and optic nerve are all present at the C level (Fig. 15.6d). Additional care must be taken in identifying the optic nerve because its diameter in the mouse is so small. Fig. 15.6e demonstrates an optic nerve apparently without cupping. However, at a deeper level of section, there is obvious cupping of the nerve (Fig. 15.6f). If the structure of the optic nerve is critical for interpretation, we recommend that regular serial sections through the entire nerve be cut and examined.

Staining of tissue with routine and special stains is beyond the scope of this chapter. Since we recommend plastic sections for the best quality ocular morphology, it should be noted that many staining procedures have been adapted for use with plastic sections and can produce results identical to those of paraffin sections (Chang 1972; Snodgrass et al. 1972).

Morphometric techniques may be used to quantitate measurable differences in cells and tissues. Many of these methods are now partially automated, utilizing sophisticated computer software. When differences between mutant and wild-type mice are subtle, morphometrics can provide statistical confirmation to support a hypothesis. These techniques have been reviewed elsewhere (Skerrow and Skerrow 1985; Sundberg and Boggess 1999).

# OCULAR PHOTOGRAPHY

The unique techniques available for producing clinical photographs of ocular structures are important adjuncts to microscopic evaluation and in many instances take the place of gross photography. The small size of the mouse eye mandates the use of a dissecting photomicroscope capable of 40× magnification for useful gross photography. The short working distance required by the high magnification makes proper lighting difficult. A more desirable approach is to utilize ophthalmic instruments that are designed for high-quality film or digital photography and that employ built-in illumination systems and suitable lenses.

The external eye, including eyelid and cornea, as well as the anterior chamber, iris, and lens are easily observed with a slitlamp biomicroscope. The ability to vary the width of the illuminating beam down to a narrow slit produces an "optical section" in which individual cells (such as those in the corneal endothelium) can be visualized. With patience and gentle restraint of the mouse, high-quality 35 mm or digital video images (Fig. 15.7a) of the anterior segment can be acquired (John et al. 1998; Khaw 1988; Holm and Holm 1991).

Clinical features of the retina and optic nerve can be photographed with a handheld or fixed fundus camera (Fig. 15.7b; DiLoreto et al. 1994). Retinal cameras specifically designed for small animal photography are available from commercial sources. Dilation of the pupil with an agent such as 1 percent cyclopentolate should be done 5–10 minutes before photography. Anesthesia is not required for successful fundus examination or photography. There is no question that abundant patience and experience are important for successful ocular photography, but the results are very useful in

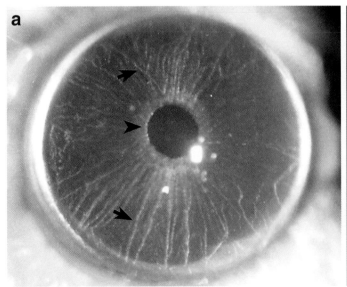
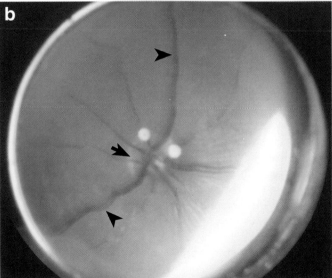

**FIGURE 15.7**  (**a**) Slitlamp photograph of a normal albino mouse eye. The iris sphincter (*arrowhead*) and individual iris vessels (*arrows*) are easily identified. (**b**) Fundus photograph of pigmented mouse demonstrating the optic nerve (*arrow*) and retinal vessels (*arrowheads*).

reaching clinicopathologic correlations as well as in providing data for publication.

## SPECIALIZED TECHNIQUES

Methods useful for detection and analysis of gene expression in other tissues are usually easily adapted to the eye. Since these are discussed at length in other chapters, this section is limited to a few specific comments about the eye. Concern is often expressed concerning penetration of fixatives into the eye. For routine fixation, it is not necessary or desirable to open the eye to allow fixative penetration. Fixation is satisfactory without this maneuver, and the risk of damage to intraocular structures is high. Immunohistochemical methodology is often useful in demonstrating gene expression, but the techniques must be specifically designed for the situation at hand. A useful summary of basic techniques is available (Sundberg and Boggess).

Ultrastructural studies of the eye require extra care during the process of fixation. Many ocular structures are highly sensitive to the osmolarity of the fixative. Satisfactory fixation of the eye is obtained by using a phosphate-buffered glutaraldehyde-paraformaldehyde mixture (Smith and Rudt 1973). The whole eye is placed in cold (4°C) fixative immediately after enucleation. For anterior segment structures, fixation is continued for 1 hour before opening the eye to produce tissue blocks. This allows time for preliminary fixation, which provides some protection from manipulation damage. The posterior part of the eye is removed, using Vannas scissors and jeweler's forceps. The lens can then be gently removed, making it and the balance of the anterior eye available for cutting into small tissue blocks. Fixation in the glutaraldehyde-paraformaldehyde fixative is continued for an additional 1–2 hours, followed by routine osmification and embedding.

The posterior segment of the eye requires a different approach. The potential space between the retina and the retinal pigment epithelium often results in an artifactual retinal detachment when attempts are made to cut small tissue blocks. Since detachment disturbs normal anatomic relationships, it must be avoided. We have found this problem particularly troublesome when there are diffuse retinal lesions, such as retinal degeneration. Better results are obtained by fixing the whole eye for 2–4 hours before opening and removing the posterior segment. The posterior segment is hemisected or cut into quarters. A clean, new razor blade is essential and often discarded after two to three cuts. This technique usually succeeds in producing 1 × 2 mm tissue blocks. These are exposed to the original fixative for an additional hour before routine processing proceeds.

## REVIEW OF OPHTHALMIC PATHOLOGY

The proliferation of publications on subjects relating to ophthalmic pathology of GEM makes it impossible to discuss all topics of interest in this chapter. References for specific mutant phenotypes are provided in Table 15.1. The four topics covered in this section provide examples of the problems and possibilities present in the development of mouse models of human disease:

1. Effects of aging and gene interaction on gene expression
2. Manipulation of human disease genes in mice
3. Background effects in ocular development
4. Effects of incomplete penetrance and genetic drift on phenotype

### Effects of Aging and Gene Interaction

Investigations of complex traits produced by interacting genes and the effects of aging on phenotype are important when analyzing GEM and are useful for obtaining information concerning human disease mechanisms. In the past, the incorrect perception has been that mice do not develop glaucoma because their eyes are anatomically different from those of primates. Glaucoma is a major public health problem that often begins in young adults. It can result in blindness in one eye of up to 27 percent of all patients after 20 years (Hattenhauer et al. 1998). With nearly 70 million people affected by glaucoma throughout the world, this is clearly an area in which a mouse model would be useful (Quigley 1996).

The strong similarities between the anatomy of mouse and human aqueous outflow pathways have been discussed earlier in the chapter and elsewhere (Smith et al. 1998). It is important to age mice to avoid missing age-related phenotypes, as illustrated by the development of glaucoma in older DBA/2J (D2) mice (Mohr et al. 1996; John et al. 1998). Affected mice develop elevated intraocular pressure (IOP), pigment dispersion, iris stromal and pigment epithelial atrophy, anterior synechias, retinal ganglion cell loss, optic nerve cupping, and optic nerve atrophy. The clinical and histopathological findings in mice resemble the findings described in human pigment dispersion and essential iris atrophy (John et al. 1998). Further studies have demonstrated that these changes are caused by two genetic loci (Chang et al. 1999).

While the D2 glaucoma model is not a GEM mouse, it serves as an illustration of the problems of analysis discussed in the previous section. Early in the study, it became apparent that plastic sections were a necessity for accurate morphologic diagnosis. In the early lesions in particular, it was necessary to develop a set of very specific definitions and a reliable and reproducible grading system (John et al. 1998). Since optic nerve cupping is an important indicator of diagnosis and progression, control of section level was essential (see Figs 15.6e and f). Finally, the presence of two genes that interact to alter the phenotype of offspring is a reminder that many diseases are affected by multiple genes. This observation is equally pertinent for both spontaneous and induced mutations as well as for GEM mice, since modifier genes from different genetic backgrounds can also have great effects on the phenotype. Thus, it is essential to use appropriately matched genetic controls. It is also important to understand that different strains can have different anatomic features, even though the basic structures are the same.

## Human Disease Genes in Mice

When a human disease gene is mapped, targeted mutagenesis of the same gene in the mouse becomes an attractive experiment to help understand disease pathology and mechanisms. In doing so it is important to carefully check different localities in the eye because of the possibility of regional variations in gene expression. Since different mouse strains have different background genes, a knockout should be studied on more than one background in order not to miss expression of a phenotype.

CYP1B1 is the gene for cytochrome P4501B1, and mutations in this gene are strongly linked in human populations with primary congenital glaucoma (Bejjani et al. 1998). Mutations have been identified that disrupt either the hinge region or the conserved core structures of cytochrome P4501B1 (Stoilov et al. 1998). The mechanisms that produce glaucoma in this mutation await explanation.

Mice that are Cyp1b1–/– (produced on a mixed genetic background) were found to demonstrate severe focal maldevelopment of the anterior chamber angle, including disorganized and hypoplastic trabecular meshwork (S.W.M. John, F. Gonzalez, and R.S. Smith, unpublished observations). These mice have normal IOP, so the deletion is currently being placed on a C57BL/6J background in an effort to produce a glaucoma phenotype. In light of the possibility of modifying genes in mice with different genetic backgrounds, it would not be surprising if a Cyp1b1–/– mouse on a different genetic background were to develop increased IOP.

Although there is little information on the histopathologic findings for human congenital glaucoma undisturbed by medical and surgical treatment, the mouse findings are consistent with what has been reported for human eyes (Spencer 1996). The failure to identify a phenotype is also consistent with human congenital glaucoma, in which patients may carry the genotype but do not develop the phenotype (Bejjani et al. 1998). The Cyp1b1 knockout mouse demonstrates the need for careful anatomic and molecular analysis in evaluating any mouse mutant.

## Ocular Development, Cataracts, and Background Effects

The effects of spontaneous and induced genetic mutations may result in unanticipated ocular effects that may be difficult to interpret. Mutations targeted to a specific ocular structure may also alter the development of other ocular structures. As understanding of the genetics of the developmental process increases, some of these effects become easier to explain. The development of the lens and the influence of diverse genes on the process represent the complexities that must be considered in evaluating GEM.

Development of the lens begins at embryonic day 10 with a thickening of the surface ectoderm that overlays the optic vesicle to form the lens placode and lens pit. Over the next 24 hours, the placode thickens and invaginates to form the lens vesicle, which is initially connected to the surface ectoderm by a stalk but becomes detached by day 11 or 12 of embryogenesis. The anterior layer of lens epithelium begins to elongate and quickly obliterates the cavity of the lens vesicle. As the lens grows, complex lens proteins (crystallins) are produced, and the lens epithelium secretes a thickened basement membrane that becomes the lens capsule. (Pei and Rhodin 1970) The apparently simple morphogenesis of the lens and its relative isolation from the rest of the eye give no hints of its relationship to general ocular development. In an ingenious experiment, the lens was removed from the developing chick eye at embryonic day 5. Growth of the entire eye was retarded, the cornea and sclera were thinner than normal, and the choroid and retinal pigment epithelium failed to fully develop, resulting in microphthalmia (Coulombre and Coulombre 1964).

Since 1964, the story has proved to be much more complex, but only a brief review is possible. Genes that control lens morphogenesis (Smith, et al. 1997; Robinson et al. 1998; Dahl et al. 1997; Eqwuagu et al. 1994b; Gotz 1995) often affect other aspects of ocular development, including induction of microphthalmia. There is strong evolutionary conservation of the many genes that control ocular development (Halder et al. 1995). Homeobox genes that control multiple aspects of ocular development, such as *Pax6,* are often expressed in the lens, and mutations of these genes can result in cataract formation (Tomarev et al. 1996; Cveki and Piatigorsky 1996; Dahl et al. 1997).

Cataracts and microphthalmia can also be induced by targeted expression of genes in the lens. Members of the fibroblast growth factor (FGF) family have important roles in embryogenesis (Fini et al. 1997) Several FGFs (FGF1,3,4,7,8,9) cause premature lens fiber differentiation, cataracts, and microphthalmia (Lovicu and Overbeek 1998; Robinson et al. 1998). Ablation or disruption of the αA-crystallin gene may cause cataracts (Brady et al. 1997) or cataracts accompanied by microphthalmia and severe retinal maldevelopment (Kaur et al. 1989).

The investigator must also be aware of the effects of genetic background, since inbred black mice have a variable incidence (1–14 percent) of microphthalmia and cataracts (Smith et al. 1994). This background effect also demonstrates the importance of environment, since the incidence of microphthalmia can be increased to as much as 50 percent by external stimuli such as fetal alcohol exposure (Cook et al. 1987).

## Effects of Incomplete Penetrance and Genetic Drift on Phenotype

In analyzing GEM it is important to be aware that the chosen background strain may carry a defect similar to the effect sought in the GEM. Findings such as retinal dysplasia have been reported with different genetic defects: *Cdkn1b* (p27$^{Kip1}$) (Nakayama et al. 1996) and *Leh* (p56$^{lck}$) (Omri et al. 1998; Rahemtulla et al. 1991) and in segmental trisomy of mouse Chr 4 and 17 (Smith et al. 1999). The common denominator in all three mice is their C57BL background. Since microphthalmia can be induced by environmental agents (Cook et al. 1987), the issue is raised of whether the retinal dysplasia is a direct genetic effect *or* an indirect effect on expression of an unknown gene in the background of the strain under investigation. The popularity of C57BL mice in GEM production suggests that the investigator must be aware of this problem when interpreting eye defects.

It is quite likely that these observations are ultimately due to the effects of one or more modifier genes present in the background of a particular inbred strain. Apart from the known problems of inbred black mice, the same gene on different genetic backgrounds can produce prominent differences in phenotype. The tumor suppressor gene *Trp53* (p53) is associated with a number of different functions, including control of the cell cycle, angiogenesis, development, and the cellular stress response (Rak et al. 1996; Stellmach et al. 1996; Brown 1997; Hopp et al. 1998). A p53-null mutant on a 129/Sv background (129/Sv-*Trp53*$^{tm1Tyj}$) was moved by backcrossing to C57BL/6J (B6) to produce a congenic B6 p53–/– line. Mice with the 129 background demonstrated no significant ocular abnormalities, while the B6 p53–/– mice developed pigmented and nonpigmented retrolental fibrous tissue, retinal folds, and focal degeneration of retinal ganglion cells and optic nerves. The difference may be explained by the presence of dominant protective alleles in the 129/Sv mice. (Ikeda et al. 1999). When differences such as this are discovered, they provide powerful tools for identifying and mapping genes that modify the effects of other genes, altering the severity of disease.

A final pitfall is the presence of genes that produce the same disease in multiple inbred mouse strains. If the investigator is unaware of this, the background disease may be interpreted as being a result of the induced mutation. An excellent example of this is the gene for retinal degeneration 1 (*rd1*). An informal survey of the inbred strains at the Jackson Laboratory revealed the presence of *rd1* in over 60 different strains. It is most widespread in C3H and FVB strains, but occurs in many others. Mice with the *rd1* mutation have normal, fully differentiated photoreceptors at birth, but beginning in the second week of life, both rod and cone photoreceptors undergo rapid apoptotic death (Bowes et al. 1990; Pittler and Baehr 1991; Hopp et al. 1998). Clearly, same age, same sex, +/+ controls of the same strain must be examined before it is concluded that a histopathological change is the result of genetic manipulation.

## REVIEW OF OCULAR DEFECTS IN GENETICALLY ENGINEERED MICE

The rapid pace of publication in areas relating to GEM with ocular defects ensures that any summary will be out of date before it is published. Many GEM have diffuse ocular and systemic defects, which make tabulation difficult. There are several recent reviews that provide useful surveys of systemically acting genes that produce ocular defects (Grindley et al. 1995; Gotz 1995; Matsuo et al. 1995; Dahl et al. 1997; Shastry 1998). Readers seeking a specific topic are advised to use any of the major search engines available on the Internet. Another useful place to start is the informatics homepage of the Jackson Laboratory [*http://www.informatics.jax.org*], which provides constantly updated information on mouse genetics as well as useful links to other sites.

The summary of references in Table 15.1 is categorized by the region of the eye affected and is intended

**TABLE 15.1. Selective introduction to ocular genetics**

| Ocular defect | Reference |
| --- | --- |
| Cornea | |
|   Fragile epithelium | Kao et al. 1996 |
|   Aberrant goblet cells | Robinson et al. 1998 |
|   Tear deficiency | McCartney-Francis et al. 1997 |
|   Hypoplastic stroma | Sanford et al. 1997 |
| Iris, ciliary body, and trabecular meshwork | |
|   Iris stromal hypoplasia | Kume et al. 1998 |
|   Anterior segment dysgenesis | Tamura et al. 1995 |
|   Tumors | Chevez-Barrios et al. 1993 |
| Lens | |
|   Microphakia | Egwuagu et al. 1994a |
|   Cataract | Balkan et al. 1992; Griep et al. 1993; Breitman et al. 1989; Khillan et al. 1987; Dunia et al. 1996; Gong et al. 1997; Brady et al. 1997 |
|   Lens tumor | Griep et al. 1993 |
|   Abnormal differentiation | Robinson et al. 1998; Lovicu and Overbeek 1998 |
|   Age-related cataract | Gilmour et al. 1998 |
| Retina/choroid | |
|   Neovascularization | Lutty et al. 1994; Okamoto et al. 1997; Favor et al. 1996; Miller 1997; Keller et al. 1994 |
|   Retinal malformation | Fantl et al. 1995 |
|   Apoptosis | Joseph and Li 1996 |
|   Inflammation | Geiger et al. 1994 |
|   Retinal tumors | Marcus et al. 1996; Reneker and Overbeek 1996 |
|   Retinal degeneration | Kedzierski et al. 1997; Humphries et al. 1997 |
|   Retinal dysplasia | Nakayama et al. 1996; Omri et al. 1998; Berger et al. 1996 |
| Diffuse effects | |
|   Microphthalmia | Egwuagu et al. 1994a; Balkan et al. 1992; Griep et al. 1993; Breitman et al. 1989; Dattani et al. 1998 |

only as a selective introduction to the topic of ocular genetics. A single keyword or phrase is associated with each reference to indicate the main subject. The references given are included with those from the balance of this chapter.

# REFERENCES

Balkan, W., Klintworth, G.K., Bock, C.B., et al. 1992. Transgenic mice expressing a constitutively active retinoic acid receptor in the lens exhibit ocular defects. Dev. Biol. 151:622–25.

Bejjani, B.A., Lewis, R.A., Tomey, K.F., et al. 1998. Mutations in CYP1B1, the gene for cytochrome P4501B1, are the predominant cause of primary congenital glaucoma in Saudi Arabia. Am. J. Hum. Genet. 62:325–33.

Berger, W., van de Pol, D., Bachner, D., et al. 1996. An animal model for Norrie disease (ND): gene targeting of the mouse ND gene. Hum. Mol. Genet. 5:51–59.

Bowes, C., Li, T., Danciger, M., et al. 1990. Retinal degeneration in the rd mouse is caused by a defect in the beta subunit of rod cGMP-phosphodiesterase. Nature 347:667–80.

Brady, J.P., Garland, D., Duglas-Tabor, Y., Robison, W.G., et al. 1997. Targeted disruption of the mouse alpha A-crystallin gene induces cataract and cytoplasmic inclusion bodies containing the small heat shock protein alpha B-crystallin. Proc. Natl. Acad. Sci. USA 94:884–89.

Breitman, M.L., Bryce, D.M., Giddens, E., et al. 1989. Analysis of lens cell fate and eye morphogenesis in transgenic mice ablated for cells of the lens lineage. Development 106:457–63.

Brown, M.A. 1997. Tumor suppressor genes and human cancer. Adv. Genet. 36:46–135.

Chang, B., Smith, R.S., Hawes, N.L., et al. 1999. Interacting loci cause severe iris atrophy and glaucoma in DBA/2J mice. Nat. Genet. 21:405–9

Chang, S.C. 1972. Hematoxylin-eosin staining of plastic-embedded tissue sections. Arch. Pathol. 93:344–51.

Chevez-Barrios, P., Schaffner, D.L., Barrios, R., et al. 1993. Expression of the rasT24 oncogene in the ciliary body pigment epithelium and retinal pigment epithelium results in hyperplasia, adenoma and adenocarcinoma. Am. J. Pathol. 43:120–28.

Cook, C.S., Nowotney, A.Z., and Sulik, K.K. 1987. Fetal alcohol syndrome: eye malformations in a mouse model. Arch. Ophthalmol. 105:1576–81.

Coulombre, A.J., and Coulombre, J.L. 1964. Lens development I. Role of the lens in eye growth. J. Exp. Zool. 156:39–48.

Cveki, A., and Piatigorsky, J. 1996. Lens development and crystallin gene expression: many roles for Pax-6. Bioessays 18:621–30.

Dahl, E., Koseki, H., and Balling, R. 1997. Pax genes and organogenesis. Bioessays 19:755–65.

Dattani, M.T., Martinez-Barbera, J., Thomas, P.Q., et al. 1998. Mutations in the homeobox gene HESX1/Hesx1 associated with septo-optic dysplasia in human and mouse. Nat. Genet. 19:125–33.

DiLoreto, D., Grover, D.A., del Cerro, C., et al. 1994. A new procedure for fundus photography and fluorescein angiography in small laboratory animal eyes. Curr. Eye Res. 13:157–61.

Dunia, I., Smit, J.J.M., van der Valk, M.A., et al. 1996. Human multidrug resistance 3-P-glycoprotein expression in transgenic mice induces lens membrane alterations leading to cataract. J. Cell. Biol. 132:701–16.

Egwuagu, C.E., Sztein, J., Chan, C.C., et al. 1994a. Ectopic expression of gamma interferon in the eyes of transgenic mice induces ocular pathology and MHC Class II gene expression. Invest. Ophthalmol. Vis. Sci. 35:332–41.

Egwuagu, C.E., Sztein, J., Chan, C.C., et al. 1994b. γ-interferon expression disrupts lens and retinal differentiation in transgenic mice. Dev. Biol. 166:557–68.

Fantl, V., Stamp, G., Andrews, A., et al. 1995. Mice lacking cyclin D1 are small and show defects in eye and mammary gland development. Genes Dev. 9:2364–72.

Favor, J., Sandulache, R., Neuhauser-Klaus, A., et al. 1996. The mouse *Pax2^1Neu* mutation is identical to a human *PAX2* mutation in a family with renal-coloboma syndrome and results in developmental defects of the brain, ear, eye, and kidney. Proc. Natl. Acad. Sci. USA 93:13870–75.

Fini, M.E., Strissel, K.J., and West-Mays, J.A. 1997. Perspectives on eye development. Dev. Genet. 20:175–85.

Folkman, J., and D'Amore, P.A. 1996. Blood vessel formation: what is its molecular basis. Cell 87:1153–55.

Geiger, K., Howes, E., Gallina, M., et al. 1994. Transgenic mice expressing IFN-γ in the retina develop inflammation of the eye and photoreceptor loss. Invest. Ophthalmol. Vis. Sci. 35:2667–81.

Gilmour, D.T., Lyon, G.J., Carlton, M., et al. 1998. Mice deficient for the secreted glycoprotein SPARC/ostonectin/BM40 develop normally but show severe age-onset cataract formation and disruption of the lens. EMBO J. 17:1860–70.

Gong, X., Li, E., Klier, G., et al. 1997. Disruption of α_3 connexin gene leads to proteolysis and cataractogenesis in mice. Cell 91:833–43.

Gotz, W. 1995. Transgenic models for eye malformations. Ophthalmic Genet. 16:85–104.

Graw, J. 1996. Genetic aspects of embryonic eye development in vertebrates. Dev. Genet. 18:181–97.

Griep, A.E., Herber, R., Jeon, S., et al. 1993. Tumorigenicity by human papillomavirus type 16 E6 and E7 in transgenic mice correlates with alterations in epithelial cell growth and differentiation. J. Virol. 67:1373–84.

Grindley, J.C., Davidson, D.R., and Hill, R.E. 1995. The role of Pax-6 in eye and nasal development. Development 121:1433–42.

Halder, G., Callaerts, P., and Gehring, W.J. 1995. Induction of ectopic eyes by targeted expression of the *eyeless* gene in *Drosophila*. Science 267:1788–92.

Hattenhauer, M.G., Johnson, D.H., Ing, H.H., et al. 1998. The probability of blindness from open-angle glaucoma. Ophthalmology 105:2099–2104.

Hero, I., Farjah, M., and Scholtz, C.L. 1991. The prenatal development of the optic fissure in colobomatous microphthalmia. Invest. Ophthalmol. Vis. Sci. 32:2622–35.

Hogan, M.J., Alvarado, J.A., and Weddell, J.E. 1971. Histology of the Human Eye. Philadelphia: W.B. Saunders Company.

Holm, A., and Holm, O. 1991. Digitizing 35mm color slides for computerized general image handling in ophthalmology. Acta Ophthalmol. 69:611–17.

Hopp, R., Ransom, M., Hilsenbeck, S.G., et al. 1998. Apoptosis in the murine *rd1* retinal degeneration is predominantly p53-dependent. Mol. Vis. 4:5.

Humphries, M.M., Rancourt, D., Farrar, G.J., et al. 1997. Retinopathy induced in mice by targeted disruption of the rhodopsin gene. Nat. Genet. 15:216–19.

Ikeda, S., Hawes, N.L., Chang, B., et al. 1999. Ocular abnormalities in C57BL/6 but not 129/Sv p53 deficient mice. Invest. Ophthalmol. Vis. Sci. 40:1874–78.

John, S.W.M.J., Smith, R.S., Savinova, O., et al. 1998. Essential iris atrophy, pigment dispersion and glaucoma in DBA/2J mice. Invest. Ophthalmol. Vis. Sci. 39:951–62.

Joseph, R.M., and Li, T. 1996. Overexpression of Bcl-2 or Bcl-X_L transgenes and photoreceptor degeneration. Invest. Ophthalmol. Vis. Sci. 37:2434–46.

Kao, W., Liu, C., Converse, R.L., et al. 1996. Keratin 12-deficient mice have fragile corneal epithelia. Invest. Ophthalmol. Vis. Sci. 37:2572–84.

Kaur, B., Key, B., Stock, J., et al. 1989. Targeted ablation of alpha-crystallin-synthesizing cells produces lens-deficient eyes in transgenic mice. Development 105:613–19.

Kedzierski, W., Lloyd, M., Birch, D.G., et al. 1997. Generation and analysis of transgenic mice expressing P216L-substituted Rds/Peripherin in rod photoreceptors. Invest. Ophthalmol. Vis. Sci. 38:498–509.

Keller, S.A., Jones, J.M., Boyle, A., et al. 1994. Kidney and retinal defects (Krd), a transgene-induced mutation with a deletion of mouse chromosome 19 that includes the Pax-2 locus. Genomics 23:309–20.

Khaw, P.T. 1988. Portable and inexpensive systems for ophthalmic photography based on the 35mm SLR camera and standard 50mm f1.8 lens. J. Audiovis. Media Med. 11:81–83.

Khillan, J.S., Oskarsson, M.K., Propst, F., et al. 1987. Defects in lens fiber differentiation are linked to *c-mos* overexpression in transgenic mice. Genes Dev. 1:1327–35.

Kume, T., Deng, K., Winfrey, V., et al. 1998. The Forkhead/winged helix gene *Mf1* is disrupted in the pleiotropic mouse mutation *congenital hydrocephalus*. Cell 93:985–96.

Leiter, E.H., Beamer, W.G., Shultz, L.D., et al. 1987. Mouse models of genetic diseases. Birth Defects 23:221–57.

Lovicu, F.J., and Overbeek, P.A. 1998. Overlapping effects of different members of the FGF family on lens fiber differentiation in transgenic mice. Development 125:3365–77.

Lutty, G.A., McLeod, D.S., Pachnis, A., et al. 1994. Retinal and choroidal neovascularization in a transgenic mouse model of sickle cell disease. Am. J. Pathol. 145:490–97.

Marcus, D.M., Lasudry, J., Carpenter, J.L., et al. 1996. Trilateral tumors in four different lines of transgenic mice expressing SV40 T-antigen. Invest. Ophthalmol. Vis. Sci. 37:392–96.

Matsuo, I., Kuratani, S., Kimura, C., et al. 1995. Mouse *Otx2* functions in the formation and patterning of rostral head. Genes Dev. 9:2646–58.

McCartney-Francis, N.L., Mizel, D.E., Frazier-Jessen, M., et al. 1997. Lacrimal gland inflammation is responsible for ocular pathology in TGF-β-1 null mice. Am. J. Pathol. 151:1281–88.

Miller, J.W. 1997. Vascular endothelial growth factor and ocular neovascularization. Am. J. Pathol. 151:13–23.

Mohr, U., Dungworth, D.L., Capen, C.C., et al. (eds.). 1996. Pathobiology of the Aging Mouse. Washington, DC: ILSI Press.

Nakayama, K., Ishida, N., Shirane, M., et al. 1996. Mice lacking p27[kip1] display increased body size, multiple organ hyperplasia, retinal dysplasia, and pituitary tumors. Cell 85:707–20.

Okamoto, N., Tobe, T., Hackett, S.F., et al. 1997. Transgenic mice with increased expression of vascular endothelial growth factor in the retina. Am. J. Pathol. 151:281–91.

Oliver, G., and Gruss, P. 1997. Current views on eye development. Trends Neurosci. 20:415–21.

Omri, B., Blancher, C., Neron, B., et al. 1998. Retinal dysplasia in mice lacking p56[lck]. Oncogene 16:2351–56.

Pei, Y.F., and Rhodin, J.A.G. 1970. The prenatal development of the mouse eye. Anat. Rec. 168:105–26.

Pittler, S.J., and Baehr, W. 1991. Identification of a nonsense mutation in the rod photoreceptor cGMP phosphodiesterase beta-subunit of the rd mouse. Proc. Natl. Acad. Sci. USA 88:8322–26.

Quigley, H.A. 1996. Number of people with glaucoma worldwide. Br. Js. Ophthalmol. 80:389–93.

Rahemtulla, A., Fung-Leung, W.P., Schith, M.W., et al. 1991. Normal development and function of CD8+ cells but markedly decreased helper cell activity in mice lacking CD4. Nature 353:180–84.

Rak, J., Filmus, J., and Kerbel, R.S. 1996. Reciprocal paracrine interactions between tumor cells and endothelial cells: the 'angiogenesis progression' hypothesis. Eur. J. Cancer 32A:2438–50.

Reme, C., Urner, U., and Aeberhard, B. 1983. The development of the chamber angle in the rat eye. Graefe's Arch. Clin. Exp. Ophthalmol. 220:139–53.

Reneker, L.W., and Overbeek, P.A. 1996. Lens-specific expression of PDGF-A in transgenic mice results in retinal astrocytic hamartomas. Invest. Ophthalmol. Vis. Sci. 37:2455–66.

Robinson, M.L., Ohtaka-Maruyama, C., Chan, C.C., et al. 1998. Disregulation of ocular morphogenesis by lens-specific expression of FGF-3/Int-2 in transgenic mice. Dev. Biol. 198:13–31.

Rugh, R. 1968. The Mouse: Its Reproduction and Development. Minneapolis, MN: Burgess Publishing Company.

Sadun, A.A., Kashima, Y., Wurdeman, A.E., et al. 1994. Morphological findings in the visual system in a case of Leber's hereditary optic neuropathy. Clin. Neurosci. 2:165–72.

Sanford, L.P., Ormsby, I., Gittenberger-de Groot, A.C., et al. 1997. TGF β-2 knockout mice have multiple developmental defects that are non-overlapping with other TGF β knockout phenotypes. Development 124:2659–70.

Schlamp, C.L., and Nickells, R.W. 1996. Light and dark causes a shift in the spatial expression of a neuropeptide-processing enzyme in the rat retina. J. Neurosci. 16:2164–71.

Schlamp, C.L., and Williams, D.S. 1996. Myosin V in the retina: localization in the rod photoreceptor synapse. Exp. Eye Res. 63:613–19.

Shastry, B.S. 1998. Gene disruption in mice: models of development and disease. Mol. Cell. Biochem. 181:163–79.

Skerrow, D., and Skerrow, C.J. (eds.). 1985. Methods in Skin Research. New York: John Wiley and Sons.

Smith, R.S., and Rudt, L.A. 1973. Ultrastructural studies of the blood-aqueous barrier. Am. J. Ophthalmol. 76:937–47.

Smith, R.S., Roderick, T.H., and Sundberg, J.P. 1994. Microphthalmia and associated abnormalities in inbred black mice. Lab. Anim. Med. 44:551–60.

Smith, R.S., Sundberg, J.P., and Linder, C.C. 1997. Mouse mutations as models for studying cataracts. Pathobiology 65:146–54.

Smith, R.S., Bechtold, L., and John, S.W.M. 1998. Ultrastructure of mouse trabecular meshwork. Invest. Ophthalmol. Vis. Sci. 39:S705.

Smith, R.S., Johnson, K.R., Hawes, N.L., et al. 1999. Lens epithelial proliferation cataract in segmental trisomy involving mouse chromosomes 4 and 17. Mamm. Genome 10:102–6.

Snodgrass, A.B., Dorsey, C.H., Bailey, G., et al. 1972. Conventional histopathologic staining methods compatible with Epon-embedded osmicated tissue. Lab. Invest. 26:329–37.

Spencer, W.H. (ed.). 1996. Ophthalmic Pathology: An Atlas and Textbook. Philadelphia: W.B. Saunders Company.

Stellmach, V., Volpert, O.V., Crawford, S.E., et al. 1996. Tumor suppressor genes and angiogenesis: The role of TP53 in fibroblasts. Eur. J. Cancer 32A:2394–400.

Stoilov, I., Akarsu, A.N., Alozie, I., et al. 1998. Sequence analysis and homology modeling suggest that primary congenital glaucoma on 2p21 results from mutations disrupting either the hinge region or the conserved core structures of cytochrome P4501B1. Am. J. Hum. Genet. 62:573–84.

Sundberg, J.P., and Boggess, B. 1999. Systematic Approach to Evaluation of Mouse Mutations. Boca Raton, FL: CRC Press.

Sundberg, J.P., and King, L.E. 1996. Mouse mutations as animal models and biomedical tools for dermatological research. J. Invest. Dermatol. 106:368–76.

Sundberg, J.P., and Shultz, L.D. 1993. Animal models of human disease: the severe combined immunodeficiency (scid) mouse. Comp. Pathol. Bull. 25:3–4.

Tamura, H., Jidoi, J., Naora, H., et al. 1995. Opaque eyes developed in transgenic mice with T-cell receptor δ Gene. Invest. Ophthalmol. Vis. Sci. 36:467–77.

Tomarev, S.I., Sundin, O., Banerjee-Basu, S., et al. 1996. Chicken homeobox gene Prox-1 related to Drosophila prospero is expressed in the developing lens and retina. Dev. Dyn. 206:354–67.

West, J.D., Hodson, B.A., and Keighran, M.A. 1997. Quantitative and spatial information on the composition of chimaeric mouse eyes from single histological sections. Dev. Growth Differ. 39:305–17.

# 16

# Strategies for Behavioral Phenotyping of Transgenic and Knockout Mice

Jacqueline N. Crawley

Transgenic and knockout mice represent a powerful new research tool for investigating genes mediating brain development, neuroanatomy, neurophysiology, neurochemistry, and behavior. Genes expressed in the central nervous system are likely to contribute to the regulation of normal behavior. Mutations in genes expressed in the central nervous system may underlie heritable neuropsychiatric diseases. Transgenic mice, overexpressing a gene in a brain pathway known to mediate a behavioral trait, can yield critical information about the function of the gene product—for example, the significance of excessively high neurotransmitter levels. Knockout mice, missing a gene in a brain pathway known to mediate a behavioral trait, can reveal the relative importance of the gene product for the behavior—for example, the specificity of a neuropeptide receptor subtype for the regulation of feeding behavior.

Conventional transgenics and knockouts express the mutation throughout ontogeny. The mutation is present from the earliest stage of development, throughout the growth of the nervous system, at birth, in juveniles, in adults, and in aged mice. This approach is excellent for animal models of human hereditary diseases. This conventional approach is also useful for studying factors mediating developmental events. However, the conventional approach is less useful for studying the role of a gene in adult animals. At an early time point during the course of development, compensatory genes may take over the function of the mutated gene. The solution to this limitation lies in "inducible mutations," a new technology that allows a mutation to be turned on and off. Currently, inducible knockouts contain a cre-lox drug-sensitive promoter that permits the expression of the gene only in the absence of a drug, such as tetracycline, which can be administered at all but a specific time

period (Mayford et al., 1996; Tsien et al., 1996). For example, an animal model of amyloid overexpression in Alzheimer's disease could best employ an inducible transgenic that turned on amyloid overexpression only in the aged mouse.

In addition, the conventional approach produces a mutation that is expressed in every gene in the body. A behavioral phenotype could result from the mutation in a peripheral organ, which confounds the interpretation of the effects of the mutation in the brain pathway of interest. The solution to this limitation lies in a new "conditional" mutation technology that allows a mutation to be selectively expressed in a discrete type of cell (Mayford et al. 1996; Tsien et al. 1996; Zhou et al. 1995). Conditional mutations are driven by promoters expressed only in specific types of cells. For example, the CamKII promoter limits gene expression to forebrain neurons in mice (Mayford et al. 1996; Tsien et al. 1996).

Over 60 transgenic and mutant mice have been developed to date for genes expressed in the central nervous system. Many of these have fascinating behavioral phenotypes, including altered social, reproductive, and parental behaviors, unusual levels of aggression, feeding disorders, learning and memory impairments, anxiety-like behaviors, or altered responses to drugs of abuse (reviewed in Campbell and Gold 1996; Nelson and Young 1998).

In the course of testing mice developed by our molecular genetics colleagues at the National Institutes of Health Intramural Research Program, our laboratory has been addressing methodological issues for behavioral phenotyping of mutant mice. Guidelines, based on the strategies that have proven successful in studying a variety of new transgenic and knockout mice in our laboratory and others, are extensively described in recent publications (Campbell and Gold 1996; Crawley et al. 1997, 1998, 2000; Crawley and Paylor 1997; Lee et al. 1996; Nelson and Young 1998; Silver 1995; Wehner and Silva 1996; Psychopharmacology 1997; Hormones and Behavior 1997; Behavioral Brain Research 1998).

# METHODOLOGICAL APPROACHES

We recommend a four-step characterization for behavioral evaluation of a new mutant mouse line (Crawley and Paylor 1997; Paylor et al. 1998): (1) initial preliminary observations of general health, (2) evaluation of simple neurological reflexes, (3) evaluation of sensory and motor abilities, (4) specific behavioral paradigms addressing the hypothesized functions of the gene. The goals behind this approach are to maximize the discoveries of important mutation-induced phenotypes, while minimizing false-positives and false-negatives. A sick mouse will yield false-positives on most behavioral tests. An animal that cannot see, hear, smell, walk, run, swim, press a lever, and so on will be unable to perform the procedures necessary for many complex behavioral tasks.

The fundamental abilities of the new mutant are first documented for general health, neurological reflexes, sensory, and motor abilities. Based on the results of these initial tests, the behavioral neuroscientist then designs several behavioral tasks specific for each hypothesized function of the gene. Specific tasks are chosen for compatibility with the documented sensory and motor abilities of the mutant mice. Multiple tasks in each behavioral domain of interest are selected, to avoid false-negatives. More than one behavioral domain, such as motor coordination, learning and memory, feeding, social behaviors, anxiety, aggression, and so on, may be relevant to the hypothesized functions of the gene of interest. Multiple tests can be conducted sequentially, with a carefully crafted experimental design. Table 16.1 summarizes the order of experiments for investigating a new transgenic or knockout mouse line.

## Initial Observations

The general examination of mice is conducted in the home cages (Crawley and Paylor 1997). Overall *health* and *condition of the fur* are recorded. *Body weight* and *body temperature* are measured. Home cage *activity, grooming, nesting,* and *sleeping patterns* are quantitated. Any unusual patterns of *locomotion, hyperreactivity to handling,* or *fighting* in the home cage are documented. Abnormal appearances and home cage

**TABLE 16.1. Order of behavioral testing of a new mutant mouse—preliminary observations and behavioral domains**

1. Initial observations
    General appearance
    Home cage behaviors
    Body weight
    Body temperature
2. Neurological reflexes
    Righting reflex
    Eye blink reflex
    Ear twitch reflex
    Whisker-orienting reflex
3. Sensory abilities
    Visual cliff response
    Acoustic startle reflex
    Von Frey hair response to touch
    Hot plate analgesia
    Olfactory location
4. Motor abilities
    Open field
    Rotarod
    Wire hang
    Pole climb
    Balance beam
    Footprint pattern
5. Behavioral domains for specific hypothesis testing
    Learning and memory
    Feeding and drinking
    Social behaviors
    Sexual behaviors
    Parental behaviors
    Aggressive behaviors
    Anxiety-related behaviors
    Depression-related behaviors
    Schizophrenia-related behaviors
    Analgesia
    Taste aversion
    Taste preference
    Drug preference

behaviors provide important clues for further experiments to define the behavioral phenotype. For example, many of the seizure-susceptible strains of mice available from the Jackson Laboratory in Bar Harbor, Maine, were derived from mice that individuals observed seizing in the home cage (Dr. Wayne Frankel, personal communication). Aggressive behaviors in nitric oxide synthase knockout mice were discovered by animal caretakers who reported fighting in the home cage (Nelson et al. 1995). Absence of normal huddled sleeping patterns in home cages led to the discovery of social interaction abnormalities in disheveled-1 knockout mice (Lijam et al. 1997).

## Neurological Reflexes

The *righting reflex* is a simple test in which the mouse is turned onto its back; the time it takes for the mouse to right itself onto all four paws is measured. The *eye blink reflex* is observed when the cornea is approached with a cotton-tip swab. The *ear twitch reflex* is tested by touching the ear with a cotton-tip swab and observing the immediate movement of the pinna. The *whisker-orienting reflex* is observed by touching the vibrissae on one side; the whiskers stop moving and the head turns to the side on which the whiskers were touched.

## Sensory and Motor Abilities

### SENSORY

Simple measures of sensory function are available for some modalities; however, better tests are needed for rapid evaluation of sensory abilities. *Visual cliff response* is conducted in a box with a horizontal surface and a vertical wall drop-off, representing an apparent ledge (Fox 1965). The inner horizontal surface of the box and vertical drop-off are covered with black-and-white checkerboard contact paper, which emphasizes the cliff-like drop-off. A piece of clear Plexiglas spans the ledge, so that there is no actual drop-off, just the visual appearance of a cliff. The mouse is placed on a platform at the border between the horizontal surface and the vertical drop-off. Normal mice will step down mostly onto the horizontal surface, to avoid the cliff that they see on the other side of the platform. Blind mice, not seeing the apparent cliff, will step down an equal number of times onto the horizontal surface and the clifflike drop-off. Another simple test of gross visual ability is the latency for a mouse to enter a dark area, when the mouse is placed in a brightly lit area. Since mice are nocturnal and prefer the dark, a mouse with normal light/dark perception will quickly enter the darkened chamber. A blind mouse will take much longer before it enters the darkened chamber. To obtain more sensitive measures of visual acuity, tasks requiring some training, using *visual stimuli* in a conditioned reward paradigm, are appropriate. Neurophysiological recording from brain structures receiving visual input is the most sensitive method for assessing visual abilities.

Gross hearing ability can be assessed by the *acoustic startle reflex*. Acoustic startle to a loud tone is evaluated by an automated startle system that measures the amplitude of whole body flinch. Sensitive measures of hearing acuity are conducted with neurophysiological recording from the auditory nerve, using the *auditory brainstem response* (Erway et al. 1993).

Touch is evaluated by the *reflexive twitch response to Von Frey hairs*, fine wires of graded thickness touched to the paw. Pain sensitivity is measured by the latency to lick or lift a hind paw in the *hot plate test* or to move the tail out of the path of an intense light beam in the *tail-flick test*.

Olfactory ability can be initially evaluated by timing the *retrieval of a buried food source*. More specific smell and taste discriminations are measured with olfactory and gustatory stimuli in *conditioned reward* and *conditioned place preference* choice paradigms.

### MOTOR

Motor activities underlie the performance of almost all behavioral tasks. If the mutation results in severe deficits in the ability of the mouse to walk, climb, balance, grip, or swim, for example, the mouse may be unable to perform the procedures necessary for more sophisticated behavioral tasks. *Open field exploratory locomotion* is measured with a photocell-equipped automated apparatus that quantitates locomotion and rearings in an empty open field. Motor coordination and balance are quantitated on an accelerating rotating cylinder, the *rotarod* automated apparatus. These two paradigms will detect major abnormalities in the spinal motor neurons and cerebellum. Measurement of *hanging wire* grip time provides an index of neuromuscular function. The ability of the mouse to climb a *pole* or to walk along a *narrow beam* provides further measures of balance and coordination. *Footprint pathway* analysis, in which the hind paws are dipped in black ink and the mouse walks across white paper through a tunnel, detects abnormal gait.

Behavioral phenotypes are often discovered during the sensory and motor analyses. Mouse models of Tay-Sachs and Sandhoff diseases, with mutations in the genes for the enzyme hexosaminidase, the enzyme that degrades gangliosides, show neurodegeneration and concomitant progressive decline in performance on the rotarod task (Sango et al. 1995), analogous to the motor deficits that characterize this human syndrome. *Atm* knockout mice, a model of ataxia-telangiectasia, are deficient on the open field and rotarod tests and show unusual footprint patterns (Barlow et al. 1996), analogous to the ataxia seen in the clinical syndrome.

## Hypothesis Testing for Complex Behavioral Traits

The goal of generating a new mutant mouse line is to test hypotheses about the function of a gene. In some cases, the gene is well-known in another species, such as *Drosophila*, and the role of the gene in mammals is then explored. Sometimes the function of the gene product is known for a peripheral tissue; when the gene is discovered to be expressed in the brain, its behavioral functions are explored. In other instances, the gene product is well-known, and the mutation is generated as a new tool to test, for example, the role of the neurotransmitter, receptor, or enzyme during development, in response to such stimuli as drug challenges. Exciting results are emerging from the fourth category, wherein the mutation is generated in mice as a model of a human hereditary disease. If the phenotype of the mutant mouse is substantively analogous to the phenotype of the human disease, the mouse model can be used as a critical research tool for developing treatments for the human disease. A robust, reliable behavioral abnormality in the mouse model provides an excellent marker to evaluate treatment efficacy.

The choice of appropriate behavioral tasks requires a clear hypothesis and a thorough understanding of the existing behavioral neuroscience literature. Obvious and testable hypotheses are readily generated for the behavioral phenotyping of mice with mutations in genes with known products (e.g., neurotransmitters, receptors, transporters). Genes expressed in discrete brain regions may be analyzed for hypotheses based on known functions of the brain pathways. Genes expressed primarily in the cerebellum would be best investigated in tasks that measure motor coordination and motor learning. Genes expressed primarily in the hypothalamus would be fruitfully evaluated in tasks involving feeding, stress responses, and sexual and parental behaviors. Genes expressed primarily in the hippocampus and cortex would be tested through learning and memory, attentional, and habituation tasks. Genes expressed primarily in the mesolimbic dopamine pathway would be investigated through motivational and appetitively rewarded tasks and through drug abuse paradigms. Genes expressed primarily in the periaqueductal gray and dorsal horn of the spinal cord may show major phenotypes for pain threshold and responses to analgesics. Figure 16.1 provides a highly simplified summary of brain regions mediating some behavioral functions in rodents.

The novice wishing to begin behavioral phenotyping experiments is encouraged to develop a collaboration with an established behavioral neuroscience laboratory. Correct choices and implementation of behavioral tasks in mice require a thorough understanding of over 50 years of scientific literature in behavioral neuroscience, knowledge of the standard methods for the basic behavioral paradigms, and familiarity with the little tricks that make any method work well. Experience with proper testing and handling of mice, to minimize stress factors and to meet the international guidelines for the care and use of laboratory rodents, can best be gained by working with a behavioral neuroscientist. Many substandard publications have emerged from molecular genetics laboratories that apply incorrect experimental designs to behavioral phenotyping of their mutant mice. Entering into a scientific collaboration with a recognized behavioral laboratory will help novice researchers to avoid the pitfalls and to move their phenotyping experiments ahead more quickly.

A wide variety of good behavioral tests are available for each of the behavioral domains of interest. Reviews cited above describe these specific methods in great

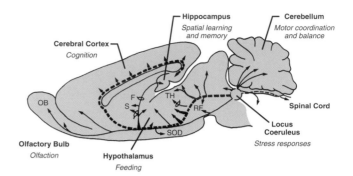

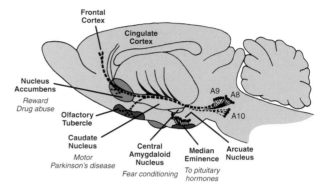

**FIGURE 16.1**   Highly simplified diagrams of the rodent brain, indicating several of the anatomical structures contributing to the regulation of some natural behaviors in rats and mice.

detail, with relevant source literature for further consultation. For example, learning and memory tests for mice include spatial navigation learning tasks such as the Morris water task, Barnes maze, radial maze, T-maze, and Y-maze; rewarded tasks such as nose-poke for a food reward in an operant chamber or a five-hole chamber on various schedules; and aversive tasks such as passive avoidance, cued and contextual conditioning, and taste aversion. Feeding tasks may involve 24-hour consumption, limited daily access, macronutrient sources, taste discrimination, and sham feeding. Parental behaviors are quantitated for latency to retrieve pups to the nest, nursing the pups, grooming the pups, and time spent in the nest. Good models of anxiety-related behaviors include the elevated plus maze, the elevated zero maze, light↔dark exploratory transitions, and the Vogel conflict test. Drug abuse tendencies can be measured with conditioned place preference, two-bottle choices, and intravenous self-administration.

# BREEDING ISSUES FOR BEHAVIORAL PHENOTYPING

Before proceeding with behavioral testing of a new transgenic or knockout mouse line, breeding of the set of mice for the behavioral experiments must be conducted in accordance with the requirements of the experimental design. To obtain statistically meaningful results, most behavioral experiments require 10–20 mice per treatment group. Treatment groups include the homozygous mutant, the heterozygous mutant litter-mates, and the wild-type littermates. If gender differences are detected, $N = 10$–20 for each gender of each genotype is required. Ages of the mice must be approximately the same across treatment groups. Adult mice in the age range of 3–8 months are relatively homogenous on most behavioral tasks. If sufficient numbers of animals are not available simultaneously, experimental groups can be split into smaller groups as litters become available. All three genotypes must be represented within each set of experiments.

Background gene issues may be critical for some behavioral tests. Two or more strains are often used to develop the set of mice for behavioral experiments. The 129/SvJ or another 129 substrain is used for the embryonic stem cells, and C57BL/6J or another inbred or outbred strain for the blastocyst donors and breeders. Varying ratios of the genetic backgrounds from each strain will be present in each offspring. Confounding interactions between the mutated gene and the background genes have been problematic in many cases, prompting suggestions for optimizing the choice of inbred strain for breeding the mutation (reviewed in Crawley et al. 1997; Wehner and Silva 1996). Congenic breeding into one inbred strain for 5–7 generations will create a more uniform genetic background, to reduce unknown gene product interactions and to reduce variability due to random assortment of parental alleles. C57BL/6J is a strain that breeds relatively well and is average on many behavioral tasks, allowing detection of increases and decreases in the behavioral scores in the mutant line bred into C57BL/6J (Silver 1995; Crawley et al. 1997).

# CONCLUSIONS

Successful applications of behavioral paradigms are seen in the growing literature on interesting new transgenic and knockout mice with mutations in genes expressed in the brain. Mouse models of Alzheimer's disease show deficits in learning and memory tasks (Hsiao et al. 1996). Obese mutant mice show unusual patterns of feeding behaviors and/or consume larger amounts of foods (Pelleymounter et al. 1995; Huszar et al. 1997). Opiate receptor knockout mice are aberrant on tests for pain responsivity, analgesic effects of morphine, morphine withdrawal responses, and conditioned place preference (Sora et al. 1997; Matthes et al. 1996). Knockouts of genes expressed primarily in the hippocampus show deficits in learning and memory

tasks (Silva et al. 1992). Estrogen receptor knockout mice are impaired in sexual behaviors (Rissman et al. 1997). Oxytocin-deficient mice fail to lactate (Young et al. 1996; Nishimori et al. 1996). Knockouts for genes expressed in the amygdala show unusual anxiety-related behaviors on stress-related tasks (Heinrichs et al. 1997).

Characterization of a new mutant mouse spans many disciplines. Pathology is one major area of phenotypic investigation. Neuroanatomy, neurochemistry, neurophysiology, and behavior are important techniques for analyzing mice with mutations in genes expressed in the brain. Our strategy of an initial neurological test battery, followed by specific, hypothesis-driven choices of a constellation of behavioral tasks, provides a useful place to start in characterizing the behavioral phenotype of a new mutant mouse. A large number of behavioral tests are available or adaptable to the needs of researchers for behavioral phenotyping of transgenic and knockout mice. Creative behavioral neuroscientists working in this field are presently developing additional and better paradigms for future use by the scientific community.

# REFERENCES

Barlow, C., Hirotsune, S., Paylor, R., et al. 1996. *Atm*-deficient mice: a paradigm of Ataxia Telangiectasia. Cell 86:159–171.

Behavioral Brain Research. 1998. Special Issue on Behavioural Neurogenetics (September) 95:1.

Campbell, I.L., Gold, L.H. 1996. Transgenic modeling of neuropsychiatric disorders. Mol. Psychiatry 1:105–120.

Crawley, J.N. 2000. What's Wrong with My Mouse? Behavioral Phenotyping of Transgenic and Knockout Mice. New York: John Wiley and Sons.

Crawley, J.N., Paylor, R. 1997. A proposed test battery and constellations of specific behavioral paradigms to investigate the behavioral phenotypes of transgenic and knockout mice. Hormones Behav. 31:197–211.

Crawley, J.N., Belknap, J.K., Collins, A., et al. 1997. Behavioral phenotypes of inbred mouse strains: implications and recommendations for molecular studies. Psychopharmacology 132:107–124.

Crawley, J.N., Gerfen, C.R., McKay, R., et al. Eds. 1998. Current Protocols in Neuroscience. New York: John Wiley and Sons.

Erway, L.C., Willott, J.F., Archer, J.R., et al. 1993. Genetics of age-related hearing loss in mice. Hear. Res. 65:125–132.

Fox, M.W. 1965. The visual cliff test for the study of visual depth perception in the mouse. Anim. Behav. 13:232–233.

Heinrichs, S.C., Min, H., Tamraz, S., et al. 1997. Anti-sexual and anxiogenic behavioral consequences of corticotropin-releasing factor overexpression are centrally mediated. Psychoneuroendocrinology 22:215–224.

Hormones and Behavior. 1997. Special Issue on Single Gene Mutations, Gene Knockouts and Behavioral Neuroendocrinology (June) 31:3.

Hsiao, K., Chapman, P., Nilsen, S., et al. 1996. Correlative memory deficits, Aβ elevation, and amyloid plaques in transgenic mice. Science 274:99–102.

Huszar, D., Lynch, C.A., Fairchild-Huntress, V., et al. 1997. Targeted disruption of the melanocortin-4 receptor results in obesity in mice. Cell 88:131–141.

Lee, M.K., Borchelt, D.R., Wong, P.C., et al. 1996 Transgenic models of neurodegenerative diseases. Curr. Opin. Neurobiol. 6:651–660.

Lijam, N., Paylor, R., McDonald, M.P., et al. 1997. Social interaction and sensorimotor gating abnormalities in mice lacking Dvl1. Cell 90:895–905.

Matthes, H.W.D., Maldonado, R., Simonin, F., et al. 1996. Loss of morphine-induced analgesia, reward effect and withdrawal symptoms in mice lacking the μ-opioid-receptor gene. Nature 383:819–823.

Mayford, M., Bach, M.E., Huang, Y.Y., et al. 1996. Control of memory formation through regulated expression of a CaMKII transgene. Science 274:1678–1683.

Nelson, R.J., Young, K.A. 1998. Behavior in mice with targeted disruption of single genes. Neurosci. Biobehav. Rev. 22:453–462.

Nelson, R.J., Demas, G.E., Huang, P.L., et al. 1995. Behavioural abnormalities in male mice lacking neuronal nitric oxide synthase. Nature 378:383–386.

Nishimori, K., Young, L.J., Guo, Q., et al. 1996. Oxytocin is required for nursing but is not essential for parturition or reproductive behavior. Proc. Natl. Acad. Sci. USA 93:11699–11704.

Paylor, R., Nguyen, M., Crawley, J.N., et al. 1998. α7 nicotinic receptor subunits are not necessary for hippocampal-dependent learning or sensorimotor gating: a behavioral characterization of Acra-7 deficient mice. Learn. Mem. 5:302–316.

Pelleymounter, M.A., Cullen, M.J., Baker, M.B., et al. 1995. Effects of the obese gene product on body weight regulation in ob/ob mice. Science 269:540–543.

Psychopharmacology. 1997. Special Issue on Behavioral and Molecular Genetics (July 11) 132:2.

Rissman, E.F., Early, A.H., Taylor, J.A., et al. 1997. Estrogen receptors are essential for female sexual receptivity. Endocrinology 138:507–510.

Sango, K., Yamanaka, S., Hoffmann, A., et al. 1995. Mouse models of Tay-Sachs and Sandhoff diseases differ in neurologic phenotype and ganglioside metabolism. Nat. Genet. 11:170–176.

Silva, A.J., Paylor, R., Wehner, J.M., et al. 1992. Impaired spatial learning in α-calcium-calmodulin kinase II mutant mice. Science 257:206–211.

Silver, L.M. 1995. Mouse Genetics. New York: Oxford University Press.

Sora, I., Takahashi, N., Funada, M., et al. 1997. Opiate receptor knockout mice define μ receptor roles in endogenous nociceptive responses and morphine-induced analgesia. Proc. Natl. Acad. Sci. USA 94:1544–1549.

Tsien, J.Z., Chen, D.F., Gerber, D., et al. 1996. Subregion- and cell type-restricted gene knockout in mouse brain. Cell 87:1317–1326.

Wehner, J.M., Silva, A. 1996. Importance of strain differences in evaluations of learning and memory processes in null mutants. Ment. Retard. Dev. Disabil. Res. Rev. 2:243–248.

Young, W.S., Shepard, E., Amico, J., et al. 1996. Deficiency in mouse oxytocin prevents milk ejection, but not fertility or parturition. J. Neuroendocrinol. 8:847–853.

Zhou, Q.Y., Quaife, C.J., Palmiter, R.D. 1995. Targeted disruption of the tyrosine hydroxylase gene reveals that catecholamines are requred for mouse fetal development. Nature 374:640–643.

# 17
# Pathologic Characterization of Neurological Mutants

Roderick T. Bronson

Many spontaneous and transgenic mutants with neurological phenotypes have been studied; many more will be discovered or produced in the next few years. Identifying lesions in the nervous systems of mutant mice can be quite difficult since you must know the basic principles of neuropathology and many of the details of neuroanatomy. Some principles of neuropathology are presented here. Neuroanatomy is so difficult that very few people have ever really mastered it. Armed with a good brain atlas (Altman and Bayer 1995; Franklin and Paxinos 1997; Sidman et al. 1971), however, almost anyone with a little diligence can identify many structures. This chapter gives a few helpful suggestions on how to study mouse neurological phenotypes.

Three main rules should be followed to ensure best results. The first rule is that discovering a phenotype requires a solid collaboration between the person who discovered or made the mutant, who knows about molecular biology but seldom knows much about mammalian biology or pathology, and a pathologist, who may know less about molecular biology. This collaborative process requires that the two look at whole mice and histological sections together. The second rule is that no one can predict what or where lesions will be found in mutant mice. Whether or not a mutant shows neurological signs, all tissues have to be examined, including brain, spinal cord, nerves, and muscles. The third rule is that wild-type mice seldom have any neurologic disease, other than the otitis media. Thus if CNS or PNS lesions are found in a mutant, they probably are caused by the mutation.

Still, you must be aware of "background" and age-related lesions. Since FVB is the background strain of many transgenic mice (Smith et al. 1997), it is important to be aware that they have a severe neurodegenerative disease, discussed in Chapter 13. A number of mouse strains, including C3H and FVB, have retinal degeneration. We have discovered that C57L/J mice have intracytoplasmic inclusions in neurons that stain with Luxol fast blue (unpublished). Hydrocephalus is quite common in C57BL/6 mice, as is microphthalamia. Total or partial agenesis of corpus callosum is seen in a number of inbred mouse strains, including BALB/cJ, I/LnJ, and 129/ReJ (Livy and Wahlsten 1991). It is not clear if all of the various 129 substrains (Simpson et al. 1997) have this lesion. Age-related lesions that occur in many mouse strains are white matter gliosis (Bronson et al. 1993a) and neuraxonal dystrophy in the spinal cord (Bronson et al. 1992). Dystrophic axons are numerous in the nucleus gracilis and cuneatus of old mice (Johnson et al. 1975), as they are in old animals of most species. The thalami of old mice often have small nodules of mineral and eosinophilic (red) intracytoplasmic inclusions in neurons. CNS tumors very rarely, if ever, occur in old mice (Bronson 1990; Bronson and Lipman 1991). We have found no neurological diseases in routine histological sections of strain 129 mice even at relatively old ages (Taverna et al. 1998; Yamasaki et al. 1996).

Some minor but important rules to follow in studying mouse mutants are

1. Study a few mutants and controls in depth, rather than study many animals superficially.
2. Make sure you study whole brains under a dissecting microscope to ensure that all externally visible parts of the brains are of normal size and shape. The reduced size and number of folia in the "cerebellar folia–deficient" mouse (Cook et al. 1997) can be appreciated grossly in Fig. 17.1.
3. Take the trouble to collect and fix tissues optimally to get the best histologic slides to study.
4. Search for lesions using conventional neurohistopathological procedures first; later, if you must, use antibodies, in situ hybridization, electron and confocal microscopy, and other procedures to

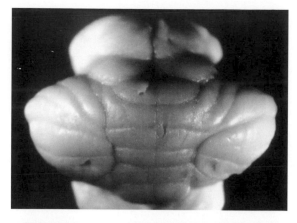

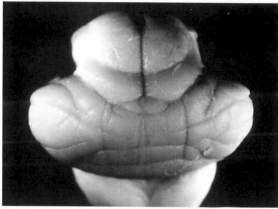

**FIGURE 17.1** Brain from a cerebellar folia–deficient mouse (bottom) and from littermate control mouse (top). Note that the cerebellum of the mutant is smaller and has fewer folia, particularly noticeable if you count folia on the midline (vermis). This is a diagnosis that can be made grossly under a dissecting microscope. To photograph brains like these, use a modern stereoscope. Ring illumination does not work for this. Adjust fiberoptic lights until you have the highlights corrected to show the hills and valleys of the image.

better define lesions that you have already identified using conventional techniques. Be very suspicious of lesions defined only by immunohistochemical staining differences between mutants and controls.

5. Plan to sacrifice mutants at different ages to study the evolution of the disease, starting with the oldest animals with the most mature lesions. It is certainly possible for animals with neurological diseases to show clinical signs before lesions develop fully.

6. Never throw any tissues away until the study is completed. Often you have to go back to check some tissue that you did not examine adequately before.

# NEUROLOGICAL EXAMINATION

A few neurological tests and observations have proven useful in studies of mouse mutants. Any mouse that has a head tilt or that spins around chasing its tail probably has a problem in the vestibular portion of its inner ears. If such a mouse is put in water, it tends to swim directly down to the bottom of the container, where it would drown. Many vestibular mutants have been discovered. Some of these are also deaf. Deafness can be diagnosed with a simple clap of the hands to induce a startle reflex, usually a very pronounced reaction in mice. Specialized auditory testing, usually using brain stem auditory–evoked potentials (Willot and Erway 1998), is necessary for detailed studies of hearing in mice. Any mouse that has a rapid tremor should be suspected to have a problem with myelination. Any mouse that lurches, staggers, sways, or leans is likely to have a cerebellar abnormality, as reflected in the names of famous cerebellar mutants like "staggerer" and "lurcher." These cerebellar mutants and all others are described in Lyon et al. 1996. Data on mutants and all genetic loci are kept up-to-date and on-line in the Mouse Locus Catalogue available on the web site of The Jackson Laboratory, [*http://www.informatics.jax.org*].

It is not easy to study reflexes in mice, but spasticity, suggestive of "upper motor neuron" disease, can be diagnosed in some mice by grasping the hind foot and flexing and extending the leg. A "spastic" mouse resists such passive manipulation (Bronson et al. 1992; Bronson et al. 1998). Mice with "lower motor neuron disease," such as the spontaneous mutation neuromuscular degeneration (Cook et al. 1995; Cox, et al. 1998), have "flaccid" paralysis. They do not resist passive manipulation, they drag their limp legs around, and importantly, they have histological evidence of neurogenic atrophy of skeletal muscles. Note that neuromuscular diseases may be generalized, but clinical signs are usually more severe in hind than in fore legs. Mice that are unable to right themselves when turned over and that exhibit writhing, uncoordinated limb and trunk movements have been found to have defects in dorsal root sensory systems (see Chap. 16). One neurological sign that is nonspecific and occurs in many neurological mutants for totally obscure reasons is clasping of the hind legs when the mouse is picked up by its tail (Sicinski et al. 1995).

A useful generalization is that if neurological abnormalities are seen in a mouse, the lesion responsible for the abnormalities is likely to be in the brain stem, cerebellum, spinal cord, nerve, or muscle. Mice with only forebrain lesions are unlikely to exhibit any neurological signs other than seizures. It is very unlikely that anyone will find a mentally retarded mouse without special testing, such as tests of performance in a water maze. In general, mice do not exhibit peculiar adventitious "extrapyramidal" movements such as tardive dyskinesia, chorea, or athetosis.

Many behavioral tests have been used in studying mutant mice. Most people who study knockout (KO) mice have heard of these tests, the most famous of which is the water maze test. Other tests include rotarod, tight wire cling, open field behavior, radial arm maze, and tail flick or hot plate tests for pain responses. One interesting but probably not very useful little test is to put red ink on the left hind foot and blue ink on the right and have the mice walk up an inclined plane. The pattern of the mouse's footprints can then be studied. A simple but effective way to evaluate a mouse's ability to smell is to bury peanut butter in the shavings of a mouse box and see if the mouse can find it. Blindness is difficult to evaluate in mice since even totally blind mice appear to behave normally. Studies of blindness in mice require use of electroretinography. It is also quite feasible to observe lesions in eyes of mice by ophthalmoscopic examination. It takes practice but can be mastered. Descriptions of quite a few mutants with such behavioral abnormalities as poor maternal nurturing (Brown et al. 1996) or aggression (Mohaghan et al., 1997) have been published. Some, like the Fos B KO, have no lesions (Brown et al. 1996); others, like the tailless gene KO, have severe lesions. In addition to defective limbic systems, tailless KO mice have small forebrains but almost normally sized cerebellums and brain stems (Mohaghan et al. 1997).

# POSTMORTEM PROCEDURES

Mutant mice can be studied immediately after death or euthanasia or hours after they have died, when of course the tissues are likely to be in poor condition. If mice are to be euthanized, you must decide if tissues are to be dissected immediately after death or after fixation. If you want to euthanize and dissect, use carbon dioxide. Do not euthanize mice by cervical dislocation. That method is considered inhumane, and much damage is done to the hindbrain when the neck is stretched. Proceed with the dissection, examining all tissues for abnormalities in size, shape, or color. Some mutants are lacking organs altogether; you may have to inventory all tissues. If the mouse is embryonic or newborn, use a dissecting microscope to observe all tissues. When you get to the brain, you have to make a decision. You can dissect the fresh brain out of the skull, but in so doing you are likely to distort it. On the other hand you will be able to examine the skull, trigeminal and optic nerves, pituitary, and bones of the skull after dissecting out the brain. These observations should not be left out of your examination. It is best to study some mice by whole dissection, as just described, and to study others by dissecting tissues after fixation, as described below.

## Fixatives

Everyone likes to argue about fixatives. A common prejudice is that aldehydes are superior to other fixatives. It is widely believed that in situ hybridization works best on formalin-fixed tissue. (Formalin is a 10 percent buffered solution of commercially available formaldehyde, which is a 37–40 percent solution of formaldehyde). This is probably true. It is also widely believed that most antibodies only work on aldehyde-fixed tissues. This is not true. Some people are so fearful of overfixation that they fix whole mouse brains for only 2 hours. That overfixation ruins antigens is probably a myth. In any case whether any particular combination of antibody and fixative works in an immunocytochemistry procedure is determined only by magic, not science, so there is no basis for anyone to be too dogmatic about what works and what does not.

An important fact that is not widely known, except to histotechnicians who have sectioned a lot of mouse tissue, is that aldehydes make mouse tissue brittle and hard to cut on the microtome. For a number of reasons I like to use Bouin's fixative. It is commercially available or can be made by mixing 160 ml 40 percent formaldehyde, 80 ml glacial acetic acid, and 1700 ml saturated aqueous picric acid. Bouin's-fixed mouse tissues do not become brittle. The acid in the fixative demineralizes tissues. After adult mouse bodies have soaked in Bouin's for a week or 10 days, the skull, spine, and limbs can be trimmed with a razor blade, and histological sections can be made that include bone and soft tissues left in their normal relationship to one another. Baby mice can be demineralized in 2–3 days. Kaufman in his monumental *Atlas of Mouse Development* (1992) gives fixation times for Bouin's fixation of mouse embryos. Although you cannot overfix adult tissue, early embryonic tissue definitely can be overfixed and overprocessed. Follow Kaufman's directions on pages 3–5 precisely. Bouin's fixative, contrary to popular opinion, does not necessarily destroy antigens. In fact antibodies to glial fibrillary acidic protein (Fig. 17.2) work very well with Bouin's-fixed tissue (Bronson et al. 1993b).

### HOLES IN WHITE MATTER
Probably the greatest virtue of Bouin's is that Bouin's-fixed brains do not develop holes in white matter, a

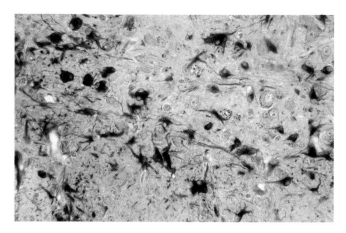

**FIGURE 17.2** Brain from an unpublished spontaneously occurring mutant with severe gliosis. The brown spiders and stars are hypertrophic astrocytes stained with an antibody to glial fibrillary acidic protein. Note that there is little background staining. This is the way you want immunohistochemical stains to behave.

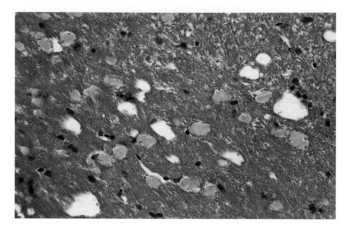

**FIGURE 17.3** Normal white matter from brain fixed in formalin. The gray blobs of material filling holes and the clear holes are artifactual. Usually the gray material, which is birefringent, is not present, but the holes are seen when mouse brains are fixed in any fixative other than Bouin's solution.

disconcerting artifact that has been misinterpreted as a real lesion in at least one experiment (Shultz et al. 1982; Woloschak et al. 1987; Xu et al. 1996). On several occasions I have had to steer people away from misinterpreting white matter holes as "status spongiosis," the lesion of such "spongiform encephalopathies" as mad cow disease and scrapie. The artifact appears as empty round holes in white matter tracts. Sometimes the holes contain pale blue material (Fig. 17.3), which is birefringent when examined under crossed polarizing lenses. It is not clear how these holes develop, but they are seen in formalin-fixed tissues. They are even larger and more numerous in a fixative used for years at the Jackson Laboratory, Tellyesniczky's or "Telly's fix," a mixture of formalin, glacial acetic acid, and ethanol. In that fix, it seems to be ethanol that causes the vacuoles. For that reason we do not transfer Bouin's fixed tissue into 70 percent ethanol, the traditional procedure used to remove the picric acid from the tissue. We remove Bouin's from tissue by washing it overnight in running water. We also store and ship Bouin's-fixed tissue in water with a little fixative to prevent bacteria from multiplying. The tissue is sealed in heat-sealed plastic bags and is good for years.

## PERFUSION TECHNIQUE

Fixation by intracardiac perfusion is essential if you want good preservation of neural tissue, particularly spinal cord. Begin by anesthetizing the mouse with Avertin (stock solution is 1 g tribromoethanol in 0.5 ml amylene hydrate, also called tert. amyl alcohol; working solution is 0.5 ml stock solution in 40 ml distilled water or saline; inject working solution IP at 0.1 ml/5 gm body weight). To anesthetize mice more quickly I overdose with an IP injection and begin the perfusion only after the leg no longer reflexly withdraws when the foot is firmly pinched with forceps. You must make sure that the mouse is really in deep, deep anesthesia, or you will inflict pain and suffering. Pin out the mouse on its back. Open the chest; cut off the right atrium; insert the tip of a 21 ga butterfly needle (26 ga in baby mice) straight down into the apex of the heart. You will be in the left ventricle at this point. With a 20 ml syringe flush in about 5 to 10 ml of saline over the course of a minute or so, change to another syringe with Bouin's, and flush in 30 to 50 ml fixative until the body is stiff and completely yellow. The whole perfusion should not take more than a few minutes. You want a fairly high rate of flow. There is no danger of blowing out blood vessels or causing hydrocephalus by forcing too much fixative through the animal too rapidly. Do not be alarmed by the twitching of muscle. That is how muscle reacts to fixation. However, if the mouse goes into a huge convulsion when the fixative first goes in, then it was not deeply enough anesthetized. Sometimes fluid flows out the nose if there has been a rupture of a blood vessel in the lungs, in which case you will not get a good perfusion. No matter, in any case proceed with the next stage, which is opening up the mouse for further fixation. Even well-perfused tissues require further fixation.

Open the abdomen completely on the midline. The abdominal and chest organs must be completely exposed. You should turn the mouse a little bit inside out to make sure everything is exposed. Then incise the skin under the neck so that fixative can get directly to salivary glands, thyroid, and lymph nodes. Turn the mouse over

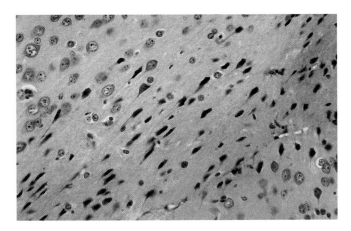

**FIGURE 17.4** Normal brain with darkly staining, shrunken neurons in the central part of the figure. This is dark neuron artifact from handling an incompletely fixed brain.

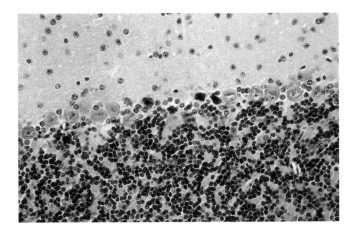

**FIGURE 17.5** Normal cerebellum showing four Purkinje cells with dark neuron artifact (in center of figure). This random distribution of dark Purkinje cells in cerebellum leads you to believe that this distribution is real and not artifactual.

and slit the skin on the midline from head to tail. Reflect the skin laterally to expose all of the muscles of the back and rump. Then carefully open the skull by following the midline and lateral sutures using a small sharp-sharp Telly's fix pair of scissors. Alternatively, cut around the sides of the skull with scissors. Do not smash the brain while you are cutting the skull. Finally, drop the whole mouse in Bouin's. If the mouse is an adult, leave it there for another week to 10 days; if it is a pup, leave it there for several days. Fixation in Bouin's solution for longer than a month should probably be avoided. After the fixation period, transfer the body to tap water with a little fixative to prevent bacteria from multiplying.

You can get a pretty good fixation by following this procedure even with a nonperfused or poorly perfused mouse. Just open everything up, and drop the mouse in fixative. Embryos and newborn mice will also fix well by immersion; the abdomen should be opened up in a newborn before putting it in fixative. Dead mice can also be opened up and put in fixative, unless they are too odiferous. When mice are found dead, it is better to do this procedure than to put them in the refrigerator pending future dissection. Refrigerated animals continue to decompose. Freezing bodies is not good either, since freezing produces ice crystals in tissues.

### DARK NEURON ARTIFACT

When you remove the skull cap from a freshly killed or perfused mouse, be very careful that you do not touch the brain with your instruments. If you do, you will cause shrinkage, leading to dark neuron artifact (Kepes et al. 1995; Ebels 1975). Both cytoplasm and nuclei will stain very darkly with any stain (Fig. 17.4). This shrinkage can occur over wide areas where the brain has been touched. More confusingly, sometimes random cells will

undergo this shrinkage. This occurs particularly commonly in Purkinje cells of the cerebellum (Fig. 17.5). This artifact can be misleading in itself. Still worse is that shrunken neurons with dark neuron artifact tend to stain nonspecifically with antibodies, potentially leading to still more misinterpretations by those not acquainted with this artifact.

### Trimming and Sectioning

A routine sampling of nervous tissue should include using a razor blade to cut cross-sectional slices through the whole head with brain in situ (Fig. 17.6). The slices should be 3 mm thick. One section should be made by cutting just behind the eye and embedding it eye side down so the section includes eyes; another through the ear holes should include inner ears and pituitary; another should be through the middle of the cerebellum. A few cross sections of the spine, epaxial muscles, and spinal cord at cervical, thoracic, and lumbar levels should be sliced. One hind leg should be sliced sagittally, and one-half embedded for sectioning. All these sections will serve as a preliminary screen. They will fit in two or three tissue cassettes. (Make sure you label cassettes with a number 2 lead pencil or with a special "HistoPrep" pen. The ink of the usual "Sharpie"-type pen comes off in xylene during processing.) Later it may be necessary to serial section the whole brain or portions of it. Serial sections should be made only on brains that have been optimally fixed. Serial sectioning a poorly fixed brain is a waste of time and money.

Neuroscience labs like to create sagittal sections; neuropathology labs like to prepare cross or coronal sections. The type of sectioning makes a difference. Learning neuroanatomy is very difficult. If you learn it

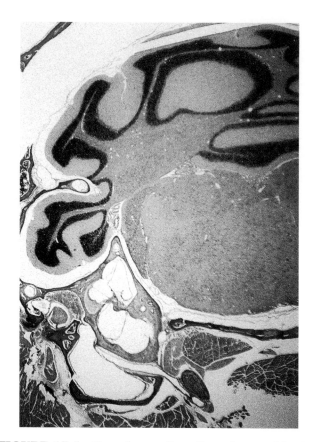

**FIGURE 17.6** Cross (coronal) section of normal brain. A wonderful advantage of studying the mouse brain is that the brain can be studied in relationship to the structures surrounding it. The petrous temporal bone with inner ear structures was demineralized as the whole head was fixed in Bouin's fixative.

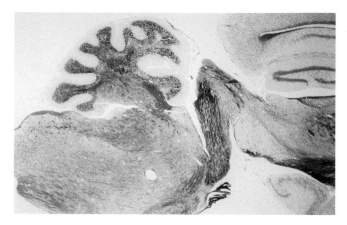

**FIGURE 17.7** Midline sagittal section of normal brain stained with Luxol fast blue to show white matter tracts and with cresyl violet to show neuronal cell bodies. At this magnification the hippocampal neurons (midleft) stain with the magenta color of cresyl violet. This plane of section is especially favored by cerebellologists because it shows the folia so well.

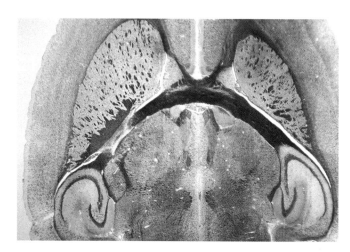

**FIGURE 17.8** Frontal (horizontal) section of normal brain stained with Luxol fast blue and cresyl violet. This plane is particularly suited to show commissures. In standard cross sections you do not appreciate how large the hippocampal commissure connecting the two hippocampi is. The brain was imperfectly oriented, so the commissure is cut off on one side.

through study of cross sections, you are unlikely to be happy trying to decipher sagittal sections and vice versa. Unfortunately since people in the two disciplines have been trained on different kinds of sections, communications between neuroscientists and neuropathologists can become strained. Actually it is best to remain flexible and to make the effort to understand the brain in both kinds of sections. Frontal sections, the third plane, can be useful too. Certainly it is clear that the cerebellar folia are best studied in sagittal sections (Fig. 17.7; Cook et al. 1995). Commissures are well defined in frontal sections (Fig. 17.8; Faseli et al. 1997). Structures close to the midline, such as nuclei of the hypothalamus (Brown et al. 1996), are best studied in cross sections. Cross sections are also required for analysis of brain symmetry. Most neoplastic, traumatic, and inflammatory diseases affect one side of the brain more than the other, leading to asymmetrical areas of swelling. In mutant pathology almost all lesions are symmetrical because the biochemical defect caused by the mutation is metabolic and affects the two sides of the brain

equally. One exception to this is the asymmetry seen in some forms of exencephaly (Fig. 17.9; Harris et al. 1997; Sah et al. 1995).

## Staining

Hematoxylin and eosin (H&E) is still the best staining method to screen all tissues for lesions. But do not forget the enormous armamentarium of classical histochemical stains for collagen, basement membranes,

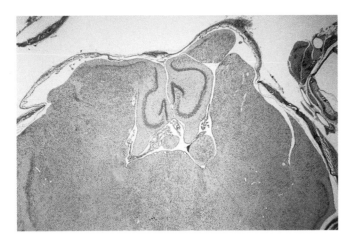

**FIGURE 17.9** Cross section of brain with exencephaly. The two sides of the brain are truly asymmetrical. Peculiar blobs of brain tissue appear on the right that are not present on the left of the midline. This asymmetry would not be apparent in sagittal sections. The hippocampi are located at the top of the brain. Such severe malformations are difficult to describe because there are no names for them.

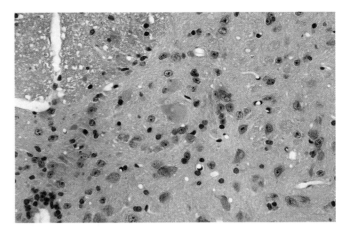

**FIGURE 17.10** Cross section of lumbar spinal cord of mouse showing "upper motor neuron" signs ("spasticity") in hind limbs. In the upper left part of the picture, the irregularly shaped red-staining structures are dystrophic axons. These are only faintly visible or not visible at all in sections stained with Luxol fast blue and cresyl violet.

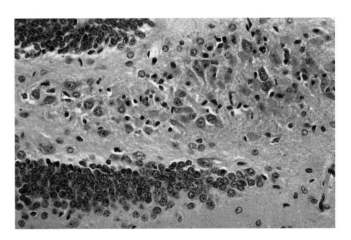

**FIGURE 17.11** Hippocampus of mouse with a seizure disorder. The dendate gyrus is at the left, above and below. The pyramidal cells of the hippocampal gyrus in the center have no nuclei, and their cytoplasms stain brightly with eosin. These are "acutely necrotic neurons," "ischemic neurons," or better yet "red-dead neurons."

cross striations in muscle, and so on (Prophet et al. 1994). Three important brain lesions show up best with H&E because they are eosinophilic (i.e., they stain red). These are swollen "dystrophic axons," which appear as red balls of various sizes (Fig. 17.10; Bronson et al. 1992); acutely necrotic neurons (red-dead neurons) that stain bright red (Fig. 17.11); and hypertrophic astrocytes, which look like splashes of red paint when a bucket of paint has been kicked over (Fig. 17.12). These lesions do not show up very well in slides stained with cresyl violet (CV), used to define cell body detail, or Luxol fast blue (LFB), used to define white matter tracts. We stain all nervous tissue with both H&E and CV-LFB. Serial sectioned brains are stained with both stains; even numbered slides with ribbons of five or six sections are stained with H&E and odd slides with CV-LFB. Sometimes we stain sections with Bodian stain, a silver stain that stains axons (Fig. 17.13). It's a pretty stain but has not been very useful as a diagnostic tool in our studies of mouse mutants. The only antibody that is useful for routine diagnosis of neurologic disease is anti–glial fibrillary acidic protein.

# DIAGNOSING NEURONAL CELL DEATH

There is widespread confusion about how to diagnose diseases occurring in neuron cell bodies. Neuronal disease is most safely diagnosed in artifact-free, well-fixed tissues stained with conventional stains. If there is no evidence of

disease in such sections, there is no disease, regardless of what immunostains show. Dead or dying neurons can have a number of different histologic appearances:

1. Acutely necrotic, red-dead neurons have been discussed. They are often seen in mice that have died with seizures, presumably from hypoxia.
2. Fading neurons, also called "ghost cells," are characteristic of motor neurons seen in "neuromuscular degeneration" (*nmd*) mutant mice (Cook et al. 1995) (Fig. 17.14).

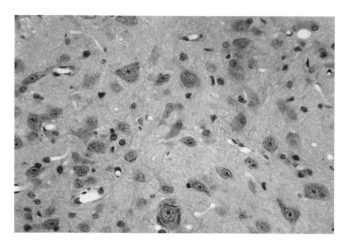

**FIGURE 17.12**  Brain stem from the same mouse shown in Figure 17.2. The red-staining cells are hypertrophic astrocytes as stained with H&E.

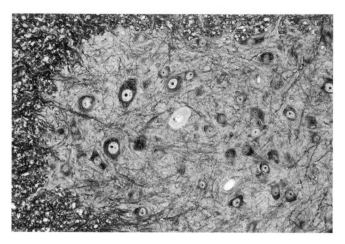

**FIGURE 17.14**  Brain from mutant mouse with neuromuscular degeneration (*nmd*). The neuron in the center of the picture is a "ghost cell." LFB-CV.

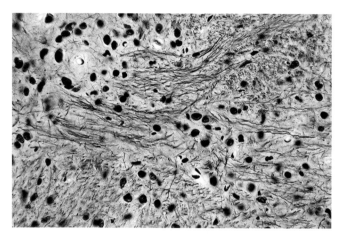

**FIGURE 17.13**  Normal brain stained with Bodian stain. This is a somewhat tricky stain that uses silver salts. The axons stain beautifully; nuclei show as black blobs. However, it is not very useful as a diagnostic tool in studies of mouse mutants.

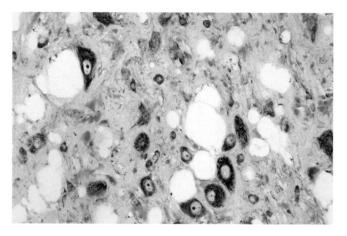

**FIGURE 17.15**  Brain from an unpublished mutant with severe vacuolization of gray matter. One neuron to the upper left has a large cytoplasmic vacuole that pushes the nucleus to one side. Beware that holes can be artifactual; if you call this "spongiform encephalopathy" you will generate widespread panic.

3. Vacuolated neurons are observed in the spongiform encephalopathies (Fig. 17.15) and in storage diseases. Vacuolated motor neurons are seen in the "wobbler" (Ishiyama et al. 1997) and "wasted" (Woloschak et al. 1987) mouse mutants that have lower motor neuron disease.
4. A lesion called "central chromatolysis" occurs in neurons whose axons have been cut. These neurons have pale cytoplasm, and the nucleus is pushed to the side. (Fig. 17.16).
5. Apoptosis occurs in some diseases. It is diagnosed in standard sections when neurons show pyknosis (shrunken nuclei) as well as karyorrhexis (fragmented nuclei) (Fig. 17.17). Apoptosis should not be diagnosed by dUDP nick end-labeling (TUNEL stain) alone unless pyknosis and karyorrhexis are also observed in standard sections. Commercially available TUNEL stains are notoriously tricky and unreliable, with lots of background staining, false-positives, and false-negatives.

6. Infarction occurs when tissues are deprived of their blood supply. Ischemic tissue first undergoes coagulation where it simply stains poorly but otherwise is morphologically entirely or nearly normal (Fig. 17.18; Kaysser et al. 1997; Wandersee et al. 1998).

All of the changes discussed so far are acute lesions, meaning that the elapsed time between the initial damage and when they are observed in sections is probably quite short—hours or days. Another type of longer-term

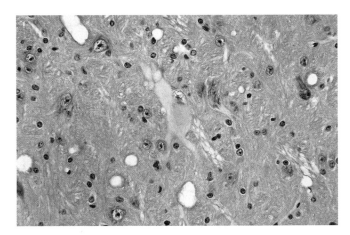

**FIGURE 17.16** Brain from unpublished mutant. The neuron in the center is enlarged, has pale-staining cytoplasm, and has an intact nucleus. This is a good illustration of "central chromatolysis."

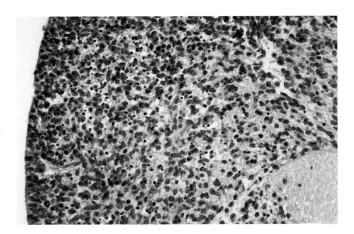

**FIGURE 17.17** Brain from a mutant that died on embryonic day 15 with extensive apoptosis of neurons. Even at this power you can see numerous tiny black dots between the larger neuronal nuclei. These small dots are pyknotic nuclei and nuclear debris.

neuronal change involves accumulation of various types of material in cytoplasm of neurons. Aged neurons have accumulated lipofuscin (wear and tear pigment). This pigment has a golden brown appearance in sections. In storage diseases, lipids accumulate in cytoplasm, giving it a vacuolated appearance. Since lipids are extracted by xylene when tissues are processed for paraffin embedding, frozen sections have to be cut and stained by lipid stains to prove that vacuolization is due to lipid accumulation. Other, nonlipid materials can also be stored in neurons. Proteolipids accumulate in neurons in the neuronal ceroid lipofuscinoses. This material stains with LFB (Fig. 17.19; Bronson et al. 1993b, 1998).

There are three kinds of long-term sequelae of neuronal disease. The first long-term sequela is typical of

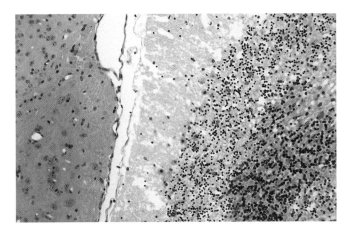

**FIGURE 17.18** Cerebellum from a mutant mouse with thrombi in the heart that have seeded off into the circulation as emboli and landed in the brain. There the emboli have occluded blood vessels and caused an infarct. Note that the strip of cerebellum in the center of the picture is pale staining. Both the Purkinje cells and granule cells are indistinct. The granule cells on the right are normal and well stained, as is the overlying cerebral cortex on the left. Very recent infarcts can be quite hard to diagnose since the affected brain stains almost normally. As the dead brain liquefies, the lesion becomes easier to diagnose.

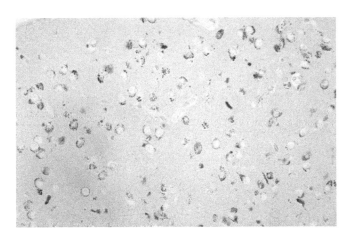

**FIGURE 17.19** Brain from a mouse with neuronal ceroid lipofuscinosis. All neurons have densely packed cytoplasmic granules that stain intensely with Luxol fast blue.

infarcts. In infarcts, both glial cells and neurons die, and the dead tissue liquefies and is removed by macrophages (Wandersee et al. 1998). Old infarcts appear as cavities containing macrophage and cell debris with blood vessels crossing through the cavity (Fig. 17.20). Embryonic brain liquefies quickly following extensive cell death (Fig. 17.21; Shen et al. 1997; Gao et al. 1998). In the second type of long-term sequela, only neurons die, but astrocytes are preserved. These lesions heal as glial scars

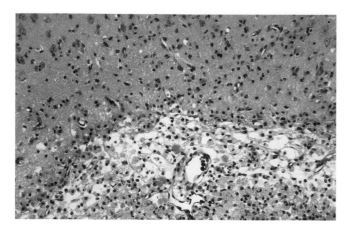

**FIGURE 17.20**   Brain from mouse with an old infarct. At the bottom of the image is a cavity containing nonstaining fluid, numerous macrophages shown as pale-staining blobs, and a few intact blood vessels. This is the cavitation that follows the liquefactive necrosis of infarction.

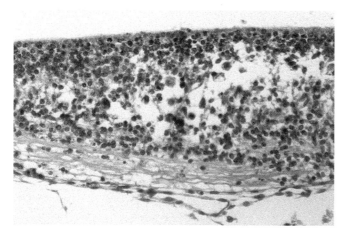

**FIGURE 17.21**   Liquefactive necrosis with cavitation in hind brain of the same mouse shown in Figure 17.17. It has been difficult to convince investigators that both apoptosis and necrosis lead to liquefaction and cavitation.

in which astrocytes are more numerous; they are enlarged, and their processes are prominent (Figs. 17.2, 17.12). The third sequela is simply neuronal cell loss, without liquefaction or gliosis. This type of lesion is most easily appreciated in mutants with Purkinje cell degeneration. In these mutants few or no Purkinje cells are seen (Fig. 17.22), whereas in normal cerebella, Purkinje cells are lined up in continuous rows (actually sheets in three dimensions).

A worrisome aspect of this third type of lesion is that simple neuronal loss is very hard to diagnose in most parts of the brain where neurons are simply scattered about without any particular orderly array. Consider the cerebral cortex. It is arranged in six layers, or lam-

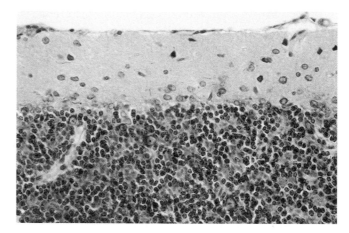

**FIGURE 17.22**   Cerebellum from an unpublished mutant. Purkinje cells have disappeared.

ina, but in most parts of the cerebrum, the layers are quite indistinct. Even in areas where certain layers are distinct, loss of 20 percent to 30 percent of the cells of any layer might not be apparent to the casual observer. Also, extensive loss of neurons in small structures such as the red nucleus would not be apparent unless you specifically studied that nucleus. Those willing to take on the unpleasant task of counting neurons (Smith et al. 1997) should be aware that neuronal counts are no more than measures of neuronal density, numbers of neurons per square unit (in single sections) or per cubic unit (in serial sections). The denominator value is affected by such artifacts as tissue shrinkage, as well as by such real entities as interstitial fluid, matrix, or glial processes. On a more positive note, in situations where neurons appear to have disappeared, it is possible that at earlier time points in the disease neurons in affected areas might have been observed to be undergoing apoptosis, vacuolization, or another significant pathologic change before disappearing.

## DEVELOPMENTAL ABNORMALITIES

Three broad categories of developmental lesions can be described. The first comprises failures of closure of neural tube or of differentiation of ventricular system. An example of a rostral neural tube defect has been mentioned (Fig. 17.9; Harris et al. 1997). Many mutants have spina bifida. Often such animals have short or kinky tails that may project dorsally from the sacral region; curly tail (*ct*) is an example (Lyon et al. 1996). Many mutants are hydrocephalic. Usually lateral and third ventricles are dilated, but aqueduct and fourth ventricles are normal (Lindeman et al. 1998). One mutant, hydrocephalus with hop gait (*hyh*), has an

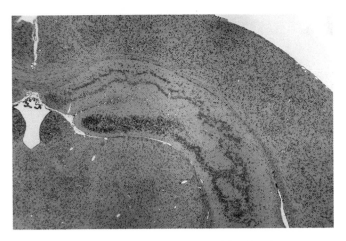

**FIGURE 17.23**  Brain from a scrambler (*scm*) mouse. Note the wavy arrangement of the hippocampus.

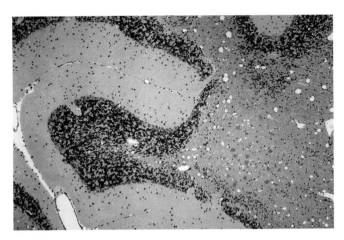

**FIGURE 17.24**  Cerebellum from a mouse with rostral cerebellar malformation (*rcm*). As you follow the granule cell layer around, note that it is absent in several places. Note holes in white matter to the right.

abnormal third ventricle as well as other abnormalities (Bronson and Lane 1990).

The second category of developmental abnormality comprises mutants with abnormal neuronal migration. This abnormality can be quite easily diagnosed if normal layering patterns are severely scrambled. Scrambler (*scm*) and reeler (*rl*) have very small cerebella, and the neurons of the hippocampi are scattered (Fig. 17.23; Sweet et al. 1996). Rostral cerebellar malformation (*rcm*) (Ackerman et al. 1998; Lane et al. 1992) has ectopic granule and Purkinje cells in the midbrain and more subtle defects in the layering pattern of cerebellum (Fig. 17.24). In reeler and scrambler the outermost cerebral cortical layer, which ordinarily is cell free, is quite cellular, making the abnormal layering pattern fairly easy to diagnose (Fig. 17.25). The cerebral cortex is not as severely disturbed morphologically in the P35 KO mouse (Chae et al. 1997). Organizational defects of

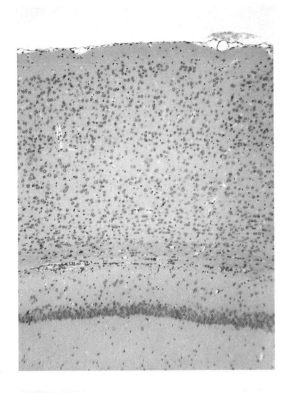

**A**

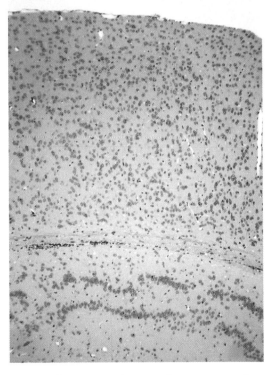

**B**

**FIGURE 17.25**  Parietal cortex from a normal mouse (**A**) and scrambler mouse (**B**). The wavy hippocampus is obvious in the mutant. The differences in the cerebra are not so obvious. Note that there is no cell-free external first layer in the mutant. With imagination, you can make out six layers in the control cortex; the layers are more scrambled in the mutant. H&E × 60.

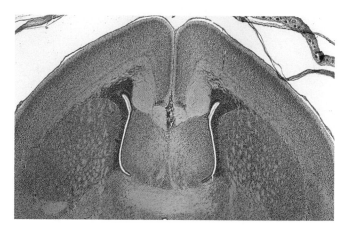

**FIGURE 17.26**   Brain from mutant mouse with absent corpus callosum. Note the prominent bundles of pale-staining white matter fibers to either side of the midline at the base of the cerebral cortex and above the septal nuclei. These are "Probst bundles," assumed to be bundles of axons that bunch up in frustration, having failed to cross the midline during development.

other parts of the brain such as nuclei of thalamus or brain stem would be very difficult to diagnose.

The third general type of defect involves abnormal axonal guidance so that white matter tracts do not develop normally. Defects of corpus callosum, rostal commissure, and hippocampal commissure have been diagnosed in many mutants (Faseli et al. 1997) as well as in inbred strains of mouse, as mentioned (Livy and Wahlsten 1991) (Fig. 17.26).

# WHITE MATTER LESIONS

Staining neural tissue with LFB is the most effective and simplest way of evaluating white matter. In studies of young mice, you must be aware that myelination is an ongoing process until 3 or 4 weeks of age. Myelination occurs in the PNS before the CNS and in spinal cord and brain stem before forebrain. Control and mutant tissues must always be stained together in the same batch, given that the intensity of LFB staining varies from batch to batch. Myelin may be slow to develop or may fail to develop, in which case mutant white matter stains less densely than control white matter (Fig 17.27; Langner et al. 1991). Myelin can begin to degenerate even before complete myelination has taken place or can degenerate after that. When myelin degenerates, it is phagocytized by macrophages, which can be observed in tissue (Fig. 17.28). Degenerating white matter often has large vacuoles containing cell debris and macrophages. Since vacuoles can also be artifactual, as discussed above, you have to beware of overinterpreting

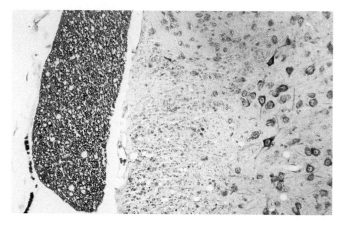

**FIGURE 17.27**   Spinal cord from a mutant with deficient CNS white matter. The blue structure to the left is spinal root, myelinated by Schwann cells. To the right is the spinal cord, whose white matter, myelinated by oligodendrogliacytes, should be as deeply staining as the root. Beware, however, that myelination develops during the first several weeks of life in mice and that the PNS myelinates before the CNS. Evaluation of myelin requires LFB staining. LFB-CV.

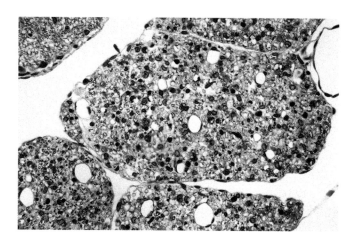

**FIGURE 17.28**   Spinal root from mouse with peripheral "radiculoneuropathy." As compared with the root in Figure 17.27, this root is obviously undermyelinated. A close look at the root reveals much magenta staining of undeveloped Schwann cells or macrophages. This lesion must be studied by electron microscopy to determine its true morphology. LFB-CR.

vacuoles. White matter lesions must be stained with Bodian stain to visualize axons. If axons are intact, the disease can be considered a disease of myelin hypomyelinization, dysmyelinization, or demyelination. If axons, as well as myelin, are degenerative, the disease is probably an axonopathy with secondary myelin degeneration. To fully define most white matter lesions, they must be studied by electron microscopy.

Remember that if there is disease in the motor neurons, roots, or peripheral nerves there may also be neurogenic atrophy of skeletal muscle. Many scattered muscle fibers as well as focal bundles of skeletal muscle fibers will be very small. Yet mice have greater variation in skeletal muscle fiber diameter than other animals, so you have to be careful not to overdiagnose "neurogenic atrophy." Be certain that if you declare a mouse to have lower motor neuron disease, you must document your diagnosis by showing neurogenic atrophy. Motor neuron degeneration (*mnd*) is probably not the only mutant incorrectly diagnosed as having lower motor neuron disease (Bronson et al. 1993b). Once mistakes get into the literature, they become self-propagating. At least three papers have been published in the last 2 years describing various aspects of *mnd/mnd* mice in which the authors still considered them models of amytrophic lateral sclerosis and not of neuronal ceroid lipofuscinosis.

# REFERENCES

Ackerman, S.L., Kozak, L.P., Przyborski, S.A., et al. 1998. The mouse rostral cerebellar malformation gene encodes an UNC-5-like protein. Nature 386:338–342.

Altman, J. and Bayer, S.A. 1995. Atlas of Prenatal Rat Brain Development. Boca Raton, FL: CRC Press.

Bronson, R.T. 1990. Rate of occurrence of lesions in 20 inbred and hybrid genotypes of rats and mice sacrificed at 6 month intervals during the first years of life. In D.E. Harrison, ed., Genetics of Aging II. Caldwell, NJ: Telford Press, pp. 278–358.

Bronson, R.T. and Lane, P.W. 1990. Hydrocephalus with hop gait (hyh), a new mutation on chromosome 7 in the mouse. Dev Brain Res 54:131–136.

Bronson, R.T. and Lipman, R.D. 1991. Reduction in rate of occurrence of age-related lesions in dietary restricted laboratory mice. Growth, Dev Aging 55:169–184.

Bronson, R.T., Sweet, H.O., Spencer, C.A., et al. 1992. Genetic and age-related models of neurodegeneration in mice: dystrophic axons. J Neurogenet 8:71–83.

Bronson, R.T., Lipman, R. and Harrison, D. 1993a. Age-related gliosis in the white matter of mice. Brain Res 609:124–128.

Bronson, R.T., Lake, B.D., Cook, S., et al. 1993b. Motor neuron degeneration of mice is a model of neuronal ceroid lipofuscinosis (Batten's disease). Ann Neurol 33:381–385.

Bronson, R.T., Donahue, L.R., Johnson, K.R., et al. 1998. Neuronal ceroid lipofuscinosis (nclf), a new disorder of the mouse linked to chromosome 9. Am J Med Genet 77:289–297.

Brown, J., Ye, H., Bronson, R.T., et al. 1996. A defect in nurturing in mice lacking the immediate early gene FosB. Cell 86:297–309.

Chae, T., Kwon, Y.T., Bronson, R.T., et al. 1997. Mice lacking p35, a neuronal specific activator of Cdk5, display cortical lamination defects, seizures and adult lethality. Neuron 18:29–42.

Cook, S.A., Johnson, K.R., Bronson, R.T., et al. 1995. Neuromuscular degeneration (nmd): a mutation on mouse chromosome 19 which causes motor neuron degeneration. Mamm Genome 6:187–191.

Cook, S.A., Bronson, R.T., Donahue, L.R., et al. 1997. Cerebellar deficient folia (cdf): a new mutation on mouse Chromosome 6. Mamm Genome 8:108–112.

Cox, G.A., Mahaffey, C.L., and Frankel, W.N. 1998. Identification of the mouse neuromuscular degeneration gene and mapping of a second site suppressor allele. Neuron 21:1327–1337.

Ebels, E.J. 1975. Dark Neurons: a significant artifact: the influence of the maturational state of neurons on the occurrence of the phenomenon. Acta Neurol (Berl) 33:271–273.

Faseli, A., Dickenson, S.L., Hermiston, M.L., et al. 1997. Phenotype of mice lacking functional deleted in colorectal cancer (Dcc) gene. Nature 386:796–804.

Franklin, K.B.J and Paxinos, G. 1997. The Mouse Brain in Stereotaxic Coordinates. New York: Academic Press.

Gao, Y., Frank, K.M., Sun, Y., et al. 1998. A critical role for DNA end-joining proteins in both lymphogenesis and neurogenesis Cell 95:891–902.

Harris, B.S., Franz, T., Ullrich, S., et al. 1997. Forebrain overgrowth (fog): a new mutation in the mouse affecting neural tube development. Teratology 55:231–240.

Ishiyama, T., Klinkosz, B., Pioro, E.P., et al. 1997. Genetic transfer of the wobbler gene to a C57BL/6J × NZB hybrid stock: natural history of the motor neuron disease and response to CNTF and BDNF cotreatment. Exp Neurol 148:247–255.

Johnson, J.E., Mehler, W.R., and Miquel, J. 1975. A fine structural study of degenerative changes in the dorsal column nuclei of aging mice. Lack of protection by vitamin E. J Gerontol 30:395–411.

Kaufman, M.H. 1992. The Atlas of Mouse Development. London: Academic Press.

Kaysser, T.M., Wandersee, N.J., Bronson, R.T., et al. 1997. Thrombosis and secondary hemachromatosis play major roles in the pathogenesis of jaundiced and spherocytic mice, murine models for hereditary spherocytosis. Blood 90:4610–4619.

Kepes, J.J., Malone, D.G., Griffin, W., et al. 1995. Surgical "touch" artifacts of the cerebral cortex. An experimental study with light and electron microscopic analysis. Clin Neuropathol 14:86–92.

Lane, P.W., Bronson, R.T., and Spencer, C.A. 1992. Rostral cerebellar malformation (rcm), a new recessive mutation on chromosome 3 of the mouse. J Hered 83:315–318.

Langner, C.A., Birkenmeier, E.H., Roth, E.A., et al. 1991. Characterization of the peripheral neuropathy in neonatal and adult mice that are homozygous for the fatty liver dystrophy (fld) mutation. J Biol Chem 266:11955–11964.

Lindeman, G., Dagnino, L., Gaubatz, S.D., et al. 1998. A specific, nonproliferative role for E2F-5 in choroid plexus function revealed by gene targeting. Genes Dev 12:1092–1098.

Livy, D.J. and Wahlsten, D. 1991. Tests of genetic allelism between four inbred mouse strains with absent corpus callosum. J Hered 82:459–464.

Lyon, M.F., Raston, S., and Brown, S.D.M. 1996. Genetic Variants and Strains of the Laboratory Mouse, vols. 1 and 2, 3rd ed. Oxford: Oxford University Press.

Mohaghan, A.P., Bock, D., Gass, P., et al. 1997. Defective limbic system in mice lacking the tailless gene. Nature 390:515–517.

Prophet, R.B., Mills, B., Arrington, J.B., et al. 1994. Laboratory Methods in Histotechnology. Washington, DC: American Registry of Pathology, Armed Forces Institute of Pathology.

Sah, V.P., Attardi, L.D., Mulligan, G.J., et al. 1995. A subset of p53 deficient embryos exhibit exencephaly. Nature Genet 10:175–180.

Shen, J., Bronson, R., Chen, D.F., et al. 1997. Skeletal and CNS defects in presenilin-1 deficient mice. Cell 89:629–639.

Shultz, L.D., Sweet, H.O., Davisson, M.T., et al. 1982 "Wasted," a new mutant of the mouse with abnormalities characteristic of ataxia telangiectasia. Nature 297:402–404.

Sicinski, P., Donaher, J.L., Parker, S.B., et al.1995. Cyclin D1 provides a link between development and oncogenesis in retina and breast. Cell 82:621–630.

Sidman, R.L., Angevine, J.B., and Pierce, E.T. 1971. Atlas of the Mouse Brain and Spinal cord. Cambridge: Harvard University Press.

Simpson, E.M., Linder, C.C., Sargent, E.E., et al. 1997. Genetic variation among 129 substrains and its impor-

tance for targeted mutagenesis in mice. Nature Genet 16:19–27.

Smith, D.J., Stevens, M.E., Sudanagunta, S.P., et al. 1997. Functional screening of 2Mb of human chromosome 21q22.2 in transgenic mice implicates minibrain in learning defects associated with Down syndrome. Nature Genet 16:28–36.

Sweet, H.O., Bronson, R.T., Johnson, K.R., et al. 1996. Scrambler, a new neurological mutation in the mouse with abnormalities of neuronal migration. Mamm Genome 7:798–802.

Taverna, D., Ullman-Cullere, M., Rayburn, H., et al. 1998. A test of the role of alpha5 integrin/fibronectin interactions in tumorgenesis. Cancer Res 58:848–853.

Wandersee, N.J., Lee, J.C., Kaysser, T.M., et al. 1998. Hematopoietic cells from α-spectrin-deficient mice are sufficient to induce thrombotic events in hematopoietically ablated recipients. Blood 92:4856–4863.

Willot, J.F., and Erway, L.C. 1998. Genetics of age-related hearing loss in mice IV. Cochlear pathology and hearing loss in 25 BXD recombinant inbred mouse strains. Hear Res 119:27–36.

Woloschak, G.E., Rodriguez, M., and Krco, C.J. 1987. Characterization of immunologic and neuropathologic abnormalities in wasted mice. J Immunol 138:2493–2499.

Xu, Y., Ashley, T., Brainerd, E.E., et al. 1996. Targeted disruption of ATM leads to growth retardation, chromosomal fragmentation during meiosis, immune defects and thymic lymphoma. Genes Dev 10:2411–2422.

Yamasaki, L., Jacks, T., Bronson, R., et al. 1996. Tumor induction and tissue atrophy in mice lacking E2F-1. Cell 85:536–548.

# 18

# Transgenic and Knockout Mice with Neuropathological Disorders

Liat Lomnitski, Abraham Nyska, and Daniel M. Michaelson

## TRANSGENIC AND KNOCKOUT MOUSE MODELS IN RESEARCH OF CNS NEURODEGENERATIVE DISORDERS

During the last few years much progress has occurred in generating transgenic (Tg) and gene knockout (KO), or targeted mutant, mice that model aspects of human neurodegenerative diseases. Recent studies, built upon the investigations of molecular geneticists who identified genetic mutations that may cause familial forms of various central nervous system disorders, have led to powerful new tools to examine the pathogenesis of Alzheimer's disease (AD) and other neurodegenerative diseases. The relatively short life of models (less than 2 years in most laboratory mice) offers advantages for investigating pathogenesis and testing novel therapeutic approaches.

In this chapter we review Tg and KO mouse models that develop clinical and pathological abnormalities resembling those occurring in the human CNS neurodegenerative disorders such as AD. Particular emphasis will be given to our experience with apolipoprotein E (apoE)-KO mice as a model for AD.

## THE GENETIC, BIOCHEMICAL, AND PATHOLOGICAL HALLMARKS OF ALZHEIMER'S DISEASE

Alzheimer's disease is diagnosed histopathologically by the combined occurrence of senile plaques and neurofibrillary tangles (NFT) in the brain. The latter are composed of the abnormal phosphorylated cytoskeletal protein, tubulin-binding protein ($\tau$), dystrophic neurites, and neuronal cell loss (Orr and Clark 1995).

Genetic studies of familial AD suggest that the etiology of this disease may be associated with several factors. These include the amyloid precursor protein (APP) gene and the allele E4 of apoE (Roses 1994), as well as the two presenilin genes PS1 and PS2 that reside, respectively, on chromosomes 1 and 14 (Levy-Lahad et al. 1995; Sherrington et al. 1995). Only apoE4 increases the risk of AD by modifying the age of onset of the disease (Roses 1994). Furthermore, the size of the senile plaques and their amyloid-$\beta$ (A$\beta$) content are greater in subjects with apoE4 than those lacking this allele (Schmechel et al. 1993).

Tg lines of mutated APP have been shown to develop A$\beta$ deposits and neuritic plaques. Tg's with presenilin, apoE4, and hyperphosphorylated $\tau$ are continuing to be developed but have not yet been shown to develop AD lesions. These various Tg mice are being developed in the hope of inducing earlier onset clinical disease with more severe pathology. Borchelt et al. (1998) stated that there is no consensus on whether these mice show several other significant features of AD including reductions in numbers of synapses and levels of transmitter markers, perturbations of the neuronal cytoskeleton,

We express appreciation to the following scientists for the contribution of figures: Dr. Greg M. Cole, UCLA, Dr. Simon Melov, Emory School of Medicine, Atlanta; Dr. Albee Messing, University of Wisconsin–Madison, Dr. Iain L. Campbell, The Scripps Research Institute, La Jolla; and Dr. S. Chapman, Tel-Aviv University, Tel-Aviv, Israel. The authors are grateful to Ms. JoAnne Johnson (NIEHS) for her helpful comments.

aberrant processing of APP by subsets of neurons that are affected in AD, death and loss of specific populations of neurons, and progressive impairments in performance of memory tasks.

## The Genetics of the Amyloid-β Precursor Protein and Presenilins

Senile plaques are a dense extracellular material formed around a core of Aβ peptide that is derived from the larger protein APP. Mutations of the APP gene may alter the normal metabolism of APP and result in amyloidogenesis (Hardy 1997). Analysis of the amyloid cores of the senile plaques led to the identification of the 40–42 long amino acid peptide Aβ that is a proteolytic fragment of the APP. Genetic studies of the familial dominant form of AD led to the identification of AD-linked mutations on the APP gene as well as in the two newly discovered genes PS1 and PS2 (Hardy 1997). All APP, PS1, and PS2 mutations analyzed thus far affect the production of Aβ peptides either by increasing the total amount of Aβ or by inducing the synthesis of the longer form of Aβ, Aβ 1–42 (Hardy 1997). These effects, which have now been reproduced in numerous cell culture and animal models (Borchelt et al. 1996, Citron et al. 1997; Johnson-Wood et al. 1997; Tomita et al. 1997), support the hypothesis that familial AD-linked APP, PS1, and PS2 mutations cause the disease by altering APP processing in a way that increases the likelihood of amyloid formation.

Aβ is generated during intracellular transport of APP by sequential cleavages by α- and β-secretases that cleave APP at the C-terminus and N-terminus, respectively. Although these enzymes have not yet been isolated, their activities and intracellular location have been studied. The α-secretase activity resides along the secretory pathway and has been found in the endoplasmic reticulum (ER), intermediate compartment (IC), trans-Golgi network (TGN), and the post-Golgi compartments as well as endosomes and the plasma membrane (Chyung et al. 1997; Haass et al. 1995). On the other hand, β-secretase activity was found mainly in the ER and, to a lesser extent, in the IC, TGN, plasma membrane, and endosomes. Nonneuronal cells secrete Aβ mainly through the plasma membrane and the endosomal systems, whereas neurons are unique in that they synthesize Aβ mainly intracellularly along the secretory pathway (Cook et al. 1997; Hartmann et al. 1997).

Analysis of the intracellular metabolism of PS1 and PS2 revealed that they are cleaved following synthesis to N- and C-terminal fragments that remain associated in vivo. The presenilin proteins reside mainly in the ER and Golgi (Kovacs et al. 1996) and thus could interact directly with APP and its breakdown peptide. Whether the physiologically relevant cross-talk between APP and

the presenilins is mediated by direct interactions between these proteins or indirectly via a signaling system is not known. Interestingly, the inactivation by targeted mutagenesis of PS1, but not of PS2, results in the loss of Aβ production.

## The Biochemistry of Neurofibrillary Tangles and τ

The NFTs are intracellular aggregates of abnormally phosphorylated microtubule-associated proteins. While the biochemical composition of the NFTs has not been completely determined, the primary component thus far identified is τ protein, a cytoskeletal protein that associates with the microtubules (Higgins et al. 1995).

The cytoskeletal protein τ exhibits abnormal phosphorylation in Alzheimer's disease (AD) and is a major constituent of neurofibrillary tangles (Grundke-Iqbal et al. 1986; Kosik and Greenberg 1994). Furthermore AD τ, unlike normal τ, does not promote the assembly of soluble tubulin into microtubules but regains this ability following dephosphorylation (Biernat et al. 1993; Bramblett et al. 1993). This finding led to the suggestion that τ hyperphosphorylation disrupts the cytoskeleton and that such a mechanism plays an important role in neurodegeneration in AD (Goedert 1993).

Mass spectroscopy analysis and the development of specific anti-τ monoclonal antibodies led to the identification and mapping of about 20 distinct serine and threonine residues that are hyperphosphorylated in AD τ. In vitro studies revealed that τ can be phosphorylated by proline-directed and second messenger–dependent kinases and dephosphorylated by numerous protein phosphatases (Billingsley and Kincaid 1997). Complementary in vivo studies revealed that inhibition of distinct phosphatases results in τ dephosphorylation (Munoz-Montano et al. 1997) and that inhibition of protein phosphatase activities results in τ hyperphosphorylation (Arendt et al. 1995). The existence of an inverse relationship between M1 muscarinic receptor activation and τ phosphorylation suggests a link between the cholinergic signal transduction system and the neuronal cytoskeleton (Sadot et al. 1996) that provides a mechanism by which cholinergic hypofunction, such as that observed in AD (Francis et al. 1994), can affect the homeostasis of the cytoskeleton and thereby enhance neurodegeneration.

## The Association of Alzheimer's Disease with the E4 Allele of Apolipoprotein E

With the identification of the APP and PS mutations, a large fraction of the familial autosomal cases were accounted for; however, a much higher number of cases is either sporadic or appears in late onset nonautosomal dominant and high-risk families. Analysis of the latter families led to the discovery of allelic segregation of the apoE gene with late onset–sporadic familial AD (Roses 1994). ApoE, which is encoded by a gene on human chromosome 19, has three major alleles that occur naturally, termed apoE2, apoE3, and apoE4; the last is associated with a higher frequency of AD (e.g., 40 percent of AD versus 15 percent of controls have apoE4). Further studies revealed that apoE4 increases the risk of AD by modifying the age of onset such that each copy of the apoE4 allele can lower the age of onset of the disease by as much as 7 to 9 years (Roses et al. 1994).

ApoE, the major brain lipoprotein, may play an important role in neuronal maintenance and repair mechanisms, as animal and cellular model studies suggest (Chapman and Michaelson 1998, Chen et al. 1997; Poirier 1994). Furthermore, some of these effects seem to be isoform specific in that apoE3 stimulates and apoE4 inhibits neurite outgrowth in culture (Bellosta et al. 1995; Nathan et al. 1995). Additional studies recently performed by our group revealed that apoE3, but not apoE4, stimulates the synthesis of membrane phospholipids (Meiri et al. 1998). This observation suggests the isoform-specific effects of apoE on neurite outgrowth may be mediated by modulation of lipid metabolism.

## Oxidative Stress, Inflammation, and Neurodegeneration

Aging is an important risk factor of AD, suggesting that the phenotypic expression of a disease-linked genotype is affected by age-dependent mechanisms. Alzheimer's disease and other neurodegenerative disorders such as amyotrophic lateral sclerosis have been linked to oxidative stress and its cumulative age-dependent effects (Brown et al. 1996, Butterfield et al. 1994, Miyata and Smith 1996). Microglial cells are emerging as a key mediating component in neurodegenerative diseases because activation of microglia and the resulting production of free oxygen radicals and reactive oxygen species may lead to neuronal death (Brown et al. 1996).

## NEUROPATHOLOGY IN TRANSGENIC AND KNOCKOUT MOUSE MODELS USED IN RESEARCH ON ALZHEIMER'S DISEASE

Pathological diagnosis of AD requires the identification of senile plaques, NFTs, dystrophic neurites, and neuronal cell loss (Orr and Clark 1995). The senile plaques are a dense extracellular material formed around a core

of Aβ peptide derived from the larger protein APP. That mutations of the APP gene alter the normal metabolism of APP resulting in amyloidogenesis has been suggested. The NFTs are intracellular aggregates of abnormally phosphorylated microtubule-associated proteins. While the biochemical composition of the NFTs has not been completely determined, the primary component thus far identified is τ protein, a cytoskeletal protein that associates with the microtubules and is abnormally phosphorylated (Higgins et al. 1995).

Identification of genes and mutations relevant to AD pathology has afforded the opportunity to make Tg mice harboring identified risk or causal factors for AD (Cole and Frautschy 1997). Transgenic lines of mutated APP develop amyloid-β deposits and neuritic plaques. Transgenic mice with the presenilin, apoE4, and τ genes are continuing to be developed but have not yet been shown to develop AD lesions. These transgenic mice are being mated with others in an attempt to induce earlier onset and more severe lesions. Borchelt et al. (1998) stated that that there is no consensus on whether these mice show several other significant features of AD.

Tables 18.1 and 18.2 present histopathological features and special pathological techniques mentioned in some of the AD models. Altered expression of cytokines and oxidative stress were observed in a variety of CNS pathologic states, such as AD, multiple sclerosis, cerebral ischemia, Parkinson's disease, and HIV encephalopathy (Campbell et al. 1997; Melov et al. 1998). Models investigating the relevance of these factors to the development of neurodegenerative diseases and AD models are presented in Tables 18.1 and 18.2. Other models are shown in Tables 18.3 and 18.4.

## APOLIPOPROTEIN E TRANSGENIC MODELS: APOLIPOPROTEIN E AND GENETIC RISK FACTORS FOR ALZHEIMER'S DISEASE

Recent studies have shown that the degree of cholinergic deficiency in AD brains, monitored by the extent of reduction in cortical and hippocampal choline acetyltransferase (ChAT) levels, correlates positively with the E4 alelle copy number (Poirier et al. 1995). These compelling findings imply that the biology of apoE is extremely relevant to the expression of AD; however, the isoform-specific cellular and molecular mechanisms that render apoE4 a major risk factor for AD are not known.

ApoE, a 34 KDa polymorphic protein, is associated with several plasma lipoproteins and particularly with the transport of cholesterol into various cells. ApoE is

**TABLE 18.1. Neuropathology in Tg models used in the research of Alzheimer's disease and related pathologies**

| Transgene and promoter | Pathological features | Reference |
|---|---|---|
| Amyloid precursor protein (APP)$_{695}$, inserted into a hamster PrP cosmid vector | Neuronal and synaptic loss and formation of amyloid-β (Aβ), Congo red+, senile plaques (neuritic plaques) with associated dystrophic neurites. Immunohistochemical + reaction for human Aβ, microtubule-associated protein τ and oxidative stress copper zinc (CuZn) superoxide dismutase (SOD) and hemoxygenase-1 (HO-1). Microglia clustered in and around plaques (Figs. 18.1, 18.2). | Frautschy et al. 1998; Pappolla et al. 1998; Smith et al. 1998 |
| APP V717F, using platelet-derived growth factor promoter | Mature neuritic plaques around Aβ core, synaptic loss, astrocytosis, microgliosis. Dystrophic neurites containing dense lamellar bodies and neurofilaments. | Games et al. 1995; Masliah et al. 1996; Orr and Clark 1995 |
| APP751, using neuron-specific enolase (NSE) promoter | Presence of Aβ and hyperphosphorylated τ protein in the distorted neurites. The Aβ immunoreactivity was extracellular. The Alz50 immunoreactivity, used to identify the τ, was noted within neurons, puncta, and processes. The frequency of both Aβ deposition and τ protein was twice as prevalent in brains from old (22 months) than young (2–3 months) β-APP751 Tg mice. The Aβ deposits were associated with GFAP (glial fibrillary acidic protein)-positive glial reaction. | Higgins and Holtzman 1994; Higgins et al. 1995 |
| (Mutant APP, Tg 2576) × (mutant presenilin, Tg PS1$_{M146L}$) | Large numbers of fibrillar Aβ deposits in cerebral cortex and hippocampus, earlier than the single Tg 2576. | Holcomb et al. 1998 |
| (PDGF-hAPP Tg) × (astrocyte-targeted expression of TGF-β Tg) | Accelerated deposition of Aβ peptide (already at 2–3 months of age). | Wyss-Coray et al. 1997 |
| Astrocyte-targeted expression of cytokines IL-6, IL-3, or TNF-α | IL-6 Tg–expressing mice: Neurodegeneration in the hippocampus and cerebellum, secondary demyelination, inflammation, reactive gliosis, angiogenesis, and blood-brain barrier disruption.<br>IL-3 Tg–expressing mice: Primary plaquelike demyelination, macrophage/microglial and mast cell accumulation, remyelination and astrocytosis.<br>TNF-α Tg–expressing mice: Meningoencephalitis and gray and white matter degeneration. | Campbell et al. 1997, 1998; Chiang et al. 1994 |
| Human AChE cDNA, using human AChE promoter | The branching of the basilar dendritic trees of layer 5 pyramidal neurons from the frontoparietal cortex totally ceased after 5 weeks of age. The dendritic arbors became smaller, and the average number of spines was significantly lower in adult transgenic mice than controls. | Beeri et al. 1997 |
| APP-C100 and Flag APP-C100, using dystrophin brain promoter | Profound degeneration of neurons and synapses in Ammon's horn and the dentate gyrus of the hippocampal formation; cerebral blood vessels with thickened basal laminae, and microglia-adjacent larger venous vessels. | Oster-Granite et al. 1996 |

synthesized in vivo in glia and subsequently taken up by neurons (Handelmann et al. 1992). In addition, in humans, unlike rodents, apoE is synthesized by neurons (Han et al. 1994). Thus, the effects of apoE on neuronal function in rodents may be mediated either extracellularly or by interactions with intracellular constituents. ApoE is unique among apolipoproteins in that its levels in the brain, unlike those of other apolipoproteins, are particularly high and are further increased following injury (Poirier 1994; Skene and Shooter 1983). Mice whose apoE gene has been inactivated by targeted mutation have basal neuronal derangements and recover from head injury less effectively than control

mice (Chen et al. 1997; Gordon et al. 1995; Masliah et al. 1995). These findings suggest that apoE plays an important, isoform-specific role in neuronal maintenance and repair.

Several mechanisms have been proposed to explain the phenotype associated with the apoE4 genotype and its age dependency. Cell culture studies revealed that apoE3 promotes, whereas apoE4 inhibits, neurite outgrowth and phospholipid synthesis (Bellosta et al. 1995; Nathan et al. 1994), and the known role of apoE in lipid transport led to the suggestion that the effects of apoE on neuronal function are mediated by isoform-specific modulation of membrane neogenesis and

**TABLE 18.2. Neuropathology in KO models used in the research of Alzheimer's disease and related disorders**

| Model | Pathological features | Reference |
|---|---|---|
| Apolipoprotein E (ApoE)$^{(-/-)}$ | Electron microscopy—extensive dendritic vacuolization and disruption of the endomembrane system and cytoskeleton. Amyloidlike protein accumulated in the protoplasmic astrocytes of the hippocampus, especially in the brains of old animals. | Kindy and Rader 1998; Laskowitz et al. 1997; Masliah et al. 1995; Robertson et al. 1998 |
| Amyloid percursor protein(APP)$^{(-/-)}$ | Reactive gliosis suggesting an impaired neuronal function; however, no evidence for neuronal cell morphological abnormalities was reported. | Zheng et al. 1995 |
| Superoxide dismutase $Sod2^{tm1Cje}$ | Symmetric spongiform degeneration of the cortex and specific brain stem nuclei associated with gliosis and intramyelinic vacuolization. Astrocytic response in areas of vacuolation (Fig. 18.3). | Melov et al. 1998 |

**TABLE 18.3. Neuropathology in Tg mice with other neuropathological disorders**

| Human disease or experimental state | Transgene | Pathological features | Reference |
|---|---|---|---|
| Familial amyotrophic lateral sclerosis | Mutant human superoxide dismutase (SOD1) | In the motor neurons of the spinal cord and brain stem: neurofilament inclusions; presence of small and large vacuoles in the motor neurons, as well as loss of these neurons; astrocytosis in spinal cord. | Hall et al. 1998; Shibata et al. 1998; Tu et al. 1996, 1997 |
| Human neurofibromatosis type 1 (NF1) | Nf1 gene was targeted by homologous recombination (Nf1/nf1) | Increased numbers of astrocytes in medial regions of the periaqueductal gray and in the nucleus accumbens and in the hippocampus. | Rizvi et al. 1999 |
| Huntington's disease (HD), caused by a cytosine-adenine-guanine (CAG)/polyglutamine expansion | Tg for a mutant version of exon 1 of the HD gene | Neuronal intranuclear inclusions (NII) that were immunoreactive for huntingtin and ubiquitin have been found in the brains of the mice developing a progressive neurological phenotype. | Bates et al. 1998 |
| Gerstmann-Sträussler-Scheinker disease (GSS), inherited neurodegenerative prion disease | Murine prion protein | Spongiform degeneration throughout the brain characterized by vacuoles and reactive gliosis, present both in the white and gray matter of the cerebral hemispheres and brain stem. | Hsiao et al. 1990; Hsiao and Prusiner 1991; Raeber et al. 1998 |
| Astrocytes-containing inclusion bodies (IB), as a model for IB, seen in Alexander's disease (Rosenthal fibers), familial myopathies, and lewy bodies in Parkinson's disease | hGFAP | Markedly hypertrophic astrocytes many of which contained IB (i.e., large eosinophilic aggregates in the perinuclear region of the cell) (Fig. 18.4). | Messing et al. 1998 |
| Human encephalopathies of unknown etiology, like Aicardi-Goutieres syndrome | GFAP interferon (IFN) -α | Progressive inflammatory encephalopathy with marked mineralization, meningoencephalitis (composed of lymphocytes), gliosis, and neurodegeneration (Fig. 18.5). | Akwa et al. 1998 |
| Overexpression of bcl-2, an apoptosis-related oncogene | Hu-bcl-2 | Increase of Purkinje cells, olivary neurons, and granule cell numbers was noted in the Tg mice. | Zanjani et al. 1996, 1997 |

**TABLE 18.4. Neuropathology in KO mice with other neuropathological disorders**

| Human disease | Gene | Pathological features | Reference |
|---|---|---|---|
| Unverricht-Lundborg disease (EPM1, an autosomal recessive inherited disorder, belongs to the progressive myclonus epilepsies group of diseases.) | Human cystatin B gene (Cstb) KO (Cstb [−/−]) | Depletion of granule cells and presence of pyknotic nuclei in the cerebellar granule cell layer. | Pennacchio et al. 1998 |
| CRASH syndrome (an inherited disease resulting from L1 mutations, characterized by corpus callosum hypoplasia, adducted thumbs, spastic paraplegia, and hydrocephalus) | L1 [−/−] | Hypoplasia of the corticospinal tract, abnormal dilatation of the ventricular system, hypoplasia of the cerebellar vermis. | Fransen et al. 1998 |
| Neurodegenerative diseases characterized by neuronal cell death caused by defects in the transport of synaptic vesicles | Monomeric neuron-specific kinesin protein (KIF1A) KO (KIF1A [−/−]) | Decreased number of synaptic vesicles; neuronal degeneration in the cerebellum, rhinencephalon, and amygdaloid areas; vacuoles surrounding the degenerated neurons; axonal degeneration in the spinal cord. | Yonekawa et al. 1998 |
| Multiple sclerosis (MS) | Inducible nitric oxide synthase (iNOS) KO (iNOS [−/−]) | The iNOS KO mice had a greater sensitivity to induced autoimmune encephalomylitis (EAE) than did wild-type control mice. | Fenyk-Melody et al. 1998 |
| Ataxia-telangiectasia (a disorder caused by mutations in the Atm protein kinase gene) | Atm [−/−] | Degeneration of neurons in the cerebellar cortex, gliosis, deterioration of neurophil structure. | Kuljis et al. 1997 |
| Zellweger syndrome (in which the inability to assemble functional peroxisomes causes multiorgan defects during fetal development) | Pxr1 [−/−] | Reduced thickness of neocortical plate. | Baes et al. 1997 Matsuda et al. 1997 |
| G(M1)-gangliosidosis. | β-galactosidase [−/−] | Periodic acid-Schiff (PAS) -positive intracytoplasmic storage in neuronal cells. | |

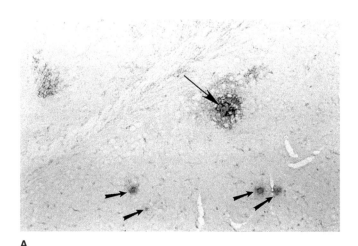
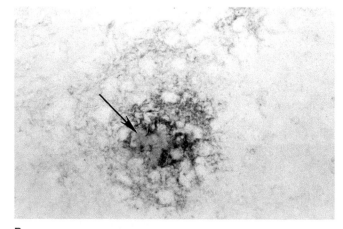

A                                    B

**FIGURE 18.1** Histology of Tg 2576 (APPsw) mouse. Relationship between Aβ immunostaining and microglia. Microglia are identified by Griffonia simlificofolia (GS) lectin labeling (stained with 3,3′-diaminobenzidine [DAB], brown) and plaques by Aβ42 immunostaining (stained blue). (**A**) Section at the level of occipital cortex and presubiculum. Small Aβ42-positive plaques contain few or no lectin-stained microglia (*thick arrows*), whereas large plaques contain prominent plaque-associated masses of lectin labeling (*thin arrow*). (**B**) The GS lectin-labeled microglia (brown, *thin arrow*) are grossly enlarged around small Aβ42-specific immunostaining (blue) and frequently wrapped around cells in the adjacent area. (Reproduced from Frautschy et al. 1998, by copyright permission)

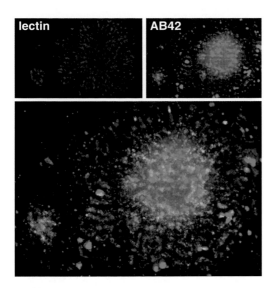

**FIGURE 18.2** Histology of Tg 2576 (APPsw) mouse. A pseudoconfocal image that depicts two β-amyloid plaques in the subiculum of a 15-month-old Tg 2576 transgene-positive mouse labeled with end-specific polyclonal anti-Aβ42 from T. Saido (red) and biotinylated GS which labels activated microglia in green. The numerous tightly plaque–associated, individual microglia are clearly resolved. Yellow overlap is limited. Original magnification ×400. (Generously given by Professor Greg M. Cole, UCLA Departments of Medicine and Neurology, University of California, Los Angeles)

synaptic modeling. Other studies revealed that apoE3 binds in vitro to cytoskeletal proteins more readily than apoE4 and suggested that apoE4 interacts less readily than apoE3 with the neuronal cytoskeleton in vivo, thereby enabling the age-dependent accumulation of excess τ phosphorylation and the consequent disruption of the cytoskeleton (Huang et al. 1994). In addition, investigations have revealed that apoE3, but not apoE4, has antioxidant activity; apoE KO mice are oxidatively stressed (Miyata and Smith 1996; Lomnitski et al. 1999a); and microglial activation can be regulated by apoE (Barger and Harmon 1997). These findings suggest that the isoform-specific effects of apoE may be mediated by oxidative and inflammatory mechanisms.

# Experimental and Histopathological Methods

## ANIMALS
Control and apoE-deficient mice derived from the same parent line (C57BL/6J) were kindly provided by Dr. J.L. Breslow (Plump et al. 1992). Fourteen-week-old male mice were used in all the studies presented here.

*Behavioral studies:* ApoE-deficient mice (*n* = 10 in each group) and age-matched controls were tested in the

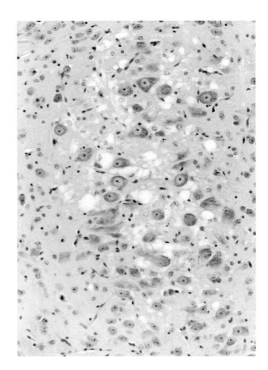

A

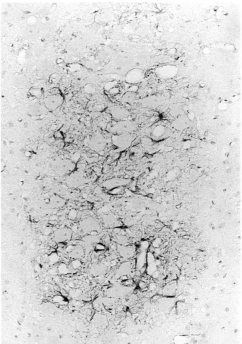

B

**FIGURE 18.3** Histology of a 15-day (Sod)$^{2tm1Cje}$(–/–) mouse treated with superoxide dismutase (SOD) mimetic compound. Similar brain lesions were noted in the untreated mice; however, the treated mice were rescued from early death, survived, and developed a striking movement disorder. (**A**) Vacuolization with relative neuronal preservation in the trigeminal motor nucleus (hematoxylin and eosin staining). (**B**) Astrocytosis is observed within this nucleus by 19 days (glial fibrillary acidic protein staining). (Reproduced from Melov et al. 1998, by copyright permission)

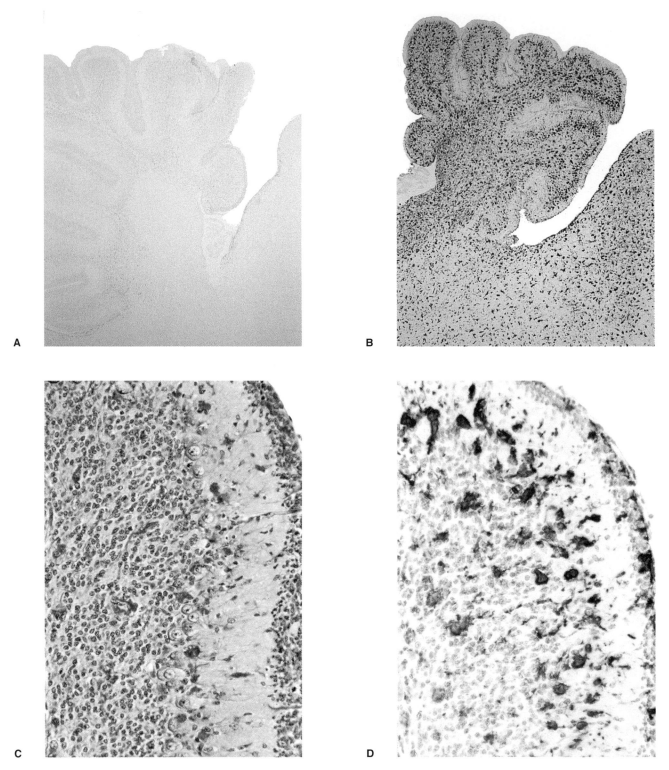

**FIGURE 18.4** Histology of mice carrying human glial fibrillary acidic protein (Tg hGFAP). **A** and **B:** Low-power photomicrographs of cerebellum from a nontransgenic littermate (**A**) and a Tg 73.1 mouse (**B**) 8 days old, stained for hGFAP (SM-21) antibody using avidin-biotin immunohistochemistry. Astrocytes immunoreactive for hGFAP are present throughout the cerebellum of the transgenic mouse, but no staining is present in the control. Magnification, ×21. **C** to **E:** High-power photomicrographs of cerebellar cortex from a Tg 73.1 mouse, 11 days old, stained with hematoxylin and eosin (**C**) or for hGFAP (**D**) or vimentin (**E**), using avidin-biotin immunohistochemistry. The numerous eosinophylic profiles in **C** correspond to the cytoplasm of enlarged astrocytes. The immunopositive profiles in **D** and **E** correspond in size and location to the eosinophilic astrocytes. Magnification, ×50. **F:** Immunostaining for nestin in the neocortex of Tg 73.8 founder, 10 days old, showing many enlarged, positive astrocytes. Magnification, ×50. (Reproduced from Messing et al. 1998, by copyright permission)

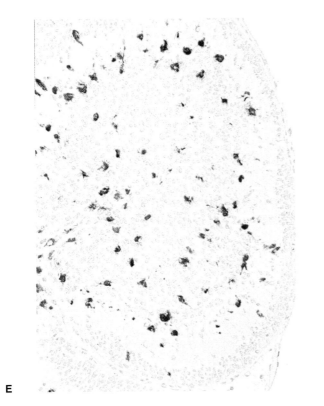

E

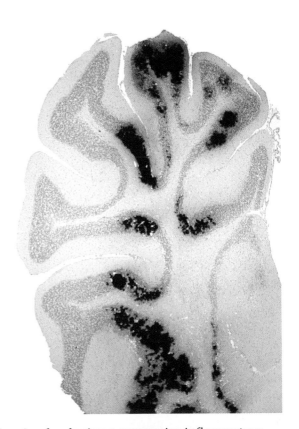

F

**FIGURE 18.4** Continued

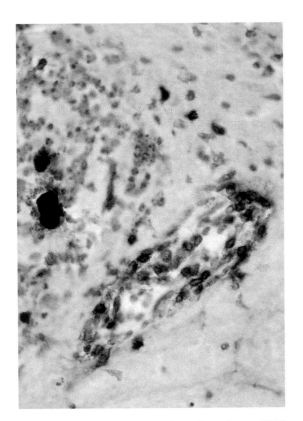

A

B

**FIGURE 18.5** Brain sections from interferon (IFN) -α transgenic mice developing a progressive inflammatory encephalopathy with marked calcium mineralization. (**A**) Immunophenotyping of cell infiltrates in brain of IFN-α mouse (age 6 months) showing the presence of CD4+ T cells. Alizarin red-S staining showing extensive calcification in the cerebellum (**B**). (Reproduced from Akwa et al. 1998, by copyright permission)

Morris water maze–working memory test described by Fisher et al. (1998). Results were analyzed for each mouse as the mean path length of the second daily trial, divided by the mean path length of the first daily trial, over a period of 10 days. The ratios obtained for each mouse represent the relative gain in performance from the first to the second trial and are thus a measure of working memory function.

*Histological studies:* The mice were sacrificed and their brains excised and rapidly frozen in a mixture of hexane and dry ice. Frozen coronal sections (20μ) were then cut, mounted on gelatin-coated glass slides, and stored at −80°C until used. The synaptic density of cholinergic neurons was determined by evaluation of acetylcholinesterase (AChE) activity and ChAT immunoreactivity. AChE activity was measured histochemically according to the method of Karnovsky and Roots (1964). The dopaminergic presynaptic transporters were visualized autoradiographically using the tritiated ligand [³H]GBR 12,935 described by Mennicken et al. (1992). Measurement of the presynaptic noradrenergic transporter was performed using the transporter-specific ligand [³H]-nisoxetine (Tejani-Butt 1992).

The serotonergic nerve terminals were autoradiographed using [³H]-paroxetine (Hardina et al. 1990).

Quantitation of the intensity of staining was performed utilizing the Cue-2 Image Analysis System (Olympus, Lake Success, NY) and the NIH Image software (NIH Image by Wayne Rasband, National Institutes of Health). Three consecutive sections for each stained area of brain were measured and averaged. The intensity of staining of control and apoE-deficient mice was analyzed by one-way ANOVA.

### CLOSED HEAD INJURY MODEL

Closed head injury was produced under anesthesia, as described by Chen et al. (1997). Following recovery from anesthesia, the mice were returned to their home cages with free access to food and water. Parallel groups of apoE-deficient and control mice were anesthetized and served as sham controls.

### PREPARATION OF BRAIN SECTIONS

Mice were sacrificed at days 3, 7, 9, and 14 postinjury, after which their brains were rapidly removed from the craniums and fixed by immersion in 10 percent phosphate-buffered formalin and then coronally trimmed at four levels. Four, 1.5–2 mm thick brain slices were taken that included the following brain sites:

- *Level 1:* frontoparietal cortex, caudate putamen, corpus callosum
- *Level 2:* frontoparietal cortex, caudate putamen, corpus callosum, lateral ventricles

- *Level 3:* frontoparietal cortex, hippocampus, thalamus, lateral ventricles
- *Level 4:* striatum, temporal cortex, hippocampus, midbrain

The brain slices were then paraffin-embedded by routine procedures, after which 5 μm thick sections were prepared.

## Morphometric Measurement of Hematoxylin and Eosin–Stained Brain Sections

After fixed brain sections were stained with hematoxylin and eosin (H&E), an image analysis system was used to determine the size of the damaged area at four different levels (L1–L4) of each brain. The remaining unaffected area of the same hemisphere and the area of the contralateral hemisphere were measured by manual tracing using an electronic pencil. The relative affected area in a given section was then calculated utilizing the following equation:

$$1 - (\text{normal area of injured hemisphere} / \text{area of contralateral hemisphere}).$$

### PERLS' PRUSSIAN BLUE STAINING

For measurement of iron-containing cells, brain sections were stained by Perls' Prussian Blue (PB) (Nyska et al. 1989), which detects protein-bound iron. The blue-black intracellular deposit detected by this method was used to quantify the number of phagocytic-glial cells that contain iron. Four brain levels (L1–L4) of each brain were stained and examined systematically at ×200 magnification. The number of iron-positive cells in each section was counted, and the average number of iron-positive cells was calculated at each of the four brain levels. The total number of iron-positive cells per brain was then calculated by summation of the values obtained at the four brain levels.

# THE EFFECTS OF APOLIPOPROTEIN E DEFICIENCY ON NEURONAL MAINTENANCE AND REPAIR

## Behavioral Studies

The cognitive performance of apoE-deficient and control mice was compared by the Morris water maze utilizing a learning and short-term memory paradigm (Gordon et al. 1995) based on the difference in performance of the mice between two daily trials over a period of 10 days. While control mice improved in performance from the first to the second daily trial, the apoE-deficient mice performed worse on their second daily trial (Gordon et al. 1995). This finding suggests that apoE-deficient mice have working memory deficits.

## Histological Studies

### CHOLINERGIC IMPAIRMENT OF APOLIPOPROTEIN E–DEFICIENT MICE

The synaptic density of basal forebrain cholinergic neurons of apoE-deficient and control mice was monitored histochemically by measurements of the levels of AChE and ChAT in distinct brain areas (Kleifeld et al. 1998). The septal area of apoE-deficient mice stained less intensely than that of the control. In contrast to the above, the level of AChE staining in the striatum of the apoE-deficient mice was unaltered and similar to that of the controls. These findings are consistent with histological and biochemical measurements of ChAT levels in brains of apoE-deficient mice (Fisher et al. 1998; Gordon et al. 1995). The data further suggest that the septohippocampal cholinergic projection is affected more extensively by apoE deficiency than the basocortical cholinergic pathway.

### COMPARISON OF CHOLINERGIC AND DOPAMINERGIC PATHWAYS

The neuronal specificity of the effects of apoE deficiency on projecting neuronal pathways was examined. The experiments focused on the nigrostriatal pathway and examining whether the density of dopaminergic nerve terminals of these neurons, like those of the cholinergic projections, is lower in apoE-deficient mice than in con-

trol. The density of dopaminergic (DA) nerve terminals was monitored by using the ligand [³H]GBR 12,935, which binds specifically to the presynaptic dopaminergic transporter, while the cholinergic synapses were monitored histochemically. We observed a marked reduction in AChE activity in the hippocampus ($33.8 \pm 5.7$ percent) of the apoE-deficient mice compared with that of the control (Fig. 18.6; Chapman and Michaelson 1998). Similar reductions were detected in the levels of ChAT immunoreactivity in the same brain areas ($27.6 \pm 3.7$ percent of control, not shown). In contrast, the density of presynaptic dopaminergic staining in the striatum of the two mice groups was similar, suggesting that cholinergic, not nigrostriatal dopaminergic, pathways are specifically susceptible to apoE deficiency. These animal model findings are compatible with clinical observations that the apoE genotype is a risk factor for Alzheimer's disease but not for Parkinson's disease, which, unlike AD, is marked by specific degeneration of the nigrostriatal dopaminergic projections.

### THE LEVEL OF NORADRENERGIC NERVE TERMINALS IN THE BRAINS OF APOLIPOPROTEIN E–DEFICIENT AND CONTROL MICE

The levels of noradrenergic nerve terminals in the brains of apoE-deficient and control mice were measured radiographically using the radioligand [³H]-nisoxetine, which binds specifically to the presynaptic noradrenergic transporter (Chapman and Michaelson 1998). The intensity of staining of the hippocampus and the parietal cortex of the apoE-deficient mice was lower than that of the corresponding control. The density of the nerve terminals was measured at different brain areas

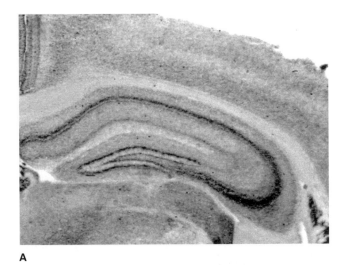

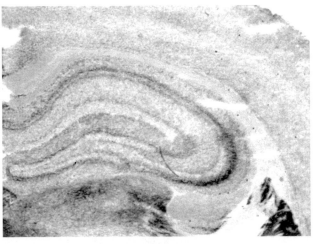

A                                                                                      B

**FIGURE 18.6**   Representative photomicrographs of frozen sections of the hippocampal cholinergic nerve terminals in apoE-deficient (**B**) and control mice (**A**). AChE histochemical staining according to Karnovsky and Roots 1964. (Reproduced from Chapman and Michaelson 1998, by copyright permission)

and quantified. This quantification revealed that the density of noradrenergic nerve terminals in areas proximal to the origin of the locus coeruleus adrenergic tract (e.g., hypothalamus and thalamus) is similar to that of controls, whereas it is markedly lower in brain areas such as the parietal cortex and the hippocampus that are located farther away from the neuronal cell bodies.

## THE LEVEL OF SEROTONERGIC SYNAPSES IN THE BRAINS OF APOLIPOPROTEIN E-DEFICIENT AND CONTROL MICE

The level of serotonergic terminals that emanate from the raphe nucleus was determined autoradiographically using [³H]-paroxetine, a specific ligand of the presynaptic serotonin transporter. The density of the serotonergic terminals in the parietal cortex of apoE-deficient mice was markedly lower than that of the control (Chapman and Michaelson 1998; data not shown). The reduction in the level of serotonergic hippocampal synapses of apoE-deficient mice was less pronounced than the reduction observed in the parietal cortex.

## τ PHOSPHORYLATION IN APOLIPOPROTEIN E-DEFICIENT AND CONTROL MICE

In apoE-deficient mice τ contains hyperphosphorylated epitopes (e.g., the epitopes recognized by mAb AT8) (Genis et al. 1995). These findings provide a unique system for studying the relationship, in vivo, between cholinergic hypofunction and τ phosphorylation and the extent to which the relationship can be modulated pharmacologically.

We investigated the effects of chronic treatment with the muscarinic agonist AF150(S) on the levels of τ phosphorylation of apoE-deficient mice and the extent to which the effects correlated with the previously published, cognitive therapeutic effects of AF150(S) (Fisher et al. 1998). This investigation was performed by immunoblot assays utilizing a panel of mAbs directed against distinct phosphorylated and nonphosphorylated τ epitopes and by comparing their immunoreactivities toward τ of apoE-deficient and control mice. In apoE-deficient mice τ contains a distinct hyperphosphorylated "hot spot" domain that is localized N-terminally to the microtubule-binding domain of τ and contains epitopes that bind to the mAbs AT8, SMI32, and SMI37. Other epitopes that are unaffected by apoE deficiency reside at the N- and C-terminals of τ. These findings suggest that apoE deficiency results in phosphorylation of a distinct τ domain. In apoE-deficient mice τ hyperphosphorylation may be due to distinct enzymatic changes that shift the balance between protein kinase and phosphatase activities. Alternatively, it may be due to changes in the accessibility of distinct τ epitopes to neuronal kinase and phosphatase. Prolonged muscarinic treatment (Genis et

al. 1999) induces epitope-specific dephosphorylation of τ, the extent of which is affected by apoE deficiency.

## ALTERED REPAIR MECHANISMS IN BRAIN OF APOLIPOPROTEIN E-DEFICIENT MICE: CLOSED HEAD INJURY CHALLENGE

Head injury is an important environmental factor that has been implicated in the neuropathology of AD (Gentleman et al. 1993). Furthermore, that subjects with the apoE4 allele are more vulnerable to head trauma than subjects who lack this apoE allele has been suggested (Poirier et al. 1995). These findings and the observation that the deleterious effects of apoE4 are apparent only late in life suggest that apoE plays a key role in neuronal maintenance and repair.

We have previously shown that apoE-deficient mice are impaired in their ability to recover neurologically and cognitively from closed head injury (Chen et al. 1997).

Histological analysis of the brain revealed that the damaged areas of the injured apoE-deficient mice are greater than those of controls in each level. While the size of the damaged brain areas of the injured control mice is subsequently diminished 14 days postinjury, such recovery was not observed in the injured apoE-deficient mice (Lomnitski et al. 1999b). Histopathologically, the decrease in the damaged areas in the control mice was interpreted as related to decreased edema.

The levels of brain iron, known to catalyze the production of free radicals through a Fenton reaction, were measured histochemically using PB staining, following head injury. We observed the existence of two stages postinjury. In the first stage (up to day 7 postinjury) the levels of iron-containing brain cells were higher in the controls than in apoE-deficient mice. In contrast, during the second phase (days 9 to 14 postinjury) the number of iron-containing cells of the controls decreased, whereas those of the apoE-deficient mice increased (Lomnitski et al. 2000). The early appearance of phagocytic cells, which express iron-binding proteins such as ferritin and transferrin, promotes the chelation of free iron and thereby reduces the iron-dependent release of reactive oxygen species. Increased susceptibility to head injury and impaired repair of the apoE-deficient mice are thus possibly, at least in part, a delayed consequence of the impaired ability of these mice to mobilize the brain iron–scavenging cells.

A synopsis of the proposed role of iron in the increased susceptibility of apoE-deficient mice to head injury is that microvascular damage following head injury results in the activation of phospholipases and different oxidases, such as xanthine oxidase and monoamine oxidase. This activation in turn triggers the generation of superoxide radicals with the accompanying edema and accumulation of phagocytes. ApoE is expressed and secreted by macrophages and is believed to play an important role in the remodeling and growth of neurons following injury (Poirier 1994). ApoE secretion is also known to be associated with elevation of macrophage colony–stimulating factor (MCSF), which can activate mature monocytes and macrophages (Clinton et al. 1992). Accordingly, the absence of apoE in the injured apoE-deficient mice results in impaired activation or migration of phagocytic cells. Such an effect is expected to be dominant at early time points during which the levels of iron in the injured brains are maximal, resulting in increased levels of free iron and reactive oxygen species (ROS) levels that, in turn, further exacerbate neuronal damage. We have previously shown that apoE-deficient mice are oxidatively stressed both prior to and following closed head injury (Lomnitski et al. 1999) and that this stress is associated with a reduced capability to generate low–molecular weight antioxidants postinjury (Lomnitski et al. 1997). Furthermore, in vitro studies revealed that apoE has an antioxidant activity related to its ability to chelate metal ions (Miyata and Smith 1996). At least part of the effects of apoE deficiency on brain iron metabolism is related to the impaired ability of their lipoproteins to scavenge free iron directly and thereby to reduce oxidative stress.

# REFERENCES

Akwa, Y., Hassett, D.E., Eloranta, M.L., et al. 1998. Transgenic expression of IFN-alpha in the central nervous system of mice protects against lethal neurotropic viral infection but induces inflammation and neurodegeneration. J. Immunol. 161:5016–5026

Arendt, T., Holzer, M., Fruth, R., et al. 1995. Paired helical filament-like phosphorylation of tau, deposition of β-A4-amyloid and memory impairment in rat reduced by chronic inhibition of phosphatase 1 and 2A. Neuroscience 69:691–698.

Baes, M., Gressens, P., Baumgart, E., et al. 1997. A mouse model for Zellweger syndrome. Nat. Genet. 17:49–57

Barger, S.W., Harmon, A.D. 1997. Microglial activation by Alzheimer amyloid precursor protein and modulation by apolipoprotein E. Nature 388:878–881.

Bates, G.P., Mangiarini L., Davies, S.W. 1998. Transgenic mice in the study of polyglutamine repeat expansion diseases. Brain Pathol. 8:699–714.

Beeri, R., Le Novere, N., Mervis, R., et al. 1997. Enhanced hemicholinium binding and attenuated dendrite branching in cognitively impaired acetylcholinesterase-transgenic mice. J. Neurochem. 69:2441–2451.

Bellosta, S., Nathan, B.P., Orth, M., et al. 1995. Stable expression and secretion of apolipoproteins $E_3$ and $E_4$ in mouse neuroblastoma cells produces differential effects on neurite outgrowth. J. Biol. Chem. 270:27063–27071.

Biernat, J., Gustke, N., Drewes, G., et al. 1993. Phosphorylation of $Ser^{262}$ strongly reduces binding of tau to micro-tubules: distinction between PHF-tau immunoreactivity and microtubule binding. Neuron 11:153–163.

Billingsley, M.L., and Kincaid, R.L. 1997. Regulated phosphorylation and dephosphorylation of tau protein: effects on microtubule interaction, intracellular trafficking and neurodegeneration. Biochem. J. 323:577–591.

Borchelt, D.R., Thinakaran, G., Eckman, C.B., et al. 1996. Familial Alzheimer's disease-linked presenilin 1 variants elevate A beta 1-42/1-40 ratio in vitro and in vivo. Neuron 17:1105–1113.

Borchelt, D.R., Wong, P.C., Sisodia, S.S., et al. 1998. Symposium: transgenic models of neurodegeneration. Transgenic mouse models of Alzheimer's disease and amyotrophic lateral schlerosis. Brain Pathol. 8:735–757.

Bramblett, G.T., Goedert, M., Jakes, R. 1993. Abnormal tau phosphorylation at $Ser^{396}$ in Alzheimer's disease recapitulates development and contributes to reduced microtubule binding. Neuron 10:1089–1099.

Brown, D.R., Schmidt, B., and Kretzschmar, H.A. 1996. Role of microglia and host prion protein in neurotoxicity of a prion protein fragment. Nature 380:345–347.

Butterfield, D.A., Hensley, K., Harris, M., et al. 1994. Beta-amyloid peptide free-radical fragments initiate synaptosomal lipoperoxidation in a sequence-specific fashion—implications to Alzheimer's-disease. Biochem. Biophys. Res. Commun. 200:710–715.

Campbell, I.L., Stalder, A.K., Chiang, C.S., et al. 1997. Transgenic models to assess the pathogenic actions of cytokines in the central nervous system. Mol. Psychiatry 2:125–129.

Campbell, I.L., Stalder, A.K., Akwa, Y., et al. 1998. Transgenic models to study the actions of cytokines in the central nervous system. Neuroimmunomodulation 5:126–135.

Chapman, S., Michaelson, D.M. 1998. Specific neurochemical derangements of brain projecting neurons in apolipoprotein E-deficient mice. J. Neurochem. 70:708–714.

Chen, Y., Lomnitski, L., Michaelson, D.M., et al. 1997. Motor and cognitive deficits in apolipoprotein E-deficient mice after closed head injury. Neuroscience 80:1255–1262.

Chiang, C.S., Stalder, A., Samimi, A., et al. 1994. Reactive gliosis as a consequence of interleukin-6 expression in the brain: studies in transgenic mice. Dev. Neurosci. 16:212–221.

Chyung, A.C., Greenberg, B.D., Cook, D.G., et al. 1997. Novel beta-secretase cleavage of beta-amyloid precursor protein in the endoplasmic reticulum intermediate compartment of NT2N cells. J. Cell Biol. 138:671–680.

Citron, M., Westaway, D., Xia, W., et al. 1997. Mutant presenilins of Alzheimer's disease increase production of 42-residue amyloid beta-protein in both transfected cells and transgenic mice. Nat. Med. 3:67–72.

Clinton, S.K., Underwood, R., Hayes, L., et al. 1992. Macrophage colony-stimulating factor gene expression in vascular cells and in experimental and human atherosclerosis. Am. J. Pathol. 140:301–316.

Cole, G.M., Frautschy, S.A. 1997. Animal Models for Alzheimer's Disease. Alzheimer's disease reviews 2:33–41.

Cook, D.G., Forman, M.S., Sung, J.C., et al. 1997. Alzheimer's A beta (1-42) is generated in the endoplasmic reticulum/intermediate compartment of NT2N cells. Nat. Med. 3:1021–1023.

Fenyk-Melody, J.E., Garrison, A.E., Brunnert, S.R., et al. 1998. Experimental autoimmune encephalomyelitis is exacerbated in mice lacking the NOS2 gene. J. Immunol. 160:2940–2946.

Fisher, A., Brandeis, R., Chapman, S., et al. 1998. M1 muscarinic agonist treatment reverses cognitive and cholinergic impairments of apolipoprotein E-deficient mice. J. Neurochem. 70:1991–1997.

Francis, P.T., Gross, A.J., and Bowen, D.M. 1994. Neurotransmitters and neuropeptides in Alzheimer's disease. In Alzheimer's Disease, R. Terry, R. Katzman, and K.L. Bick, eds. New York: Raven Press, pp. 247–261.

Fransen, E., D'Hooge, R., Van Camp, G., et al. 1998. L1 knockout mice show dilated ventricles, vermis hypoplasia and impaired exploration patterns. Hum. Mol. Genet. 7:999–1009.

Frautschy, S.A., Yang, F.S., Irrizarry, M., et al. 1998. Microglial response to amyloid plaques in APPsw transgenic mice. Am. J. Pathol. 152:307–317.

Games, D., Adams, D., Alessandrini, R., et al. 1995. Alzheimer-type neuropathology in transgenic mice overexpressing V717F beta-amyloid precursor protein. Nature 373:523–527.

Genis, I., Gordon, I., Sehayek, E., et al. 1995. Phosphorylation of tau in apolipoprotein E-deficient mice. Neurosci. Lett. 199:5–8.

Genis, I., Fisher, A., Michaelson, D.M. 1999. Site-specific dephosphorylation of tau of apolipoprotein E-deficient and control mice by M1 muscarinic agonist treatment. J. Neurochem. 72:206–213.

Gentleman, S.M., Graham, D.I., Roberts, G.W., et al. 1993. Molecular pathology of head—altered beta-APP metabolism and the etiology of Alzheimer's-disease. Prog. Brain Res. 96:237–246.

Goedert, M. 1993. Tau protein and the neurofibrillary pathology of Alzheimer's disease. Trends Neurosci. 16:460–465.

Gordon, I., Grauer, E., Genis, I., et al. 1995. Memory deficits and cholinergic impairment in apolipoprotein E-deficient mice. Neurosci. Lett. 199:1–4.

Grundke-Iqbal, I., Iqbal, K., Tung, Y.C. 1986. Abnormal phosphorylations of the microtubule-associated protein tau in Alzheimer cytoskeletal pathology. Proc. Natl. Acad. Sci. USA 83:4913–4917.

Haass, C., Lemere, C.A., Capell, A., et al. 1995. The Swedish mutation causes early-onset Alzheimer's disease by beta-secretase cleavage within the secretory pathway. Nat. Med. 1:1291–1296.

Hall, E.D., Oostveen, J.A., Gurney, M.E. 1998. Relationship of microglial and astrocytic activation to disease onset and progression in a transgenic model of familial ALS. Glia 23:249–56

Han, S.H., Hulette, C., Saunders, A.M., et al. 1994. Apolipoprotein-E is present in hippocampal-neurons without neurofibrillary tangles in Alzheimer's disease and in age-matched controls. Exp. Neurol. 128:13–26.

Handelmann, G.E., Boyles, J.K., Weisgraber, K.H., et al. 1992. Effects of apolipoprotein-E, beta-very low-density

lipoproteins, and cholesterol on the extension of neurites by rabbit dorsal-root ganglion neurons in vitro. J. Lipid Res. 33:1677–1688.

Hardina, P.D., Foy, B., Hepner, A., et al. 1990. Antidepressant binding sites in brain: autoradiographic comparison of [3H] paroxetine and [3H] imipramine localization and relationship to serotonin transporter. J. Pharmacol. Exp. Ther. 252:410–418.

Hardy, J. 1997. Amyloid, the presenilins and Alzheimer's disease. Trends Neurosci. 20:154–159.

Hartmann, T., Bieger, S.C., Bruhl, B., et al. 1997. Distinct sites of intracellular production for Alzheimer's disease A beta 40/42 amyloid peptides. Nat. Med. 3:1016–1020.

Higgins, L.S., Holtzman, D.M. 1994. Transgenic mouse brain histopathology resembles early Alzheimer's disease. Ann. Neurol. 35:598–607.

Higgins, L.S., Rodems, J.M., Catalano, R., et al. 1995. Early Alzheimer's disease-like histopathology increases in frequency with age in mice transgenic for beta-APP751. Proc. Natl. Acad. Sci. USA 92:4402–4406.

Holcomb, L., Gordon, M.N., McGowan, E., et al. 1998. Accelerated Alzheimer-type phenotype in transgenic mice carrying both mutant amyloid precursor protein and presenilin transgenes. Nat. Med. 4:97–100.

Hsiao, K., Prusiner, S.B. 1991. Molecular-genetics and transgenic model of Gertsmann-Straussler-Scheinker disease. Alzheimer Dis. Assoc. Disord. 5:155–162.

Hsiao, K.K., Scott, M., Foster, D., et al. 1990. Spontaneous neurodegeneration in transgenic mice with mutant prion protein. Science 250:1587–1590.

Huang, D.Y., Goedert, M., Jakes, R. 1994. Isoform-specific interactions of apolipoprotein-E with the microtubule-associated protein MAP2C—implications for Alzheimer's-disease. Neurosci. Lett. 182:55–58.

Johnson-Wood, K., Lee, M., Motter, R., et al. 1997. Amyloid precursor protein processing and A beta (42) deposition in a transgenic mouse model of Alzheimer's disease. Proc. Natl. Acad. Sci. USA 94:1550–1555.

Karnovsky, M.J., Roots, L. 1964. A "direct coloring" thiocholine method for cholinesterases. J. Histochem. Cytochem. 12:219.

Kindy, M.S., Rader, D.J. 1998. Reduction in amyloid A amyloid formation in apolipoprotein-E-deficient mice. Am. J. Pathol. 152:1387–1395.

Kleifeld, O., Diebler M.J., Chapman, S., et al. 1998. The effect of apolipoprotein E deficiency on brain cholinergic neurons. Int. J. Dev. Neurosci. 16:755–762.

Kosik, K.S., Greenberg, S.M. 1994. Tau protein and Alzheimer's disease. In Alzheimer's Disease, R.D. Terry, P. Katzmann, and K.L. Bick, eds. New York: Raven Press, pp. 335–344.

Kovacs, D.M., Fausett, H.J., Page, K.J., et al. 1996. Alzheimer-associated presenilins 1 and 2: neuronal expression in brain and localization to intracellular membranes in mammalian cells. Nat. Med. 2:224–229.

Kuljis, R.O., Xu, Y., Aguila, M.C., et al. 1997. Degeneration of neurons, synapses, and neuropil and glial activation in a murine Atm knockout model of ataxia-telangiectasia. Proc. Natl. Acad. Sci. USA 94:12688–12693.

Laskowitz, D.T., Sheng, H., Bart, R.D., et al. 1997. Apolipoprotein E-deficient mice have increased susceptibility to focal cerebral ischemia. J. Cereb. Blood Flow Metab. 17:753–758.

Levy-Lahad, E., Wasco, W., Poorkaj, P., et al. 1995. Candidate gene for the chromosome 1 familial Alzheimer's disease locus. Science 269:973–977.

Lomnitski, L., Kohen, R., Chen, Y., et al. 1997. Reduced levels of antioxidants in brains of apolipoprotein E-deficient mice following closed head injury. Pharmacol. Biochem. Behav. 56:669–673.

Lomnitski, L., Chapman, S., Hochman, A., et al. 1999a. Antioxidant mechanisms in apolipoprotein E-deficient mice prior to and following closed head injury. Biochim. Biophys. Acta 1453:359–368.

Lomnitski, L., Nyska, A., Shohami, E., et al. 2000. Increased levels of intracellular iron in the brains of apoE-deficient mice with closed head injury. Exp. Toxicol. Pathol. 52:(in press).

Masliah, E., Mallory, M., Ge, N. 1995. Neurodegeneration in the central nervous system of apoE-deficient mice. Exp. Neurol. 13:107–122.

Masliah, E., Sisk, A., Mallory, M., et al. 1996. Comparison of neurodegenerative pathology in transgenic mice overexpressing V717F beta-amyloid precursor protein and Alzheimer's disease. J. Neurosci. 16:5795–5811.

Matsuda, J., Suzuki, O., Oshima, A., et al. 1997. Beta-galactosidase-deficient mouse as an animal model for G(M1)-gangliosidosis. Glycoconj. J. 14:729–736.

Meiri, G., Shiboleth, A., Michaelson, D.M. 1998. Isoform specific effects of apolipoprotein E on neuronal phospholipid biosynthesis. Neurosci. Lett. 51:S29.

Melov, S., Schneider, J.A., Day, B.J., et al. 1998. A novel neurological phenotype in mice lacking mitochondrial manganese superoxide dismutase. Nat. Genet. 18:159–163.

Mennicken, F., Savasta, M., Peretti-Renucci, R., et al. 1992. Autoradiographic localization of dopamine uptake sites in the rat brain with 3H-GBR 12935, J. Neural Transm. 87:1–14.

Messing, A., Head, M.W., Galles, K., et al. 1998. Fatal encephalopathy with astrocyte inclusions in GFAP transgenic mice. Am. J. Pathol. 152:391–398.

Miyata, M., Smith, J.D. 1996. Apolipoprotein E allele-specific antioxidant activity and effects on cytotoxicity by oxidative insults and beta-amyloid peptides. Nat. Genet. 14:55–61.

Munoz-Montano, J.R., Moreno, F.J., Avila, J., et al. 1997. Lithium inhibits Alzheimer's disease-like protein phosphorylation in neurons. FEBS Lett. 411:183–188.

Nathan, B.P., Bellosta, S., Sanan, D.A. 1994. Differential-effects of apolipoproteins E3 and E4 on neuronal growth invitro. Science 264:850–852.

Nathan, B.P., Chang, K.C., Bellesta, S., et al. 1995. The inhibitory effect of apolipoprotein E4 on neurite outgrowth is associated with microtubule depolymerization. J. Biol. Chem. 270:19791–19799.

Nyska, A., Waner, T., Scolnik, M., et al. 1989. Splenic hemosiderosis: a quantitative evaluation of hemosiderin by means of an automatic image analyzer. Hum. Vet. Toxicol. 31:218–221.

Orr, T.H., Clark H.B. 1995. Genetic approaches to pathogenesis of neurodegenerative diseases. Lab. Invest. 73:161–171.

Oster-Granite, M.L., McPhie, D.L., Greenan, J., et al. 1996. Age-dependent neuronal and synaptic degeneration in mice transgenic for the C terminus of the amyloid precursor protein. J. Neurosci. 16:6732–6741.

Pappolla, M.A., Chyan, Y.J., Omar R.A., et al. 1998. Evidence of oxidative stress and in vivo neurotoxicity of beta-amyloid in a transgenic mouse model of Alzheimer's disease: a chronic oxidative paradigm for testing antioxidant therapies in vivo. Am. J. Pathol. 152:871–877.

Pennacchio, L.A., Bouley, D.M., Higgins, K.M., et al. 1998. Progressive ataxia, myoclonic epilepsy and cerebellar apoptosis in cystatin B-deficient mice. Nat. Gen. 20:251–258.

Plump A.S., Smith J.D., Hayek T. 1992. Severe hypercholesterolemia and atherosclerosis in apolipoprotein E-deficient mice created by homologous recombination in ES cells. Cell 71:343–353.

Poirier, J. 1994. Apolipoprotein-E in animal-models of CNS injury and in Alzheimer's-disease. Trends Neurosci. 17:525–530.

Poirier, J., Delisle, M.C., Quirion, R., et al. 1995. Apolipoprotein E4 allele as a predictor of cholinergic deficits and treatment outcome in Alzheimer's disease. Proc. Natl. Acad. Sci. USA 92:12260–12264.

Raeber, A.J., Brandner, S., Klein, M.A., et al. 1998. Transgenic and knockout mice in research on prion diseases. Brain Pathol. 8:715–733.

Rizvi, T.A., Akunuru, S., de Courten-Myers, G., et al. 1999. Region-specific astrogliosis in brains of mice heterozygous for mutations in the neurofibromatosis type 1 (Nf1) tumor suppressor. Brain Res. 816:111–123

Robertson, T.A., Dutton, N.S., Martins, R.N., et al. 1998. Age-related congophilic inclusions in the brains of apolipoprotein E-deficient mice. Neurosci. 82:171–180.

Roses, A.D. 1994. Apolipoprotein E is a genetic locus that affects the role of Alzheimer's disease expression: β-amyloid burden is a secondary consequence dependent on apoE genotype and duration of disease. J. Neuropathol. Exp. Neurol. 53:429–437.

Sadot, E., Gurwitz, D., Barg, J., et al. 1996. Activation of M1 muscarinic acetylcholine receptor regulates the phosphorylation in transfected PC12 cells. J. Neurochem. 66:877–880.

Schmechel, D.E., Saunders, A.M., Strittmatter W.J., et al. 1993. Increased amyloid beta-peptide eposition in cerebral-cortex as a consequence of apolipoprotein-E genotype in late-onset Alzheimer's-disease. Proc. Nat. Acad. Sci. USA 90:9649–9653.

Sherrington, R., Rogaev, E.I., Liang, Y., et al. 1995. Cloning of a gene bearing missense mutations in early-onset familial Alzheimer's-disease. Nature 375:754–760.

Shibata, N., Hirano, A., Kobayashi, M., et al. 1998. Presence of Cu/Zn superoxide dismutase (SOD) immunoreactivity in neuronal hyaline inclusions in spinal cords from mice carrying a transgene for Gly93Ala mutant human Cu/Zn SOD. Acta Neuropathol. (Berl.) 95:136–142.

Skene, J.H., Shooter, E.M. 1983. Denervated sheath cells secrete a new protein after nerve injury. Proc. Natl. Acad. Sci. USA 80:4169–4173.

Smith, M.A., Hirai, K., Hsiao, K., et al. 1998. Amyloid-beta deposition in Alzheimer transgenic mice is associated with oxidative stress. J. Neurochem. 70:2212–2215.

Tejani-Butt, S.M. 1992. [$^3$H] Nisoxetine: a radiolig and for quantitation of norepinephrine uptake sites by autoradiography or by homogenate binding. J. Pharmacol. Exp. Ther. 260:427–436.

Tomita, T., Maruyama, K., Saido, T.C., et al. 1997. The presenilin 2 mutation (N141I) linked to familial Alzheimer's disease (Volga German families) increases the secretion of amyloid beta protein ending at the 42nd (or 43rd) residue. Proc. Natl. Acad. Sci. USA 94:2025–2030.

Tu, P.H., Raju, P., Robinson, K.A., et al. 1996. Transgenic mice carrying a human mutant superoxide dismutase transgene develop neuronal cytoskeletal pathology resembling human amyotrophic lateral sclerosis lesions. Proc. Natl. Acad. Sci. USA 93:3155–3160.

Tu, P.H., Gurney, M.E., Julien, J.P., et al. 1997. Oxidative stress, mutant SOD1, and neurofilament pathology in transgenic mouse models of human motor neuron disease. Lab. Invest. 76:441–456.

Wyss-Coray, T., Masliah, E., Mallory, M., et al. 1997. Amyloidogenic role of cytokine TGF-beta1 in transgenic mice and in Alzheimer's disease. Nature 389:603–606.

Yonekawa, Y., Harada, A., Okada, Y., et al. 1998. Defect in synaptic vesicle precursor transport and neuronal cell death in KIF1A motor protein-deficient mice. J. Cell Biol. 141:431–441.

Zanjani, H.S., Vogel, M.W., Delhaye-Bouchaud, N., et al. 1996. Increased cerebellar Purkinje cell numbers in mice overexpressing a human bcl-2 transgene. J. Comp. Neurol. 374:332–341.

Zanjani, H.S., Vogel, M.W., Delhaye-Bouchaud, N., et al. 1997. Increased inferior olivary neuron and cerebellar granule cell numbers in transgenic mice overexpressing the human Bcl-2 gene. J. Neurobiol. 32:502–516.

Zheng, H., Jiang, M., Trumbauer, M.E., et al. 1995. Beta-amyloid precursor protein-deficient mice show reactive gliosis and decreased locomotor activity. Cell 81:525–531.

# 19
# Pathology of the Gastrointestinal Tract of Genetically Engineered and Spontaneous Mutant Mice

Michael Mähler, Björn Rozell, Joel F. Mahler, Glenn Merlino, Deborah Devor-Henneman, Jerrold M. Ward, and John P. Sundberg

The gastrointestinal tract (GI) is composed of the oral cavity, esophagus, stomach, and small and large intestines. Numerous lesions have been reported in the GI tract of spontaneous mutant and genetically engineered mice. Some of these, especially the spontaneous mutants, closely resemble genetically based human diseases, while many others are relatively unique, providing useful tools to dissect mechanisms associated with the normal development and pathology of these organs. This chapter reviews methodology specifically useful for investigating abnormalities of the GI tract and describes selected lesions to provide guidelines on how to approach interpreting changes observed in novel mutant mice.

## PROTOCOL FOR EVALUATION OF THE MOUSE GASTROINTESTINAL TRACT

### Oral Cavity

The oral cavity consists of the buccal and gingival mucosa, tongue, teeth, bones, and associated glands. Each major structure should be examined carefully for abnormalities. The oral cavity in mice is difficult to visualize unless opened. Following appropriate euthanasia, the mucocutaneous/muscular wall forming the cheek can be cut with scissors parallel to the length of the mandible. The temporomandibular joint can be dissected to sepa-

rate the mandible, or it can be cut with heavy scissors at the ramus. Upon completion, the oral cavity can be examined for gross abnormalities such as cleft palate, tooth malformations, tumors, erosions, or other types of lesions. The tongue should be examined carefully on the dorsal and ventral surfaces. Very subtle lesions, such as vesicles (Montagutelli et al. 1997), can occur in this location. The tongue should be collected in toto and trimmed lengthwise. Representative sections of the oral cavity will be evident in three coronal sections of the skull trimmed to include (1) the nasal cavity, (2) the eyes and pituitary gland, and (3) the middle ear. Decalcification of bones is required prior to tissue processing (Relyea et al. 1999). Many fixatives are available and are suitable for these structures (Sundberg et al. 1998a; Relyea et al. 1999).

### TECHNIQUES TO STUDY MUTATIONS AFFECTING THE TEETH

Except for malocclusions resulting from overgrowth of the incisors, changes involving teeth often are not readily apparent. It is possible to study the incisors in live mice to determine if there is a missing tooth and to identify variations in, for example, size, color, and shape. Molars are relatively inaccessible. Under general anesthesia or after euthanization, mice should be radiographed to determine if any skeletal abnormalities are present. Lateral radiographs of intact mouse skulls are very difficult to evaluate because radiographs reveal overlapping rows of teeth, thus obscuring detail

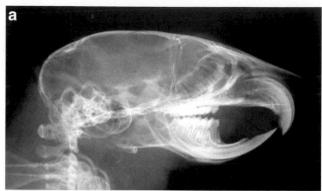

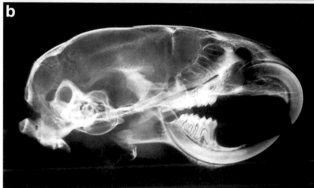

**FIGURE 19.1** Radiographs of intact (**a**) and bisected (**b**) skulls. Notice the increased detail when only one set of teeth and bones is examined in the bisected skull (**b**).

(Fig. 19.1). Radiographs are best done using bisected skulls with skin removed. Using single-edged razor blades, the skull is bisected following a midsagittal plane starting between the incisors. In certain strains of mice (e.g., C3H), this may be difficult to accomplish due to a denser, more calcified bone structure (Beamer et al. 1996; Rosen et al. 1997; Rogers et al. 1997; Dimai et al. 1998; Linkhart et al. 1999). In very young mice the softness of the skeleton may also prove to be a hindrance. In the latter case, bisection is more easily accomplished with a pair of scissors.

Small X-ray machines (Faxitron, Faxitron X-ray Corporation, Buffalo Grove, IL) are well suited for radiographic investigations of mice. If carefully made, the films may be used for morphometric analysis of tooth size and its relationship to other craniofacial structures (Tracey and Roberts 1985). It is possible to follow tooth formation from birth, although the exposure conditions may have to be adjusted to compensate for size and stage of mineralization.

To study isolated teeth, mechanically remove teeth from the alveolar bone, and then digest with papain to remove adherent soft tissue. This allows for careful study of both the crown and roots (Sofaer 1979). Using stereomicroscopes, strain differences in both cuspal patterns and root morphology have been described

(Gruneberg 1965). Recently the crown morphology of mouse molars was also studied by scanning electron microscopy (Lyngstadaas et al. 1998)

For histological investigations of teeth (Figs. 19.2, 19.3) and jaws, the specimens should be sectioned in a buccolingual direction. In very young individuals the entire skull may be embedded and frontal sections produced. For careful study, serial sections are preferred. An additional advantage of serial sections is that three-dimensional reconstructions can be created, which may be of great value, especially during the formative periods of tooth development (Peterkova et al. 1996).

The fixatives chosen for preservation of teeth and jaws are dependent upon the goal of the investigation. If jaws from adult animals are to be studied histologically, a rapidly penetrating fixative, such as acid-alcohol-formalin, should be used (Sundberg et al. 1998a). If the aim is to achieve good preservation of the pulp, it is better to fix via vascular perfusion, using a buffered formalin solution. This is especially important since fully formed molars have only a narrow opening at the root apex, limiting access of the fixative. For electron microscopic investigations of pulp cell populations, a glutaraldehyde-based fixative, like Karnovsky's, should be perfused (Bechtold 1999; Relyea et al. 1999). So that the gingiva is fully preserved and intact, a glutaraldehyde-based fixative should also be used when teeth are to be viewed in situ by scanning electron microscopy. Skull and intact jaws from prenatal mice can be fixed in either Bouin's solution or neutral buffered formalin (Sundberg et al. 1998a). Neonatal mice are also relatively easy to cryosection, a procedure that may be favorable for immunohistochemistry or in situ hybridization studies.

Since the mature tooth is a composite tissue, made up of several differentially mineralized tissues, it will, in most cases, have to be demineralized. Several demineralizing solutions are available, the choice of which is dependent upon the goal of the investigation. For routine histology, a combination of hydrochloric acid and EDTA may be used, but this will probably limit the usefulness of the specimens for immunohistochemical analysis. An alternative, to preserve both antigenicity and nucleic acids, is to use a buffered EDTA solution. This latter approach is also necessary for transmission electron microscopy.

Mature enamel requires special precautions to be taken. Less than 5 percent of organic material is retained in enamel, resulting in complete removal of this structure during demineralization (Sasaki et al. 1990); therefore, enamel is usually studied in ground sections. Specialized equipment is available, making the production of 10 μm thick sections possible (Donath and Breuner 1982; Exakt Technologies, Inc., Oklahoma City, OK). These sections may be viewed by ordinary bright-field

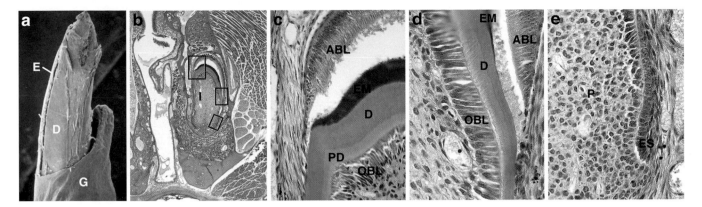

**FIGURE 19.2** (**a**) Eruption of an incisor in a 14-day-old C57BL/6J normal mouse. **c–e** represent higher magnification of boxed areas in **b** (counterclockwise). Ameloblast layer (*ABL*), dentin (*D*), epithelial sheath (*ES*), enamel (*E*), gingiva (*G*), odontoblast layers (*OBL*), predentin (*PD*), and pulp (*P*).

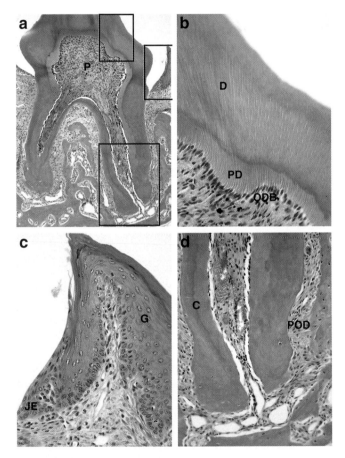

**FIGURE 19.3** Low magnification of a molar (**a**) illustrates the shape of the tooth and the pulp (*P*). Boxed areas magnified exhibit, in (**b**), the dentin (*D*), predentin (*PD*), and odontoblasts (*ODB*); in (**c**), the junctional epithelium (*JE*) and gingiva (*G*) of the adjacent mucosa; and, in (**d**), the cementum (*C*) and periodontium (*POD*).

microscopy, but more information may be gained when viewed under polarized light. Furthermore, ground sections of undecalcified teeth may be examined using microradiography. This approach makes it possible to estimate the mineral density in the different tooth compartments. More detailed information can be obtained by doing densitometry on the microradiographs. Mineral content of teeth may also be determined using scanning electron microscopy and energy dispersive X-ray analyses (Moinichen et al. 1996).

## Esophagus and Stomach

Following euthanasia, the skin is excised on the ventral surface of the mandible. The mandibular symphysis can be cut if the oral cavity has not been opened in another manner for other studies. Gentle retraction of the tongue permits easy and rapid dissection of the trachea and esophagus to the thoracic inlet. Removal of the ribs permits continuation of the dissection to the diaphragm. The esophagus can be cut here, laid out on the dissection board, and examined. A variety of procedures can be done at this point depending upon the project goals. For initial evaluation, the esophagus should be opened lengthwise to look for small tumors and ulcers, among other things. For detailed studies, the esophagus can be dissected lengthwise with half being fixed for histopathology and the remainder frozen for molecular studies. If lesions are known to occur at specific regions, transverse sections can be cut and used alternately for histopathology or molecular/immunohistochemical studies. Lastly, the esophagus can be inflated with fixative and coiled in a "Swiss roll" or left straight on an unlined index card (Relyea et al. 1999).

Several different protocols can be used to collect the stomach to suit the needs of the investigation. Most methods inflate the stomach with fixative. The stomach can then be immersed in fixative overnight to harden and then cut lengthwise with a sharp, single-edged razor blade (Sundberg et al. 1992; Mähler et al. 1998). An alternative method inflates the stomach with 10 percent neutral buffered formalin at the time of necropsy. After 5 minutes, the stomach is opened, laid flat on the dissection board, stapled between two pieces of filter paper, and returned to the fixative for several days. The stomach is trimmed into the sections shown in Figure 19.4 and placed into cassettes (Tamano et al. 1995).

## Intestines and Cecum

The intestine is first examined from the serosal surface to check for lesions, especially enlargement of Peyer's patches (an early site of lymphoma), and any irregularities or masses within the lumen. Opening of the entire length of the small and large intestine is desirable to search for tumors, especially small polyps, adenomas, and early invasive carcinomas. Individual tumors can be identified, counted, and placed in separate vials for fixation and embedding. Representative sections of selected portions of the intestine can also be sampled.

Inflammatory lesions of the intestines can be very segmental in nature, and if semiquantitative grading is used for quantitative trait locus analysis, it is important

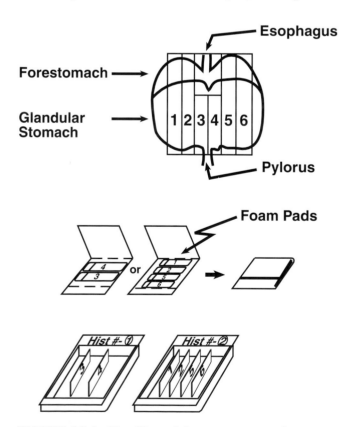

**FIGURE 19.4** Handling of the mouse stomach at necropsy, its trimming and placing into cassettes for embedding in paraffin.

to examine the entire length of the intestine that is affected. Some approaches focus on specific regions. The specimen can be taken as a cross section of the bowel at a defined distance from an anatomic structure, such as a number of centimeters proximal to the anus. We have found that intestinal "Swiss" rolls provide continuous segments of bowel suitable for reproducible grading (Moolenbeek and Ruitenberg 1981; Mähler et al. 1999). These are prepared by removing the intestines intact and dividing them into units that, when coiled, will fit into a histology cassette. These units may be duodenum and jejunum, jejunum and ileum, cecum, and colon. Each intestinal segment is gently expressed to remove feces, and the fixative of choice is injected into the lumen by needle and syringe to maximize luminal integrity. The segment is then rolled around a wooden stick, placed on an unlined index-type card, and fixed by immersion (Sundberg et al. 1994).

# GI LESIONS IN GENETICALLY ENGINEERED MICE

## Oral Cavity

### ORAL MUCOSA

As mentioned above, tumors, ulcers, structural abnormalities such as cleft palate, and other obvious abnormalities can be identified occasionally in all inbred colonies of laboratory mice (Mohr et al. 1996). Consistent findings associated with specific mutations, regardless of the cause of the mutation, need to be investigated carefully.

Lesions of the mucous membranes are being identified in mutant mice. One group of very important mutations is due to different mutations within the desmoglein-3 gene, an important adhesion molecule found in stratified squamous epithelium. Mice affected by these mutations have blister formation affecting the ventral tongue as well as the foot pads, mucocutaneous junction of the eyelids, and separation of the root sheaths of hair follicles. These lesions are morphologically identical to pemphigus vulgaris in humans and other mammals. These are illustrated in Chapter 14. It is interesting to note that the first three mutations occurred spontaneously in different inbred mouse colonies (Davisson, et al. 1994; Sundberg 1994; Montagutelli et al. 1997; Sundberg et al. 1998b). Although the mutated gene was identified as a candidate by traditional gene-mapping approaches (Montagutelli et al. 1997), creation of the targeted mutation of desmoglein-3 defined the gene (Koch et al. 1997).

Keratins 4 and 13 are coexpressed in internal stratified epithelia and form heterodimers. Mutations in either keratin 4 or 13 are known to cause White Sponge Nevus in humans (Richard et al. 1995; Rigg et al. 1995). Recently a targeted mutation of mouse keratin 4 was reported (Ness et al. 1998). Null mutants have lesions on the tongue, esophagus, and cornea characterized histologically by hyperplasia, lack of maturation, hyperkeratosis, nuclear atypia, perinuclear clearing, and cellular degeneration. In contrast to humans, no changes were found in the buccal mucosa of mice.

## TEETH

Tooth eruption is a complex process, starting before complete formation of both crowns and roots (Figs. 19.2, 19.3). Two simultaneous processes are coordinated: resorption and remodeling of surrounding bone. During penetration of the oral mucosa, an epithelial lining must be formed, a process mediated by a fusion of the reduced enamel and oral epithelia. It is known that several regulatory molecules are expressed in the developing tooth: parathyroid hormone–like peptide (Pthlh) (Philbrick et al. 1998), colony-stimulating factor-1 (Csf1) (Grier et al. 1998), and monocyte chemoattractant protein (Que and Wise 1998). During fusion of the oral mucosa and reduced enamel epithelia, the cell adhesion molecule C-CAM is specifically expressed in this location (Luning et al. 1995).

Several spontaneous and targeted mutations leading to failure of eruption of teeth have been described (Table 19.1). A common feature in most of these mutant mice is osteopetrosis. In several mutants this leads to both disturbances in tooth formation as well as to delayed eruption. In the gray-lethal mouse (gl), all teeth are retained (Gruneberg 1935), while in the microoph-

thalmic mutation (mi), eruption of molars is delayed. The mutations in Mitf are known to be caused by mutation in a basic-helix-loop-helix-zipper protein (Hodgkison et al. 1993). The osteopetrotic Csfm mutant develops osteopetrosis due to a null mutation in Csf1 (Yoshida, et al. 1990).

By in situ hybridization, expression of Pthlh has been demonstrated in the enamel epithelium. Its receptor, the type I PTH/PTHrP receptor, is expressed both in the dental follicle and adjacent alveolar bone (Philbrick et al. 1998). Null mutants at the Pthlh locus develop a chondodystrophic phenotype and die at birth. This phenotype can be partially rescued by expressing the Pthlh gene in chondrocytes. The rescued phenotype has a life span of about 6 months and is characterized by small stature, cranial chondrodystrophy, and failure of tooth eruption. Expression of Pthlh in the enamel epithelium permits a normal eruption of teeth. This points to a unique role of Pthlh in tooth eruption (Philbrick et al. 1998).

**Mice with Spontaneous Mutations Affecting Teeth.** A search of the Mouse Locus Catalog [*http://www. informatics.jax.org*] yielded relatively few spontaneous mutations with phenotypes known to affect teeth. In 1965 Gruneberg presented an extensive survey of first molar crown and root morphology in a number of inbred mouse strains. Clear differences were noted. In addition to the interstrain variability, a number of spontaneous mouse mutants with phenotypes involving the teeth have been described. The different mutations are listed in Table 19.2.

The tabby mutant mouse is one of the best known spontaneous mutations. It belongs to a group of mutant mice with very similar phenotypes that are homologous to the human anhidrotic ectodermal dysplasias:

**TABLE 19.1. Mouse mutations with delayed or failed tooth eruption**

| Gene symbol | Chr. | Name | Reference |
|---|---|---|---|
| Csfm (op) | 3 | Colony-stimulating factor, macrophage (formerly osteopetrosis) | Marks and Lane 1976 |
| Fos | 12 | FBJ osteosarcoma oncogene | Johnson et al. 1992 |
| gl | 10 | Gray-lethal | Gruneberg 1935 |
| Mitf | 6 | Microophthalmia-associated transcription factor | Hertwig 1942 |
| oc | 19 | Osteosclerotic | Dickie 1967 |
| Pthlh | 6 | Parathyroid hormone–like peptide | Philbrick et al. 1998 |
| Src | 2 | Rous sarcoma oncogene | Soriano et al. 1991 |
| Tnfsf11 | 14 | Tumor necrosis factor (ligand) superfamily, member 11 | Kong et al. 1999 |

Note: Chr. = mouse chromosome number.

**TABLE 19.2. Spontaneous mouse mutations with abnormalities of the teeth**

| Gene symbol | Chr. | Name |
|---|---|---|
| Cd | 6 | Crooked(-tail) |
| cr | 13 | Crinkled |
| di | Unmapped | Duplicate incisors |
| din | 16 | Dense incisors |
| dl, dl$^{sl}$ | 10 | Downless, sleek |
| Iac | Unmapped | Iris anomaly with cataract |
| It | X | Irregular teeth |
| jb | 7 | Juvenile bare |
| Phex$^{Gy}$ | X | Gyro |
| Phex$^{Hyp}$ | X | Hypophosphatemia |
| Lep$^{ob}$ | 6 | Obese |
| Ta | X | Tabby |
| tl | Unmapped | Nonerupted teeth (extinct) |

Note: Chr. = mouse chromosome number.

tabby (*Ta*), crinkled (*cr*), downless (*dl*), and sleek (*dl^Sl*). Tabby is the prototypical mutant for the X-linked anhidrotic ectodermal dysplasia in mice and is also a model for the human condition in which mutations occur in the same gene in both species, ectodysplastin (*Eda*) (Srivastava et al. 1997; Montonen et al. 1998). In mice, the *Eda* gene is expressed in the oral and outer enamel epithelium at cap stage (Srivastava et al. 1997). Downless and sleek are allelic mutations. Both map to the same autosome, the former is recessive, while the latter is dominant. These mice all exhibit the same general phenotype, at least for teeth, although the extent of lesions varies (Sofaer 1977b). Sofaer (1969a, 1969b) described the development of Tabby teeth. In both homo- and hemizygotes, the incisors are either reduced or absent. The first or second molars are reduced in size, while the third molars may be totally missing. In rare instances, fourth molars are detected, a phenomenon that Gruneberg termed "twinning." It is probable that the reduction in size is due to reduced growth rate and delayed histodifferentiation. Crosses between tabby and crinkled mice augment the changes, although these mutations involve different genes on different chromosomes (Sofaer 1979). Since the function of the ectodysplastin gene is not known, further speculation will have to await more experiments to elucidate the role of this gene in development. The gene responsible for the downless and sleek allelic mutations has not been identified, but recently a yeast artificial chromosome (YAC) was found to rescue both phenotypes in mice when made transgenic (Majumder et al. 1998).

The mutation crooked (*Cd*) produces anomalies in the axial skeleton, microophthalmia, and small molars where the cusp pattern is simplified (Sofaer 1977a). During tooth development, the dental lamina will proliferate, which has been interpreted as competing with the adjacent tooth, thereby effectively reducing its size. The skeletal abnormalities of crooked mice have been attributed to defective somite formation, suggesting a defect in mesenchymal differentiation. No gene responsible for this mutation has been identified.

Dense incisors (*di*) is a new recessive locus on mouse Chromosome 16 (Sweet et al. 1996). The mutation is characterized by a defect in incisor eruption after the initial eruptive phase, reduced body size, reduction of pinnae, and coat color dilution. Incisors of older mice exhibit an enlarged dentin layer with reduction in size of the pulp chamber. Molars are unaffected. No changes were found in the skeleton excluding osteopetrosis as the cause.

Juvenile bare (*jb*) was recently described as a new mutation with effects on skin and incisors (Lane et al. 1998). In affected mice, hair follicles follow irregular pathways and become dystrophic by the time mice are 23 days of age. This is concomitant with almost complete hair loss starting anterior to the dorsal skin (tail head) region. Mice older than 1 month of age have a normal hair coat, albeit thinner compared with controls. Breeding, but not virgin, females may exhibit overgrowth and breakage of the incisors. The skin condition is thought to be due to a systemic response, since full thickness skin transplants do not become affected. The tooth changes have not been characterized.

The hypophosphatemia mutations (phosphate-regulating neutral endopeptidase gene; hypophosphatemia, *Phex^Hyp,* and gyro, *Phex^Gy*) are allelic mutations in the *Pex* gene, located on mouse Chromosome X, leading to the development of hypophosphatemic rickets (Beck et al. 1997). *Phex* thereby provides mouse models for human X-linked hypophosphatemias (Strom et al. 1997; HYP Consortium 1995). The function of the PEX protein is still not understood (Turner and Tanzawa 1997). The dental changes in these mutant mice involve dentin, with a widened pulp chamber due to a thin dentin wall, a broad predentin zone, and the formation of interglobular dentin (Abe et al. 1989). *Pex* mRNA has been demonstrated in both odonto- and osteoblasts (Fig. 19.5; Ruchon et al. 1998).

A very common background lesion found around teeth in mice is foreign body periodontitis. Mice groom themselves and each other constantly and often get hair fibers embedded between the teeth and gingiva (Fig. 19.6). This begins as a focal ulceration but often leads to a foreign body granuloma or extends to a more serious osteomyelitis. The frequency and severity of this lesion may change with some of the spontaneous or induced mutant mice, but it also occurs very commonly in most normal background strains used, so care must be taken in the interpretation of this lesion.

**Targeted Mutations Affecting Tooth Development.** To date there are probably more publications on targeted mutations in genes involved in tooth development compared with what has been published about induced or spontaneous phenotypes. During the last decade an intense effort has been focused on elucidating the mechanism involved in the epithelial mesenchymal interactions involved in the differentiation pathways that will eventually form fully functional amelo- and odontoblasts capable of making the tooth proper. Several of these pathways have been worked out in detail.

Initiation of tooth formation is mediated by a series of reciprocal interactions between the dental epithelium and the dental mesenchyme, the latter derived from cranial neural crest cells. Before embryonic day (E) 11.5 no morphological changes are evident, but recombination experiments show the dental epithelium carries information for tooth formation since nondental mesenchyme

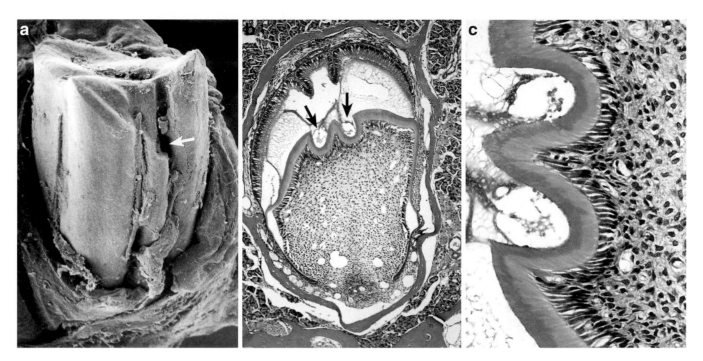

**FIGURE 19.5**   The mutation hypophosphatemia (B6C3H-*Phex^Hyp*) causes hypophosphatemic rickets (Strom et al. 1997). Teeth have parallel grooves (*arrows*) in the incisors, as seen by scanning electron microscopy (**a**) and histology (**b, c**).

will be reprogrammed. After E11.5 this ability switches to the dental mesenchyme. Experiments during the last 10 years have elucidated some of the mechanisms involved in initiation. A recent review by Peters and Balling (1999) summarized available data. The dental epithelium expresses several diffusible factors that influence gene expression in the mesenchymal cells. Sonic hedgehog (*Shh*) will induce patched (*Ptch*) and GLI-Kruppel family member GLI (*Gli1*). Bone morphogenetic protein 4 (*Bmp4*) up-regulates expression of *Msx1* while depressing *Pax9*. Mesenchymal expression of bone morphogenetic protein 2 (*Bmp2*) acts synergistically with *Bmp4* and fibroblast growth factor 8 (*Fgf8*) to induce *Msx1*, while also repressing *Pax9*. Data also indicate that *Bmp4* signaling is repressed in *Pax9*-deficient mice. Lymphoid enhancer–binding factor 1 (*Lef1*) is also a downstream target of *Bmp4*. Thus, *Lef1* may integrate the different signaling pathways involved in the initiation of odontogenesis. Furthermore, several homeobox genes are involved in these early events.

Fibroblast growth factor receptor 2b-HFc, a novel secreted kinase-deficient receptor, specific for a defined subset of the FGF superfamily, caused agenesis of teeth and severe dysgenesis of kidney, lung, specific cutaneous structures, exocrine and endocrine glands, and craniofacial and limb abnormalities (Celli et al. 1998). Studies revealed that this dominant-negative mutant disrupted early inductive signaling in affected tissues.

1. *Targeted mutations of homeobox-containing genes.* Tooth development is known to be governed by reciprocal epithelial-mesenchymal interactions (Thesleff and Sharpe 1997; Peters et al. 1998). Recombination studies done decades ago demonstrated that before embryonic day 11.5 (E11.5), oral epithelium could direct nonoral mesenchyme to initiate tooth formation. At later stages this potential switched to the mesenchyme. Thus, it was clear that diffusible factors must be present that directed these formative events. Several signaling pathways are presently at the verge of being fully understood (Peters et al. 1998). In addition, several classes of homeobox-containing proteins have been studied and found to affect early stages of odontogenesis. Null mutants in several of these developmentally regulated genes are tabulated in Table 19.3.

Several members of the homeobox class distal-less are expressed during tooth formation (i.e., *Dlx1, 2, 3,* and *5*) (Robinson and Mahon 1994; Weiss et al. 1995; Davideau et al. 1999). In humans, mutations in *Dlx3* have been shown to be responsible for the tricho-dento-osseous syndrome featuring both taurodontism and enamel hypoplasia (Price et al. 1998). A targeted mutation of *Dlx3* in mice results in early embryonic lethality due to a defect in placentation (Morasso et al. 1999). In contrast, mice with combined null mutations in both *Dlx1*

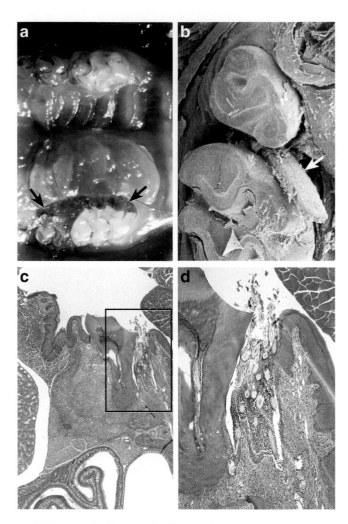

**FIGURE 19.6** Foreign body (hair) periodontitis is a common finding in all mouse strains including this 4.5-month-old female C57BL/6J *Cybb*^tm1^ mutant mouse. Ulcers (**a,** *arrows*) are often associated with the foreign body (**b,** *arrow*), which can be better seen by scanning electron microscopy (**b**) or histology (**c, d**).

and *Dlx2* show severe disturbances in odontogenesis, resulting in a complete lack of maxillary molars, while the incisors and mandibular molars are normally developed (Thomas et al. 1997). The mutant results in a block at the earliest detectable event in odontogenesis, a thickening of the oral epithelium (Kaufman and Bard 1999). The adjacent mesenchyme fails to condense and instead develops into cartilage. The epithelium has been shown to express relevant signaling proteins, but the mesenchyme is not programmed to respond (Thomas et al. 1997). These findings and others indicate that a unique homeobox code may exist that specifies patterning of teeth (Sharpe 1995; Thesleff and Sharpe 1997). Additional evidence for this hypothesis has come

**TABLE 19.3. Induced mutations of genes involved in tooth development**

| | Consequence |
|---|---|
| **Targeted mutations** | |
| Activin βA | Maxillary space molars are normal in homozygotes; development of incisors and mandibular molars blocked at bud stage. |
| *Dlx1/Dlx2* | No maxillary molars. Failure in mesenchyme programming leads to formation of ectopic cartilage. Epithelial thickening with normal signaling events but failure to reach bud stage. |
| Follistatin | Abnormal lower incisors as well as delayed eruption of incisors. |
| *Gli2* | In heterozygotes, the upper incisors are fused. Homozygotes lack all teeth, intermediate phenotype in *Gli2* –/– *Gli3* +/– double mutants. |
| *Lef1* | Homozygous mutants lack all teeth with arrest at bud stage; failure in dental papilla formation. |
| *Msx1* | All teeth are absent. Humans with missense mutations show oligodontia. |
| *p53* | Fused maxillary incisors combined with exencephaly. |
| *p63* | Organs dependent upon epithelial mesenchymal interactions absent. Teeth, hair follicles, and mammary glands absent, truncated or absent limbs, skin at an early developmental stage without stratification. |
| *Pax9* | Homozygotes lack all teeth; tooth formation is arrested in early bud stage. |
| **Transgenic mice** | |
| Fibroblast growth factor receptor 2b-Hfc (dominant-negative mutant) | No embryonic tooth development. |
| Urokinase-type plasminogen receptor in enamel organ | Fragile incisors, with chalky appearance and a granular surface; disorganized ameloblast layer. |

from studies on *Barx1*, a homeodomain transcription factor, only expressed in mouse molar mesenchyme (Tissier-Seta et al. 1995; Tucker et al. 1998). Furthermore, ectopic expression of *Barx1* will induce incisor tooth germs to develop into molars (Tucker et al. 1998).

The Msx class of homeobox proteins are thought to influence inductive events during organogenesis. Homozygous null mutants in the *Msx1* gene lack all teeth (Chen et al. 1996). Odontogenesis is blocked at bud stage, at the beginning of dental lamina formation. Abortive odontogenesis is a feature of the mouse maxillary diastema, where the dental lamina undergoes apoptosis. Recently *Msx1* was shown to be necessary for the induction of patched by *Shh* during early tooth development (Zhang et al. 1999). Missense mutations in *Msx1* in humans are known to cause oligodontia (Vastardis et al. 1996).

2. *Targeted mutations of genes in the signaling pathways.* Several signaling pathways are known to integrate the epithelial-mesenchymal interactions that regulate odontogenesis (Thesleff and Sharpe 1997; Peters and Balling 1999). *Lef1*-null mutants lack several organs that depend upon epithelial mesenchymal interactions during their formation (i.e., teeth, vibrissae, hair, and mammary glands) (van Genderen et al. 1994). Tooth development is arrested at the bud stage. Expression of bone morphogenetic protein 4 (*Bmp4*) in the dental mesenchyme is a key regulator of *Lef1* expression, as has also been demonstrated in hair follicle development (Kratochwil et al. 1996). *Lef1* is also a strong candidate for being an integrative part of several signaling pathways (Peters and Balling 1999).

**Neoplastic Diseases of the Teeth.** The process of odontogenesis involves a complex orchestration of signaling and induction events between epithelial and mesenchymal cells, undoubtedly requiring the interactions of numerous genes as described above. Given this complexity, disorders of the tooth, including neoplasms, are surprisingly rare in normal mice but, not unexpectedly, may be common findings in genetically altered mice. An illustrative example is the striking array and frequency of proliferative odontogenic lesions observed in lines of dual transgenic mice expressing both *ras* and *myc* oncogenes (Gibson et al. 1992). Tumors appear in mice as early as 4 weeks of age and with frequencies up to 100 percent. Three morphological types are described with various mixtures of epithelial and mesenchymal cells and hard tissue (matrix) components.

Another *ras*-expressing transgenic mouse line (Tg.AC) develops a similar spectrum of odontogenic tumor types. These occur with reported frequencies ranging from approximately 15 percent in heterozygotes (Mahler et al. 1998) to 36 percent in homozygotes (Wright et al. 1995). The lesser frequency in this line compared with the *ras/myc* bitransgenic line suggests cooperation between these two genes in the development of odontogenic neoplasms. Odontogenic tumors in Tg.AC mice

may appear as early as 10 weeks of age and are grossly evident as firm masses of the mandible or, less commonly, the maxilla. Three basic microscopic phenotypes correspond to those previously described in transgenic mice (Gibson et al. 1992). One type appears to arise from the periodontal ligament and is composed of mesenchymal-type cells embedded in a dense eosinophilic matrix (Fig. 19.7a, b). Another tumor phenotype resembling true odontomas forms abortive tooth structures with enamel, dentin, and well-differentiated ameloblasts and odontoblasts (Fig. 19.7c). A third type consists of anastomosing cords of squamous epithelial cells interspersed by loose stroma (Fig. 19.7d) with occasional palisading of basal cell nuclei suggestive of ameloblastoma. Mixed tumors composed of more than one histologic type may be seen.

## Esophagus

Esophageal dilatation (megaesophagus) has been reported in some lines of mice (Randelia and Lalithia 1988). We recently identified a syndrome in transforming growth factor α transgenic mice on a CD-1 background (line MT42, Jhappan et al. 1990) characterized by runting from 15–50 weeks of age. Most cases occurred by 20 weeks of age. By 50 weeks of age 11/20 (55 percent) transgenic males and 8/23 (35 percent) transgenic females developed the condition, compared with 0/20 male CD-1 and 0/21 female CD-1 mice. The major cause of the progressive illness and death in the transgenic MT42 mice up to 50 weeks of age was runting (progressive severe body weight loss) due to natural starvation and/or dehydration from esophageal, and possibly gastric, constriction. In the mice, esophageal distension occurred ≤ 10 mm above the stomach junction (Fig. 19.8). Grossly, the constricted portion was pale due to the tight lumenal folding. Histologically, marked hyperkeratosis and epithelial hyperplasia occurred (Fig. 19.9). The epithelia of the forestomach was often hyperplastic, and there was frequent localized papillomatous to sessile lesions (Fig. 19.10). In a few severe cases, the entire stomach is grossly thickened with a very small lumen. The cause of this syndrome has not been determined. Expression of the transgene in the squamous epithelium of the esophagus and forestomach apparently causes epithelial hyperplasia and hyperkeratosis leading to the lesions, in part. Abnormalities in innervation of the esophageal nerves may also occur. Gastric forestomach hyperplasia may involve the esophagus in a number of spontaneous mutant mice, some of which have scaly skin disease as another phenotype. The most notable of these is chronic proliferative dermatitis (*cpdm*) (Gijbels et al. 1996). Others are described below under Stomach.

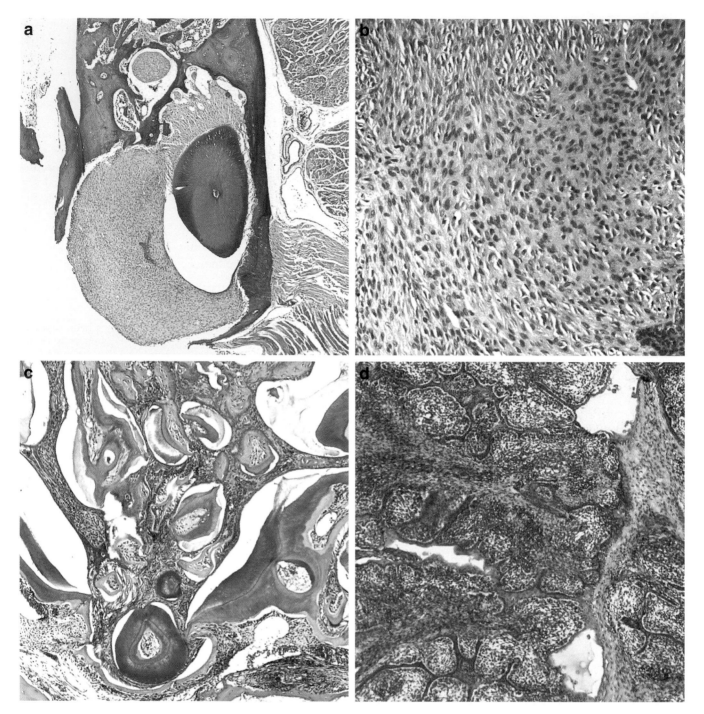

**FIGURE 19.7** (**a**) Odontogenic tumor arising around a mandibular incisor in a Tg.AC mouse. (**b**) Higher magnification of the tumor in **a** showing mesenchymal-type cells embedded in a dense matrix. (**c**) Odontogenic tumor in a Tg.AC mouse composed of multiple abortive tooth structures. (**d**) Odontogenic tumor in a Tg.AC mouse composed of anastomosing cords of epithelial cells with occasional cyst formation and intervening loose stromal cells.

## Stomach

The murine stomach is composed of two regions, the squamous forestomach into which the esophagus empties and the glandular stomach that itself empties into the duodenum. The glandular stomach is a specialized organ composed of two regions (body and antrum) with several differentiated epithelial cell types that synthesize products (enzymes, acids) important for digestion. The epithelial differentiation pattern follows a specific well-defined mode (Matsukura et al. 1985; Ghoshal and Bal 1989; Karam et al. 1997).

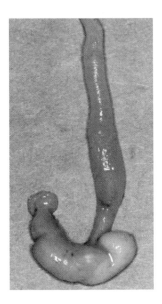

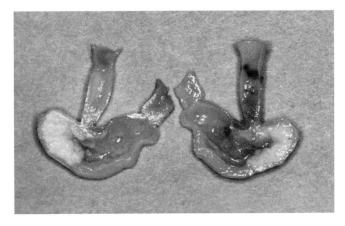

**FIGURE 19.10**  Gross appearance of sectioned forestomach and esophagus showing grossly thickened squamous epithelium.

**FIGURE 19.8**  Gross appearance of dilated esophagus above gastric junction.

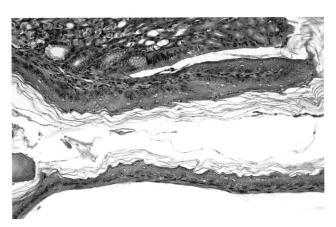

**FIGURE 19.9**  Histologically, the squamous epithelium at the esophagus-forestomach junction is hyperplastic with hyperkeratosis.

Proliferative changes of the stratified squamous epithelium are found associated with a number of spontaneous mouse mutations that also have proliferative changes in the skin including flaky skin (*fsn*) (Sundberg et al. 1992, 1997) and chronic proliferative dermatitis (*cpdm*) (Gijbels et al. 1996). Others appear to be clinically normal but have proliferative, ulcerative, or both types of lesions of the forestomach. These include steel-Dickie (*Mgf^{Sl}/Mgf^{Sl-d}*) (Sundberg et al. 1992; Mähler et al. 1998), some of the white-spotting mutants (*W/W^v*) (Kitamura et al. 1980), and viable motheaten (*me^v/me^v*) (Shultz and Sundberg 1994).

A variety of growth factors and oncogenes have been expressed as transgenes in the gastric mucosa with consequent effects (Table 19.4). Typically, overexpression of these transgenes induces hyperplasia of the glandular

stomach and/or nonglandular compartment (forestomach) and, depending on the promoter used, occasionally stimulates the formation of tumors. In some instances, however, the transgene acts in a dominant fashion to disrupt the normal pattern of differentiation of the glandular epithelium. A few homozygous (–/–) or heterozygous (+/–) lines of "knockout" mice have also developed gastric lesions. Some examples are given in Table 19.4 and in the following paragraphs.

Transforming growth factor α (*Tgfα*) elicits a wide variety of biological activities, including cellular proliferation, differentiation, and survival by binding to and activating the epidermal growth factor (*Egf*) receptor (reviewed by Salomon et al. 1990). In the stomach, Tgfα and Egf inhibit gastric acid secretion and stimulate mucosal growth and mucin production (see references in Sharp et al. 1995). Tgfα is elevated in the gastric mucosa of patients with Ménétrier's disease (Coffey et al. 1992), a human syndrome characterized by diffuse thickening of the gastric wall due to extensive foveolar hyperplasia, cystic dilatation of gastric glands, and predisposition to gastric carcinoma (Scharschmidt 1977). Transgenic mice overexpressing *Tgfα* in the gastric mucosa develop gastric lesions that grossly (Figs. 19.11-19.13) and microscopically resemble those seen in Ménétrier's patients (Takagi et al. 1992; Dempsey et al. 1992).

In one *Tgfα* transgenic line on an FVB/N genetic background (line MT100)(FVB/N-TgN(MtTGFA) 100Lmb), mice develop severe adenomatous hyperplasia (Fig. 19.12), resulting in nodular thickening or hypertrophy of the gastric mucosa that is overtly analogous to the prominent giant rugal folds characteristic of Ménétrier's disease (Takagi et al. 1992). The dramatic enlargement of the gastric mucosa resulted in a three- to six-fold increase in stomach mass and severely constricted the lumen, which contained viscous, mucus-laden

**TABLE 19.4.   Examples of targeted mutagenesis (Tm) and transgenic (Tg) mutant mice with gastric lesions**

|  | Nonneoplastic lesions | Neoplastic lesions | Reference |
|---|---|---|---|
| **Tm (genotype)** |  |  |  |
| GF1 (+/–) | Glandular stomach pyloric hyperplasia, polyps |  | Boivin et al. 1996 |
| CYP1A2 (–/–) | Glandular stomach fundic gastric plaques |  | Kimura et al. 1999; Ennulat et al. 1998 |
| α-Inhibin (–/–) | Altered differentiation |  | Li et al. 1998 |
| **Tg (promoter)** |  |  |  |
| TGF (MT) | Glandular stomach hyperplasias/Dysplasias |  | Sharp et al. 1995; Bockman et al. 1995; Takagi et al. 1992; Goldenring et al. 1996; Tamano et al. 1995; Dempsey et al. 1992 |
| IGF-1 (-smooth muscle actin) | Smooth muscle hyperplasia |  | Lund 1998; Wang et al. 1997 |
| IGFBP-4 (-smooth muscle actin) | Smooth muscle hypoplasia |  | Wang et al.1998 |
| SV40Tag(ATPase β) | Parietal cell loss, altered differentiation |  | Karam et al. 1997; Li et al. 1995 |
| SV40Tag (amylase) | Hyperplasia | Carcinoma, metastatic | Ceci et al. 1991 |
| Cyclin D1(Epstein-Barr virus) | Forestomach dysplasia |  | Nakagawa et al. 1997 |
| Papillomavirus 16 early region (keratin 6) | Hyperplasia, dysplasia | Carcinoid, metastatic | Searle et al. 1994 |
| Adenovirus 12 E1A/E1B (MMTV-LTR) |  | Carcinoma | Ullrich et al. 1994 |
| Adenovirus 12 (MMTV-LTR) | Hyperplasia | Adenocarcinoma | Koike et al. 1989 |
| Myxoma growth factor (MT) | Hyperplasia |  | Strayer et al. 1993 |
| Shope growth factor(RSV-LTR) | Epithelial atypia | Papillary tumors | Strayer et al. 1993 |

Note: ATPase , adenosinetriphosphatase β-subunit; *IGF-I,* insulinlike growth factor I; *IGFBP-4,* insulinlike growth factor–binding protein-4; LTR, long terminal repeat; MT, metallothionein; MMTV, mouse mammary tumor virus; RSV, Rous sarcoma virus; SV40, Simian virus 40; Tag, SV40 T antigen; *TGF,* transforming growth factor; +/–, heterozygous mutant; –/–, homozygous mutant.

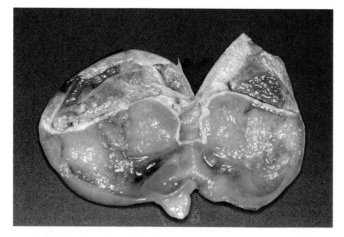

**FIGURE 19.11**   Gross diffuse epithelial thickening in the glandular stomach of FVB/N-TgN(MtTGFA)100Lmb mouse. Note thickest zones near the forestomach junction.

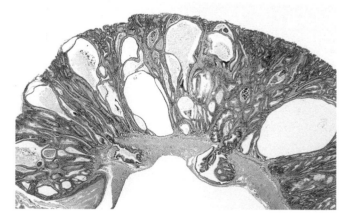

**FIGURE 19.12**   Diffuse hyperplasia and focal cystic hyperplasia in stomach of FVB/N-TgN(MtTGFA)100Lmb mouse. Note cystic epithelial structures within tunica muscularis encroaching on the serosa (herniation).

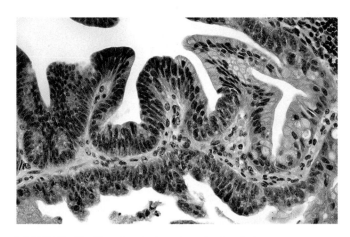

**FIGURE 19.13** Cystic herniated glandular structure within tunica muscularis of FVB/N-TgN(MtTGFA)100Lmb mouse. Note dysplastic hyperchromatic epithelium.

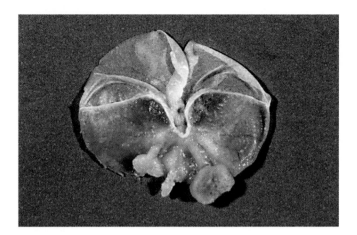

**FIGURE 19.14** Pyloric polyps in mouse glandular stomach.

secretions. Histologic analysis revealed that this was due to an expansion of the mucin-secreting, periodic acid-Schiff (PAS) -positive, columnar epithelia. This hyperplastic change is accompanied by a gradual deterioration of the glandular base. Mature parietal and chief cells were specifically depleted from the glandular mucosa, as judged by an obvious decrease in expression of specific markers (Sharp et al. 1995). The loss of parietal cells compromises gastric acid secretion in the MT100 stomach and compromises the ability to respond to gastrin. *Tgfα* overexpression disrupts the normal program of gastric cell differentiation in the gastric mucosa and may play an important role in the normal regulation of epithelial cell renewal (Sharp et al. 1995; Bockman et al. 1995; Goldenring et al. 1996). Moreover, this pathologic condition enhances the susceptibility of the MT100 mice to the insult of chemicals such as N-nitrosomethylurea, which induces gastric carcinogenesis (Tamano et al. 1995). The MT100 mouse also demonstrates other phenotypes, including a lesion resembling chronic pancreatitis (Jhappan et al. 1990; Bockman and Merlino 1992).

## PYLORIC POLYPS IN *Tgfβ1* (+/–) AND *Ahr* (–/–) MICE

Proliferative lesions have been found in the glandular stomach of transforming growth factor β-1 heterozygous (+/–) mice on a 129 × CF1 background (Boivin et al. 1996). The incidence was 10/15 (67 percent) in aging mutant and 0/8 in wild-type mice. Mutant mice had lesions in the lesser curvature from the limiting ridge to the pylorus. The sex of the mice was not noted. Cystic and diverticular lesions were seen. Similar pyloric lesions were found in high frequency (10/14, 71 percent) by 13 months of age in *Ahr*-null mice on a B6,129

(B6,129/Sv-*Ahr*<sup>tm1Gonz</sup>) background, but none were found in 42 *Ahr* controls (+/– or +/+) (Fernandez-Salguero et al. 1997). Pyloric lesions were often associated with inflammatory lesions but not *Helicobacter* spp. The largest pyloric lesions were large polyps that appeared to be inflammatory in origin. Dilated glands within submucosa (mucosal herniations/diverticula) were observed in both *Ahr*-null and *Tgfβ1* heterozygous mice (Fig. 19.14–19.16). When serial sections were prepared, one could see the connection of diverticula to the surface epithelium, a connection that is not seen in carcinomas. These lesions resembled ones that were not transplantable and described in some old strains of mice not used today (Kaplan 1949). Recently, it was reported that developmental abnormalities in midgestation of *Cdx2* –/– mice lead to colonic hamartomas that resemble the unusual proliferative lesions of these targeted mutants (Tamai et al. 1999). It is possible that unusual proliferative lesions in both *Ahr*-null and *Tgfα1* heterozygous mice may arise from developmental defects.

## OTHER GLANDULAR STOMACH PROLIFERATIVE LESIONS

Dysplastic changes of the glandular stomach are progressive in the spontaneous mutation known as flaky skin (*fsn*). Other proliferative lesions in *fsn* mice affect the skin and forestomach. Mice do not live long enough to determine whether or not the glandular stomach changes progress to metastatic disease (Sundberg et al. 1997).

Spontaneous plaquelike lesions in the fundus of the glandular stomach (Figs. 19.17–19.20) were found in C57BL/NCr × 129/SvTer (B6,129) and 129/SvTer mice (5–20 percent in aging wild-type mice). The *CYP1A2*-null mice on that segregating background have very high frequency of this lesion (70–90 percent) by 20 months of age (Ennulat et al. 1998; Kimura et al.

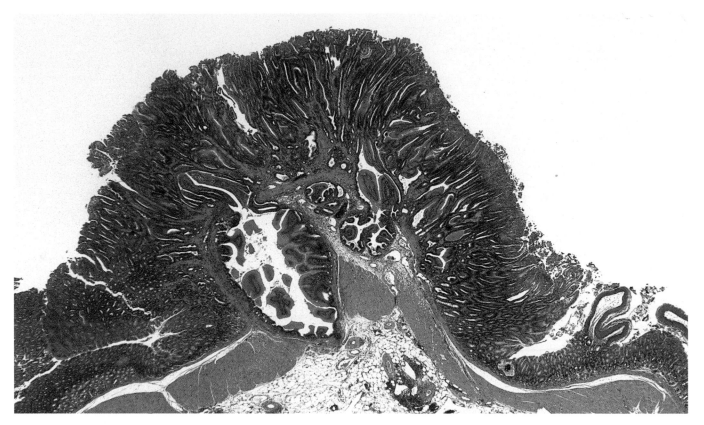

**FIGURE 19.15** Pyloric polyp showing broad base, "invasive" lesions (diverticula, herniation) into tunica muscularis and serosal inflammation in *Ahr* –/– mouse.

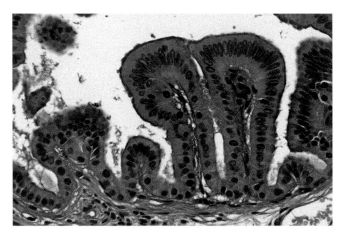

**FIGURE 19.16** Higher magnification of pyloric polyp in *Ahr* –/– mouse. The epithelium is well organized with mild dysplasia evident.

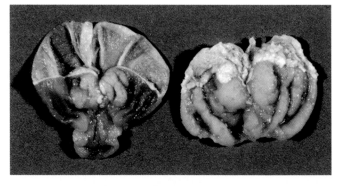

**FIGURE 19.17** Glandular stomach plaques at the forestomach junction in a *CYP1A2* –/– mouse.

1999). Lesions are characterized by diffuse epithelial hyperplasia (Fig. 19.17), altered epithelial differentiation, eosinophilic cytoplasmic inclusions in chief cells (Figs. 19.18-19.20) associated with extracellular eosinophilic crystals (Fig. 19.20), and herniation/diverticula of the epithelium into the tunica muscularis and serosa

(Fig. 19.18). These diverticula resembled those seen in *Ahr*-null mice (Fernandez-Salguero et al. 1997).

## Small Intestines

Meckel's diverticulum is a rare, noninherited, congenital anomaly characterized by an outpouching of the antimesenteric border of the ileum. It is also known as an ileal diverticulum. It results from the incomplete closure and disappearance of the omphalomesenteric duct that is the embryonic connection between the primitive

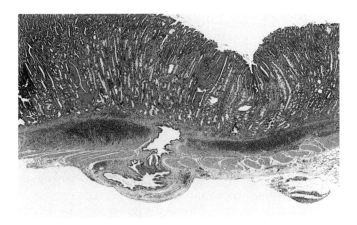

**FIGURE 19.18** Portion of gastric plaque in *CYP1A2* –/– mouse. Note diffuse hyperplasia, eosinophilic areas, lymphocyte foci in submucosa, and herniated glands (diverticula) within tunica musclaris and serosa.

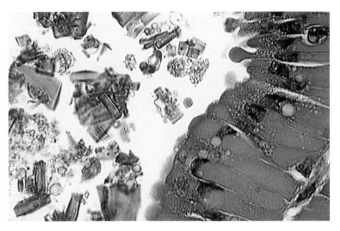

**FIGURE 19.19** Portion of gastric plaque in *CYP1A2* –/– mouse showing hyaline eosinophilic cytoplasm of epithelial cells and various eosinophilic crystals within the lumen.

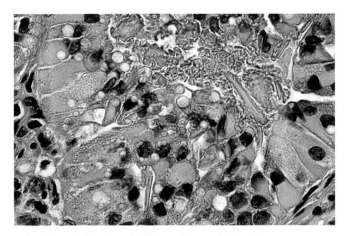

**FIGURE 19.20** Hyalinized cytoplasm of gastric epithelium and abundant protein and crystals in the lumen of *CYP1A2* –/– mouse.

gut and yolk sac. This anomaly occurs rarely in most inbred mouse strains and should not be misinterpreted as a mutant phenotype unless all mice with the mutant gene exhibit this change (Sundberg 1989).

Colorectal carcinoma is a genetically complex disease in humans, influenced by environmental factors, heritable predisposing genes, and somatic genetic mutations. Of these factors, somatic genetic mutations have been most extensively characterized, including inactivation of several tumor suppressor loci (Fearon and Vogelstein 1990; Steele 1993). One frequently mutated gene is adenomatous polyposis coli (*Apc*), which has been implicated as an initiating event in colonic epithelium transformation (Levy et al. 1994; Luongo et al. 1994). The APC protein is physically associated with β-catenin, suggesting that the loss of APC function may transform cells through cell adhesion or contact-mediated growth inhibitory pathways (Rubinfeld et al. 1993). Animal models for investigating the role of *Apc* in polyp initiation and carcinoma progression have been developed, including the multiple intestinal neoplasia (*Min*) mutation in the mouse (Moser et al. 1990) that results from a non-sense mutation in the *Apc* gene (Su et al. 1992). $Apc^{Min}$ confers a phenotype of susceptibility to intestinal tumors that is dominantly inherited and 100 percent penetrant on the C57BL/6J inbred background. Generation of a null allele of the *Apc* gene has confirmed the *Min* phenotype (Fodde et al. 1994). Creation of the double mutant, $Apc^{Min}/+$, $Prkdc^{scid}/Prkdc^{scid,}$ which has both severe combined immunodeficiency and multiple intestinal neoplasia phenotypes, indicated that tumor induction was independent of the immune system status (Dudley et al. 1996). Mutant mice available for investigating this phenomenon are listed in Table 19.5.

The first model for human familial adenomatous polyposis (FAP) was developed by a chemically induced (ethylnitrosourea) germline mutation resulting in the multiple intestinal neoplasia (*Min*) mutation (Moser et al. 1990). On the C57BL/6J background, *ApcMin/+* mice typically develop 50 or more adenomas throughout the intestinal tract. Tumors occur primarily in the small intestines in $Apc^{Min}/Apc+$, unlike FAP patients in which lesions are predominantly in the colon and rectum. Small intestine tumors in $Apc^{Min}/+$ mice are grossly visible on the mucosal surface as circular raised lesions 1 to several mm in diameter (Fig. 19.21a). Colon tumors tend to be larger and more polypoid than those in the small bowel. Microscopically the tumors are typical exophytic adenomas (Fig. 19.21b) with irregular glands lined by dark-staining atypical enterocytes. Clear invasion into the submucosa or muscularis (Fig. 19.21c) and scirrhous response are the most reliable indicators of conversion to malignancy with intestinal epithelial neoplasms, since even preneoplastic lesions may be composed of severely dysplastic cells (Fig. 19.21).

**TABLE 19.5.  Selected examples of genetically altered mice with proliferative intestinal phenotypes**

| Mutation or transgene | Phenotype | Reference |
|---|---|---|
| *Apc1638N* | Small and large intestines<br>Mostly adenomas<br>~5 tumors/mouse | Fodde et al. 1994 |
| *Apc* $^{Min}$ | Small and large intestines<br>Mostly adenomas<br>~50 tumors/mouse | Moser et al. 1990 |
| *Apc* $^{\Delta716}$ | Small and large intestines<br>Mostly adenomas<br>>200 tumors/mouse | Oshima et al. 1995 |
| *Mlh1* +/–, –/– | Small and large intestines<br>Adenomas and carcinomas<br>< 5 tumors/mouse | Edelmann et al. 1999 |
| *Smad3* –/– | Colorectal tumors<br>Mostly carcinomas<br>1–6 tumors/mouse | Zhu et al. 1998 |
| *Pten/Mmac1* +/– | Mixed lymphoepithelial polyps | Podsypanina et al. 1999 |
| SV40 Tag/*K-ras* | Small and large intestines<br>Dysplasia | Kim et al. 1993 |
| *Cdx2* | Colonic hamartomas | Tamai et al. 1999 |

Since the description of the *Apc*$^{Min}$/+ phenotype, two other *Apc* mutant strains have been generated through gene-targeting technology, designated as *Apc*$^{716}$ (Oshima et al. 1995) and *Apc*$^{1638N}$ (Fodde et al. 1994). Tumors in these mutants are morphologically similar to those in *Min* mice, although quantitatively there are dramatic differences in tumor multiplicity, with the *Apc*$^{716}$ and *Apc*$^{1638N}$ mutants having significantly greater and fewer tumors respectively than the *Apc*$^{Min}$/+ mouse.

Differences in *Apc* mutant tumor phenotype may not only be due to the specific genetic lesion induced but also to the genetic background on which the mutation is maintained. For example, intestinal tumor multiplicities are markedly reduced when both the *Apc*$^{Min}$/+ and *Apc*$^{1638N}$ mutations are carried on strains other than the C57BL/6 (Dietrich et al. 1993; van der Houven van Oordt et al. 1999). This intestinal phenotype variability clearly indicates the presence of modifying genetic factors. It should also be noted that, similar to humans with mutations in the *Apc* gene, induced *Apc* mouse mutants have several extraintestinal phenotypes including glandular stomach tumors, mammary tumors, desmoid tumors, and epidermoid cysts (Moser et al. 1993; Smits et al. 1998).

The *Apc* mutant tumor phenotype has proven to be an excellent model for the study of modulating factors in intestinal tumorigenesis. For example, to support findings of protective effects of nonsteroidal anti-inflammatory drugs (NSAIDs) in patients with FAP, treatment of *Apc*$^{Min}$/+ mice with various NSAIDs was shown to significantly reduce the development of tumors (Beazer-Barclay et al. 1996). This was presumed to be due to the inhibitory effect of NSAIDs on cyclo-oxygenase (*Cox*) and prostaglandin synthesis, and accordingly crossing *Apc*$^{716}$ mice with *Cox*-deficient mice resulted in markedly reduced intestinal tumor burdens (Oshima et al. 1996). Alternatively, tumor numbers in *Apc* mutants may be increased by exposure to X rays (van der Houven van Oordt et al. 1999), chemicals (Sorensen et al. 1997)), diet (Yang et al. 1998), or synergistic mutations (Edelmann et al. 1999; Takaku et al. 1998; Baker et al. 1998).

## Large Intestines and Cecum

Several strains of mice with genes inserted or selectively deleted by genetic manipulation spontaneously develop chronic intestinal inflammation. They represent models for the study of human inflammatory bowel diseases (IBDs). Most of these models have involved deletion of genes encoding for a protein with known immunologic functions, that is, interleukin (IL-2) (Sadlack et al. 1993), IL-2$\alpha$ receptor (IL-2R) chain (Willerford et al. 1995), IL-10 (Kühn et al. 1993), T cell receptor (*TCR*) $\alpha$ or $\beta$ chain (Mombaerts et al. 1993), and the G (for "guanine nucleotide–binding") protein $\alpha_{i2}$ subunit (Rudolph et al. 1995). IBD also develops in transgenic mouse chimeras expressing a dominant-negative N-cadherin mutant (NCAD$\Delta$) in small intestinal epithelial cells along the entire crypt-villus axis (Hermiston and Gordon 1995) and in multiple lines of transgenic mice carrying murine IL-7 cDNA and SR$\alpha$ promoter (Watanabe et al. 1998). It should be noted that the immune-gene deletions resulting in chronic intestinal inflammation represent only a small fraction of the total number of immunological genes that have been deleted, which argues that they represent critical nonredundant mechanisms of mucosal homeostasis. Most of these mutations affect T cell function in some way; others may have a predominant effect on the epithelium.

In several of the genetically engineered mouse models of IBD, disease expression is strongly influenced by two factors. First, a critical role for the enteric microbial flora in the pathogenesis of IBD is demonstrated by the absence of disease under germ-free conditions and by the attenuation of disease under specific pathogen-free conditions in multiple models of IBD (Bristol et al. 1997; Dianda et al. 1996; Kühn et al. 1993; Sadlack et

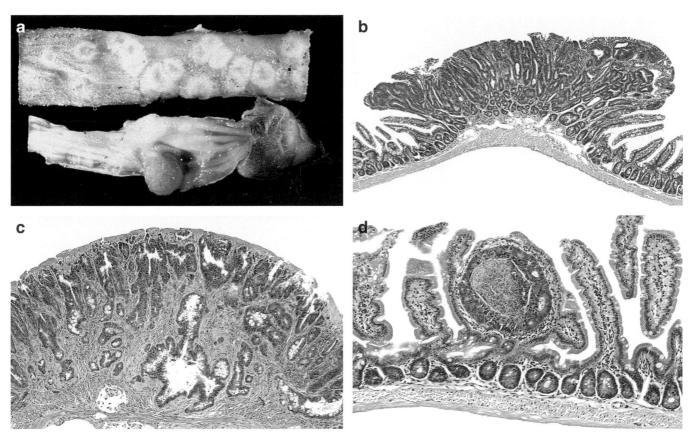

**FIGURE 19.21** (**a**) Gross appearance of intestinal tumors in an *Apc^{Min}*/+ mouse. There are numerous circular sessile tumors in the small bowel (top) and a single polypoid tumor in the colon (bottom). (**b**) Exophytic intestinal adenoma from an *Apc^{Min}*/+ mouse. (**c**) Invasive adenocarcinoma with scirrhous response in an *Apc^{Min}*/+ mouse. (**d**) Focal dysplasia in an *Apc^{Min}*/+ mouse. The focal dysplasia is characterized by an abnormal gland lined by atypical multilayered and dark-staining enterocytes.

al. 1993; see also Chap. 20). The microbial antigen(s) driving the disease is, as yet, unknown. Second, the frequency and severity of disease are highly dependent on the genetic background strain carrying the mutation, thus indicating the presence of modifier genes (Berg et al. 1996; Bristol et al. 1998; Hörnquist et al. 1997; Mähler et al. 1996; Mombaerts et al. 1993; Sadlack et al. 1995). Interestingly, certain strains are consistently susceptible or resistant to intestinal inflammation, independent of the mutation leading to IBD. Strains 129, BALB/c, and C3H/He confer disease susceptibility whereas strain C57BL/6 confers resistance.

Selected clinical and histopathological features of the genetically engineered mice with IBD are summarized in Table 19.6. Data are based on the original reports (Hermiston and Gordon 1995; Kühn et al. 1993; Mombaerts et al. 1993; Rudolph et al. 1995; Sadlack et al. 1993; Watanabe et al. 1998; Willerford et al. 1995), most of which were obtained from mutants on a mixed genetic background (C57BL/6 × 129). Important fea-

tures not originally reported have been added, with the particular reference noted. Frequent clinical signs of IBD are weight loss, diarrhea, rectal prolapse (Fig. 19.22), and (occult) intestinal bleeding. On gross inspection, severely affected portions of the bowel are enlarged (dilated, thick walled) and rigid (Fig. 19.23). Histologically, the majority of mutants exhibit diffuse mucosal to submucosal inflammation that preferentially involves the large intestine. The inflammatory infiltrates are primarily composed of lymphocytes, plasma cells, neutrophils, and macrophages. Other histological findings include mucosal hyperplasia, distortion of the crypt architecture, goblet cell depletion, crypt abscesses, epithelial erosions, and ulcerations. Of note, three of the mutants develop intestinal neoplasms at an advanced stage of disease (Fig. 19.24; Berg et al. 1996; Hermiston and Gordon 1995; Rudolph et al. 1995), which is also a typical feature in human IBD. Metastases have not been observed. The mechanism(s) of tumor induction are unknown.

**TABLE 19.6. Clinical and histopathological features of genetically engineered mice with IBD**

| Model | Time Course | Area of involvement | Distribution of inflammation | Depth of inflammation | Anorectal lesions | Intestinal neoplasia | Other lesions |
|---|---|---|---|---|---|---|---|
| IL-2 deficiency | Onset 6–15 wk of age, 50% mortality. By 9 wk of age (severe anemia) progressive to death within 10–25 wk | Large intestine (distal > proximal), small intestine and stomach (late)[a] | Diffuse | Mucosal to submucosal | Prolapse | No | Autoimmune disease (multiorgan inflammation[a,b], hemolytic anemia, splenomegaly, lymphadenopathy), amyloidosis |
| IL-2Rα deficiency | Onset 12–16 wk of age, 25% mortality by 20 wk of age (severe anemia) | Large intestine | Diffuse[c] | Mucosal to transmural[c] | Prolapse[c] | No | Autoimmune disease (hemolytic anemia, splenomegaly, lymphadenopathy) |
| IL-10 deficiency | Onset 3–8 wk of age, progressive, 30% mortality by 3 mo of age, 60% develop adenocarcinoma by 6 mo of age[d] | Entire intestinal tract (predominantly proximal colon, proximal small intestine) | Segmental | Mucosal to transmural | Prolapse, ulceration[e] | Adenocarcinoma[d] | Anemia |
| TCRα deficiency TCRβ deficiency | Onset 3–4 mo of age, progressive to death between 6 and 12 mo of age | Large intestine (distal > proximal) | Diffuse | Mucosal to submucosal | Prolapse | No | Focal hepatitis (in some TCRα deficient mice) |
| Gα_i2 deficiency | Onset 8–13 wk of age, progressive, 75% mortality by 36 wk of age, 31% develop adenocarcinoma by 36 wk of age | Large intestine (distal > proximal) | Diffuse | Mucosal | Prolapse | Adenocarcinoma | No |
| NCADΔ chimera | Onset by 3 mo of age, progressive, adenomas at 3–9 mo of age | Small intestine | Focal | Mucosal to transmural | No | Adenoma | No |
| IL-7 transgenic mouse | Onset 1–3 wk of age (acute colitis) and 4–12 wk of age (chronic colitis), progressive, 60% develop colitis by 16 wk of age | Large intestine (distal > proximal), ileum | Diffuse | Mucosal | Prolapse | No | Dermatitis (in one transgenic line) |

[a]Mähler et al. 1996.
[b]Sadlack et al. 1995.
[c]D.M. Willerford, 1999, personal communication.
[d]Berg et al. 1996.
[e]M. Mähler, unpublished observation.

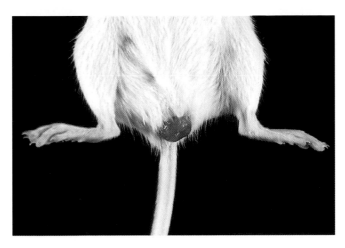

**FIGURE 19.22** Rectal prolapse in an 8-month-old female B6,129-*Il10^{tm1Cgn}* mouse with inflammatory bowel disease.

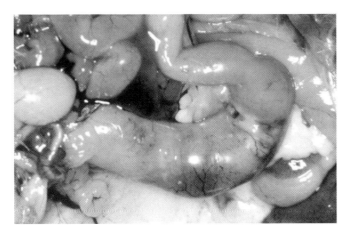

**FIGURE 19.23** Colon of a 27-week-old male Gα_{i2}-deficient mouse showing marked dilation, thickening, and congestion. In the region of the splenic flexure, there is suppurative exudation and a small perforation of the wall at the mesenteric attachment site. (Rudolph et al. 1995. Used with permission from Nature America, Inc.)

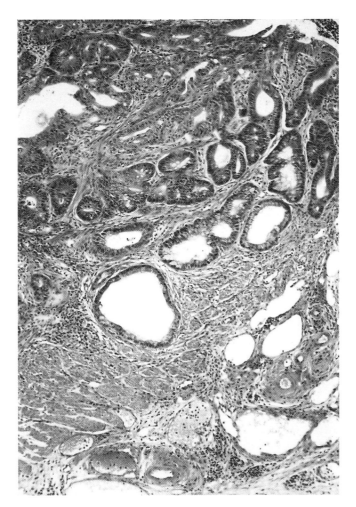

**FIGURE 19.24** Colonic adenocarcinoma of a 13-week-old female C3H/HeJBir-*Il10^{tm1Cgn}* mouse.

The following sections focus on the intestinal pathology of mutant mice with targeted disruptions of the *Il2*, *Il10*, and *Tcrα* genes. They represent three of the most widely used mouse models of IBD.

## IL-2–DEFICIENT MOUSE

IL-2 is a regulatory cytokine that promotes growth and expansion of T cells, differentiation of B cells, and activation of macrophages, lymphokine-activated killer cells, and natural killer (NK) cells (Smith 1992). It is mainly produced by activated T helper 1 (Th1) cells.

Mice homozygous for the null mutation of the *Il2* gene (*Il2^{tm1Hor}*) completely lack IL-2 activity (Horak et al. 1995; Schorle et al. 1991). Homozygous mutants on the mixed C57BL/6 × 129/Ola genetic background develop normally up to 4 weeks of age (Sadlack et al. 1993). About 50 percent of these mice die between 4 and 9 weeks after birth with splenomegaly, lymphadenopathy, and a severe hemolytic anemia if maintained in a conventional (non–germ-free) environment. All of the remaining mice develop progressive inflammation of the large intestine. In addition, generalized amyloidosis frequently occurs. Clinical signs of IBD are diarrhea, remittent intestinal bleeding, and frequent rectal prolapse. Gross findings include colonic thickening and enlarged mesenteric lymph nodes. There is diffuse inflammation in the mucosa and submucosa of the large intestine with infiltration by lymphocytes, plasma cells, and granulocytes (Fig. 19.25a). Other histologic findings include

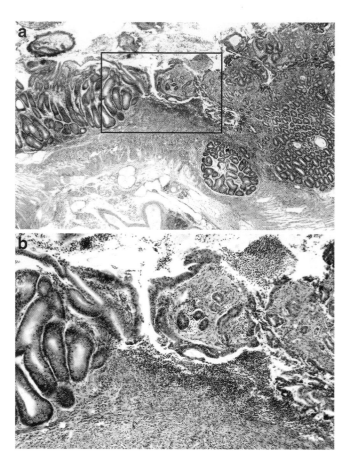

**FIGURE 19.25** (**a**) Colon of an 18-week-old female C57BL/6J-*Il2^{tm1Hor}* mouse. (**b**) Higher magnification of boxed area in **a** shows mucosal hyperplasia adjacent to a large ulcer.

ulcerations (Fig. 19.25b), crypt abscesses, epithelial hyperplasia with crypt distortion, and goblet cell depletion. Lesions are most severe in the distal colon. In the later stages, the small intestine and stomach may also be affected (Mähler et al. 1996). Immunologic alterations include a high number of activated T cells (CD44+, CD69+) and B cells, elevated immunoglobulin (IgA, IgG1) secretion, anticolon antibodies, and aberrant expression of class II major histocompatibility complex (MHC) molecules on colonic epithelium (Sadlack et al. 1993). When *Il2^{tm1Hor}* mutant mice are maintained germ-free, they do not develop bowel inflammation. The viability and disease development of *Il2^{tm1Hor}* mice are strongly dependent on their genetic background. Mutant mice crossed onto a BALB/c background develop a generalized autoimmune disease and die within 5 weeks of age (Sadlack et al. 1995). The disease is manifested by severe hemolytic anemia and mononuclear inflammatory cell infiltrates in multiple organs. This multiorgan disease has also been observed in *Il2^{tm1Hor}* mutants on C3H/HeJCrlBR and C57BL/6J genetic

backgrounds, with the digestive system being most severely affected (Mähler et al. 1996). Interestingly, C57BL/6 × 129 mice deficient in both IL-2 and β2-microglobulin develop IBD as well as colonic adenocarcinoma between 6 and 12 months of age, with an incidence of 32 percent (Shah et al. 1998). The occurrence of colonic adenocarcinoma in these mice may be explained by the lack of CD8+ T cells (which may have an immunosurveillance or cytotoxic function against early tumors) and/or the lack of major histocompatibility class I expression (which may allow the tumors to escape detection by the immune system) as a result of the targeted disruption of the *β2m* gene. Because *Il2^{tm1Hor}* mice have a much higher mortality rate than the double-mutant mice, it is also possible that *Il2^{tm1Hor}* mice do not live long enough to develop colonic cancer as a complication of IBD.

Experimental crosses of *Il2^{tm1Hor}* mutant mice with various immunodeficient mutants indicate that CD4+ T cells are required for the development of colitis associated with IL-2 deficiency (Simpson et al. 1995), while anemia is dependent on B cells (Ma et al. 1995). There is evidence that IBD occurring in *Il2^{tm1Hor}* mice is due to a dysregulated Th1 cell–mediated immune response (high production of interferon-γ) to exogenous antigens (Autenrieth et al. 1997; Ehrhardt et al. 1997; Lúdvíksson et al. 1997; McDonald et al. 1997). The pathogenic Th1 cell in *Il2^{tm1Hor}* mice may result from an impaired production of the suppressor cytokine transforming growth factor α (Lúdvíksson et al. 1997). Stimulation of mucosal macrophages by Th1 cytokines and the subsequent release of inflammatory cytokines such as IL-1, IL-6, and tumor necrosis factor α (TNFα) presumably contribute to the tissue damage (Autenrieth et al. 1997; McDonald et al. 1997). In addition to the failure in down-regulating autoreactive Th1 cells, *Il2^{tm1Hor}* mice might have a defect in eliminating such Th1 cell clones by FAS-mediated apoptosis, further contributing to bowel inflammation and other autoimmune phenomena in *Il2^{tm1Hor}* mice (Kneitz et al. 1995).

## IL-10–DEFICIENT MOUSE

IL-10 is a regulatory cytokine that suppresses effector functions of macrophages, Th1 cells, and NK cells (Moore et al. 1993). In addition, IL-10 augments proliferation and differentiation of B cells. It is mainly produced by Th2 cells.

Mice homozygous for the null mutation of the *Il10* gene (*Il10^{tm1Cgn}*) completely lack IL-10 activity (Kühn et al. 1993). Homozygous mutants on the mixed genetic background C57BL/6 × 129/Ola (B6,129-*Il10^{tm1Cgn}*) are growth retarded by 3–4 weeks of age and anemic by 7–11 weeks of age. They spontaneously develop chronic

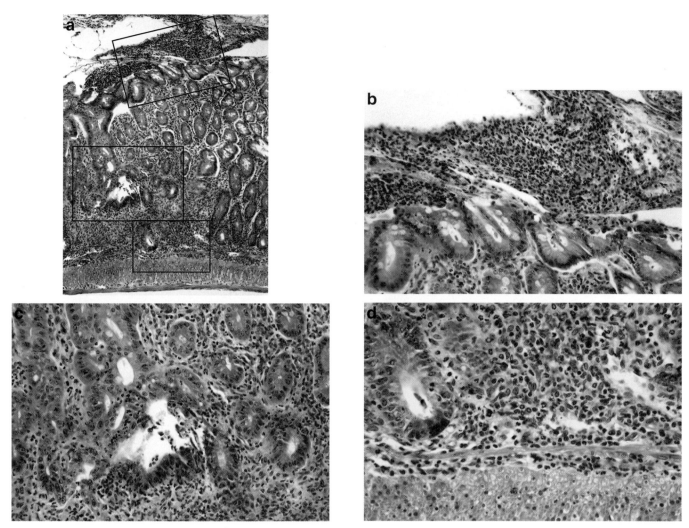

**FIGURE 19.26**    (**a**) Colon of a 6-week-old female C3H/HeJBir-*Il10^{tm1Cgn}* mouse with mixed inflammatory cell infiltrates in the lamina propria, mucosal hyperplasia, and cellular debris in the lumen. Higher magnifications of boxed areas in **a** show surface inflammation (**b**), dilation and ulceration of crypts (**c**), and inflammatory cells within the lamina propria and submucosa (**d**).

IBD, which can affect the entire intestinal tract if housed under conventional conditions (Berg et al. 1996; Kühn et al. 1993; Löhler et al. 1995). By 3 months of age, the incidence of IBD is 100 percent, and mortality is about 30 percent. The type of anorectal lesion in *Il10^{tm1Cgn}* mutant mice is influenced by genetic factors. C57BL/6J-*Il10^{tm1Cgn}* and B6,129-*Il10^{tm1Cgn}* mice frequently develop rectal prolapse (Fig. 19.22), whereas C3H/HeJBir-*Il10^{tm1Cgn}* mice exhibit perianal ulceration in the same environment (M. Mähler, unpublished observation). Intestinal pathology is characterized by a regionally variable pattern of chronic mucosal inflammation associated either with hyperplastic or degenerative lesions of the intestinal epithelia (Berg et al. 1996; Kühn et al. 1993; Löhler et al. 1995). The duodenum, proximal jejunum, cecum, and proximal colon are most severely affected. The bowel lesions consist of epithelial

hyperplasia (Fig. 19.26a) with abnormal crypt and villous structures, goblet cell depletion, erosion and desquamation of superficial epithelia, focal ulcerations, crypt abscesses (Fig. 19.27a, b), inflammatory cell infiltration in the mucosa and submucosa (Fig. 19.26a, b), and focal transmural inflammation (Fig. 19.28a, b). Inflammatory cell infiltrates are composed predominantly of lymphocytes, plasma cells, and macrophages but also contain small-to-moderate numbers of neutrophils, eosinophils, and multinucleated giant cells. There is increased expression of MHC class II molecules on the epithelium of the small and large intestines. In addition, 60 percent of B6,129-*Il10^{tm1Cgn}* mice develop colorectal adenocarcinomas by 6 months of age (Berg et al. 1996) (Fig. 19.24). Intestinal lesions are most severe in *Il10^{tm1Cgn}* mutants on 129/SvEv, BALB/c, and C3H/HeJBir backgrounds, of intermediate severity in

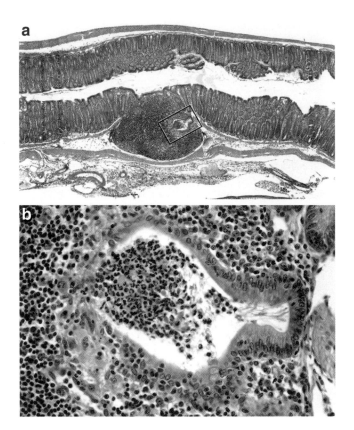

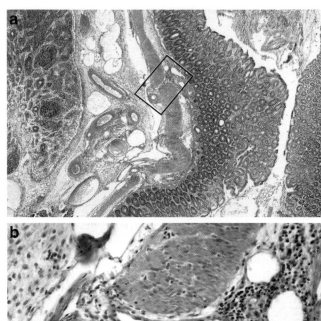

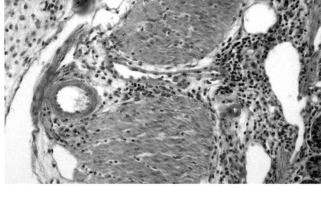

**FIGURE 19.27** (**a**) Crypt abscess in the colon of a 6-week-old female C3H/HeJ-*Il10^{tm1Cgn}* mouse. (**b**) Higher magnification of boxed area in **a**.

**FIGURE 19.28** (**a**) Colon of a 6-week-old female mouse B6,129-*Il10^{tm2Cgn}* showing transmural inflammation. (**b**) Higher magnification of boxed area in **a** showing inflammatory cells adjacent to vessels transversing muscular wall.

C57BL/6 × 129/Ola outbred mutants, and least severe in C57BL/6J mutants (Berg et al. 1996; Bristol et al. 1998). B6,129-*Il10^{tm1Cgn}* mice kept under specific pathogen-free conditions exhibit only local inflammation confined to the proximal colon (Kühn et al. 1993; Löhler et al. 1995); germ-free mutants do not develop IBD (Sellon et al. 1997). Infection with the pathogen *Helicobacter hepaticus* is not required for the development of IBD in *Il10^{tm1Cgn}* mice (Czinn et al. 1998; Dieleman et al. 1998), although Kullberg et al. (1998) showed that IL-10–deficient mice developed no IBD when they were cleared of *Helicobacter* infections and infection of clean mice with *Helicobacter* caused IBD.

Cell transfer experiments and antibody treatment studies have shown that IBD in *Il10^{tm1Cgn}* mice is predominantly mediated by CD4+ Th1 cells (Berg et al. 1996; Davidson et al. 1996). Collectively, the data indicate that the pathogenic mechanism is an enhanced mucosal Th1 response to antigens of the enteric bacterial flora due to the lack of IL-10 that normally downregulates such T cell reactivity. This leads to macrophage activation and production of inflammatory mediators such as IL-1, IL-6, TNFα, and nitric oxide,

all of which have been demonstrated in the inflamed tissue (Berg et al. 1996).

## TCRα-DEFICIENT MOUSE

T cells recognize antigens via a heterodimeric surface receptor made up of an α and β chain (αβ T cell receptor) or a γ and δ chain (γδ T cell receptor) (Penninger et al. 1991).

Mice homozygous for the null mutation of the *Tcrα* gene (*Tcrα^{tm1Mom}*) are selectively deficient in αβ T cells (Mombaerts et al. 1992). Homozygous mutants on various genetic backgrounds develop progressive inflammation of the large intestine after 3–4 months of age (Mombaerts et al. 1993). Clinically, the disease presents as nonbloody diarrhea and wasting often associated with rectal prolapse. Macroscopic findings include marked dilation and thickening of the large intestine as well as enlarged mesenteric lymph nodes. Histopathologic changes are characterized by hyperplasia and dis-

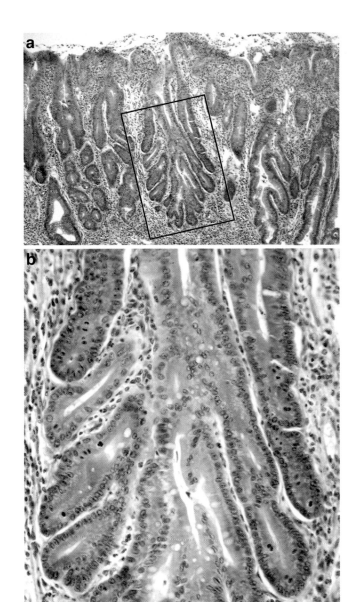

**FIGURE 19.29** (**a**) Colon of an 11-month-old female B6,129-*Tcrα*^tm1Mom^ mouse with marked hyperplasia of the mucosa. Higher magnification of boxed area in **a** showing marked crypt hyperplasia with arborization (**b**).

tortion of epithelial crypts (Fig. 19.29), goblet cell depletion, diffuse infiltration of the mucosa and submucosa by lymphocytes, plasma cells and neutrophils, occasional crypt abscesses, and rare, focal ulcerations.

Lesions are most severe in the rectum. The numbers of γδ T cells and B cells are increased in the large intestine. In diseased mice there is also an increase in the production of serum and mucosal antibodies of various isotypes directed against food and self-antigens, such as the cytoskeletal protein tropomyosin (Mizoguchi et al. 1996, 1997; Takahashi et al. 1997). The genetic background of the mutant mice again plays a role in the incidence and severity of IBD, with strain 129/Sv-*Tcrα*^tm1Mom^ being most severely affected (Mombaerts et al. 1993). Germfree *Tcrα*^tm1Mom^ mice do not develop IBD (Dianda et al. 1996).

The development of IBD in *Tcrα*^tm1Mom^ mice is mediated by a unique subset of CD4+ TCR αβ T cells (Takahashi et al. 1997). The exact mechanism of tissue injury remains unknown. In contrast to the pathogenic Th1 response occurring in many mouse models of IBD (Davidson et al. 1996; Ehrhardt et al. 1997; Hörnquist et al. 1997; Watanabe et al. 1998), *Tcrα*^tm1Mom^ mice with IBD exhibit a Th2-predominant cytokine profile characterized by high IL-4 production (Mizoguchi et al. 1996; Takahashi et al. 1997). Interestingly, histopathology of the large bowel lesions observed in *Tcrα*^tm1Mom^ mice is somewhat similar to those of models with a Th1 cell–driven response, indicating that the histopathologic features are not good predictors of the immune mechanisms involved in the bowel lesions.

# REFERENCES

Abe, K., Ooshima, T., Masatomi, Y., et al. 1989. Microscopic and crystallographic examinations of teeth of the X-linked hypophosphatemic mouse. J. Dent. Res. 68:1519–1524.

Autenrieth, I.B., Bucheler, N., Bohn, E., et al. 1997. Cytokine mRNA expression in intestinal tissue of interleukin-2 deficient mice with bowel inflammation. Gut 41:793–800.

Baker, S.M., Harris, A.C., Tsao, J.L., et al. 1998. Enhanced intestinal adenomatous polyp formation in *Pms2–/–;Min* mice. Cancer Res. 58:1087–1089.

Beamer, W.G., Donahue, L.R., Rosen, C.J., et al. 1996. Genetic variability in adult bone density among inbred strains of mice. Bone 18:397–403.

Beazer-Barclay, Y., Levy, D.B., Moser, A.R., et al. 1996. Sulindac suppresses tumorigenesis in the *Min* mouse. Carcinogenesis 17:1756–1760.

Bechtold, L.S. 1999. Ultrastructural evaluation of mouse mutations. In: Systematic Characterization of Mouse Mutations, ed. Sundberg, J.P., Boggess, D. Boca Raton, FL: CRC Press, pp. 121–129.

Beck, L., Soumounou, Y., Martel, J., et al. 1997. PEX/PHEX tissue distribution and evidence for a deletion in the 3′ region of the *Pex* gene in X-linked hypophosphatemic mice. J. Clin. Invest. 99:1200–1209.

Berg, D.J., Davidson, N., Kühn, R., et al. 1996. Enterocolitis and colon cancer in interleukin10-deficient mice are associated with aberrant cytokine production and CD4⁺ TH1-like responses. J. Clin. Invest. 98:1010–1020.

Bockman, D.E. and Merlino, G. 1992. Cytological changes in the pancreas of transgenic mice overexpressing transforming growth factor alpha. Gastroenterology 103:1883–1892.

Bockman, D.E., Sharp, R., and Merlino, G. 1995. Regulation of terminal differentiation of zymogenic cells by transforming growth factor α in transgenic mice. Gastroenterology 108:447–454.

Boivin, G.P., Molina, J.R., Ormsby, I., et al. 1996. Gastric lesions in transforming growth factor beta1 heterozygous mice. Lab. Invest. 74:513–518.

Bristol, I.J., Mähler, M., Leiter, E.H., et al. 1997. *Il10^{tm1Cgn,}* an interleukin-10 gene targeted mutation. Jax Notes 471:2–4.

Bristol, I.J., Mähler, M., Sundberg, J.P., et al. 1998. Severe, early colitis in C3H/HeJBirIL10-deficient mice. Gastroenterology 114:A943.

Ceci, J.D., Kovatch, R.M., Swing, D.A., et al. 1991. Transgenic mice carrying a murine amylase 2.2/SV40 T antigen fusion gene develop pancreatic acinar cell and stomach carcinomas. Oncogene 6:323–332.

Celli, G., LaRochelle W.J., Mackem, S., et al. 1998. Soluble dominant-negative receptor uncovers essential roles for fibroblast growth factors in multi-organ induction and patterning. EMBO J. 17:1642–1655.

Chen, Y., Bei, M., Woo, I., et al. 1996. *Msx1* controls inductive signalling in mammalian tooth morphogenesis. Development 122:3035–3044.

Coffey, R.J., Romano, M., Polk, W.H., et al. 1992. Roles for transforming growth factor-alpha in gastric physiology and pathophysiology. Yale J. Biol. Med. 65:693–704.

Czinn, S.J., Zagorski, B.M., Spencer, D.M., et al. 1998. Superinfection with *Helicobacter hepaticus* does not alter the natural course of colitis in IL10 deficient mice. Gastroenterology 114:A958.

Davideau, J.L., Demri, P., Gu, T.T., et al. 1999. Expression of DLX5 during human embryonic craniofacial development. Mech. Dev. 81:183–186.

Davidson, N.J., Leach, M.W., Fort, M.M., et al. 1996. T helper cell 1-type CD4+ T cells, but not B cells, mediate colitis in interleukin 10-deficient mice. J. Exp. Med. 184:241–251.

Davisson, M.T., Cook, S.A., Johnson, K.R., et al. 1994. Balding: a new mutation on mouse chromosome 18 causing hair loss and immunological defects. J. Hered. 85:134–136.

Dempsey, P.J., Goldenring, J.R., Soroka, C.J., et al. 1992. Possible role of transforming growth factor alpha in the pathogenesis of Menetrier's disease: supportive evidence from humans and transgenic mice. Gastroenterology 103:1950–1963.

Dianda, L., Hanby, A.M., Wright, N.A., et al. 1996. T cell receptor-deficient mice fail to develop colitis in the absence of a microbial environment. Am. J. Pathol. 150:97–98.

Dickie, M.M. 1967. Osteosclerotic (*oc*). Mouse News Lett. 36:39.

Dieleman, L.A., Tonkonogy, S.L., Sellon, R.K., et al. 1998. *Helicobacter hepaticus* does not potentiate colitis in interleukin-10 deficient mice. Gastroenterology 114:A965.

Dietrich, W.F., Lander, E.S., Smith, J.S., et al. 1993. Genetic identification of Mom-1, a major modifier locus affecting Min-induced intestinal neoplasia in the mouse. Cell 75:631–639.

Dimai, H.P., Linkhart, T.A., Linkhart, S.G., et al. 1998. Alkaline phosphatase levels and osteoprogenitor cell numbers suggest bone formation may contribute to peak bone density differences between two inbred strains of mice. Bone 22:211–216.

Donath, K. and Breuner, G. 1982. A method for the study of uncalcified bones and teeth with attached soft tissues. The Sage-Schliff (sawing and grinding) technique. J. Oral Pathol. 11:318–326.

Dudley, M.E., Sundberg, J.P., and Roopenian, D.C. 1996. Frequency and histological appearance of adenomas in multiple intestinal neoplasia mice are unaffected by severe combined immunodeficiency (*scid*) mutation. Int. J. Cancer 65:249–253.

Edelmann, W., Yang, K., Kuraguchi, M., et al. 1999. Tumorigenesis in *Mlh1* and *Mlh1/Apc1638N* mutant mice. Cancer Res. 59:1301–1307.

Ehrhardt, R.O., Lúdvíksson, B.R., Gray, B., et al. 1997. Induction and prevention of colonic inflammation in IL2-deficient mice. J. Immunol. 159:566–573.

Ennulat, D., Kawabe, M., Kudo, G., et al. 1998. Hyperplastic gastric mucosal lesions with eosinophilic cytoplasmic inclusions in aging C57BL × 129 and Sv/129 mice. Vet. Pathol. 35:456.

Fearon, E.R. and Vogelstein, B. 1990. A genetic model for colorectal tumorigenesis. Cell 61:759–767.

Fernandez-Salguero, P., Ward, J.M., Sundberg, J.P., et al. 1997. Lesions of arylhydrocarbon receptor-deficient mice. Vet. Pathol. 34:605–614.

Fodde, R., Edelmann, W., Yang, K., et al. 1994. A targeted chain-termination mutation in the mouse *Apc* gene results in multiple intestinal tumors. Proc. Natl. Acad. Sci. USA 91:8969–8973.

Ghoshal, N.G. and Bal, H.S. 1989. Comparative morphology of the stomach of some laboratory mammals. Lab. Anim. 23:21–29.

Gibson, C.W., Lally, E., Herold, R.C., et al. 1992. Odontogenic tumors in mice carrying albumin-*myc* and albumin-*ras* transgenes. Calcif. Tissue Int. 51:162–167.

Gijbels, M., Zurcher, C., Kraal, G., et al. 1996. Pathogenesis of skin lesions in mice with chronic proliferative dermatitis (*cpdm/cpdm*). Am. J. Pathol. 148:941–950.

Goldenring, J.R., Ray, G.S., Soroka, C.J., et al. 1996. Overexpression of transforming growth factor-alpha alters differentiation of gastric cell lineages. Dig. Dis. Sci. 41:773–784.

Grier, R.L., Zhao, L., Adams, C.E., et al. 1998. Secretion of CSF-1 and its inhibition in rat dental follicle cells: implications for tooth eruption. Eur. J. Oral Sci. 106:808–815.

Gruneberg, H. 1935. A new sub-lethal color mutation in the house mouse. Proc. R. Soc. B 118:321–342.

Gruneberg, H. 1965. Genes and genotypes affecting the teeth of the mouse. J. Embryol. Exp. Morphol. 14:137–159.

Hardcastle, Z., Mo, R., Hui, C.C., et al. 1998. The *Shh* signaling pathway in tooth development: defects in Gli2 and Gli3 mutants. Development 125:2803–2811.

Hermiston, M.L. and Gordon, J.I. 1995. Inflammatory bowel disease and adenomas in mice expressing a dominant negative Ncadherin. Science 270:1203–1207.

Hertwig, P. 1942. Sechs neue mutationen bei der hausmaus in ihrer bedeutung fur allgemeine vererbungsfragen. Z. Menschl. Vererb. Konstitutions 26:1–21.

Hodgkison, C.A., Moore, K.J., Nakayama, A., et al. 1993. Mutations at the mouse microophthalmia locus are associated with defects in a gene encoding a basic-helix-loop-helix-zipper protein. Cell 74:395–404.

Horak, I., Löhler, J., Ma, A., et al. 1995. Interleukin-2 deficient mice: a new model to study autoimmunity and self-tolerance. Immunol. Rev. 148:35–44.

Hörnquist, C.E., Lu, X., RogersFani, P.M., et al. 1997. Gi2-deficient mice with colitis exhibit a local increase in memory CD4+ T cells and proinflammatory Th1-type cytokines. J. Immunol. 158:1068–1077.

HYP Consortium. 1995. A gene (*Pex*) with homologies to endopeptidases is mutated in patients with X-linked hypophosphatemic rickets. Nat. Genet.11:130–136.

Jhappan, C., Stahle, C., Harkins, R.N., et al. 1990. TGF alpha overexpression in transgenic mice induces liver neoplasia and abnormal development of the mammary gland and pancreas. Cell 61:1137–1146.

Johnson, R.S., Spiegelman, B.M., and Papaioannou, V. 1992. Peliotropic effects of a null mutation in the c-fos proto-oncogene. Cell 71:577–586.

Kaplan, H.S. 1949. Lesions of the gastric mucosa in Strong strain NHO mice. J. Natl. Cancer Inst. 10:407–421.

Karam, S.M., Li, Q., and Gordon, J.I. 1997. Gastric epithelial morphogenesis in normal and transgenic mice. Am. J. Physiol. 272:G1209–G1220.

Kaufman, M.H. and Bard, J.B.L. 1999. The Anatomical Basis of Mouse Development. San Diego: Academic Press. 291 pp.

Kim, S.H., Roth, K.A., Moser, A.R., et al. 1993. Transgenic mouse models that explore the multistep hypothesis of intestinal neoplasia. J. Cell Biol. 123:877–893.

Kimura, S., Kawabe, M., Ward, J.M., et al. 1999. CYP1A2 is not the primary enzyme responsible for 4-amino-biphenyl-induced hepatocarcinogenesis in mice. Carcinogenesis 20:1825–1830.

Kitamura, Y., Yokoyama, M., Matsuda, H., et al. 1980. Coincidental development of forestomach papilloma and prepyloric ulcer in nontreated mutant mice of W/W$^v$ and SL/SL$^d$ genotypes. Cancer Res. 40:3392–3397.

Kneitz, B., Herrmann, T., Yonehara, S., et al. 1995. Normal clonal expansion but impaired Fas-mediated cell death and anergy induction in interleukin-2-deficient mice. Eur. J. Immunol. 25: 2572–2577.

Koch, P.J., Mahoney, M.G., Ishikawa, H., et al. 1997. Targeted disruption of the pemphigus vulgaris antigen (desmoglein 3) gene in mice causes loss of keratinocyte cell adhesion with a phenotype similar to pemphigus vulgaris. J. Cell Biol. 137:1091–1102.

Koike, K., Hinrichs, S.H., Isselbacher, K.J., et al. 1989. Transgenic mouse model for human gastric carcinoma. Proc. Natl. Acad. Sci. USA 86:5615–5619.

Kong, Y.Y., Yoshida, H., Sarosi, I., et al. 1999. OPGL is a key regulator of osteoclastogenesis, lymphocyte development and lymph-node organogenesis. Nature 397:315–323.

Kratochwil, K., Dull, M., Farinas, I., et al. 1996. Lef1 expression is activated by BMP-4 and regulates inductive tissue interactions in tooth and hair development. Genes Dev. 10:1382–1394.

Kühn, R., Löhler, J., Rennick, D., et al. 1993. Interleukin-10-deficient mice develop chronic enterocolitis. Cell 75:263–274.

Kullberg, M.C., Ward, J.M., Gorelick, P.L., et al. 1998. *Helicobacter hepaticus* triggers colitis in specific-pathogen-free interleukin-10 (IL10)-deficient mice through an IL12- and gamma interferon-dependent mechanism. Infect. Immun. 66:5157–5166.

Lane, P.W., Bronson, R.T., Cook, S.A., et al. 1998. Juvenile Bare: A new hair loss mutation on chromosome 7 of the mouse. J. Hered. 89:254–257.

Levy, D.B., Smith, K.J., Beazer-Barclay, Y., et al. 1994. Inactivation of both *APC* alleles in human and mouse tumors. Cancer Res. 54:5953–5958.

Li, Q., Karam, S.M., and Gordon, J.I. 1995. Simian virus 40 T antigen-induced amplification of preparietal cells in transgenic mice. Effects on other gastric epithelial cell lineages and evidence for a p53-independent apoptotic mechanism that operates in a committed progenitor. J. Biol. Chem. 270:15777–15788.

Li, Q., Karam, S.M., Coerver, K.A., et al. 1998. Stimulation of activin receptor II signaling pathways inhibits differentiation of multiple gastric epithelial lineages. Mol. Endocrinol. 12:181–192.

Linkhart, T.A., Linkhart, S.G., Kodama, Y., et al. 1999. Osteoclast formation in bone marrow cultures from two inbred strains of mice with different bone densities. J. Bone Miner. Res. 14:39–46

Löhler, J., Kühn, R., Rennick, D., et al. 1995. Interleukin-10-deficient mice: a model of chronic mucosal inflammation. In: Inflammatory Bowel Diseases, ed. Tytgat, G.N.J., Bartelsman, J.F.W.M., Deventer, S.J.H. Dordrecht, Germany: Kluwer Academic Publishers, pp. 401–407.

Lúdvíksson, B.R., Ehrhardt, R.O., and Strober, W. 1997. TGFα production regulates the development of the 2,4,6-trinitrophenol-conjugated keyhole limpet hemocyanin-induced colonic inflammation in IL2-deficient mice. J. Immunol. 159:3622–3628.

Lund, P.K. 1998. The alpha-smooth muscle actin promoter: a useful tool to analyze autocrine and paracrine roles of mesenchymal cells in normal and diseased bowel. Gut 42:320–322.

Luning, C., Wroblewski, J., Obrink, B., et al. 1995. C-CAM expression in odontogenesis and tooth eruption. Connect. Tissue Res. 32:201–207.

Luongo, C., Moser, A.R., Gledhill, S., et al. 1994. Loss of *Apc⁺* in intestinal adenomas from Min mice. Cancer Res. 54:5947–5952.

Lyngstadaas, S.P., Moinichen, C.B., and Risnes, S. 1998. Crown morphology, enamel distribution and enamel in mouse molars. Anat. Rec. 250:268–280.

Ma, A., Datta, M., Margosian, E., et al. 1995. T cells, but not B cells, are required for bowel inflammation in interleukin 2-deficient mice. J. Exp. Med. 182:1567–1572.

Mahler, J.F., Flagler, N.D., Malarkey, D.E., et al. 1998. Spontaneous and chemically induced proliferative lesions in Tg.AC transgenic and p53-heterozygous mice. Toxicol. Pathol. 26:501–511.

Mähler, M., Serreze, D., Evans, R., et al. 1996. *Il2^{tm1Hor}*, an interleukin-2 gene targeted mutation. Jax Notes 467:2–4.

Mähler, M., Hogan, M.E., Bedigian, H.G., et al. 1998. Gastric ulcers in steelDickie (*Mgf^{sl}/Mgf^{sl-D}*) mutant mice are not associated with *Helicobacter* infections. J. Exp. Anim. Sci. 38:159–164.

Mähler, M., Sundberg, J.P., Birkenmeier, E.H., et al. 1999. Genetic analysis of susceptibility to dextran sulfate sodium-induced colitis in mice. Genomics 55:147–156.

Majumder, K., Shawlot, W., Schuster, G., et al. 1998. Overbeek PA YAC rescue of downless locus mutations in mice. Mam. Genome 9:863–868.

Marks, S.C. and Lane, P.W. 1976. Osteopetrosis, a new recessive skeletal mutation on chromosome 12 of the mouse. J. Hered. 67:11–18.

Matsukura, N., Shirota, A., and Asano, G. 1985. Anatomy, histology, ultrastructure, stomach, rat. In: Digestive System. Monographs on Pathology of Laboratory Animal, ed. Jones, T.C., Mohr, U., Hunt, R.D. Heidelberg, Germany: Springer-Verlag, pp. 281–288.

Matzuk, M.M., Lu, N., Vogel, H., et al. 1995. Multiple defects and perinatal death in mice deficient in follistatin. Nature 374:360–363.

McDonald, S.A.C., Palmen, M.J.H.J., Van Rees, E.P., et al. 1997. Characterization of the mucosal cell-mediated immune response in IL2 knockout mice before and after the onset of colitis. Immunology 91:73–80.

Mizoguchi, A., Mizoguchi, E., Chiba, C., et al. 1996. Cytokine imbalance and autoantibody production in T cell receptor mutant mice with inflammatory bowel disease. J. Exp. Med. 183:847–856.

Mizoguchi, E., Mizoguchi, A., Chiba, C., et al. 1997. Antineutrophil cytoplasmic antibodies in T-cell receptor-deficient mice with chronic colitis. Gastroenterology 113:1828–1835.

Mohr, U., Dungworth, D.L., Capen, C.C., et al. 1996. Pathobiology of the Aging Mouse. Vol. 2. Washington, DC: ILSI Press.

Moinichen, C.B., Lyngstadaas, S.P., and Risnes, S. 1996. Morphological characteristics of mouse incisor enamel. J. Anat. 189:325–333.

Mombaerts, P., Clarke, A.R., Rudnicki, M.A., et al. 1992. Mutations in T-cell antigen receptor genes and block thymocyte development at different stages. Nature 360:225–231.

Mombaerts, P., Mizoguchi, E., Grusby, M.J., et al. 1993. Spontaneous development of inflammatory bowel disease in T cell receptor mutant mice. Cell 75:275–282.

Montagutelli, X., Lalouette, A., Boulouis, H.G., et al. 1997. Vesicle formation and follicular root sheath separation in mice homozygous for deleterious alleles in the balding (*bal*) locus. J. Invest. Dermatol. 109:324–328.

Montonen, O., Ezer, S., Saarialho-Kere, U.K., et al. 1998 The gene defective in anhidrotic ectodermal dysplasia is expressed in the developing epithelium, neuroectoderm, thymus and bone. J. Histochem. Cytochem. 46:281–289.

Moolenbeek, C. and Ruitenberg, E.J. 1981. The "Swiss roll": a simple technique for histological studies of the rodent intestine. Lab. Anim. 15:57–59.

Moore, K.W., O'Garra, A., de Waal Malefyt, R., et al. 1993. Interleukin-10. Annu. Rev. Immunol. 11:165–190.

Morasso, M.I., Grinberg, A., Robinson, G., et al. 1999. Placental failure in mice lacking the homeobox gene Dlx3. Proc. Natl. Acad. Sci. USA 96:162–167.

Moser, A.R., Pitot, H.C., and Dove, W.F. 1990. A dominant mutation that predisposes to multiple intestinal neoplasia in the mouse. Science 247:322–324.

Moser, A.R., Mattes, E.M., Dove, W.F., et al. 1993. *Apc^{Min}*, a mutation in the murine *Apc* gene, predisposes to mammary carcinogenesis and focal alveolar hyperplasias. Proc. Natl. Acad. Sci. USA 90:8977–8981.

Nakagawa, H., Wang, T.C., Zukerberg, L., et al. 1997. The targeting of the cyclin D1 oncogene by an EpsteinBarr virus promoter in transgenic mice causes dysplasia in the tongue, esophagus and forestomach. Oncogene 14:1185–1190.

Ness, S.L., Edelmann, W., Jenkins, T.D., et al. 1998. Mouse keratin 4 is necessary for internal epithelial integrity. J. Biol. Chem. 273:23904–23911.

Oshima, M., Oshima, H., Kitagawa, K., et al. 1995. Loss of Apc heterozygosity and abnormal tissue building in nascent intestinal polyps in mice carrying a truncated Apc gene. Proc. Natl. Acad. Sci. USA 92:4482–4486.

Oshima, M., Dinchuk, J.E., Kargman, S.L., et al. 1996. Suppression of intestinal polyposis in Apc716 knockout mice by inhibition of cyclooxygenase 2 (COX-2). Cell 87:803–809.

Penninger, J., Wallace, V.A., Kishihara, K., et al. 1991. Molecular organization, ontogeny and expression of murine alpha beta and gamma delta T cell receptors. Exp. Clin. Immunogenet. 8:57–74.

Peterkova, R., Lesot, H., Vonesch, J.L., et al. 1996. Mouse molar morphogenesis revisited by three dimensional reconstruction. I. Analysis of initial stages of the first upper molar development revealed two transient buds. Int. J. Dev. Biol. 40:1009–1016.

Peters, H. and Balling, R. 1999. Teeth where and how to make them. Trends Genet. 15:59–65.

Peters, H., Neubuser, A., Kratochwil, K., et al. 1998. *Pax9*-deficient mice lack pharyngeal pouch derivatives and teeth and exhibit craniofacial and limb abnormalities. Genes Dev. 12:2735–2747.

Philbrick, W.M., Dreyer, B.E., Nakchbandi, I.A., et al. 1998. Parathyroid hormone-related protein is required for tooth eruption. Proc. Natl. Acad. Sci. USA 95:11846–11851.

Podsypanina, K., Ellenson, L.H., Nemes, A., et al. 1999. Mutation of *Pten/Mmac1* in mice causes neoplasia in multiple organ systems. Proc. Natl. Acad. Sci. USA 96:1563–1568.

Price, J.A., Bowden, D.W., Wright, J.T., et al., 1998. Identification of a mutation in DLX3 associated with tricho-dento-osseous (TDO) syndrome. Hum. Mol. Genet. 7:563–569.

Que, B.G. and Wise, G.E. 1998. Tooth eruption molecules enhance MCP-1 gene expression in the dental follicle of the rat. Dev. Dyn. 212:346–351.

Randelia, H.P. and Lalithia, V.S. 1988. Megaoesophagus in ICRC mouse. Lab. Anim. 22:23–26.

Relyea, M.J., Miller, J., Boggess, D., et al. 1999. Necropsy methods for laboratory mice: biological characterization of a new mutation. In: Systematic Approach to Evaluation of Mouse Mutations, ed. Sundberg, J.P., Boggess, D. Boca Raton, FL: CRC Press, pp. 57–90.

Richard, G., De Laurenzi, V., Didona, B., et al. 1995. Keratin 13 point mutation underlies the hereditary mucosal epithelia disorder white sponge nevus. Nat. Genet. 11:453–455.

Rigg, E.L., McLean, W.H.I., Allison, W.E., et al. 1995. A mutation in mucosal keratin K4 is associated with oral white sponge nevus. Nat. Genet. 11:450–452.

Robinson, G.W. and Mahon, K.A. 1994. Differential and overlapping expression domains of D1x-2 and D1x-3 suggest distinct roles for Distal-less homeobox genes in craniofacial development. Mech. Dev. 48:199–215.

Rogers, J., Mahaney, M.C., Beamer, W.G., et al. 1997. Beyond one gene-one disease: alternative strategies for deciphering genetic determinants of osteoporosis. Calcif. Tissue Int. 60:225–228.

Rosen, C.J., Dimai, H.P., Vereault, D., et al. 1997. Circulating and skeletal insulin-like growth factor-I (*IGFI*) concentrations in two inbred strains of mice with different bone mineral densities. Bone 21:217–223

Rubinfeld, B., Souza, B., Albert, I., et al. 1993. Association of the *APC* gene product with beta-catenin. Science 262:1731–1734.

Ruchon, A.F., Marcinkiewicz, M., Siegfried, G., et al. 1998. *Pex* mRNA is localized in developing mouse osteoblasts and odontoblasts. J. Histochem. Cytochem. 46:459–468.

Rudolph, U., Finegold, M.J., Rich, S.S., et al. 1995. Ulcerative colitis and adenocarcinoma of the colon in Gi2-deficient mice. Nat. Genet. 10:143–150.

Sadlack, B., Merz, H., Schorle, H., et al. 1993. Ulcerative colitis-like disease in mice with a disrupted interleukin-2 gene. Cell 75:253–261.

Sadlack, B., Löhler, J., Schorle, H., et al. 1995. Generalized autoimmune disease in interleukin-2-deficient mice is triggered by an uncontrolled activation and proliferation of CD4+ T cells. Eur. J. Immunol. 25:3053–3059.

Salomon, D.S., Kim, N., Saeki, T., et al. 1990. Transforming growth factor-alpha: an oncodevelopmental growth factor. Cancer Cells 2:389–397.

Sasaki, T., Goldberg, M., Takuma, S., et al. 1990. Cell biology of tooth formation. Monogr. Oral Sci. 14:1–204.

Scharschmidt, B.F. 1977. The natural history of hypertrophic gastrophy (Menetrier's disease). Report of a case with 16 year followup and review of 120 cases from the literature. Am. J. Med. 63:644–652.

Schorle, H., Holtschke, T., Hünig, T., et al. 1991. Development and function of T cells in mice rendered interleukin-2 deficient by gene targeting. Nature 352:621–624.

Searle, P.F., Thomas, D.P., Faulkner, K.B., et al. 1994. Stomach cancer in transgenic mice expressing human papillomavirus type 16 early region genes from a keratin promoter. J. Gen. Virol. 75:1125–1137.

Sellon, R.K., Tonkonogy, S.L., Grable, H., et al. 1997. Development of spontaneous colitis in IL-10 knockout mice requires normal enteric bacterial flora. Gastroenterology 112:A1088.

Shah, S.A., Simpson, S.J., Brown, L.F., et al. 1998. Development of colonic adenocarcinoma in a mouse model of ulcerative colitis. Inflam. Bowel Dis. 4:196–202.

Sharp, R., Babyatsky, M.W., Takagi, H., et al. 1995. Transforming growth factor α disrupts the normal program of cellular differentiation in the gastric mucosa of transgenic mice. Development 121:149–161.

Sharpe, P.T. 1995. Homeobox genes and orofacial development. Connect. Tissue Res. 32:17–25.

Shultz, L.D. and Sundberg, J.P. 1994. The motheaten (*me*) and viable motheaten (*me^v*) mutations, chromosome 6. In: Handbook of Mouse Mutations with Skin and Hair Abnormalities: Animal Models and Biomedical Tools, ed. Sundberg, J.P. Boca Raton, FL: CRC Press, pp. 351–358.

Simpson, S.J., Mizoguchi, E., Allen, D., et al. 1995. Evidence that CD4+, but not CD8+ T cells, are responsible for murine interleukin-2-deficient colitis. Eur. J. Immunol. 25:2618–2625.

Smith, K.A. 1992. Interleukin-2. Curr. Opin. Immunol. 4:271–276.

Smits, R., van der Houven van Oordt, W., Luz, A., et al. 1998. Apc1638N: a mouse model for familial adenomatous polyposis-associated desmoid tumors and cutaneous cysts. Gastroenterology 114:275–283.

Sofaer, J.A. 1969a. Aspects of the tabby-crinkled-downless syndrome I. The development of tabby teeth. J. Embryol. Exp. Morphol. 22:181–205.

Sofaer, J.A. 1969b. Aspects of the tabby-crinkled-downless syndrome II. Observations on the reaction to changes of genetic background. J. Embryol. Exp. Morphol. 22:207–227.

Sofaer, J.A. 1977a. Tooth development in the "crooked" mouse. J. Embryol. Exp. Morphol. 41:279–287.

Sofaer, J.A. 1977b. The teeth of the "sleek" mouse. Arch. Oral Biol. 22:299–301.

Sofaer, J.A. 1979. Additive effects of the genes tabby and crinkled on tooth size in the mouse. Genet. Res. 33:169–174.

Sorensen, I.K., Kristiansen, E., Mortensen, A., et al. 1997. Short-term carcinogenicity testing of a potent murine intestinal mutagen, 2-amino-1-methyl-6-phenylimidazo(4,5-b)pyridine (PhIP), in Apc1638N transgenic mice. Carcinogenesis 18:777–781.

Soriano, P., Montgomery, C., Geske, R., et al. 1991. Targeted mutations of the c-src proto-oncogene leads to osteopetrosis in mice. Cell 64:693–702.

Srivastava, A.K., Pispa, J., Hartung, A.J., et al. 1997. The Tabby phenotype is caused by mutation in a mouse homologue of the EDA gene that reveals novel mouse and human exons and encodes a protein (ectodysplasin-A) with collagenous domains. Proc. Natl. Acad. Sci. USA 94:13069–13074.

Steele, G., Jr. 1993. Accomplishments and promise in the understanding and treatment of colorectal cancer. Lancet 342:1092–1096.

Strayer, D.S., Yang, S., and Schwartz, M.S. 1993. Epiderminal growth factor-like growth factors. I. Breast malignancies and other epithelial proliferations in transgenic mice. Lab. Invest. 69:660–673.

Strom, T.M., Francis, F., Lorenz, B., et al. 1997. Pex gene deletions in Gy and Hyp mice provide mouse models for X-linked hypophosphatemia. Human Mol. Genet. 6:165–171.

Su, L.-K., Kinzler, K.W., Vogelstein, B., et al. 1992. Multiple intestinal neoplasia caused by a mutation in the murine homologue of the APC gene. Science 256:668–670.

Sundberg, J.P. 1989. Meckel's diverticulum in laboratory mice. Jax Notes 439:3–4.

Sundberg, J.P. 1994. The balding (bal) mutation, chromosome 18. In: Handbook of Mouse Mutations with Skin and Hair Abnormalities. Animal Models and Biomedical Tools, ed. Sundberg, J.P. Boca Raton, FL: CRC Press, pp. 187–191.

Sundberg, J.P., Kenty, G.A., Beamer, W.G., et al. 1992. Forestomach papillomas in flaky skin and steelDickie mutant mice. J. Vet. Diagn. Invest. 4:312–317.

Sundberg, J.P., Elson, C.O., Bedigian, H., et al. 1994. Spontaneous, heritable colitis in a new substrain of C3H/HeJ mice. Gastroenterology 107:1726–1735.

Sundberg, J.P., France, M., Boggess, D., et al. 1997. Development and progression of psoriasiform dermatitis and systemic lesions in the flaky skin (fsn) mouse mutant. Pathobiology 65:271–286.

Sundberg, J.P., Montagutelli, X., and Boggess, D. 1998a. Systematic approach to evaluation of mouse mutations with cutaneous appendage defects. In: Molecular Basis of Epithelial Appendage Morphogenesis, ed. Chuong, C.M. Austin: R.G. Landes Company, pp. 421–435.

Sundberg, J.P., Shultz, L.D., King, L.E., et al. 1998b. The spontaneous balding and desmoglein 3 null mutations: mouse models for pemphigus vulgaris. Comp. Pathol. Bull. 30:3–4.

Sweet, H.O., Marks, S.C., MacKay, C.A., et al. 1996. Dense incisors (din): a new mouse mutation on chromosome 16 affecting tooth eruption and body size. J. Hered. 87:162–167.

Takagi, H., Jhappan, C., Sharp, R., et al. 1992. Hypertrophic gastropathy resembling Menetrier's disease in transgenic mice overexpressing transforming growth factor α in the stomach. J. Clin. Invest. 90:1161–1167.

Takagi, H., Fukusato, T., Kawaharada, U., et al. 1997. Histochemical analysis of hyperplastic stomach of TGFα transgenic mice. Dig. Dis. Sci. 42:91–98.

Takahashi, I., Kiyono, H., and Hamada, S. 1997. CD4+ T-cell population mediates development of inflammatory bowel disease in T-cell receptor chain-deficient mice. Gastroenterology 112:1876–1886.

Takaku, K., Oshima, M., Miyoshi, H., et al. 1998. Intestinal tumorigenesis in compound mutant mice of both Dpc4 (Smad4) and Apc genes. Cell 92:645–656.

Tamai, Y., Nakajima, R., Ishikawa, T., et al. 1999. Colonic hamartoma development by an anomalous duplication in Cdx2 knockout mice. Cancer Res. 59:2965–2970.

Tamano, S., Jakubczak, J., Takagi, H., et al. 1995. Increased susceptibility to N-nitrosomethylurea gastric carcinogenesis in transforming growth factor alpha transgenic mice with gastric hyperplasia. Jap. J. Cancer Res. 86:435–443.

Thesleff, I. and Sharpe, P.T. 1997. Signaling networks regulating dental development. Mech. Dev. 67:111–123.

Thomas, B.L., Tucker, A.S., Qiu, M., et al. 1997. Role of Dlx-1 and Dlx-2 genes in patterning of the murine dentition. Development 124:4811–4818.

Tissier-Seta, J.P., Mucchielli, M.L., Mark, M., et al. 1995. Barx1, a new mouse homeodomain transcription factor expressed in cranio-facial ectomesenchyme and the stomach. Mech. Dev. 51:3:15.

Tracey, C. and Roberts, G.J. 1985. A radiographic study of dental development in the hypopituitary dwarf mouse. Arch. Oral Biol. 11/12:805–811.

Tucker, A.S., Matthews, K.L., and Sharpe, P.T. 1998. Transformation of tooth type by inhibition of BMP signalling. Science 282:1136–1138.

Turner, A.J. and Tanzawa, K. 1997. Mammalian membrane metalloendopeptidases: NEP, ECE, KELL, and PEX. F.A.S.E.B. J. 11:355–364.

Ullrich, S.J., Zeng, Z.Z., and Jay, G. 1994. Transgenic mouse models of human gastric and hepatic carcinomas. Semin. Cancer Biol. 5:61–68.

van der Houven van Oordt, C.W., Smits, R., Schouten, T.G., et al. 1999. The genetic background modifies the spontaneous and X-ray-induced tumor spectrum in the Apc1638N mouse model. Genes Chromosomes Cancer 24:191–198.

van Genderen, C., Okamura, R.M., Farinas, I., et al. 1994. Development of several organs that require inductive epithelial-mesenchymal interactions is impaired in Lef-1-deficient mice. Genes Dev. 8:2691–2703.

Vastardis, H., Karimbux, N., Guthua, S.W., et al. 1996. A human MSX1 homeodomain missense mutation causes selective tooth agenesis. Nat. Genet. 13:417–421.

Wang, J., Niu, W., Nikiforov, Y., et al. 1997. Targeted overexpression of IGF-I evokes distinct patterns of organ remodeling in smooth muscle cell tissue beds of transgenic mice. J. Clin. Invest. 100:1425–1439.

Wang, J., Niu, W., Witte, D.P., et al. 1998. Overexpression of insulinlike growth factor-binding protein-4 (IGFBP-4) in smooth muscle cells of transgenic mice through a smooth muscle alpha-actin-IGFBP-4 fusion gene induces smooth muscle hypoplasia. Endocrinology 139:2605–2614.

Watanabe, M., Ueno, Y., Yajima, T., et al. 1998. Interleukin 7 transgenic mice develop chronic colitis with decreased interleukin 7 protein accumulation in the colonic mucosa. J. Exp. Med. 187:389–402.

Weiss, K.M., Ruddle, F.H, Bollekens, J. 1995. D1x and other homeobox genes in the morphological development of the dentition. Connect. Tissue Res. 32:35–40.

Willerford, D.M., Chen, J., Ferry, J.A., et al. 1995. Inter-leukin-2 receptor chain regulates the size and content of the peripheral lymphoid compartment. Immunity 3:521–530.

Wright, J.T., Hansen, L., Mahler, J., et al. 1995. Odontogenic tumours in the v-Ha-ras (TG.AC) transgenic mouse. Arch. Oral Biol. 40:631–638.

Yang, K., Edelmann, W., Fan, K., et al. 1998. Dietary modu-lation of carcinoma development in a mouse model for human familial adenomatous polyposis. Cancer Res. 58:5713–5717.

Yoshida, H., Hayashi, S., Kunisada, T., et al. 1990. The murine mutation osteopetrosis is in the coding region of the macrophage colony stimulating factor gene. Nature 345:442–444.

Zhang, Y., Zhao, X., Hu, Y., et al. 1999. Msx1 is required for the induction of Patched by Sonic hedgehog in the mam-malian tooth germ. Dev. Dyn. 215:45-53.

Zhu, Y., Richardson, J.A., Parada, L.F., et al. 1998. Smad3 mutant mice develop metastatic colorectal cancer. Cell 94:703–714.

# 20

# Inflammatory Bowel Disease in Mouse Models: Role of Gastrointestinal Microbiota as Proinflammatory Modulators

James G. Fox, Charles A. Dangler, and David B. Schauer

Inflammatory bowel disease (IBD), an idiopathic, chronic disease, has been recognized as a serious clinical entity since the early 1900s. Although manifestations of IBD may vary, two major syndromes have been classified into Crohn's disease (CD) and ulcerative colitis (UC). Crohn's disease is defined as a chronic transmural inflammation that may affect any portion of the gastrointestinal tract, whereas in ulcerative colitis, the inflammation is restricted to the large intestine and the inflammation is largely confined to the mucosa. The prevalence of UC in the human population approaches 0.03–0.08 percent whereas in CD the prevalence is approximately 0.01–0.08 percent. Interestingly, there is an increasing incidence of CD being recognized in developed countries (Montgomery et al. 1999).

Though poorly defined, IBD is considered to be the result of a combination of genetic and environmental factors. Microbial flora are undoubtedly an important component of the disease process, in which microbial antigens are thought to initiate and promote inflammation, particularly in the presence of immune dysregulation or an impaired mucosal barrier in the susceptible host (Fiocchi 1998; Panwala et al. 1998).

Given the experimental limitations of studying IBD in humans, animal models have been used with some success in attempting to unravel and comprehend this complex disease process. Spontaneous IBDs in animals, most notably a UC-like syndrome in the cotton-top tamarin, have assisted in this process, but their limited availability has curtailed their use (Johnson et al. 1996; Saunders et al. 1999). Chemically induced IBD rodent models have also been used, but they do not mimic the full spectra of IBD observed in humans (Elson et al. 1995). However, with the introduction and widespread use of genetically engineered mice, many of which have dysregulated immune responses, IBD, an unexpected phenotype, was noted. The disease, in retrospect, could have been predicted in some mice (e.g., IL-10$^{-/-}$) but not in others (IL-2$^{-/-}$). The purpose of this chapter is (1) to discuss the advantages of using defined microflora mice to study gastrointestinal disease, (2) to review the murine data on experimentally induced persistent gastric *Helicobacter* spp. infection in the context of a model of persistent mucosal inflammation, and (3) to highlight mouse models of IBD with particular emphasis on the role that enterohepatic murine *Helicobacter* spp. play in the development and progression of this disease (Tables 20.1 and 20.2).

## INTESTINAL FLORA OF THE MOUSE

The gastrointestinal tract of mice as well as other mammals is colonized with a diverse microecosystem. The ceca of mice contain multiple microbial species and can reach levels of $10^{11}$ bacteria/g of feces (Schaedler et al. 1965b; Schaedler and Orcutt 1983). These microorganisms provide essential nutrients for their host (e.g.,

This work, was supported, in part, by NIH Grants R01DK52413, R01CA67529, and PO1CA26731.

**TABLE 20.1.  Characteristics of formally named rodent *Helicobacter* species**

| Taxon | Catalase production | Nitrate reduction | Alkaline phophatase hydrolysis | Urease | Indoxyl acetate hydrolysis | γ-glutamyl transpeptidase | Growth at 42°C |
|---|---|---|---|---|---|---|---|
| *H. rodentium* | + | + | − | − | − | − | + |
| *H. trogontum* | + | + | − | + | ND | + | + |
| *H. muridarum* | + | − | + | + | + | + | − |
| *H. hepaticus* | + | + | ND | + | + | ND | − |
| *H. bilis* | + | + | ND | + | − | ND | + |
| "*H. rappini*" | + | − | − | + | ND | + | + |
| *H. cinaedi* | + | + | − | − | − | − | − |
| *H. cholecystus* | + | + | + | − | − | − | + |

| Taxon | Growth with 1% glycine | Susceptibility to Nalidixic acid (30 µg disc) | Cephalothin (30 µg disc) | Periplasmic fibers | Number of flagella | Distribution of flagella | G + C content (mol %) |
|---|---|---|---|---|---|---|---|
| *H. rodentium* | + | R | R | − | 2 | Bipolar | ND |
| *H. trogontum* | ND | R | R | + | 5–7 | Bipolar | ND |
| *H. muridarum* | − | R | R | + | 10–14 | Bipolar | 34 |
| *H. hepaticus* | + | R | R | − | 2 | Bipolar | ND |
| *H. bilis* | + | R | R | + | 3–14 | Bipolar | ND |
| "*H. rappini*" | − | R | R | + | 10–20 | Bipolar | 34 |
| *H. cinaedi* | + | S | I | − | 1–2 | Bipolar | 37–38 |
| *H. cholecystus* | + | I | R | − | 2 | Bipolar | ND |

Source: Data were obtained from Versalovic and Fox 1999.

Note: Symbols and abbreviations: +, positive reaction; −, negative reaction; S, susceptible; R, resistant; I, intermediate; ND, not determined.

**TABLE 20.2.  *Helicobacter hepaticus* and other novel *Helicobacter* spp.–associated IBD in mice**

| Genetic status of mice | Type of defect | Pathology | Pathogenesis CD4[+] |
|---|---|---|---|
| CD45RB[high]-reconstituted SCIDs | Reconstitution with naïve CD4[+] T cell | Typhlocolitis | Mediated by CD4[+] T cells ↑ IFN-γ ↑TNFα |
| TCR-defined flora |  |  |  |
| SCID ICR-defined flora[a] | Lack T and B cell | Typhlocolitis | Macrophage |
| IL-10[−/− b] | Knockout | Typhlocolitis | ↑ Th1, CD4[+] T cells involved |
| RAG -2[−/−] | Knockout | Typhlocolitis | MHC class II ↑ |
|  |  |  | Lack T and B cells macrophage infiltration WBC ↑ |
| IL-7[−/−]/RAG-2[−/−] | Double knockout | None | Lack T and B cells and IL-7 |
| A/JCr | Normal | Typhlitis | Th1 ↑ IFN-γ ↑ |
| Swiss-Webster gnotobiotic | Normal | Enterocolitis | ND |

Note: In mice of same genetic status that had *H. hepaticus* (or other *Helicobacter* spp.)–negative microflora, no intestinal disease was noted. ND = not determined.

[a]Mice infected with *H. bilis* (Shomer et al. 1997).

[b]IBD also produced in IL-10[−/−] mice experimentally infected with a novel urease-negative *Helicobacter* sp. (Fox et al. 1999).

vitamin K) and colonize mucosal niches in which their presence, in part, helps protect the host against microbial pathogens (Thompson 1978; Schaedler and Orcutt 1983; Steffen and Berg 1983; Hentges et al. 1985; Kennedy and Volz 1985; Wells et al. 1987).

Numerous studies have demonstrated the increased susceptibility of germ-free mice to a variety of infectious agents when compared with mice with the normal complement of microorganisms (Gordon and Pesti 1971). For example, conventionalization with normal fecal flora of germ-free BALB/c mice monocolonized with *Campylobacter jejuni* eliminated viable *C. jejuni* from the ceca (Yrios and Balish 1986). Interestingly, in the context of IBD in mice, IL-10[−/−] mice prone to develop IBD at an early age are protected from colitis if *Lactobacillus* spp. are orally inoculated into neonatal mice.

The authors stated that normalizing *Lactobacillus* spp. levels reduced colonic mucosal adherent and translocated bacteria and prevented colitis (Madsen et al. 1999). In contrast, C$_3$H/HeOuJ mice either infected with *Serpulina hyodysenteriae*, the etiological cause of swine dysentery, or exposed to the β hemolysin of *S. hyodysenteriae* induced cecal lesions 30 hours postinfection. Ultrastructural changes consisted of loss of microvilli and terminal webs, plus necrosis and exfoliation of epithelial cells. Translocation of *Helicobacter*-like organisms, present as luminal bacteria prior to experimental infection with *S. hyodysenteriae*, appeared to play a unique role in lesion development in this mouse model (Hutto and Wannemuehler 1999). Thus, the ecology of bacterial flora in the lower bowel is critical in terms of assessing and predicting intestinal inflammation (Falk et al. 1998).

# DEFINED MURINE MICROFLORA (ALTERED SCHAEDLER FLORA)

Gnotobiotic animals colonized with known microbiota have been extensively used for biomedical research (Gordon and Pesti 1971). For specific studies, it is particularly desirable to colonize germ-free mice with a defined microbiota. Three decades ago, germ-free mice were colonized with selected bacteria isolated from "normal" mice (Schaedler et al. 1965a). Schaedler, who developed this microbial model system, subsequently supplied commercial animal breeders with these microorganisms (Baker 1966) for use in colonizing their rodent colonies. Defined microbial flora consisted of the easier-to-grow aerobic bacteria along with some of the less oxygen-sensitive anaerobic bacteria. The EOS (extremely oxygen-sensitive) fusiform-shaped bacteria, which make up the vast majority of the normal microbiota of rodents, were not included due to the technical difficulties in isolating and cultivating EOS bacteria (Lee et al. 1968). Of the defined microbiota subsequently utilized in gnotobiotic experiments, the "Schaedler Flora" was the most popular. It contained eight bacteria, designated *Streptococcus faecalis*, *Lactobacillus acidophilus*, *L. salivarius*, Group N *Streptococcus*, *Bacteroides distasonis*, a *Clostridium* sp., *Escherichia coli* var. *mutabilis*, and an EOS fusiform-shaped bacterium.

The "Schaedler Flora" or "cocktail" of eight bacteria was later reconstituted in 1978 in order to standardize the microbiota to be used in colonizing axenic (germ-free) rodents. The new defined microbiota (i.e., the "Altered Schaedler Flora" [ASF]) consisted of four members of the original "Schaedler Flora" (the two lactobacilli, *Bacteroides,* and the EOS fusiform-shaped

bacterium), a spiral-shaped bacterium, and three new fusiform-shaped EOS bacteria (Orcutt et al. 1987). The altered "Schaedler Flora" specifically excluded *E. coli* to avoid confusion in experiments designed to define the pathogenic potential of *E. coli* serotypes and other closely related bacteria.

Although very important, it is difficult to monitor a gnotobiotic mouse colony with a defined microbiota. The validation process requires that the mouse colony is free of any adventitious microorganisms, but it must also be demonstrated that the microorganisms of the specified microbiota are present. Historically, the monitoring of gnotobiotic rodents relied on examining the morphology of the microorganisms and a limited evaluation of the organisms, biochemical traits, and growth characteristics of the organisms.

Because of the limitations of the monitoring system used to identify the bacteria in ASF, we recently characterized their phylogenetic positions relative to known bacteria by utilizing 16S rRNA sequence analysis (Dewhirst et al. 1999). Three strains previously identified on phenotypic criteria as *L. acidophilus* (ASF 360), *L. salivarius* (ASF 361), and *B. distasonis* (ASF 519) differed from their original identification when 16S rRNA analysis was used. Strain ASF 361 has an identical 16S rRNA sequence with the type strains of *L. murinus* and *L. animalis* (each isolated from mice), indicating that all strains likely represent a single species (Fig. 20.1). Strain ASF 360 represents a novel lactobacillus clustering with *L. acidophilus* and *L. lactis*. Strain ASF 519 falls into an unnamed genus with [*Bacteroides*] *distasonis*, [*Bacteroides*] *merdae*, [*Bacteroides*] *forsythus*, and CDC group DF-3. This unnamed genus is in the *Cytophaga/Flavobacterium/Bacteroides* phylum, most closely related to the genus *Porphyromonas*. The spiral-shaped strain, ASF 457, is in the *Flexistipes* phylum and has sequence identity with rodent isolates of Robertson (1998). The remaining four ASF extremely oxygen-sensitive fusiform-shaped bacteria group phylogenetically into the low G + C Gram-positive bacteria (*Firmicutes, Bacillus/ Clostridium* group). ASF 356, ASF 492, and ASF 502 fall into *Clostridium* cluster XIV of Collins et al. (1994). Morphologically, ASF 492 resembles members of this cluster, *Roseburia cecicola*, and *Eubacterium plexicaudatum*. The 16S rRNA sequence for ASF 492 is identical to that of *Eu. plexicaudatum*. Strain ASF 492 is a candidate for a neotype strain. Strain ASF 500 branches deeply in the low G + C Gram-positive phylogenetic tree but is not closely related to any organisms whose 16S rRNA sequences are currently in GenBank. This 16S rRNA sequence information will allow rapid identification of ASF strains and will permit detailed analysis of the interactions of ASF organisms in the development

(% Difference)

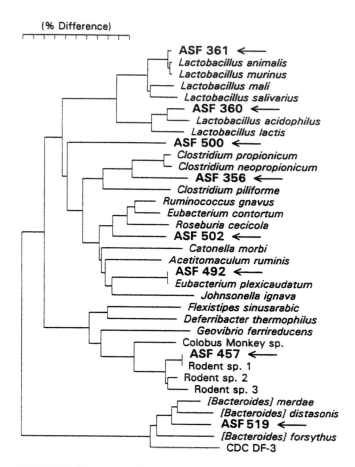

**FIGURE 20.1** Dendogram depicting taxonomic classification of Altered Schaedler Flora.

of IBD in mice co-infected with a variety of known or suspected pathogenic microorganisms.

# EXPERIMENTAL MOUSE MODELS OF *HELICOBACTER*-INDUCED GASTRIC DISEASE

The discovery of *Helicobacter pylori* as a cause of chronic, persistent gastritis and peptic ulcer disease, and more recently the bacterium's association with gastric adenocarcinoma and mucosa-associated lymphoid tissue lymphoma, are classic examples of how previously unrecognized microbial agents are critical to our understanding of poorly defined disease processes.

Germ-free mice were the first rodents to be successfully colonized with *H. felis* (Lee et al. 1990). Fortunately, conventional and SPF mice also can be persistently infected with *H. felis*. In the first description of *H. felis* gastritis in the germ-free mouse, along with an acute inflammatory response, a moderate degree of glandular epithelial cell hyperplasia was evident at

4 weeks postinfection in portions of the gastric mucosa. This was characterized by an overall increase in thickness of the mucosa in areas of inflamed tissue (Lee et al. 1990). The changes included lack of epithelial cell maturation and differentiation, increased basophilia, and increased nuclear to cytoplasmic ratio. Also of interest was the enlargement of individual glands and the presence of columnar-type epithelium versus cuboidal epithelium. Occasional branching of glands was noted as well as luminal epithelium forming small pseudovillous projections (Lee et al. 1990). These lesions persisted for the duration of the 8-week study. It is now known that persistent, active, chronic gastritis occurs for at least 1 year in germ-free and SPF mice infected with *H. felis* (Fox et al. 1993). Studies of 72- to 76-week colonization of conventional and SPF mice have provided additional clues on progression of the lesions in the stomach of infected mice. Furthermore, conventional mice, persistently infected with either *H. felis* or *H. heilmannii* and also cocolonized with *H. muridarum* in the lower bowel and stomach, had more significant lesions than the SPF mice, which had either *H. felis* or *H. heilmannii* infection only (Lee et al. 1993). Indeed, the conventional mice co-infected with enterohepatic and gastric helicobacters showed significant glandular atrophy of the gastric corpus and in some cases apparent dysplasia of the glandular element (Lee et al. 1993).

Studies of the role of genetic factors in the pathogenesis of *Helicobacter*-associated gastritis have taken advantage of the wide range of inbred and other types of genetically defined mice. Three inbred strains of mice inoculated with *H. felis* had varying levels of intensity of inflammation: in BALB/c mice inflammation was minimal, in C3H/He moderate, and in C57BL/6 most severe when examined up to 11 weeks postinfection (Mohammadi et al. 1996b). The authors also stated that C57BL/6 mice had mucous cell hyperplasia and parietal cell loss in gastric fundic glands. Furthermore, the study demonstrated that by using congenic strains of the BALB/c and C57BL/6 background both MHC and non-MHC genes contributed to *H. felis*–associated gastritis.

Results of analyzing the effect of chronic *H. felis* infection on p53 heterozygous C57BL/6 and their wild-type counterpart C57BL/6 also have been published (Fox et al. 1996a). One year after infection with *H. felis*, the wild-type and p53 heterozygous mice showed severe adenomatous and cystic hyperplasia of the gastric pit or foveolar epithelium. BrdU incorporation and PCNA staining were markedly increased in both sets of infected mice compared with controls, and infected p53 hemizygous mice had a higher proliferative index than the infected wild-type mice. Perhaps the most surprising finding was the effect of *H. felis* infection on the wild-type C57BL/6 mouse. Previous studies

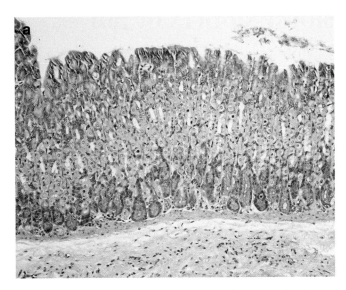

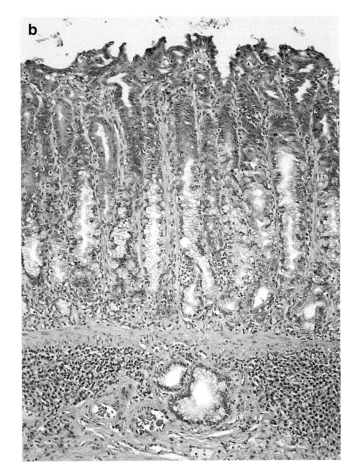

**FIGURE 20.2** Chronic gastric helicobacter infection in C57BL/6 mice results in marked inflammation and mucosal alterations focused largely on the gastric corpus. (**a**) Normal corpus mucosal histology. (**b**) Chronic gastric infection with *H. felis* in a C57BL/6 mouse. Intense chronic inflammation in the submucosa and mucosa is accompanied by marked mucosal changes. Within the corpus mucosa, the parietal cells and chief cells in the glandular zone have been replaced by a hypertrophic metaplastic mucous epithelium. The gastric pit epithelium is hyperchromic and extends down into the superficial glandular zone. A focus of invasive epithelial hyperplasia is present in the submucosa. The invasive glandular nest is lined by the metaplastic mucous epithelium.

in which *H. felis* was inoculated in Swiss-Webster mice revealed chronic active inflammation with minimal hyperplasia, but the histological changes did not approach the severity of gastric disease shown by the presence of extensive proliferation, gastritis, mucous metaplasia, glandular atrophy, and invasive hyperplasia (Fig. 20.2) in the C57BL/6 mice after *H. felis* infection. However, previous investigators have pointed out that the gastric phenotype is strongly influenced by the genetic background of the mouse. For example, overexpression of transforming growth factor α in inbred FVB/N mice leads to much more severe cystic hyperplasia compared with that observed in the outbred Swiss mice (Takagi et al. 1992).

Importantly, recent studies showed that only the C57BL/6 strain, not the BALB/c and C3H/HeJ, had increased proliferation and apoptosis in the gastric corpus epithelium in response to *H. felis* infection (Wang et al. 1998). In addition, the C57BL/6 mouse showed a marked loss of parietal and chief cells, along with a marked expansion of gastric cell lineage that stained positive for spasmolytic polypeptide. In contrast, no significant change in these cell types was observed in BALB/c and C3H/HeJ strains. Increased expression of the secreted form of type II phospholipase $A_2$ ($sPLA_2$) was observed in BALB/c and C3H/HeJ after *H. felis* infection, whereas $sPLA_2$ expression was absent in C57BL/6 mice. These studies demonstrate that *H. felis* infection leads to increased apoptosis and altered cellular differentiation in the C57BL/6 mouse, a strain that lacks gastric $sPLA_2$ expression. Because $sPLA_2$ has recently been identified as the MOM1 (modifier of the multiple intestinal neoplasia) locus that influences polyp formation in the colon, these studies suggest that $sPLA_2$ may also influence the gastric epithelial response to *Helicobacter* infection (Wang et al. 1998). Thus, studies indicating that particular inbred strains of mice have differing severities of *H. felis*–induced gastritis point to the importance of the genetic makeup in determining the response to chronic *Helicobacter* infection in the stomach as well as the lower gastrointestinal tract.

## Immune Response in Gastric *Helicobacter* Infection

What role cell-mediated immunity plays in protection against chronic colonization with *Helicobacter* or in the progression of *Helicobacter*-associated gastric lesions has not been clearly delineated. Mononuclear cells obtained from the blood of *H. pylori*–infected patients had a lower in vitro proliferative index to *H. pylori* antigens than similar cells isolated from control patients (Karttunen 1991; Knipp et al. 1993). This data suggested that *H. pylori* may suppress host cell–mediated immune responses by production of an inhibitory factor (Knipp et al. 1996). However, inhibition of cell-mediated immune responses was not found in *H. felis*–infected mice, where mononuclear cell proliferation was positively correlated with infection (Mohammadi et al. 1996a). A Th1-like immune response to *H. pylori* in humans and *H. felis* infection in mice is manifested by the presence of inflammatory cells that produce interferon-γ (IFN-γ) in excess over interleukin-4 (Karttunen et al. 1995; Mohammadi et al. 1996a; D'Elios et al. 1997). Also, *H. pylori*–associated gastritis and ulcers in humans are considered by some to result from a Th1-type delayed hypersensitivity response (D'Elios et al. 1997; Bamford et al. 1998).

Mice with immune dysregulation are beginning to be utilized in studying gastric disease induced by *Helicobacter* spp. For example, IL-10⁻/⁻ mice on a 129/SvEv background that were infected with *H. felis* developed severe hyperplastic gastritis, including a profound loss of parietal and chief cells within 4 weeks postinfection (Berg et al. 1998). Thus, in the absence of IL-10, the inflammatory and immunological responses in the mouse to *H. felis* infection evolve very rapidly and create significant gastric lesions.

Undoubtedly with time, more transgenic and targeted mutagenesis models will become available that have specifically targeted genetic alterations of the gastric mucosa. Of particular importance will be the identification of genes that modulate the mucous neck cells of glands colonized by where *Helicobacter* spp. tend to colonize; indeed, it may be these gastric cells that undergo malignant transformation. The knowledge gained from *Helicobacter*-associated gastritis of mice has particular relevance in studying *Helicobacter*-associated IBD in murine models. For example, given that most immune dysregulated mice with targeted gene disruption are on a C57BL/6 background, the *H. felis* infection studies in the C57BL/6 mouse may help explain proliferative and inflammatory intestinal lesions observed in immune dysregulated mice on this genetic background in response to enteric helicobacter infection.

# MOUSE MODELS OF IBD

Since the original descriptions of IBD in several knockout mice such as IL-10⁻/⁻, IL-2⁻/⁻, TCR-α⁻/⁻, and TCR-β⁻/⁻, the list of genetically engineered mice with IBD has continually grown (Table 20.3; Fig. 20.3; Kuhn et al. 1993; Mombaerts et al. 1993; Sadlack et al. 1993). Many of these mouse models of IBD have an immune dysregulation, whereas in other mice, for example those deficient in keratin 8 and transgenic mice expressing a dominant-negative N-cadherin, there is a defect in intestinal barrier function (Baribault et al. 1994; Hermiston and Gordon 1995). Mice lacking trefoil factor are susceptible to colitis after mild mucosal injuries, strengthening the argument that an impaired mucosal defense mechanism predisposes the intestine to inflammation (Mashimo et al. 1996). Similarly, mice lacking a multidrug resistance gene (*Mdr1a*) also develop a spontaneous IBD syndrome (Foltz et al. 1997; Panwala et al. 1998).

Berg et al. also showed that inheritable factors strongly influenced the expression of IBD in IL-10⁻/⁻ mice on varying genetic backgrounds (Berg et al. 1996). In 3-month-old mutants, intestinal lesions were most severe in the 129 and BALB/c/SvEv background, intermediate severity was noted in the IL-10⁻/⁻ 129 × C57Bl /6J, and the least severe lesions were recorded in IL-10⁻/⁻ C57BL/6J mice.

Furthermore, the development of IBD in several mouse models after transfer of various T cell subsets have clearly defined the importance of T cells in modulating intestinal inflammation. Generalized autoimmune disease, including colitis in IL-2⁻/⁻, is a B cell–independent but T cell–dependent mechanism that triggers an activation and proliferation of CD4⁺ T cells (Ma et al. 1995; Sadlack et al. 1995). Many of these other IBD mouse models also have intestinal inflammation directly linked with CD4⁺ T cells and a Th1-like (i.e., interferon-γ and tumor necrosis factor α) inflammatory response (Powrie et al. 1993, 1994; Kullberg et al. 1998). Studies in Tac:Icr:Ha(ICR)-*scid*/DF and RAG–2–deficient mice infected with *Helicobacter* spp., with marked macrophage infiltration in the lamina propria, and elevated production of iNOS in *H. hepaticus*–infected IL-10⁻/⁻ mice, strongly suggest a pivotal role for macrophages in development of colitis and typhlitis in the IBD murine model (Kullberg et al. 1998; von Freeden-Jeffry et al. 1998). T cell function abnormalities in mouse models of IBD may or may not be developmental defects. For example, appendectomy of TCR-α⁻/⁻ mice at 6 weeks of age prevented the subsequent development of IBD as well as eliminated the IBD-associated antibody response to the intestinal microflora (Mizo-

**TABLE 20.3. Inflammatory bowel disease in mutant mice**

| Targeted gene or gene product | Type of defect | Pathology | Microflora influence | Immunologic abnormalities | Genetic background effect |
|---|---|---|---|---|---|
| IL-2 | Knockout | Anemia; acute and chronic colitis in entire colon (severe distal) | Required | Cytokine imbalance, not B cell mediated, CD4⁻ T cells involved autoimmune-mediated generalized disease | Likely |
| IL-2 receptor α | Knockout | Anemia; colitis | Unknown | Lymphoproliferation, lack of cell death? | Likely |
| IL-10 | Knockout | Enterocolitis | Required | Increased Th1, CD4⁺ T cells involved | Yes |
| Gα$_{i2}$ | Knockout | Colitis, distal to proximal; adenocarcinoma | Unknown | Abnormal thymic development; IgG2α and IgM increased; mature T cells increased | Yes |
| N-cadherin | Transgenic chimera | Focal enteritis, neoplasms | Unknown | Crypt epithelium disruption | Unknown |
| TCR-α⁻ or β⁻ | Knockout | Colitis, milder for TCR-β⁻ × δ⁻ | Required | Unrestrained humoral response, IL-4 dependent, IFN-γ independent | Yes |
| MHC class II | Knockout | Acute colitis, distal to proximal | Unknown | B cells involved? | Unknown |
| CD3ε26 reconstituted | Transgenic | Colitis after marrow transplantation | Unknown | Lack of thymic selection; increased IFN-γ, CD4⁺ cells involved | Unknown |
| IL-7 RAG | Knockout | Colitis | Required | Macrophage required | Unknown |
| CD45RB-reconstituted SCID | Reconstitution of immunodeficient mouse with purified lymphoid populations | Enterocolitis | Required | Mediated by CD45RB$^{hi}$ | Unknown |
| mdrla⁻/⁻ | Knockout | Colitis | Required | Intestinal epithelial barrier defect | Unknown |

guchi et al. 1996). However, if the appendix was removed in the mutant mice older than 12 weeks, the colitis and associated sera antibody responses were not abrogated, suggesting that bacterial antigen interaction with the mouse immune system (i.e., appendix) at an early age is requisite for induction of IBD in this particular model (Mizoguchi et al. 1996). A particular T cell subset, CD4⁺ TCR-α–negative B+ T cell, was defined as particularly important in expression of the colitis observed in these mice (Mizoguchi et al. 1996).

## Pathology of Murine IBD

Spontaneous inflammatory bowel disease develops progressively in adult mice and is manifested clinically by poor body condition and soft stools. Rectal prolapse may also be observed in some mouse strains associated with histologic evidence of a localized proctitis or a more generalized lower-bowel distribution (Fig. 20.4).

The entire colon and cecum may be involved or, alternatively, the lesion is segmental, being in part dependent on the nature of the IBD syndrome. The strain of mouse, duration of disease, and microflora composition are major determinants. Differences in distribution and character of intestinal lesions have been noted in various mouse models of IBD (Strober and Ehrhardt 1993). Mombaerts reported intestinal lesions in TCR-deficient mice that closely resembled ulcerative colitis, with lesions primarily confined to the distal colon and rectum (Mombaerts et al. 1993). However, Foltz et al. also noted segmental lesions in the proximal colon in some TCR-α/β–deficient mice infected with *H. hepaticus* (Foltz et al. 1998). IL-2–deficient mice have lesions consistent with ulcerative colitis where the entire colon is involved, with progressively severe involvement in the distal colon (Sadlack et al. 1993). IL-10–deficient mice have panenteritis when maintained under conventional housing conditions and a proximal colitis

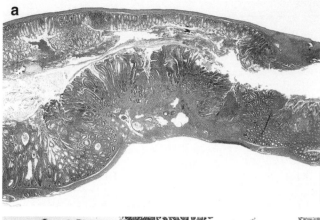

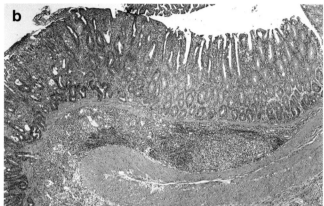

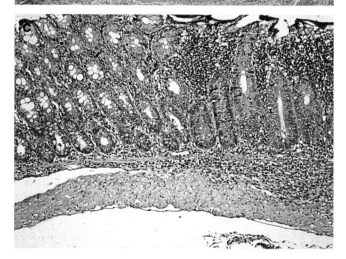

**FIGURE 20.3** Inflammatory bowel disease in several genetically engineered mouse strains with immunologic or mucosal barrier defects. (**a**) IBD in an IL-2⁻/⁻ mouse. The mucosa has marked segmental adenomatous hyperplasia and inflammation. (**b**) IBD in an IL-10⁻/⁻ mouse. Colonic crypt epithelial hyperplasia is accompanied by extensive chronic mucosal and submucosal inflammation. (**c**) IBD in a mdr1a⁻/⁻ mouse. The transition between unaffected (left) and affected (right) segments can be abrupt. Goblet cell differentiation is often attenuated in markedly hyperplastic crypt epithelium.

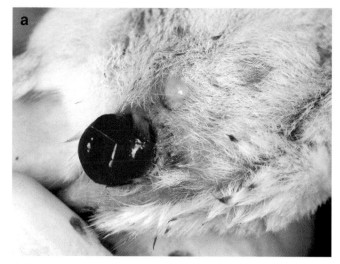

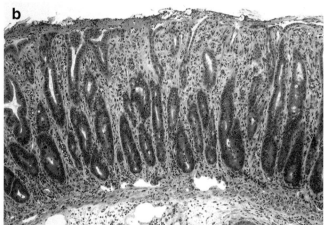

**FIGURE 20.4** Rectal prolapse may be observed clinically in association with IBD. (**a**) The prolapsed rectal mucosa is hyperemic and edematous and may be subjected to secondary trauma. (**b**) Proctitis is associated with rectal prolapse and may be an early manifestation of IBD prior to more extensive lower-bowel involvement. Superficial mucosal erosion and formation of a fibrinonecrotic membrane may occur in tandem with the more common mucosal and submucosal inflammation, mucosal fibrosis, and crypt epithelial hyperplasia.

when maintained under specific pathogen-free conditions (Kuhn et al. 1993; Berg et al. 1996). We have observed that there is relative sparing of the cecum in syndromes that do not involve *Helicobacter* infection (Ward et al. 1996; Cahill et al. 1997; Shomer et al. 1997; Foltz et al. 1998; Haines et al. 1998; Kullberg et al. 1998; Li et al. 1998; Panwala et al. 1998; Shomer et al. 1998a; Fox et al. 1999; Chin et al. submitted); however, *Helicobacter* infection is associated with both cecal and colonic lesions. Similarly, some IBD syndromes appear to initiate in either the distal or proximal colon, suggesting some regional factors' (e.g., microflora)

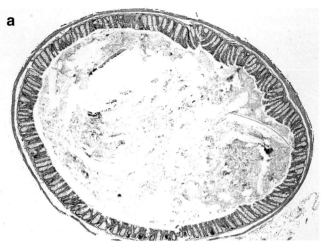

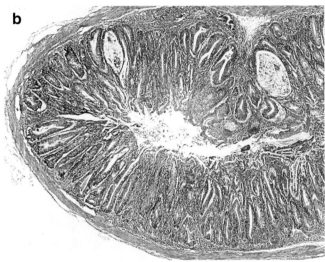

**FIGURE 20.5** Marked proliferative colitis is a hallmark lesion of murine IBD. (**a**) Normal transverse section of colon from a *scid* mouse. (**b**) Marked crypt hyperplasia with cystic dilation, diminished goblet cell differentiation, and inflammation are common changes in murine IBD. This specimen was from a *scid* mouse naturally infected with two species of *Helicobacter* (*H. bilis* and *H. rodentium*).

impact on lesion initiation. Accurate appraisal of the distribution of lower-bowel lesions, particularly during early stages of disease, requires extensive sampling at all levels. Longitudinal sections of the lower bowel yield a greater appreciation of lesion distribution and transitions between affected and unaffected segments.

The primary histopathologic changes are chronic inflammation and marked crypt hyperplasia of the lower bowel, as illustrated in the majority of figures in this chapter (Fig. 20.5). Inflammation commonly involves the mucosa and submucosa, but transmural extension may be seen in some syndromes, often associated with local mucosal necrosis or juxtaposed to the mesenteric border (Fig. 20.6). Inflammation may extend

along the serosal surface or into the mesentery. Local perforations of the bowel wall obviously have more far-reaching implications for peritonitis and extraintestinal infections. Inflammatory infiltrates are characteristically composed of a chronic mixed mononuclear cell infiltrate. Lymphocytes, plasma cells, and macrophages predominate in many syndromes; however, the composition of the infiltrate is clearly impacted by the genetic background of the mouse (e.g., *scid* mice lack a prominent lymphoid component). Granulocytes, primarily neutrophils, are less consistently observed but may be present in large numbers usually associated with sites of epithelial disruption (i.e., erosions and mucosal ulcers) (Fig. 20.6). Giant cells are variably present within the mucosa or extramucosal sites of inflammation, in which macrophages are present (Fig. 20.6).

Proliferation of the crypt epithelium begins as a relatively subtle elongation of the crypts; however, the changes become quite distinctive as the disease progresses. The crypt epithelium becomes notably hyperchromic, which is further accentuated by a decline in goblet cell differentiation (Fig. 20.5). With increasing severity of epithelial hyperplasia, crypt growth deviates from normal architecture to form branching, tortuous, or adenomatous patterns. Invasive hyperplasia through the muscularis mucosae into the submucosa are often associated with intense mucosal hyperplasia. Extensions of epithelium into the submucosa often penetrate into submucosal lymphoid foci (Fig. 20.7); however, some invasive foci induce a prominent fibrous response, suggestive of neoplastic invasion. Leakage of mucin from invasive glandular foci, particularly in the rectum, results in microscopic "lakes" of mucin in the submucosa. Preneoplastic changes are generally infrequent but may occur as dysplastic foci, which are further distorted in architecture and manifest some degree of atypia (Fig. 20.7). Adenocarcinomas resulting from IBD-associated hyperplasia have been reported in IL-10$^{-/-}$ on a C57BL × 129 background at the relatively young age of 6 months (Berg et al. 1996). CD3ε transgenic (Tgε26) and Gα$_{i2}$ mutants have also been proposed as models of colitis and adenocarcinoma (Gα$_{i2}$), (Hollander et al. 1995; Rudolph et al. 1995).

In association with marked IBD lesions in the lower bowel, lesions may be observed in other tissues. Phlebothrombosis may be observed within the mesentery and liver, as well as within the lower-bowel tissues (Fig. 20.8). A likely pathogenetic basis of these lesions is septic spread into the portal circulation. Even in the absence of obvious vascular lesions, foci of hepatic necrosis, hepatitis, and portal inflammatory infiltrates may be profound in mice with IBD (Fig. 20.8).

Chronic proliferative gastritis is often seen in association with severe IBD (Fig. 20.9). Gastritis appears to develop subsequent to the lower-bowel lesions. Proliferative

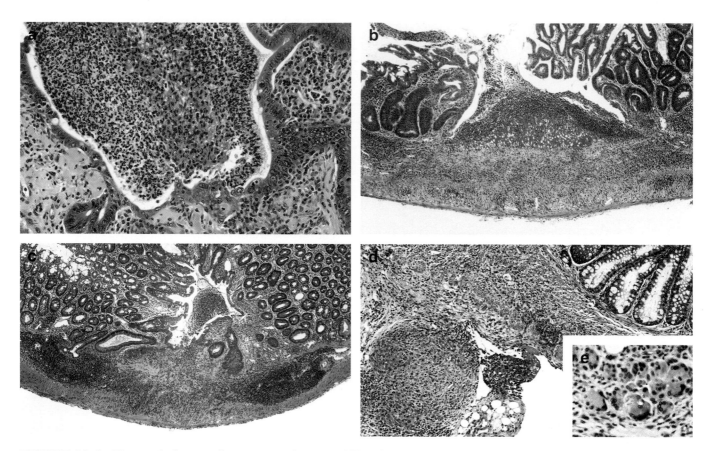

**FIGURE 20.6**  Histopathologic inflammatory changes of IBD. (**a**) Infiltration and exudation of neutrophils may be observed commonly in sites of epithelial erosion. (**b**) Mucosal ulceration occurs with variable frequency depending on the IBD syndrome. Prior to healing, the defects fill with fibrinonecrotic material, and intense local inflammation arises in the adjacent tissues, penetrating laterally and transmurally. (**c**) Transmural inflammation is also observed variably dependent on mouse genotype, and it arises frequently in association with mucosal necrosis. (**d**) Inflammation, frequently granulomatous in composition, may extend into the mesenteric tissue. (**e**) Multinucleate giant cells occurring in the inflammatory infiltrate.

antral gastritis is more commonly observed, characterized by marked thickening of the antral mucosa and inflammation of the deep mucosa and submucosa. Gastritis may extend proximally to involve the corpus mucosa, resulting in loss of parietal and chief cells, hyperplasia and hypertrophy of a mucous epithelium within the glands, and inflammation similar to that in the antrum. The corpus changes resemble those observed in C57BL/6 mice infected with gastric helicobacters, suggesting a microbial etiology as well as implicating the C57BL/6 genetic background. Of interest is the observation that urease-positive intestinal helicobacters (e.g., *H. muridarum* ) can also colonize the gastric mucosa and elicit gastritis (Queiroz et al. 1992).

Clearly differences in the type and distribution of intestinal lesions, host genotype, as well as microbial flora will be important in dissecting the pathogenesis of IBD as these mouse models become more fully characterized.

## *Helicobacter*-Associated IBD in Mice

Numerous mouse models have been developed to help understand the complex interaction between the immune system and intestinal antigens—particularly bacteria—that appear to be involved in the pathogenesis of IBD. For example, when IL-2– and IL-10–deficient mice are rederived by hysterectomy and maintained under specific pathogen-free (SPF) or germ-free conditions, they exhibit no clinical signs of disease. The SPF IL-2$^{-/-}$ animals did have mild histopathological changes, but lesions were completely absent from the colonic tissue of IL-2$^{-/-}$ germ-free animals, up to 20 weeks of age (Sadlack et al. 1993). Similarly IL-10$^{-/-}$ and TCR-$\alpha^{-/-}$ mice maintained as germ-free do not develop IBD (Dianda et al. 1997). In each report of the original descriptions of IBD in targeted mutagenesis, animals were examined for known pathogenic agents and were reported to be free from known pathogens

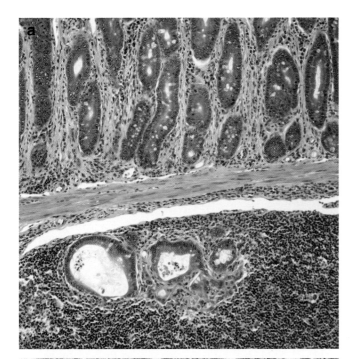

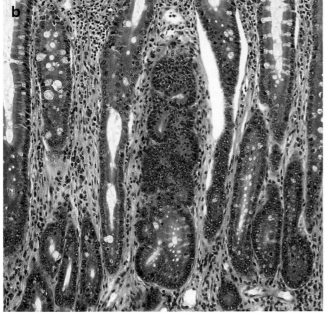

**FIGURE 20.7** Severe, chronic crypt hyperplasia is associated with deviations from normal mucosal architecture. (**a**) Invasive hyperplasia results from extension of crypt epithelium through the muscularis mucosae, forming discrete glandular foci in the submucosa, often within lymphoid foci. The invasive glandular epithelium is typically regarded as lacking in atypia, and by convention the invasive foci are regarded as nonneoplastic. (**b**) Discrete foci of dysplasia, characterized by cellular atypia and architectural distortion, can be observed with marked crypt hyperplasia of chronic duration.

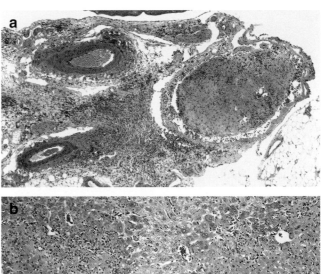

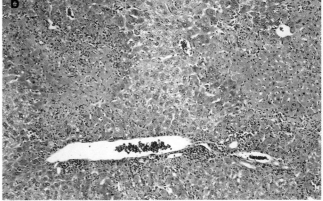

**FIGURE 20.8** Marked IBD lesions in the bowel may be associated with secondary involvement of the portal circulation. (**a**) Phlebothrombosis may be observed in the mesenteric vessels associated with perivascular inflammation and serositis. (**b**) Liver lesions, including multifocal necrosis with associated inflammation and portal and periportal hepatitis, are common in mice with IBD, probably due to sepsis of the portal blood flow.

(Kuhn et al. 1993; Mombaerts et al. 1993) (Table 20.3). However, at the time these studies were conducted, *Helicobacter* spp. were not recognized as murine pathogens. *Helicobacter hepaticus* as well as several other novel *Helicobacter* spp. have now been identified in mice from several commercial vendors (Shames et al. 1995; Fox et al. 1998) and are enzootic in many institutional mice colonies around the world (Table 20.2).

*Helicobacter hepaticus* was first isolated from livers in some strains of mice with hepatitis, hepatic adenoma, and hepatocellular carcinoma (Fox et al. 1994; Ward et al. 1994a). However, the primary sites of colonization of many enterohepatic helicobacters are the cecum and colon in these strains of mice that develop liver lesions, as well as in resistant strains of mice that do not develop liver lesions (Fox et al. 1994). In some immune-deficient strains of mice (Athymic NCr-nu, BALB/cAnNCr-nu, C57BL/6NCr-nu, *scid*/NCr), *H. hepaticus* has been associated with chronic proliferative typhlitis, colitis,

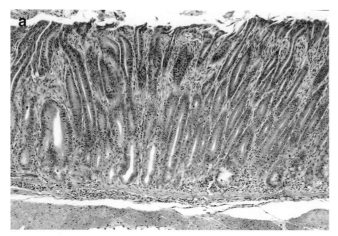

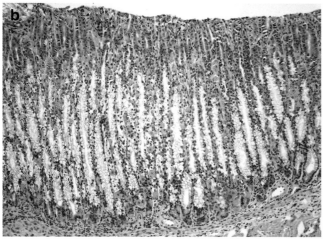

**FIGURE 20.9** Proliferative gastritis is often associated with chronic murine IBD. (**a**) Marked elongation of the antral pits is associated with moderate multifocal inflammation. (**b**) With increasing severity, gastritis extends into the corpus region of the stomach, resulting in loss of parietal and chief cells and mucous cell hyperplasia.

and proctitis characteristic of IBD (Ward et al. 1996; Li et al. 1998). A/J mice, a strain particularly susceptible to *H. hepaticus*–induced liver disease, also develop a typhlitis after natural or experimental infection with *H. hepaticus* (Ward et al. 1994b; Whary et al. 1998). These mice developed a cell-mediated Th1 immune response with a predominant IgG2a antibody response and in vitro production of γ-IFN in excess of IL-4 or IL-5 (Whary et al. 1998). Rectal prolapse and proliferative bowel disease in multiple lines of genetically altered mice within our facilities were also infected with *H. hepaticus* (Foltz et al. 1998). An outbreak of IBD has also been noted in a *scid* mouse colony naturally infected with *H. bilis* and *H. rodentium* (Fox et al. 1995; Shen et al. 1997; Shomer et al. 1998a).

## IBD Experimentally Induced by *Helicobacter* Species

Germ-free Swiss-Webster mice monocolonized with *H. hepaticus* developed both hepatitis and, in selected animals, enterocolitis (Fox et al. 1996b). Also we have recently demonstrated that *H. hepaticus* inoculated into defined flora *scid* mice reconstituted with CD45RB[high] T cells resulted in severe IBD, similar to that noted with human disease (Table 20.2; Cahill et al. 1997). The expression of typhlitis and colitis in defined flora *scid* mice that had been reconstituted with T cells but not infected with *H. hepaticus* was statistically less severe than in reconstituted *scid* mice infected with *H. hepaticus* (Fig. 20.10; Powrie et al. 1993, 1994; Cahill et al. 1997). Also, mice infected with *H. hepaticus* experienced more morbidity when compared with uninfected reconstituted *scid* mice (Cahill et al. 1997).

Another intestinal helicobacter, *H. bilis* (Fig. 20.11), recovered from diseased livers when inoculated into Tac:Icr:Ha(ICR)-*scid*/DF mice without reconstitution of CD45RB[high] T cells, produces severe lower-bowel disease with marked infiltration of macrophages into inflamed tissue (Fox et al. 1995; Shomer et al. 1997). In addition, *H. bilis* has been isolated from nude rats suffering from colitis and typhlitis. Experimental inoculation of *H. bilis* into noninfected nude rats reproduced the same clinical and histological findings (Haines et al. 1998).

Although IBD has been characterized in IL-10[-/-] mice, previous reports had implicated that "normal" enteric bacteria were responsible for eliciting the proinflammatory response (Kuhn et al. 1993; Berg et al. 1996). Recently, however, a study indicated that *Helicobacter*-free IL-10[-/-] mice inoculated either intraperitoneally (ip) or orally with *H. hepaticus* developed severe IBD, whereas those free of *H. hepaticus* did not (Kullberg et al. 1998). Also of interest is the development of IBD in RAG-2[-/-] mice infected with *H. hepaticus* (von Freeden-Jeffry et al. 1998). We have also isolated and characterized a novel urease-negative *Helicobacter* sp. in IL-10[-/-] mice with IBD. Experimentally, this urease-negative *Helicobacter* sp. induced IBD in several different strains of helicobacter-free mice including IL-10[-/-] (Fox et al. 1999).

Similar to observations of rederived (or germ-free–maintained) IL-2 and IL-10 knockout mice, we have noted a decreased incidence of rectal prolapse among β₂-microglobulin–deficient mice and a delay of disease onset among urokinase-type plasminogen activator (u-PA) –deficient mice when lines have been rederived into *H. hepaticus*–free conditions (data not shown). T cell receptor (TCR) mutant mice, which remained disease-free for up to 4 months, gradually developed chronic diarrhea (Mombaerts et al. 1993),

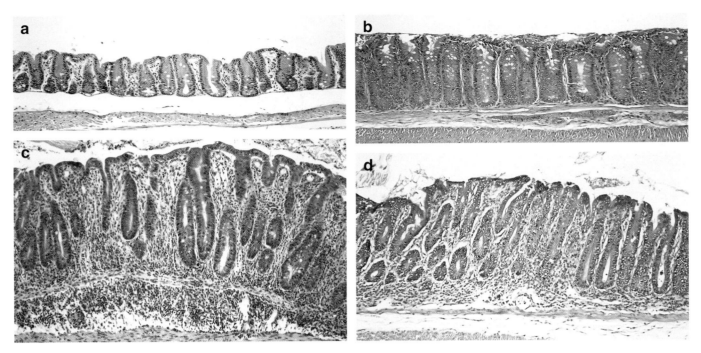

**FIGURE 20.10** Experimental infection with *H. hepaticus* induces significant exacerbation of IBD in *scid* mice reconstituted with CD45Rb^high T cells. (**a, b**) The cecum and colon (respectively) of reconstituted *scid* mice not infected with *H. hepaticus* have relatively limited lower-bowel lesions. (**c, d**) *Helicobacter hepaticus* infection is associated with a significant increase in mucosal hyperplasia and inflammation of the cecum and colon in reconstituted *scid* mice.

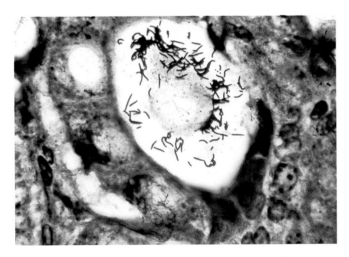

**FIGURE 20.11** Illustration of a colony of *H. bilis* within a colonic crypt of an infected *scid* mouse. The characteristic slender, curved to spiral morphology of the bacteria can be examined with argyrophilic stains (e.g., Warthin-Starry).

lesions in the large bowel, and a wasting syndrome usually associated with rectal prolapse. The average life span for the mice ranged from 6 months to 1 year. In our laboratory, using the embryo transfer rederivation technique, all known *Helicobacter* spp. were eliminated from the intestinal microbiota of TCR-α and TCR-β

mutant mice. None of the *Helicobacter*-free TCR mutant mice (α or β chain deficient) shows signs of inflammatory bowel disease through 4 months of age. In a subsequent experiment, in which either TCR-α or TCR-β mutant mice were experimentally inoculated with *H. hepaticus,* all of the infected mice once again developed cecal and colonic lesions of IBD (Fig. 20.12). While infection with *H. hepaticus* is sufficient to induce IBD in TCR mutant mice, it does not appear to be necessary, since TCR-α mutant mice, but not TCR-β mutant or TCR-α-β double mutant mice, do develop IBD of the distal colon that is independent of *Helicobacter* infection. The *Helicobacter*-independent colitis in TCR-α mutant mice was observed in older animals, beyond 6 months of age.

## CONCLUSION

Genetically engineered mice have provided a unique opportunity to begin unraveling the immune mechanisms responsible for induction and progression of IBD. Use of defined microflora in these mouse models plus experimental inoculation of specific bacteria with proinflammatory antigens will also allow us to dissect the importance of particular antigens in eliciting and maintaining IBD in these models.

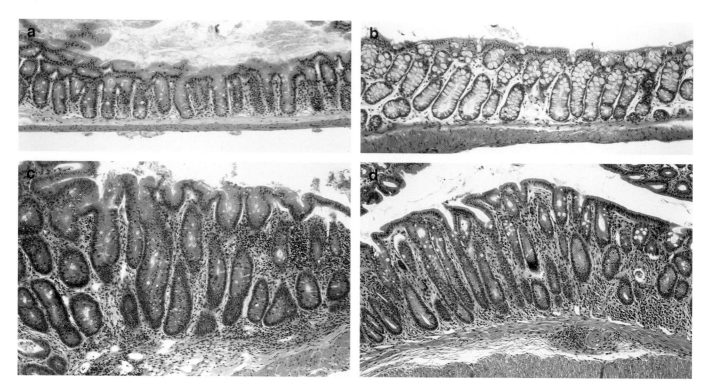

**FIGURE 20.12**   Experimental infection with *H. hepaticus* induces significant IBD in TCR mutant mice. (**a, b**) The cecum and colon (respectively) of TCR-β⁻/⁻ mice not infected with *H. hepaticus* have limited lower-bowel lesions. (**c, d**) *Helicobacter hepaticus* infection is associated with induction of significant IBD affecting the cecum and colon in TCR-β⁻/⁻ mice.

# REFERENCES

Baker, D.E. 1966. The commercial production of mice with a specified flora. Natl. Cancer Inst. Mongr. 20: 161–166.

Bamford, K.B., Fan, X., Crow, S.E., et al. 1998. Lymphocytes in the human gastric mucosa during *Helicobacter pylori* have a T helper cell 1 phenotype. Gastroenterology 114: 482–492.

Baribault, H., Penner, L., Lozzo, R.V., et al. 1994. Colorectal hyperplasia and inflammation in keratin 8-deficient FVB/N mice. Genes Dev. 8: 2964–2973.

Berg, D.J., Davidson, N., Kuhn, R., et al. 1996. Enterocolitis and colon cancer in interleukin 10 deficient mice are associated with aberrant cytokine production and CD₄+ Th1-like response. J. Clin. Invest. 98: 1010–1020.

Berg, D.J., Lynch, N.A., Lynch, R.G., et al. 1998. Rapid development of severe hyperplastic gastritis with gastric epithelial dedifferentiation in *Helicobacter felis*-infected IL-10⁻/⁻ mice. Am. J. Pathol. 152: 1377–1386.

Cahill, R.J., Foltz, C.J., Fox, J.G., et al. 1997. Inflammatory bowel disease: an immune mediated condition triggered by bacterial infection with *Helicobacter hepaticus*. Infect. Immun. 65: 3126–3131.

Chin, E.Y., Dangler, C.A., Schauer, D.B., et al. Submitted. *Helicobacter hepaticus* triggers inflammatory bowel disease in T cell receptor (TCR) deficient mice.

Collins, M.D., Lawson, P.A., Willems, A., et al. 1994. The phylogeny of the genus *Clostridium*: proposal of five new genera and eleven new species combinations. Int. J. Syst. Bacteriol. 44: 812–826.

D'Elios, M., Manghetti, M., De Carla, M., et al. 1997. T helper 1 effector cells specific for *Helicobacter pylori* in the gastric antrum of patients with peptic ulcer disease. J. Immunol. 158: 962–967.

Dewhirst, F.E., Chien, C.C., Paster, B.J., et al. 1999. Phylogeny of the defined murine microbiota: altered Schaedler flora. App. Environ. Microbiol. 65: 3287–3292.

Dianda, L., Hanby, A.M., Wright, N.A., et al. 1997. T cell receptor-alpha beta-deficient mice fail to develop colitis in the absence of a microbial environment. Am. J. Pathol. 150: 91–97.

Elson, C.O., Sartor, R.B., Tennyson, G.S., et al. 1995. Experimental models of inflammatory bowel disease. Gastroenterology 109: 1344–1367.

Falk, P.G., Hooper, L.V., Midtvedt, T., et al. 1998. Creating and maintaining the gastrointestinal ecosystem: what we know and need to know from gnotobiology. Microbiol. Mol. Biol. Rev. 62: 1157–1170.

Fiocchi, C. 1998. Inflammatory bowel disease: etiology and pathogenesis. Gastroenterology 115: 182–205.

Foltz, C.J., Morgan, T.J., Dangler, C.A., et al. 1997. Inflammatory bowel disease spontaneously arising in multidrug resistant gene knockout (mdr 1a) mice (abstract). Vet. Pathol. 34: 509.

Foltz, C.J., Fox, J.G., Cahill, R.J., et al. 1998. Spontaneous inflammatory bowel disease in multiple mutant mouse lines: association with colonization by *Helicobacter hepaticus*. Helicobacter 3: 69–78.

Fox, J.G., Blanco, M., Murphy, J.C., et al. 1993. Local and systemic immune response in murine *Helicobacter felis* active chronic gastritis. Infect. Immun. 61: 2309–2315.

Fox, J.G., Dewhirst, F.E., Tully, J.G., et al. 1994. *Helicobacter hepaticus* sp. nov, a microaerophilic bacterium isolated from livers and intestinal mucosal scrapings from mice. J. Clin. Microbiol. 32: 1238–1245.

Fox, J.G., Yan, L., Dewhirst, F.E., et al. 1995. *Helicobacter bilis* sp. nov., a novel *Helicobacter* isolated from bile, livers, and intestines of aged, inbred mouse strains. J. Clin. Microbiol. 33: 445–454.

Fox, J.G., Li, X., Cahill, R.J., et al. 1996a. Hypertrophic gastropathy in *Helicobacter felis* infected wildtype C57BL/6 mice and p53 hemizygous transgenic mice. Gastroenterology 110: 155–166.

Fox, J.G., Yan, L., Shames, B., et al. 1996b. Persistent hepatitis and enterocolitis in germfree mice infected with *Helicobacter hepaticus*. Infect. Immun. 64: 3673–3681.

Fox, J.G., MacGregor, J., Shen, Z., et al. 1998. Comparison of methods to identify *Helicobacter hepaticus* in B6C3F$_1$ used in a carcinogenesis bioassay. J. Clin. Microbiol. 36: 1382–1387.

Fox, J.G., Gorelick, P.L., Kullberg, M.C., et al. 1999. A novel urease-negative helicobacter species associated with colitis and typhlitis in IL-10-deficient mice. Infect. Immun. 67: 1757–1762.

Gordon, H.A. and Pesti, L. 1971. The gnotobiotic animals as a tool in the study of host microbial relationships. Bacteriol. Rev. 35: 390–429.

Haines, D.C., Gorlick, P.L., Battles, J.K., et al. 1998. Natural and experimental inflammatory large bowel disease in immunodeficient rats infected with *Helicobacter bilis*. Vet. Pathol. 35: 202–208.

Hentges, D.J., Stein, A.J., Casey, S.W., et al. 1985. Protective role of intestinal flora against infection with *Pseudomonas aeruginosa* in mice: influence of antibiotics on colonization resistance. Infect. Immun. 47: 118–122.

Hermiston, M.L. and Gordon, J.I. 1995. Inflammatory bowel disease and adenomas in mice expressing a dominant negative N-cadherin. Science 270: 1203–1207.

Hollander, G.A., Simpson, S.J., Mizoguchi, E., et al. 1995. Severe colitis in mice with aberrant thymic selection. Immunity 3: 27–38.

Hutto, D.L. and Wannemuehler, M.J. 1999. A comparison of the morphologic effects of *Serpulina hyodysenteriae* or its beta-hemolysin in the murine cecal mucosa. Vet. Pathol. 36: 412–422.

Johnson, L.D., Ausman, L.M., Sehgal, P.K., et al. 1996. A prospective study of the epidemiology of colitis and colon cancer in cotton-top tamarins (*Saguinus eodipus*). Gastroenterology 110: 102–115.

Karttunen, R. 1991. Blood lymphocyte proliferation, cytokine secretion and appearance of T cells with activation surface markers in cultures with *Helicobacter pylori*. Clin. Exp. Immunol. 83: 396–400.

Karttunen, R., Karttunen, T., Ekre, H.P., et al. 1995. Interferon gamma and interleukin 4 secreting cells in the gastric antrum in *Helicobacter pylori* positive and negative gastritis. Gut 36: 341–345.

Kennedy, M.J. and Volz, P.A. 1985. Ecology of *Candida albicans* gut colonization: inhibition of *Candida* adhesion, colonization, and dissemination from the gastrointestinal tract by bacterial antagonism. Infect. Immun. 49: 654–663.

Knipp, U., Birkholz, S., Kaup, W., et al. 1993. Immune suppressive effects of *Helicobacter pylori* on human peripheral blood mononuclear cells. Med. Microbiol. Immunol. 182: 63–76.

Knipp, U., Birkholz, S., Kaup, W., et al. 1996. Partial characterization of a cell proliferation inhibiting protein produced by *Helicobacter pylori*. Infect. Immun. 64: 3491–3496.

Kuhn, R., Lohler, J., Rennick, D., et al. 1993. Interleukin-10-deficient mice develop chronic enterocolitis. Cell 75: 263–274.

Kullberg, M.C., Ward, J.M., Gorelick, P.L., et al. 1998. *Helicobacter hepaticus* triggers colitis in specific pathogen free interleukin-10 (IL-10) deficient mice through an IL-12 and gamma interferon-dependent mechanism. Infect. Immun. 66: 5157–5166.

Lee, A., Gordon, J., and Dubos, R. 1968. Enumeration of the oxygen sensitive bacteria usually present in the intestine of healthy mice. Nature (Lond.) 220: 1137–1139.

Lee, A., Fox, J.G., Otto, G., et al. 1990. A small animal model of human *Helicobacter pylori* active chronic gastritis. Gastroenterology 99: 1315–1323.

Lee, A., O'Rourke, J., Dixon, M., et al. 1993. Helicobacter-induced gastritis: look to the host. Acta Gastro-Enterol. Belg. 56: 61.

Li, X., Fox, J.G., Whary, M.T., et al. 1998. Scid/NCr mice naturally infected with *Helicobacter hepaticus* develop progressive hepatitis, proliferative typhlitis and colitis. Infect. Immun. 66: 5477–5484.

Ma, A., Datta, M., Margosian, E., et al. 1995. T cells, but not B cells, are required for bowel inflammation in interleukin 2-deficient mice. J. Exp. Med. 182: 1567–1572.

Madsen, K.L., Doyle, J.S., Jewell, L.D., et al. 1999. *Lactobacillus* species prevents colitis in interleukin 10 gene-deficient mice. Gastroenterology 116: 1107–1114.

Mashimo, H., Wu, D.C., Podolsky, D.K., et al. 1996. Impaired defense of intestinal mucosa in mice lacking intestinal trefoil factor. Science 274: 262–265.

Mizoguchi, A., Mizuguchi, E., Chiba, C., et al. 1996. Role of appendix in the development of inflammatory bowel disease in TCR-alpha mutant mice. J. Exp. Med. 184: 707–715.

Mohammadi, M., Czinn, S., Redline, R., et al. 1996a. Helicobacter-specific cell-mediated immune responses display a predominant Th1 phenotype and promote a delayed-type hypersensitive response in the stomachs of mice. J. Immunol. 156: 4729–4738.

Mohammadi, M., Redline, R., Nedrud, J., et al. 1996b. Role of the host in pathogenesis of Helicobacter-associated gastritis: *H. felis* infection of inbred and congenic mouse strains. Infect. Immun. 64: 238–245.

Mombaerts, P., Mizoguchi, E., Grusby, M.J., et al. 1993. Spontaneous development of inflammatory bowel disease in T cell receptor mutant mice. Cell 75: 274–282.

Montgomery, S.M., Morris, D.L., Pounder, R.E., et al. 1999. Paramyxovirus infections in childhood and subsequent inflammatory bowel disease. Gastroenterology 116: 796–803.

Orcutt, R.P., Gianni, F.J., and Judge, R.J. 1987. Development of an "Altered Schaedler Flora" for NCI gnotobiotic rodents. Microecol. Ther. 17: 59.

Panwala, C.M., Jones, J.C., and Viney, J.L. 1998. A novel model of inflammatory bowel disease: mice deficient for the multiple drug resistance gene, mdrla, spontaneously develop colitis. J. Immunol. 161: 5733–5744.

Powrie, F., Leach, M., Mauze, S., et al. 1993. Phenotypically distinct subsets of CD4+ T cells induce or protect from intestinal inflammation in C.B-17 scid mice. Int. Immunol. 5: 1461–1471.

Powrie, F., Leach, M., Mauze, S., et al. 1994. Inhibition of Th1 response prevents inflammatory bowel disease in scid mice reconstituted with CD45RB hi CD4+ T cells.

Queiroz, D.M.M., Contigli, C., Coimbra, R.S., et al. 1992. Spiral bacterium associated with gastric, ileal and caecal mucosa of mice. Lab. Anim. 26: 288–294.

Robertson, B.R. 1998. The molecular phylogeny and ecology of spiral bacteria from the mouse gastrointestinal tract. Ph.D. thesis. The University of New South Wales, Sydney, Australia.

Rudolph, U., Finegold, M.J., Rich, S.S., et al. 1995. Ulcerative colitis and adenocarcinoma of the colon in G alpha i2-deficient mice. Nature Genet. 10: 143–150.

Sadlack, B., Merz, H., Schorle, H., et al. 1993. Ulcerative colitis-like disease in mice with a disrupted interleukin-2 gene. Cell 75: 253–261.

Sadlack, B., Lohler, J., Schorle, H., et al. 1995. Generalized autoimmune disease in interleukin-2 deficient mice is triggered by an uncontrolled activation and proliferation of CD4+ T cells. Eur. J. Immunol. 25: 3053–3059.

Saunders, K.E., Shen, Z., Dewhirst, F.E., et al. 1999. A novel intestinal *Helicobacter* species isolated from cotton-top tamarins (*Saguinus oedipus*) with chronic colitis. J. Clin. Microbiol. 37: 146–151.

Schaedler, R.W. and Orcutt, R.P. 1983. Gastrointestinal microflora. *In* The Mouse in Biomedical Research, vol. III, eds. H.L. Foster et al., pp. 327–345. New York: Academic Press.

Schaedler, R.W., Dubos, R., and Costello, R. 1965a. Association of germfree mice with bacteria isolated from normal mice. J. Exp. Med. 122: 77–82.

Schaedler, R.W., Dubos, R., and Costello, R. 1965b. The development of the bacterial flora in the gastrointestinal tract of mice. J. Exp. Med. 122: 59–66.

Shames, B., Fox, J.G., Dewhirst, F.E., et al. 1995. Identification of widespread *Helicobacter hepaticus* infection in feces in commercial mouse colonies by culture and PCR assay. J. Clin. Microbiol. 33: 2968–2972.

Shen, Z., Fox, J.G., Dewhirst, F.E., et al. 1997. *Helicobacter rodentium* sp. nov., a urease negative *Helicobacter* species isolated from laboratory mice. Intern. J. Syst. Bacteriol. 47: 627–634.

Shomer, N.H., Dangler, C.A., and Fox, J.G. 1997. *Helicobacter bilis* induced inflammatory bowel disease (IBD) in defined flora *scid* mice. Infect. Immun. 65: 4858–4864.

Shomer, N.H., Dangler, C.A., Marini, R., et al. 1998a. *Helicobacter bilis/Helicobacter rodentium* co-infection associated with diarrhea in a colony of scid mice. Lab. Anim. Sci. 48: 455–459.

Shomer, N.H., Dangler, C.A., Schrenzel, M.D., et al. 1998b. A novel urease-negative intestinal *Helicobacter* species causes severe proliferative typhlocolitis in *scid* mice with defined flora (abstract). Lab. Anim. Sci. 48: 408.

Steffen, E.K. and Berg, R.D. 1983. Relationship between cecal population levels of indigenous bacterial and translocation to the mesenteric lymph nodes. Infect. Immun. 39: 1252–1259.

Strober, W. and Ehrhardt, R.O. 1993. Chronic intestinal inflammation: an unexpected outcome in cytokine or T cell receptor mutant mice. Cell 75: 203–205.

Takagi, H., Jhappan, C., Sharp, R., et al. 1992. Hypertrophic gastropathy resembling Menetrier's disease in transgenic mice overexpressing transforming growth factor α in the stomach. J. Clin. Invest. 90: 1161–1167.

Thompson, G.E. 1978. Control of intestinal flora in animals and humans: implications for toxicology and health. J. Environ. Pathol. Toxicol. 1: 113–123.

Versalovic, J. and Fox, J.G. 1999. Helicobacter. *In* Manual of Clinical Microbiology, eds. P.R. Murray et al., pp. 727–738. Washington, DC: ASM Press.

von Freeden-Jeffry, U., Davidson, N., Wiler, R., et al. 1998. IL-7 deficiency prevents development of a non-T cell non-B cell-mediated colitis. J. Immunol. 15: 5673–5680.

Wang, T.C., Goldenring, J.R., Ito, S., et al. 1998. Mice lacking secretory phospholipase A2 show altered apoptosis and differentiation with *Helicobacter felis* infection. Gastroenterology 114: 675–689.

Ward, J.M., Fox, J.G., Anver, M.R., et al. 1994a. Chronic active hepatitis and associated liver tumors in mice caused by a persistent bacterial infection with a novel *Helicobacter* species. J. Nat. Cancer Inst. 86: 1222–1227.

Ward, J.M., Anver, M.R., Haines, D.C., et al. 1994b. Chronic active hepatitis in mice caused by *Helicobacter hepaticus*. Am. J. Pathol. 145: 959–968.

Ward, J.M., Anver, M.R., Haines, D.C., et al. 1996. Inflammatory large bowel disease in immunodeficient mice naturally infected with *Helicobacter hepaticus*. Lab. Anim. Sci. 46: 15–20.

Wells, C.L., Maddaus, M.A., Reynolds, C.M., et al. 1987. Role of anaerobic flora in the translocation of aerobic and facultative anaerobic intestinal bacteria. Infect. Immun. 55: 2689–2694.

Whary, M.T., Morgan, T.J., Dangler, C.A., et al. 1998. Chronic active hepatitis induced by *Helicobacter hepaticus* in the A/JCr mouse is associated with a Th1 cell-mediated immune response. Infect. Immun. 66: 3142–3148.

Yrios, J.W. and Balish, E. 1986. Colonization and infection of athymic and euthymic germfree mice by *Campylobacter jejuni* and *Campylobacter* fetus subsp. fetus. Infect. Immun. 53: 378–383.

# 21
# Hepatic Pathology in Genetically Engineered Mice

Maria L.Z. Dagli, Jerrold M. Ward, Glenn Merlino, Akiko Enomoto, and Robert R. Maronpot

Mice have long been used as models to study liver diseases, and a large amount of knowledge has been acquired on these animals, especially on their susceptibility to developing spontaneous or induced liver cancers. Many models to study liver diseases have been created, using different chemicals, protocols, or surgical procedures, to detect pathological or molecular alterations.

The study of the pathogenesis of liver lesions has benefited enormously from the advent of transgenic technology. The genetic manipulation of mice represents another step of biological discovery, in which the genetic defect is known: foreign genes can be introduced into the genome, or endogenous genes can be silenced (Merlino 1994a, b). The goal of genetic manipulation is to evaluate the effects on animal or organ behavior; the obtained responses can validate or even change current concepts.

Aberrant gene expression is frequently found in human cancers. Overexpression of genes, mutations in some genes, mutations that abolish the expression of genes important for cell growth control, or even translocations that generate new genes have all been implicated as genetic defects found in cancer cells. It is known that chronic viral hepatitis (hepatitis B and C) is associated with the majority of hepatocellular carcinomas worldwide. However, there are many individuals in whom no obvious cause of hepatocellular carcinoma (HCC) can be identified. Some inherited diseases are well-known to be risk factors for the development of HCC. Among them are hemochromatosis, α-1-antitrypsin deficiency, glycogen storage disease, porphyria cutanea tarda, and tyrosinemia. Alcoholic cirrhosis may result in HCC, although it is not clear whether alcohol is intrinsically carcinogenic or associated hepatocellular injury and regeneration, iron accumulation, or coexistent infection with the hepatitis C virus (HCV) is required (Di Bisceglie et al. 1998).

Transgenic and knockout models have been developed to answer these and other critical questions about human HCC, aberrant gene effects, and gene-environmental interactions (Merlino 1994a, b). By combining transgenic and embryonic stem cell technologies, it is possible to explore many of the critical questions regarding the mechanisms of liver growth regulation in the intact animal. (Sandgren and Merlino 1995). Several transgenic mouse models have been developed in which introduction of transgene constructs leads to development of HCC (Gordon 1994). This chapter summarizes some genetically engineered mouse models in which liver lesions have been described.

## PATHOLOGY PROTOCOL FOR MOUSE LIVER

The study of liver pathology begins before performing the necropsy. A complete report should be available for each mouse, indicating strain and mating data, date of birth, special treatments, clinical signs, and all other useful information. Each animal should be carefully weighed. It may be necessary to decide if the animal weight will be recorded (1) before or after exsanguination and (2) after an overnight fast (Carr and Maurer 1998).

At necropsy, the liver can be easily accessed by opening the ventral skin, sectioning the abdominal muscle overlying the abdominal cavity, and detaching the liver from the sternum and diaphragm. The adult mouse liver is made up of four lobes: the left lobe, the median lobe (subdivided into two portions by a fissure in which the gallbladder is located), the right lobes (anterior and posterior), and the two caudate lobes. The liver should be carefully excised, washed in saline solution, briefly blotted on a paper towel, and weighed. The relative liver weight may be calculated using the following formula:

$$\text{Relative liver weight (percent)} = \frac{\text{liver weight} \times 100}{\text{body weight}}$$

As with other parenchymal organs, the liver should be grossly described with respect to size, color, consistency, and appearance of cut surfaces. The individual liver lobes should be examined and sectioned every 2–3 mm.

Specifically for cancer studies, grossly visible focal or nodular lesions (Fig. 21.1) should be measured and recorded separately for each liver lobe. Small nodules (generally <1 cm) are usually adenomas, while larger nodules with irregular borders and prominent vascularization are usually carcinomas. In addition, larger gross lesions should be examined for evidence of local invasion. Other organs, like lungs or kidneys, should be examined for the presence of metastases when a potential neoplasm has been observed in the liver.

Representative slices of each liver lobe should be excised and immediately immersed in an appropriate fixative. It is important to consistently sample from the same positions in the liver lobes, especially when comparative quantification will be undertaken (e.g., quantitation of altered foci or measurement of replicative DNA synthesis from histologic sections).

Several fixatives are available for the liver, depending on which component is necessary to preserve for the study. The most commonly used fixatives are neutral buffered 10 percent formalin and Bouin's. However, if it is necessary to preserve the hepatic glycogen, nonaqueous alcoholic (coagulative) fixatives are preferred. The proper choice of fixative and prompt embedment may be critical for subsequent immunohistochemistry or in situ hybridization staining. In general, a good tactic is to fix separate and contiguous liver slices in one of at least two alternative fixatives, followed by embedment in paraffin as soon as the slices are fixed. Methacarn (60 percent methylic alcohol, 30 percent chloroform, and 10 percent acetic acid) is an excellent fixative for the immunostaining of intermediate filaments in hepatic or stromal cells, as well as for other immunohistochemical stains. For some studies, it may be necessary to have frozen liver slices for immunostaining or enzymatic histochemistry (e.g., glucose-6-phosphatase staining). Frozen liver slices may also be collected and kept at –80°C for molecular analyses.

# HEPATIC PATHOLOGY INCLUDING CLASSIFICATION OF HEPATIC PRENEOPLASTIC AND NEOPLASTIC LESIONS

As was indicated above, a careful gross examination is the first step in evaluating liver lesions. The liver may be enlarged due to excessive cell proliferation or degenerative processes, such as fatty change, or passive congestion. Primary liver neoplasms or neoplastic dissemination to the liver, as in the case of lymphomas or leukemias, may also cause hepatomegaly. On the other hand, the liver can be reduced in size due to several reasons, the most common being fibrosis and cirrhosis. In this case, the consistency of the liver will also be altered. A yellow and friable liver is highly suggestive of fatty change. An enlarged and deeply red liver is consistent with congestion. A prominent lobular pattern may represent chronic passive congestion, associated with necrotic areas adjacent to central veins. Malformations should be also considered when performing necropsies on genetically engineered mice. Definitive diagnosis of liver lesions ultimately requires histologic confirmation of grossly observed and appropriately sampled abnormalities.

Foci of cellular alteration are potential preneoplastic lesions, representing the earliest visible stage of the formation of neoplasia in mice (Frith et al. 1994; Harada et al. 1996, 1999), as in rats. While these lesions cannot be definitively diagnosed grossly, they are quite distinguishable from the surrounding liver in hematoxylin and eosin–stained slides. Eosinophilic, basophilic, vacuolated, clear cell, or mixed lesions can be recognized and classified according to the predominant hepatocyte cytoplasmic changes (Harada et al. 1999). In contrast to

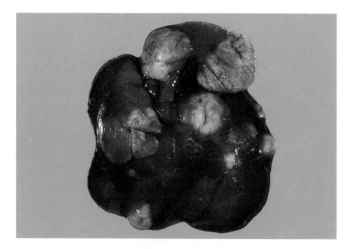

**FIGURE 21.1** Gross appearance of hepatocellular neoplasms in a mouse. Small nodules are hepatocellular adenomas, and large masses with prominent vasculature are hepatocellular carcinomas.

the rat liver, where preneoplastic lesions are typically identified by positive enzyme staining for γ-glutamyl transpeptidase (GGT), or the immunostaining for the placental form of the glutathione-S-transferase (GST-P), the most commonly used marker for both preneoplastic and neoplastic liver lesions in mice is the reduction or absence of the activity of the enzyme glucose-6-phosphatase, although some authors have reported positivity for GGT in some preneoplastic liver lesions of mice (Lipsky et al. 1984). Several publications (Frith et al. 1994; Harada et al. 1996, 1999) have classified and defined the histological types of liver tumors in mice (Table 21.1). Hepatic preneoplastic and neoplastic lesions in transgenic mice are often morphologically different (e.g., increased cellularity and pleomorphism, cytologic atypia, increased basophilia) from those that occur naturally in conventional mice.

# TRANSGENIC MICE WITH HEPATIC LESIONS

A variety of hepatic lesions documented in transgenic mice are summarized in Table 21.2 and discussed below.

**TABLE 21.1. Preneoplastic and neoplastic hepatic lesions in mice**

Lesions of hepatocytes
  Preneoplastic foci of cellular alteration
    Acidophilic (Eosinophilic)
    Basophilic
    Vacuolated
    Clear cell
    Mixed
  Hepatocellular adenoma
    Acidophilic (Eosinophilic)
    Basophilic
    Vacuolated
    Mixed
  Hepatocellular carcinoma
    Trabecular
    Solid
    Glandular
  Hepatocellular carcinoma arising in an adenoma
  Hepatoblastoma

Other primary hepatic neoplasms
  Cholangioma
  Cholangiocarcinoma
  Hepatocholangioma
  Hepatocholangiocarcinoma
  Hemangioma
  Hemangiosarcoma
  Ito cell tumor
  Kupffer's cell sarcoma
  Histiocytic sarcoma
  Sarcoma

Source: Modified from Frith et al. 1994; Harada et al. 1996, 1999.

## Viral Transgenes

### HEPATITIS B VIRUS

The hepatitis B virus (HBV) is an enveloped virus with a circular double-stranded DNA genome. This virus causes acute and chronic necroinflammatory liver disease and hepatocellular carcinoma. It's accepted that HBV is noncytopathic, and the disease is mostly caused by the immune response to viral antigens, expressed by infected hepatocytes. Hepatocarcinogenesis is attributed to the deregulation of cellular growth control genes by integrated viral DNA sequences, to the increased cellular turnover in the inflamed liver, or to the viral X protein, which acts as a transcriptional transactivator of host genes (Chisari 1995). More than 10 strains of hepatitis virus transgenic mice have been created (summarized by Chisari 1995), and these apparently have different characteristics. Many of them develop hepatitis, and some of them present with hepatocellular carcinoma. The contribution of these transgenic mouse models to our understanding of HBV biology, immunobiology, and the pathogenesis of HCC has been reviewed (Chisari 1996). In the transgenic mouse models, it has been established that HBV-induced disease has an immunological basis and that cytotoxic T lymphocytes (CTL) play a central role in this process. When CTL recognize viral antigen in hepatocytes, they cause the hepatocytes to undergo apoptosis, forming the acidophilic Councilman's bodies characteristic of viral hepatitis. The same activated CTL and the cytokines they secrete can cause down-regulation of HBV gene expression and possibly even control viral replication. Huang and Chisari (1995) studied two strains of mice overexpressing the HBV large envelope protein that retains the filamentous hepatitis B surface antigen (HBsAg) particles in the endoplasmic reticulum, resulting in the formation of ground glass hepatocytes. Abundant HBsAg was found within hepatocytes (Figs. 21.2, 21.3), and foci were deficient in antigen (Fig. 21.3). The higher-expressing lineage (50-4) strain develops a necro-inflammatory liver disease that progresses to HCC; the lower-expressing lineage (107-5) shows only ground glass hepatocytes. Increased hepatocyte proliferation was observed in the higher-expressing HBV strain, but not in the lower, and thus it was concluded that hepatocyte proliferation precedes the development of HCC. However, hepatocyte proliferation alone is probably not sufficient to cause HCC. Hepatitis B transgenic mice develop hepatocellular foci (Fig. 21.3), adenomas (Fig. 21.4), and carcinomas similar to those in other types of mice.

Hepatocellular carcinomas in humans exposed to aflatoxin B1(AFB1) frequently have a p53ser249 mutation. Hepatitis B surface antigen transgenic mice were crossed with mice expressing the p53ser246 mutant

**TABLE 21.2. Transgenic mice with liver lesions**

| Transgene | Liver lesions and related changes | Age of first appearance | Reference |
| --- | --- | --- | --- |
| Hepatitis B virus (HBV) large envelope protein | Hepatocellular foci, adenomas, and carcinomas; increased hepatocyte proliferation | — | Huang and Chisari 1995; Chisari 1995 |
| Hepatitis C virus core protein | Hepatic steatosis | 3 months | Moriya et al. 1998 |
|  | Hepatocellular adenomas and carcinomas | 16 months | |
| SV40 T antigen (TAg) | High density of hepatocytes | 1 week | Enomoto et al. 1998a |
|  | Increased mitosis and apoptosis, slight hepatocyte dysplasia | 2 weeks | |
|  | Hepatocyte dysplasia, nuclear enlargement and pleomorphism, multinucleated hepatocytes, biliary cysts | 1 month | Cullen et al. 1993 |
|  | Preneoplastic foci of cellular alteration, biliary adenomas | 2 months | |
|  | Multiple hepatocellular adenomas and carcinomas, cholangiocarcinomas | 3 months | |
| BK virus/HIV-1 Tat | Hyperplastic and dysplastic hepatocytes, hepatomas and hepatocarcinomas, hemangiomas | — | Altavilla et al. 1999 |
| Hepatocyte growth factor/scatter factor (HGF/SF) | Increased hepatocyte proliferation | 4 weeks | Sakata et al. 1996 |
|  | Hepatocyte heterogeneity | 10 weeks | |
|  | Hepatocellular adenoma and carcinoma, hemangiosarcoma | 12 months | |
| TGFα (rat TGFα) | Centrilobular hypertrophy | 4 weeks | Enomoto et al. 1998a |
|  | Diffuse hepatocyte hyperplasia | 2 months | Sandgren et al. 1990 |
|  | Hepatocellular adenomas and carcinomas | 6 months | Sandgren et al. 1993 |
| TGFα (human TGFα) | Centrilobular hypertrophy, cell proliferation | 1 month | Jhappan et al. 1990 |
|  | Pleomorphic hepatocytes | 2 months | |
|  | Heterogeneity in cell size, cellular dysplasia | 7 months | |
|  | Hepatocellular neoplasms | 10 months | Jhappan et al. 1990; Lee et al. 1992; Takagi et al. 1992 |
| c-myc | Increased apoptosis, centrilobular hypertrophy | 4 weeks | Enomoto et al. 1998a |
|  | Hepatocellular adenomas | 15 months | Sandgren et al. 1989 |
| PML-RARα protein | Hepatocyte hyperplasia; preneoplastic and neoplastic lesions | — | David et al. 1997 |
| TAg × c-myc | Preneoplastic lesions of hepatocytes and biliary cells | 1 week | Enomoto et al. 1998a |
|  | Hepatocellular and biliary tumors leading to death by 1–2 months | 3 weeks | Sandgren et al. 1989 |
| TAg × TGFα (rat) | Preneoplastic lesions of hepatocytes and biliary cells | 4–6 weeks | Enomoto et al. 1998a |
|  | Hepatocellular and biliary tumors leading to death by 3– 4 months | 4–6 weeks | Sandgren et al. 1993 |
| TGFα (rat or human) × c-myc | Hepatocyte dysplasia | 2 months | Santoni-Rugiu et al. 1996 |
|  | Preneoplastic foci | 2 months | Murakami et al. 1993 |
|  | Hepatocellular tumors leading to death by 9 months | 4 months | Sandgren et al. 1993 |
| TGFα × HBsAg | Hepatocellular carcinoma, increased cell proliferation | 8 months | Jakubczak et al. 1997 |
| HBV × p53⁻/⁻ + aflatoxin | High-grade hepatocellular carcinomas, hepatocholangiocarcinomas, adenocarcinomas, and undifferentiated carcinomas | 13 months | Gherbranious and Sell 1998a, 1998b |

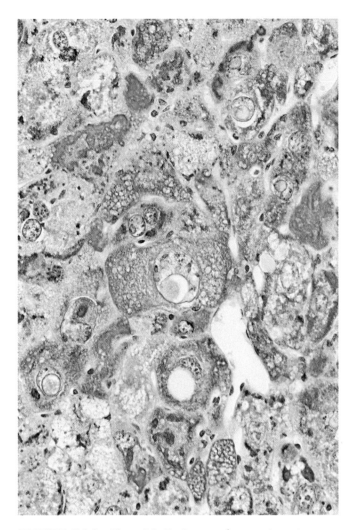

**FIGURE 21.2**  Hepatitis B virus surface antigen in hepatocytes of an HBV transgenic mouse. ABC immunohistochemistry.

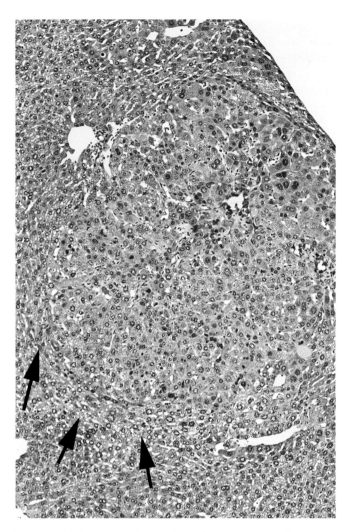

**FIGURE 21.4**  Hepatocellular adenoma in the liver of an HBV transgenic mouse. The adenoma has produced slight compression (*arrows*) of the adjacent normal hepatic parenchyma.

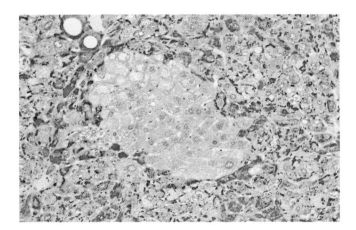

**FIGURE 21.3**  Deficiency of hepatitis B surface antigen in a preneoplastic focus from an HBV transgenic mouse. ABC immunohistochemistry, hematoxylin.

protein (Gherbranious and Sell 1998a, 1998b). Offspring were treated with AFB1. At 13 months of age, 100 percent of the p53-null male mice expressing HBsAg and treated with AFB1 developed HCC. The incidence of these carcinomas was lower if one of three factors (i.e., HBsAg, p53ser246 mutation, male gender) was absent. The presence of the p53ser246 mutation increased the cocarcinogenic effect of AFB1 and HBsAg and also increased the tumorigenesis in AFB1-treated p53 heterozygous and homozygous mice not expressing the HBsAg. Females presented similar results, except that the incidence of HCC was not 100 percent. Interestingly, some liver tumors in mice with more than one risk factor were of unusual types (e.g., hepatocholangiocarcinomas, adenocarcinomas, and undifferentiated carcinomas). These studies emphasize the utility of genetically engineered mouse models in studying the interaction of multiple factors that contribute to the development of HCC.

## HEPATITIS C VIRUS

Epidemiological data point to a strong association between chronic hepatitis C infection and development of hepatocellular carcinoma. However, the role of this virus in hepatocarcinogenesis is still unclear. It has been postulated that HCV can induce continuous cell death followed by regeneration and indirectly lead to HCC development, or alternatively, viral products might be directly involved in the regulation of cell proliferation. Two lines of transgenic mice each expressing a fragment of HCV core gene were created and evaluatd for the development of spontaneous liver lesions (Moriya et al. 1998). These mice developed steatosis, one of the characteristics of chronic hepatitic C, as early as 3 months of age. Hepatic nodules, histologically classified as hepatocellular adenomas, were seen in 16-month-old mice. One-fourth of male transgenic mice between 16 and 19 months of age presented with hepatic nodules that developed into HCC. It is noteworthy that transgenic mice expressing the envelope genes of HCV did not develop neoplastic lesions in the liver. Core HCV protein, which has been demonstrated by immunoelectronmicroscopy in the nuclei, mitochondria, and lipid droplets, apparently can act as a transcriptional regulator affecting the proliferative ability of the cells, thus contributing to hepatocarcinogenesis.

## SIMIAN VIRUS 40 T ANTIGEN

Simian virus 40 T antigen (TAg) is a potent viral oncogene that binds to two tumor suppressor gene products, p53 and pRb, and inhibits their functions. Although there is no normal counterpart of this viral gene in the mammalian genome, it has been proven to be a useful tool for the in vivo study of carcinogenesis because it induces tumors in a variety of tissues (Enomoto et al. 1998a). Morphological changes of the liver from mice expressing albumin-enhancer-promoter/SV40 T antigen (AL-TAg) were examined at several ages (Cullen et al. 1993). One-month-old transgenic mice showed increased relative liver weight as compared with controls; histologically, the liver was characterized by marked hepatocyte pleomorphism. Two-month-old mice had an even larger relative liver weight; their livers contained numerous grossly visible cysts, as well as histologically evident multiple preneoplastic foci of hepatocytes, cystic and hyperplastic bile ducts, and biliary adenomas. At three months of age, transgenic mice had trabecular, glandular, and anaplastic hepatocellular carcinomas, as well as benign and malignant biliary neoplasms.

## BK VIRUS

Several viral infections may participate in AIDS-associated oncogenesis; among them is the BK virus (BKV). Mice transfected with the BKV early region gene and the HIV-1 Tat gene develop nonneoplastic, dysplastic, and hyperplastic lesions as well as neoplasms in many organs (Altavilla et al. 1999). In the liver, moderate to severe hyperplasia or dysplasia in hepatocytes is found. Kupffer's cell hyperplasia is also observed. Neoplasms of different origins, such as epidermal squamous cell carcinomas, leiomyosarcomas, hepatomas, hepatocarcinomas, and hepatic cavernous hemangiomas, were diagnosed in 29 percent of the transgenic mice. Many of these findings are comparable to the lesions in AIDS patients, suggesting a role of BKV and Tat in the pathogenesis of AIDS.

# Growth Factors

## HEPATOCYTE GROWTH FACTOR

Hepatocyte growth factor (HGF), also called scatter factor (SF) and initially called hepatopoietin A, is an Mr87.000 polypeptide considered the most potent mitogen for hepatocytes in vitro, as well as for various other cell types such as epithelial cells, melanocytes, and endothelial cells (Zarnegar and Michalopoulos 1995). It was also discovered that HGF/SF possesses mitogenic and morphogenic properties. HGF is dramatically increased after partial hepatectomy or the administration of hepatotoxins. Transgenic mice were created that overexpress HGF/SF under the control of a metallothionein promoter (Takayama et al. 1996; Sakata et al. 1996). The liver of adult HGF/SF transgenic mice is enlarged up to two times the liver weight of control mice, hepatocytes are pleomorphic, and many small hepatocytes are also seen. The DNA labeling index is also increased in 4-week-old mice. Most transgenic mice develop hepatocellular adenomas and/or carcinomas by the age of 1.5 years. Following a 70 percent hepatectomy, the liver of HGF/SF transgenic mice regenerated nearly three times faster than that of their wild-type counterparts.

## TRANSFORMING GROWTH FACTOR α

Transforming growth factor α (TGFα) is a polypeptide containing 50 amino acids and has been detected in many human and animal neoplasms. TGFα is consistently associated with neoplastic transformation of cells in culture and is a member of the epidermal growth factor family of proteins.

Using a metallothionein (MT) promoter and similar research strategies, lines of transgenic mice overexpressing TGFα have been created by two different groups

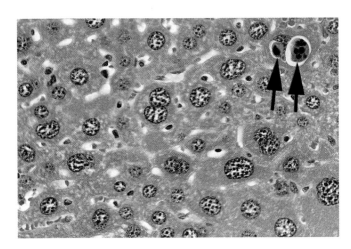

**FIGURE 21.5** Hepatocytomegaly in TGFα transgenic mouse liver. Many hepatocyte nuclei are enlarged. Note apoptotic bodies (*arrows*).

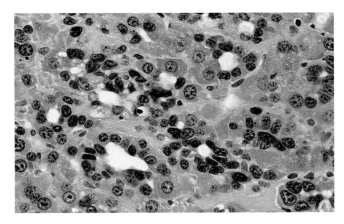

**FIGURE 21.7** Portion of hepatocellular adenoma showing small hepatocytes forming glandular/acinar structures in a TGFα transgenic mouse treated with diethylnitrosamine.

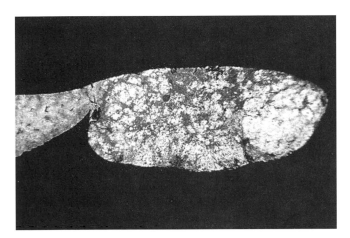

**FIGURE 21.6** Expression of TGFα within normal hepatocytes in a lobular pattern (left side) and within a hepatocellular carcinoma. Note intense areas of expression within the carcinoma. In situ hybridization.

(Sandgren et al. 1990; Jhappan et al. 1990). Both groups concluded that TGFα is a potent mitogen in several tissues and is involved in oncogenesis in some of these tissues. Jhappan et al. (1990) found progressive liver lesions in MT42 transgenic mice. Pleomorphic hepatocytes were found, with cytomegaly and karyomegaly (Fig. 21.5), in mice over 2 months of age; mice necropsied between 10 and 15 months had solid or trabecular hepatocellular carcinomas. High expression of TGFα mRNA was found in these liver tumors, and lower levels of expression were found in nonneoplastic hepatocytes (Fig. 21.6). Sandgren et al. (1993) reported that about 59 percent (16/27) of their TGFα transgenic

mice, the MT-TGFα 1745-8 line, developed hepatic tumors between 6 and 24 months of age, compared with 5 percent (1/20) in the control mice.

In a two-stage hepatocarcinogenesis protocol consisting of injection of 15-day-old mice with diethylnitrosamine (DEN) and subsequent treatment with phenobarbital in drinking water, MT42 transgenic mice developed hepatocellular carcinomas earlier (after 23 weeks of treatment) than the control CD1 mice (after 37 weeks of treatment) (Tamano et al. 1994; Takagi et al. 1992). Adenomas and carcinomas often had focal aggregates of small anaplastic hepatocytes and acinar formation (Fig. 21.7), an unusual finding in mouse hepatocarcinogenesis. In 4-week-old MT42 mice, there was higher hepatocyte proliferative activity and liver enlargement in comparison with controls (Webber et al. 1994).

In contrast, mice in which TGFα had been targeted (homozygous TGFα knockout mice) were submitted to a hepatocarcinogenesis protocol, consisting of initiation with DEN and promotion with phenobarbital. Both control and transgenic mice developed liver nodules by 9 months of age, suggesting that TGFα is not required in early events leading to chemically induced hepatocarcinogenesis (Russell et al. 1996). However, tumors in control animals were larger than those diagnosed in the TGFα⁻/⁻ mice.

## PML-RARα

In order to study the effect of the chimeric protein expressed by the PML-RARα gene, which is generated in promyelocytic leukemia cells after the translocation t(15;17), transgenic mice were created (David et al.

1997). The gene is driven by the MT promoter, and after 5 days of zinc stimulation, 26 out of 54 MT135 mice developed liver preneoplasia and neoplasia with an incidence significantly higher than the non–zinc-treated controls. Moreover, hepatocytes expressing PML-RARα had a higher proliferative response, and the gene was expressed in preneoplastic or neoplastic tissue at much higher levels than in the surrounding tissue. This abnormal protein was able to increase cell proliferation and induce tumorigenesis in vivo.

## Double Transgenics

### SV40 T ANTIGEN + C-*MYC* OR TGFα

The effects of c-*myc* or TGFα on hepatocarcinogenesis induced by TAg were studied using bitransgenic mice (Sandgren et al. 1989, 1993; Enomoto et al. 1998a, 1998b). Most of the AL-TAg mice crossed with AL-*myc* mice showed hepatocyte dysplasia (marked karyomegaly) (Fig. 21.8) and increased cell proliferation in

normal as well as karyomegalic hepatocytes (Fig. 21.9). Most of these mice developed preneoplastic biliary and hepatocellular lesions (Figs. 21.10–21.12) by 2 weeks of age and died at 1 to 2 months with multiple biliary and hepatocellular tumors (Figs. 21.12-21.19). There was an enhanced persistence of predominantly centrilobular ductular structures with both biliary and hepatocellular features in the AL-TAg × c-*myc* bitransgenic mice prior to or during tumor development, but these ductular formations could not be unequivocally identified as progenitor cells for either biliary or hepatocellular tumors

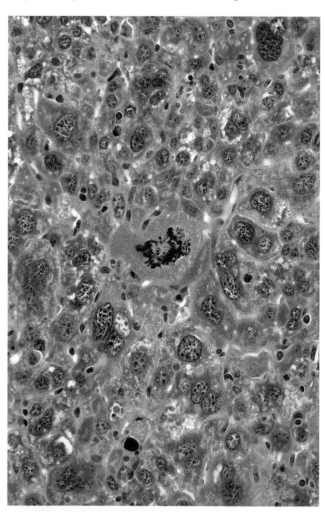

**FIGURE 21.8** Hepatocytomegaly and bizarre nuclei and a mitotic figure in a 39-day-old AL-TAg × AL-*myc* transgenic mouse.

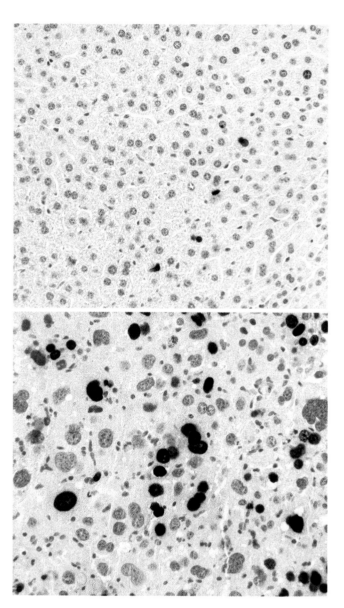

**FIGURE 21.9** BrdU immunohistochemistry showing a low labeling index in normal liver (top) and a high labeling index in hepatocytes of a 39-day-old AL-TAg × AL-*myc* transgenic mouse. Note that several normal-sized as well as cytomegalic hepatocytes are highly labeled.

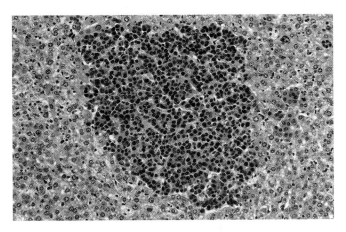

**FIGURE 21.10** Basophilic preneoplastic focus of hepatocytes in the liver of a 4-week-old AL-TAg × AL-*myc* transgenic mouse. Note the small size of focus cells.

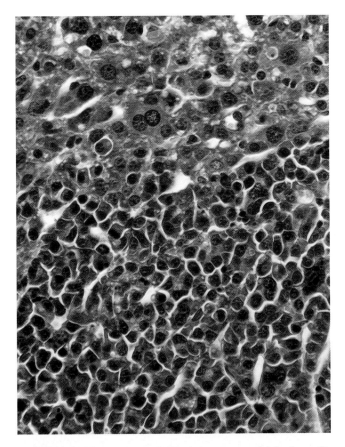

**FIGURE 21.11** A basophilic focus composed of small dense hyperchromatic preneoplastic hepatocytes in a 4-week-old AL-TAg × AL-*myc* transgenic mouse. More normal-appearing hepatic parenchyma is present in the upper third.

(Enomoto et al. 1998b). Biliary lesions appeared to progress from cystic hyperplasias to adenomas or carcinomas (Figs. 21.14–21.16, 21.19).

In AL-TAg mice crossed with MT–TGFα mice, biliary and hepatocellular tumors developed by 4–6 weeks of age, and the animals died at 3–4 months with multiple liver tumors. Tumors in these bitransgenic mouse lines were histologically similar to the ones that developed in the mice carrying AL-TAg alone; no specific effects of c-*myc* or TGFα could be observed on tumor morphology in these bitransgenic mice. However, the accelerated development of liver tumors in the bitransgenic mice indicates a cooperative interaction between c-*myc* or TGFα and TAg during development and growth of liver tumors.

## TGFα × C-*MYC*

When TGFα mice were crossed with c-*myc* transgenic mice, two-thirds of the mice developed one to three large liver lesions beginning at 62 weeks of age (Sandgren et al. 1993). Among these hepatic lesions, 62 percent were solid or trabecular carcinomas, 23 percent were adenomas, and about 15 percent were hyperplastic foci.

Murakami et al. (1993) reported that coexpression of c-*myc* and TGFα in the mouse liver resulted in the acceleration of neoplastic development as compared with the expression of either of these transgenes alone. A comparison between the evolution of spontaneous liver cancer in c-*myc* and double transgenic TGFα × c-*myc* has been performed by Santoni-Rugiu et al. (1996). Mice were examined monthly until 20 months of age. Most double transgenics died at the age of 12 months. Moreover, they exhibited a dramatic acceleration in extent and severity of hepatic lesions when compared with c-*myc* alone. Hepatocyte dysplasia, preneoplastic foci, hepatocellular adenomas, and hepatocellular carcinomas appeared much earlier than in c-*myc* mice, demonstrating a synergistic effect of these transgenes. The acceleration of c-*myc*–induced hepatocarcinogenesis in the double transgenic mice was subsequently shown to be associated with TGFβ1 signaling disruption (Santoni-Rugiu et al. 1999).

The molecular characteristics of liver tumors that developed in c-*myc* or double transgenic (TGFα × c-*myc*) mice were studied (Ohgaki et al. 1996). High expression of TGFα was found in 64 percent of liver tumors in double transgenic mice; c-*myc* expression was also found in most of the liver tumors, but at lower levels. These results confirm the cooperative activity between these genes, but c-*myc*–expressing cells may have a growth disadvantage in later stages of hepatocarcinogenesis.

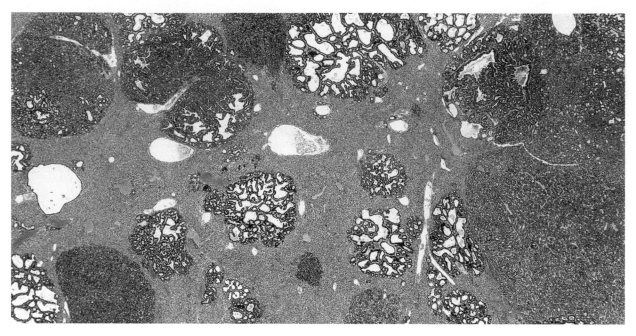

**FIGURE 21.12**  Low magnification of many focal hyperplastic and neoplastic lesions of biliary and hepatocellular origins in a 4-week-old AL-TAg × AL-*myc* transgenic mouse.

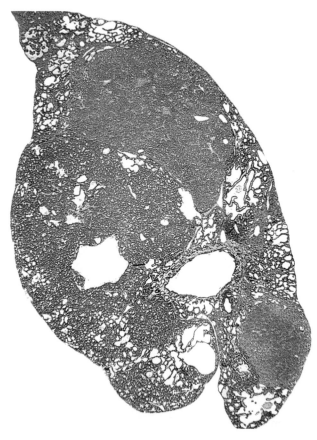

**FIGURE 21.13**  Low magnification of confluent biliary and hepatocellular neoplasms totally occupying the left liver lobe from a 4-week-old AL-TAg × AL-*myc* transgenic mouse.

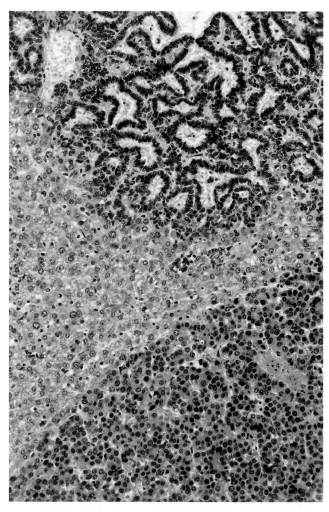

**FIGURE 21.14**  Hepatocellular adenoma (bottom) and bile duct carcinoma (top) in a 4-week-old AL-TAg × AL-*myc* transgenic mouse.

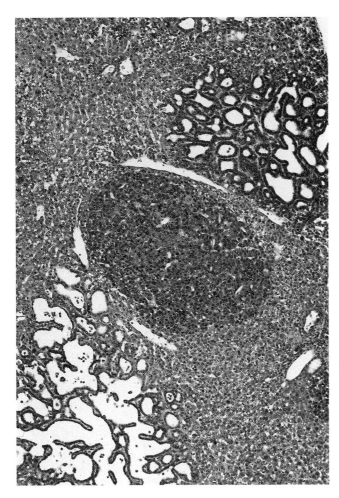

**FIGURE 21.15** A proliferative cystic biliary lesion (lower left), solid basophilic adenoma (center), and bile duct adenoma (upper right) in a 4-week-old AL-TAg × AL-*myc* transgenic mouse.

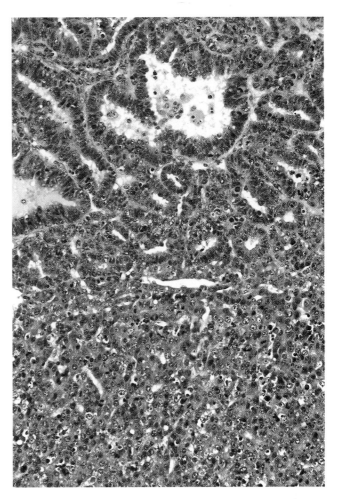

**FIGURE 21.16** Bile duct adenocarcinoma (upper half) and solid hepatocellular adenoma with small glandular formations (lower half) in a 4-week-old AL-TAg × AL-*myc* transgenic mouse.

The same double transgenic mice, TGFα × c-*myc*, have been recently used to clarify the mechanism of phenobarbital (PB) action as a nongenotoxic liver tumor promoter. Treatment with PB in these double transgenic mice resulted in an increase in liver mass, mostly due to hepatocyte hypertrophy, and an associated decrease in apoptosis. An increase in cell death and decrease in liver mass were observed when PB was withdrawn (Sanders and Thorgeirsson 1999). The technique of fluorescent in situ hybridization has been used to analyze chromosomal alterations in 11 hepatocellular carcinomas from the TGFα × c-*myc* transgenic mice (Sargent et al. 1999). Many nonrandom cytogenetic alterations have been found, among them a balanced translocation t(5:6)(G1;F2), with a breakpoint near the c-*myc* transgene site of integration.

## TGFα × HBV

HBV transgenic mice represent an experimental model for the human HBV disease, including degenerative changes, hepatocyte hyperplasia, and neoplasms. TGFα transgenic mice also show increased hepatocyte proliferation and liver cancer rates. In TGFα × HBV surface antigen (HBsAg) double transgenics, hepatocytes that express both transgenes exhibited an increased proliferation rate when compared with each transgene alone (Jakubczak et al. 1997). Moreover, males expressing both transgenes also present a dramatic increase in appearance of hepatocellular carcinomas, demonstrating synergistic activity between TGFα and HBsAg. This situation may mimic pathogenesis of human HCC development.

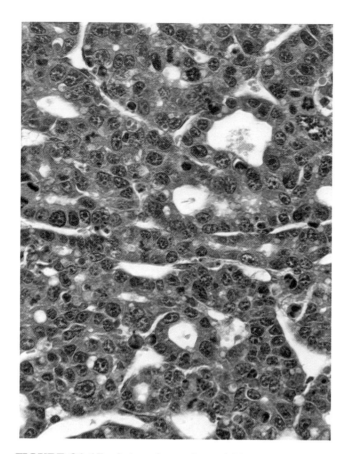

**FIGURE 21.17** Acinar formation within a hepatocellular carcinoma in an AL-TAg × AL-*myc* transgenic mouse.

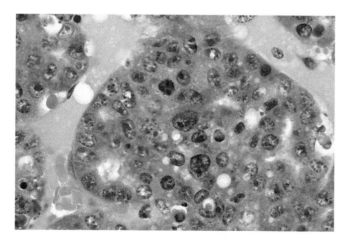

**FIGURE 21.18** Portion of hepatocellular carcinoma in a 4-week-old AL-TAg × AL-*myc* transgenic mouse. Note anaplastic cytology and poorly formed acini.

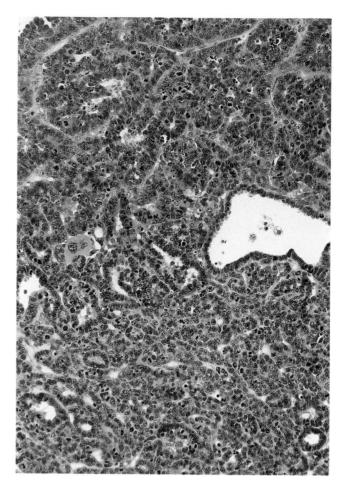

**FIGURE 21.19** Cholangiocarcinoma (upper half) and more solid adenomatous lesion with hepatocyte cytological features (lower half) in a 4-week-old AL-TAg × AL-*myc* transgenic mouse.

# TARGETED MUTANT (KNOCKOUT) MICE WITH HEPATIC LESIONS

Liver lesions documented in targeted mutant mice are summarized in Table 21.3 and discussed below.

## p53

Because the p53 tumor supressor gene is frequently altered in human tumors, it has been receiving much attention. Kemp (1995) treated p53 (homozygous or heterozygous) -deficient mice with DEN at 12 days of age. At 15 weeks of age, six among seven null p53 mice presented tumors. Two of them had hemangiosarcomas, but none had hepatocellular adenoma or carcinoma. It was concluded that p53 may favor development of hepatic hemangiosarcoma.

**TABLE 21.3. Knockout mice with liver lesions**

| Gene | Liver lesions and related changes | Age of first appearance | Reference |
|------|-----------------------------------|-------------------------|-----------|
| AHR | Portal tract fibrosis, hypercellularity, smaller hepatocytes concentrated in the centrilobular area of the liver | 3–4 weeks | Fernandez-Salguero et al. 1995, 1997 |
| Connexin 32 | Interference with cell communication capacity, low level of connexin 26 in hepatocytes | — | Nelles et al. 1996 |
| | Reduced mobilization of glucose from glycogen stores after sympathetic nerve and hormonal stimulation | — | Nelles et al. 1996; Stumpel et al. 1998 |
| | Higher BrdU labeling index in quiescent livers of male and female mice | — | Temme et al. 1997 |
| | Twenty-five–fold higher incidence of spontaneous liver tumors in males and eightfold higher incidence of spontaneous tumors in females | 1 year | (Note: No histological examination reported) |
| | DEN-induced tumors in males | 3 months | (Note: No histological examination reported) |
| | DEN-induced tumors in females | 6 months | (Note: No histological examination reported) |
| IL-10 | Increased inflammation, fibrosis, and proliferative responses to CCl4 treatment | — | Louis et al. 1998 |
| mdr2 glycoprotein | Mice unable to secrete phospholipids into bile | — | Mauad et al. 1994 |
| | Nonsuppurative cholangitis with ductular proliferation, preneoplastic foci, and nodules | 4–6 months | |
| acyl-CoA oxidase | Incapacity to metabolize long-chain fatty acids; steatohepatitis; increased hydrogen peroxide levels; hepatocellular regeneration | 6–8 months | Cy et al. 1998 |
| | Adenomas and carcinomas | 15 months | |
| TGFα | Similar incidence of liver lesions induced by DEN as in wild-type controls, but tumors are smaller | 9 months | Russell et al. 1996 |
| IkB kinase 2 | Severe liver degeneration and apoptosis, leading to death | Embryos (E12.5 to E13.5) | Li et al. 1999 |

Note: BrdU = bromodeoxyuridine.

The interaction of HBsAg and mutated p53 was discussed earlier (See "Hepatitis B Virus"). The presence of a p53ser246 mutation increased the cocarcinogenic effect of AFB1 and HBsAg and also increased hepatic tumorigenesis in AFB1-treated p53 heterozygous and homozygous mice not expressing the HBsAg (Gherbranious and Sell 1998a, 1998b).

## Arylhydrocarbon Receptor

The arylhydrocarbon receptor (AHR) is a transcription factor that mediates the effects of some harmful environmental chemicals such as dioxin, the cigarette smoke by-product benzo(a)pyrene, and the products of other combustion processes. AHR-null mice have decreased lymphocyte populations in lymphoid organs and a 50 percent reduction in liver weight compared with $Ahr^{+/+}$ mice (Fernandez-Salguero et al. 1995, 1997). Histologically, hypercellularity and small hepatocytes concentrated around central veins were seen. Periportal fibrosis, observed in $Ahr^{-/-}$ livers as early as 3 weeks of age, was a prominent finding in these livers. A defect in hepatocyte growth or differentiation could be responsible for these alterations in liver growth and possible impaired liver function.

## Connexin 32

Gap junctions permit the passage of chemical or electrical signals from one cell to another and are found in most animal tissues and in practically all animal species. They permit the coupling of the cells both metabolically and electrically. This feature has functional implications, since it is essential for maintenance of tissue homeostasis.

Alterations in gap junctions have been associated with oncogenesis (Yamasaki 1990; Trosko et al. 1990; Krutovskikh et al. 1991, 1995; Yamasaki and Naus 1996) Almost all malignant cells show altered homologous and/or heterologous gap junction intercellular communication (GJIC). These alterations are often associated with aberrant expression or localization of connexins. As an example of the importance of gap junctions in various physiological functions, deletion of different connexin genes from mice results in various disorders, including cancers, heart malformation or conduction abnormality, and cataract (Yamasaki et al. 1999).

In hepatocytes, connexin 32 (Cx32) and connexin 26 (Cx26) proteins are located in the same gap junctional plaque. The channels so formed can be homomeric or heteromeric. Surprisingly, Cx32-null mice also have considerably lower Cx26 protein, and smaller gap junction plaques, although the amount of Cx26 mRNA appears to be the same as in wild-type mice (Nelles et al. 1996). This suggests that Cx32 stabilizes the level of Cx26 in mouse liver.

Due to defects in liver connexins, electrical stimulation of sympathetic nerves in the Cx32-deficient liver triggers a lower amount of glucose mobilization from glycogen stores (Nelles et al. 1996). This shows that Cx32–containing gap junctions are essential for the intercellular propagation of the noradrenaline signal from the periportal to perivenous areas. When noradrenaline or glucagon were directly infused into Cx32-deficient livers of mice, these mice showed reduced glucose release when compared with wild-type mice (Stumpel et al. 1998). This suggests that gap junctions are involved in both nervous and hormonal signal propagation in the mouse liver.

When cell proliferation was evaluated in quiescent livers, bromodeoxyuridine incorporation was higher in both male and female Cx32$^{-/-}$ mice when compared with their wild-type counterparts. GJIC evaluated in embryonic hepatocytes by the transfer of Lucifer yellow dye was 60–70 percent lower than in wild-type cells (Temme et al. 1997).

One-year-old male and female Cx32-deficient mice had 25-fold and eightfold higher incidences of spontaneous liver cancer, respectively, when compared with wild-type mice. When 15-day-old mice were treated with DEN, male and female Cx32-deficient mice showed two- to threefold higher glucose-6-phosphatase–deficient putative preneoplastic lesions than wild-type mice after 1 year. These data suggest that the presence of functional gap junctions in hepatocytes can inhibit the development of spontaneous and chemically induced tumors in mouse liver (Temme et al. 1997).

An alternative method to study the effects of alterations in gap junction or connexin genes on cell proliferation and cancer is the dominant-negative approach. Mice with a mutated Cx32 gene linked to the albumin promoter (alb-V139M) express Cx32 specifically in the liver. This mutant Cx32 exerts a dominant-negative effect on the wild-type hepatocyte Cx32. These mice present moderately reduced GJIC capacity in the liver and delayed regeneration after 30 percent hepatectomy (Dagli et al. 1999). The susceptibility of these mice to liver cancer is currently under investigation.

## Interleukin 10

Inflammation in liver is known to be initiated and perpetuated by the hepatic macrophages, Kupffer's cells. These cells are also important in hepatic injury produced by agents such as CCl4 and acetaminophen. Uncontrolled inflammatory response is involved in many liver diseases and results in tissue damage, fibrosis, and cirrhosis. Interleukin 10 (IL-10) is an anti-inflammatory cytokine that inhibits a range of macrophage effector functions; it has been detected in different cells including T cells, monocytes/macrophages, ultraviolet-activated keratinocytes, and stromal cells. IL-10–deficient mice, and their wild-type counterparts, were treated with CCl4 (Louis et al. 1998). The levels of TNFα and TGFβ1 were significantly higher in IL-10–deficient mice. These mice also had more prominent neutrophilic infiltration, higher PCNA-expressing hepatocytes, but only a marginal alteration in centrilobular necrosis. As expected, repeated CCl4 injections lead to more severe liver fibrosis after 7 weeks. Studies in IL-10–deficient mice have permitted the clarification of the role of IL-10 in liver response to treatment with CCl4.

## Mdr2 Glycoprotein

MDR genes encode for cell membrane proteins known as P-glycoproteins. The mdr2 P-glycoprotein is the homologue of the MDR3 human gene product, is present in high concentration in the bile canalicular membrane of hepatocytes, and plays a role in biliary excretion. Mice of the 129/OlaHsd strain have homozygous disruption of the mdr2 gene and lack the mdr2 P-glycoprotein in the canalicular membrane (Mauad et al. 1994). These mice are unable to secrete phospholipids into bile. Due to this incapacity, a hepatic disease develops starting soon after birth and progresses for 3 months, becoming stable afterwards. Animals develop a nonsuppurative cholangitis with ductular proliferation. Bile canaliculi are wide and relatively smooth; this immature phenotype persists in mdr2$^{-/-}$ mice. At 4–6 months of age, mdr2$^{-/-}$ mice start to develop preneoplastic foci that progress to neoplastic lesions, some of which can metastasize. These mice represent an interesting model for study of chronic cholangitis and liver cancer.

## Acyl-CoA Oxidase

The enzyme acyl-CoA oxidase (AOX) participates in the peroxisomal β-oxidation system that metabolizes very long chain fatty acids. Mice deficient in AOX show steatohepatitis, increased hepatic levels of hydrogen peroxide, and hepatocellular regeneration (Cy et al. 1998). The fatty change reverts completely at 6–8 months of age. Spontaneous peroxisome proliferation and increased levels of mRNA from genes regulated by peroxisome proliferator–activated receptor α are seen in the liver of $AOX^{-/-}$ mice. Tumors have also been observed in these animals by 15 months of age.

## IkB Kinase 2

IkB are proteins associated with the transcription factor NF-kB, which are phosphorylated, ubiquinated, and degraded when cells are stimulated by TNFα or interleukin 1 (IL-1), thereby allowing the NF-kB to translocate to the nucleus and activate transcription. The IkB kinases (IKK1 and IKK2) are important for the phosphorylation of IkB. The gene coding for IKK2 has been inactivated in a mouse strain (Li et al. 1999). Heterozygous IKK2 mice had normal phenotypes, but homozygous mutant mice showed embryonic lethality. Necropsy of embryonic day (E) 12.5 to E13.5 embryos revealed severe liver degeneration and death after massive liver hemorrhage. The large number of TUNEL-positive cells in the livers in this study suggests that lethality was caused by a massive hepatocyte apoptosis.

# GENETICALLY ENGINEERED MICE WITH ALTERATIONS IN HEPATIC REGENERATION

The liver has the capacity to rapidly regenerate after resection or loss of functional mass. Regeneration is a complex process involving many steps and elements (Michalopoulos and DeFrances 1997). Regeneration may be an important factor for the development of liver cancer.

A frequently used model for the study of liver regeneration is the two-thirds partial hepatectomy, first described in rats (Higgins and Anderson 1931) but also applicable in mice. In mice, resection of the left liver lobe is used as a model of one-third hepatectomy. Removal of the middle lobe, including the gall bladder, plus the left liver lobe, is used as a model of two-thirds hepatectomy. Partial hepatectomy is preferred by some investigators over other treatments (e.g., CCl4) because it is not associated with chemically induced tissue injury and inflammation, and the initiation of the regenerative stimulus is precisely defined (Michalopoulos and DeFrances 1997).

An interesting model of hepatic regeneration is represented by transgenic mice for albumin-urokinase–type plasminogen activator (Alb-uPA) (Sandgren et al. 1991). Plasminogen activators are known to catalyze the proteolytic cleavage and activation of plasminogen to plasmin that degrades fibrin clots. Urokinase receptors appear in the hepatocyte membrane, and urokinase activity increases within 1 to 5 minutes after partial hepatectomy. This is considered one of the triggering mechanisms of liver regeneration. In one line of Alb-uPA transgenic mice, pups died soon after birth due to hemorrhage. In another line of these transgenics, half of the mice survived, and plasma uPA gradually increased and returned to normal by time mice were 2 months old. This is attributed to DNA rearrangement in some hepatocytes, abolishing the expression of the transgene. The transgene–deficient hepatocytes selectively proliferate, and this process culminates in repopulation of the liver with clonal hepatocyte nodules derived from transgene-deficient cells. Alb-uPA mice have been used in another series of experiments in which the transgenic livers can be repopulated with transplanted xenogeneic hepatocytes, for example from rats (Rhim et al. 1994, 1995).

Many transgenic or targeted mutant (knockout) mouse models have been tested for liver regenerative capacity. Table 21.4 summarizes some of these models.

**TABLE 21.4. Examples of transgenic or knockout (KO) mice with alterations in liver regeneration after partial hepatectomy**

| Gene | Protocol for liver regeneration | Time points evaluated | Proliferation marker | Pattern of liver regeneration | Reference |
|---|---|---|---|---|---|
| TGFα transgenic | 2/3 hepatectomy | 24, 30, 39, and 48 hours | [³H]-thymidine (1 hour before sacrifice) | Higher incorporation of [³H]-thymidine in transgenic mice at all the time points; peak at 39 hours | Webber et al. 1994 |
| TGFα KO | 2/3 hepatectomy | 36 and 48 hours | [³H]-thymidine (2 hours before sacrifice) | No differences between knockout and wild-type | Russell et al. 1996 |
| TGFα + c-myc | 2/3 hepatectomy | 1–96 hours | Intraperitoneal BrdU (1 hour before sacrifice) | Higher BrdU labeling index when compared with WT mice; 4-week-old mice showed much higher values than 10-week-old mice | Factor et al. 1997 |
| HGF transgenic | 2/3 hepatectomy | 1, 3, 5, 7, 10, and 14 days | DNA quantification in the excised liver and in regenerating liver; intraperitoneal BrdU (1 hour before sacrifice) | Higher fraction of regenerated liver in transgenic mice beginning 1 day after partial hepatectomy | Shiota et al. 1994; Sakata et al. 1996 |
| p21 transgenic | 1/3 hepatectomy or 2/3 hepatectomy | 24, 36, 48, and 60 hours | Intraperitoneal BrdU (1 hour before sacrifice) | Smaller fraction of BrdU-labeled hepatocytes in all time points when compared with WT mice | Wu et al. 1996 |
| Type 1 TNFR KO | 2/3 hepatectomy | 24, 26, 34, 36, 40, 44, 48, 50, and 64 hours | Intraperitoneal BrdU (2 hours before sacrifice) | Reduced BrdU labeling index from the peak of S-phase at 40 hours until 64 hours when compared with WT mice | Yamada et al. 1997 |
| Type 1 TNFR or type 2 TNFR KO | 2/3 hepatectomy | 40 hours | Intraperitoneal BrdU (2 hours before sacrifice) | Reduced BrdU labeling index in type 1 TNFR but not in type 2 TNFR mice when compared with WT mice | Yamada et al. 1998 |

Note: WT = wild-type; BrdU = bromodeoxyuridine; TNFR = tumor necrosis factor receptor.

# REFERENCES

Altavilla, G., Trabanelli, C., Merlin, M., et al. 1999. Morphological, histochemical, immunohistochemical and ultrastructural characterization of tumors and dysplastic and non-neoplastic lesions arising in BK Virus/tat transgenic mice. Am. J. Pathol. 154: 1231–1244.

Carr, G.J., Maurer, J.K. 1998. Precision of organ and body weight data: additional perspective. Toxicol. Pathol. 26: 321–333.

Chisari, F.V. 1995. Hepatitis B virus transgenic mice: insights into the virus and the disease. Hepatology 22: 1316–1325.

Chisari, F.V. 1996. Hepatitis B virus transgenic mice: models of viral immunobiology and pathogenesis. Curr. Top. Microbiol. Immunol. 206: 149–173.

Cullen, J.M., Sandgren, E.P., Brinster, R.L., et al. 1993. Histologic characterization of hepatic carcinogenesis in transgenic mice expressing SV40 T-antigens. Vet. Pathol. 30: 111–118.

Cy, F., Pan, J., Usuda, N., et al. 1998. Steatohepatitis, spontaneous peroxisome proliferation and liver tumors in mice lacking peroxisomal fatty acyl-CoA oxidase. Implications for peroxisome proliferator-activated receptor alpha natural ligand metabolism. J. Biol. Chem. 273: 15639–15645.

Dagli, M.L.Z., Omori, Y., Krutovskikh, V., et al. 1999. Reduced GJIC capacity and delayed initiation of liver regeneration in liver-specific transgenic mice with a dominant-negative mutant of connexin 32. Proceedings of the 90th Annual Meeting of the American Association for Cancer Research 40: 462–463.

David, G., Terris, M., Marchio, A., et al. 1997. The acute promyelocytic leukemia PML-RAR alpha protein induces hepatic preneoplastic and neoplastic lesions in transgenic mice. Oncogene 14: 1547–1554.

Di Bisceglie, A.M., Carithers, R.L., Gores, G.J. 1998. Hepatocellular carcinoma. Hepatology 28:1161–1165.

Enomoto, A., Sandgren, E.P., Maronpot, R.R. 1998a. Interactive effects of c-myc and transforming growth factor alpha transgenes on liver tumor development in Simian virus 40 T antigen transgenic mice. Vet. Pathol. 35: 283–291.

Enomoto, A., Sandgren, E.P., Maronpot, R.R. 1998b. Altered differentiation of hepatocytes in a transgenic mouse model of hepatocarcinogenesis. Toxicol. Pathol. 26: 570–578.

Factor, V.M., Jensen, M.R., Thorgeirsson, S.S. 1997. Coexpression of c-myc and transforming growth factor alpha in the liver promotes early replicative senescence and diminishes regenerative capacity after partial hepatectomy in transgenic mice. Hepatology 26: 1434–1443.

Fernandez-Salguero, P., Pineau, T., Hilbert, D.M., et al. 1995. Immune system impairment and hepatic fibrosis in mice lacking the dioxin-binding Ah receptor. Science 268: 722–726.

Fernandez-Salguero, P.M., Ward, J.M., Sundberg, J.P., et al. 1997. Lesions of aryl-hydrocarbon receptor deficient mice. Vet. Pathol. 34: 605–614.

Frith, C.H., Ward, J.M., Turusov, V.S. 1994. Tumors of the liver. In: Pathology of Tumors in Laboratory Animals, vol. 2, Tumors of the Mouse, 2nd edition, ed. Turusov, V.S. and Mohr, U., pp. 223–269, Lyon: IARC Scientific Publications.

Gherbranious, N., Sell, S. 1998a. Hepatitis B injury, male gender, aflatoxin and p53 expression each contribute to hepatocarcinogenesis in transgenic mice. Hepatology 27: 383–391.

Gherbranious, N., Sell, S. 1998b. The mouse equivalent of the human p53ser249 mutation p53ser246 enhances aflatoxin hepatocarcinogenesis in hepatitis B surface antigen transgenic and p53 heterozygous null mice. Hepatology 27: 967–973.

Gordon, J.W. 1994. Transgenic mouse models of hepatocellular carcinoma. Hepatology 19: 538–539.

Harada, T., Maronpot, R.R., Enomoto, A., et al. 1996. Changes in the liver and gall bladder. In: Pathobiology of the Aging Mouse, vol. 2, ed. Mohr, U., Dungworth, D.L., Capen, C.C., et al., pp. 207–241. Washington, DC: ILSI Press.

Harada, T., Enomoto, A., Boorman, G.A., et al. 1999. Liver and gallbladder. In: Pathology of the Mouse, ed. Maronpot, R.R., Boorman, G.A., Gaul, B.W., pp. 119–183. Vienna, IL: Cache River Press.

Higgins, G.M., Anderson, R.M. 1931. Experimental pathology of the liver: restoration of the liver of the white rat following partial surgical removal. Arch. Pathol. 12: 186.

Huang, S.-N., Chisari, F.V. 1995. Strong, sustained hepatocellular proliferation precedes hepatocarcinogenesis in hepatitis B surface antigen transgenic mice. Hepatology 21: 620–626.

Jakubczak, J.L., Chisari, F.V., Merlino, G. 1997. Synergy between transforming growth factor alpha and hepatitis B virus surface antigen in hepatocellular proliferation and carcinogenesis. Cancer Res. 57: 3606–3611.

Jhappan, C., Stahle, C., Harkins, R.N., et al. 1990. TGF alpha overexpression in transgenic mice induces liver neoplasia and abnormal development of the mammary gland and pancreas. Cell 61: 1137–1146.

Kemp, C.J. 1995. Hepatocarcinogenesis in p53-deficient mice. Mol. Carcinog. 12:132–136.

Krutovskikh, V., Oyamada, M., Yamasaki, H. 1991. Sequential changes of gap-junctional intercellular communications during multistage rat liver carcinogenesis. Direct measurement of communication in vivo. Carcinogenesis 12: 1701–1706.

Krutovskikh, V., Mesnil, M., Mazzoleni, G., et al. 1995. Inhibition of rat liver gap junction intercellular communication by tumor-promoting agents in vivo: association with aberrant localization of connexin proteins. Lab. Invest. 72: 571–575.

Lee, G.-H., Merlino, G., Fausto, N. 1992. Development of liver tumors in transforming growth factor alpha transgenic mice. Cancer Res. 5: 5162–5170.

Li, Q., Van Atwerp, D., Mercurio, F., et al. 1999. Severe liver degeneration in mice lacking the IkappaB kinase 2 gene. Science 284: 321–325.

Lipsky, M.M., Tanner, D.C., Hinton, D.E., et al. 1984. Reversibility, persistence and progression of safrole-induced mouse liver lesions following cessation of exposure. In: Mouse Liver Neoplasia, Current Perspectives, ed. Popp, J.A., p. 161. Washington, DC: Hemisphere.

Louis, H., Van Laethem, J.-L., Wu, W., et al. 1998. Interleukin-10 controls neutrophilic infiltration, hepatocyte proliferation, and liver fibrosis induced by carbon tetrachloride in mice. Hepatology 28: 1607–1615.

Mauad, T.H., Van Niewerk, C.M.J., Dingemans, K.P., et al. 1994. Mice with homozygous disruption of the mdr2 P-glycoprotein gene. A novel animal model for studies of nonsuppurative inflammatory cholangitis and hepatocarcinogenesis. Am. J. Pathol. 145: 1237–1245.

Merlino, G. 1994a. Transgenic mice as models for tumorigenesis. Cancer Invest. 12: 203–213.

Merlino, G. 1994b. Transgenic mice: designing genes for molecular models. In: The Liver: Biology and Pathobiology, 3rd edition, ed. Arias, I.M., Boyer, N., Fausto, W.B., et al., p. 1579–1589. New York: Raven Press.

Michalopoulos, G.K., DeFrances, M.C. 1997. Liver regeneration. Science 276: 60–66.

Moriya, K., Fujie, H., Shintani, Y., et al. 1998. The core protein of hepatitis C virus induces hepatocellular carcinoma in transgenic mice. Nat. Med. 4: 1065–1067.

Murakami, H., Sanderson, N.D., Nagy, P., et al. 1993. Transgenic mouse model for synergistic effects of nuclear oncogenes and growth factors in tumorigenesis: interaction of c-myc and transforming growth factor alpha in hepatic oncogenesis. Cancer Res. 53: 1719–1723.

Nelles, E., Butzler, C., Jung, D., et al. 1996. Defective propagation of signals generated by sympathetic nerve stimulation in the liver of connexin 32-deficient mice. Proc. Natl. Acad. Sci. USA 93: 9565–9570.

Ohgaki, H., Sanderson, N., Ton, P., et al. 1996. Molecular analyses of liver tumors in c-myc transgenic mice and c-myc and TGFα double transgenic mice. Cancer Lett. 106: 43–49.

Rhim, J.A., Sandgren, E.P., Degen, J.L., et al. 1994. Replacement of diseased mouse liver by hepatic cell transplantation. Science 263: 1149–1152.

Rhim, J.A., Sandgren, E.P., Palmiter, R.D., et al. 1995. Complete reconstitution of mouse liver with xenogeneic hepatocytes. Proc. Natl. Acad. Sci. USA 92: 4942–4946.

Russell, W.E., Kaufmann, W.K., Sitaric, S., et al. 1996. Liver regeneration and hepatocarcinogenesis in transforming growth factor alpha-targeted mice. Mol. Carcinog. 15: 183–189.

Sakata, H., Takayama, H., Sharp, R., et al. 1996. Hepatocyte growth factor/scatter factor overexpression induces growth, abnormal development, and tumor formation in transgenic mouse livers. Cell Growth Differ. 7: 1513–1523.

Sanders, S., Thorgeirsson, S.S. 1999. Phenobarbital promotes liver growth in c-myc/TGFα transgenic mice by inducing hypertrophy and inhibiting apoptosis. Carcinogenesis 20: 41–49.

Sandgren, E.P., Merlino, G. 1995. Hepatocarcinogenesis in transgenic mice. Prog. Clin. Biol. Res. 391: 213–222.

Sandgren, E.P., Quaife, C.J., Pinkert, C.A., et al. 1989. Oncogene-induced liver neoplasia in transgenic mice. Oncogene 4: 715–724.

Sandgren, E.P., Luetteke, N.C., Palmiter, R.D., et al. 1990. Overexpression of TGF alpha in transgenic mice: induction of epithelial hyperplasia, pancreatic metaplasia and carcinoma of the breast. Cell 61: 1121–1135.

Sandgren, E.P., Palmiter, R.D., Heckel, J.L., et al. 1991. Complete hepatic regeneration after somatic deletion of an albumin-plasminogen activator transgene. Cell 66: 245–256.

Sandgren, E.P., Luetteke, N.C., Qiu, T.H., et al. 1993. Transforming growth factor alpha dramatically enhances oncogene-induced carcinogenesis in transgenic mouse pancreas and liver. Mol. Cell Biol. 13: 320–330.

Santoni-Rugiu, E., Nagy, P., Jensen, M.R., et al. 1996. Evolution of neoplastic development in the liver of transgenic mice co-expressing c-myc and transforming growth factor-alpha. Am. J. Pathol. 149: 407–428.

Santoni-Rugiu, E., Jensen, M.R., Factor, V.M., et al. 1999. Acceleration of c-myc-induced hepatocarcinogenesis by co-expression of transforming growth factor (TGF)-α in transgenic mice is associated with TGF-β1 signaling disruption. Am. J. Pathol. 154: 1693–1700.

Sargent, L.M., Zhou, X., Keck, C.L., et al. 1999. Nonrandom cyogenetic alterations in hepatocellular carcinoma from transgenic mice overexpressing c-myc and transforming growth factor-alpha in the liver. Am. J. Pathol. 154: 1047–1055.

Shiota, G., Wang, T.C., Nakamura, T., et al. 1994. Hepatocyte growth factor in transgenic mice: effects on hepatocyte growth, liver regeneration and gene expression. Hepatology 19: 962–972.

Stumpel, F., Ott, T., Willecke, K., et al. 1998. Connexin 32 gap junctions enhance stimulation of glucose output by glucagon and noradrenaline in mouse liver. Hepatology 28: 1616–1620.

Takagi, H., Sharp, R., Hammermeister, C., et al. 1992. Molecular and genetic analysis of liver oncogenesis in transforming growth factor alpha transgenic mice. Cancer Res. 52: 5171–5177.

Takayama, H., LaRochelle, W.J., Anver, M., et al. 1996. Scatter factor/hepatocyte growth factor as a regulator of skeletal muscle and neural crest development. Proc. Natl. Acad. Sci. USA 93: 5866–5871.

Tamano, S., Merlino, G.T., Ward, J.M. 1994. Rapid development of hepatic tumors in transforming growth factor alpha transgenic mice associated with increased cell proliferation in precancerous hepatocellular lesions initiated by N-nitrosodiethylamine and promoted by phenobarbital. Carcinogenesis 15: 1791–1798.

Temme, A., Buchmann, A., Gabriel, H.D., et al. 1997. High incidence of spontaneous and chemically induced liver tumors in mice deficient for connexin 32. Curr. Biol. 7: 713–716.

Trosko, J.E., Chang, C.C., Madhukar, B.V., et al. 1990. Chemical, oncogene and growth factor inhibition of gap-junction intercellular communication: an integrative hypothesis of carcinogenesis. Pathobiology 58: 265–278.

Webber, E.M., Wu, J.C., Wang, L., et al. 1994. Overexpression of transforming growth factor-alpha causes liver enlargement and increased hepatocyte proliferation in transgenic mice. Am. J. Pathol. 145: 398–408.

Wu, H., Wade, M., Krall, L., et al. 1996. Targeted in vivo expression of the cyclin-dependent kinase inhibitor p21 halts hepatocyte cell-cycle progression, postnatal liver development and regeneration. Genes Dev. 10: 245–260.

Yamada, Y., Kirillova, I., Peschon, J.J., et al. 1997. Initiation of liver growth by tumor necrosis factor: deficient liver regeneration in mice lacking type I tumor necrosis factor receptor. Proc. Natl. Acad. Sci. USA 94:1441–1446.

Yamada, Y., Webber, E.M., Kirillova, I., et al. 1998. Analysis of liver regeneration in mice lacking type 1 or type 2 tumor necrosis factor receptor: requirement for type 1 but not type 2 receptor. Hepatology 28: 959–970.

Yamasaki, H. 1990. Gap junction intercellular communication and carcinogenesis. Carcinogenesis 11: 1051–1058.

Yamasaki, H., Naus, C.C.G. 1996. Role of connexin genes in growth control. Carcinogenesis 17: 1199–1213.

Yamasaki, H., Krutovskikh, V., Mesnil, M., et al. 1999. Role of connexin (gap junction) genes in cell growth control and carcinogenesis. C.R. Acad. Sci. Paris/Life Sci. 322: 151–159.

Zarnegar, R., Michalopoulos, G.K. 1995. The many faces of hepatocyte growth factor: from hepatopoiesis to hematopoiesis. J. Cell. Biol. 129: 1177–1180.

# 22
# Pathology of the Reproductive System in Genetically Engineered and Spontaneous Mutant Mice

Joel F. Mahler

It is appropriate that a distinction is made between the reproductive tract and the reproductive system. The tract itself is composed of those anatomical parts needed for the basic performance of reproductive function (ovary, oviduct, uterus, and vagina in the female; testis, excurrent ducts, and accessory sex glands in the male). However, in the broader sense, the reproductive system is more anatomically diverse and encompasses multiple tissue levels of control and interaction, in particular those involving the hypothalamus and pituitary gland (referred to as the hypothalamic-pituitary-gonadal axis). The anatomical complexity is matched at the molecular level by the bewildering interactions and feedback mechanisms between numerous hormones and growth factor peptides, mediated by hormonal, autocrine, paracrine, and neurocrine mechanisms, that are essential for proper development and function of this system. Distinctions between the reproductive and endocrine systems also become blurred in view of the fact that the gonads are endocrine organs themselves, producing the steroid sex hormones, and that the mammalian brain and pituitary are clearly target organs of these hormones (McEwen 1992; Stefaneanu 1997). The field of sex hormone biology is a particularly dynamic one with a broadening scope, as exemplified by the growing list of nonreproductive tissues in which estrogen has been shown to be critical for homeostasis (Couse and Korach 1998, 1999).

The purpose of this chapter is to present an overview of the major spontaneous and induced mouse mutants with reproductive phenotypes. This overview focuses on gonadal phenotypes but also includes mutants whose effects are primarily at the level of the hypothalamus or pituitary and lead to changes in reproductive function or structure. Due to the overwhelming amount of literature on this topic, this discussion cannot be totally comprehensive but rather is intended to give the reader a sense of the diversity of phenotypes that may be found and the variety of pathogenetic mechanisms involved. A brief summary of the key anatomical features and chemical mediators of the hypothalamic-pituitary-gonadal axis is presented below, but for further details, the reader is referred to basic texts on these subjects. In addition to the normal, it is also particularly important for the investigator to know the spectrum of background lesions that may occur in these tissues in order to distinguish these from possible phenotypic effects of the mutation. For this purpose, the reader is referred to mouse pathology texts describing the lesions often found in these organs in nonmutant mice (e.g., Davis et al. 1999b; Radovsky et al. 1999; Mahler and Elwell 1999). A description of the background lesions observed specifically in mouse strains commonly used for the generation of genetically engineered animals is provided in a separate chapter of this book (Chap. 13).

## THE HYPOTHALAMIC-PITUITARY-GONADAL AXIS

The hypothalamus is the interface between the central nervous system and the endocrine system (pituitary). Hypothalamic hormonal factors that act as pituitary-releasing or -inhibiting factors are delivered to the pituitary by the specialized blood vessels of the hypothalamo-hypophyseal portal system. The anterior pituitary is composed of distinct cell types that produce and secrete various hormones in response to cell-specific hypothalamic factors, and most important to reproductive function are the pituitary gonadotrophs that secrete follicle-stimulating hormone (FSH) and luteinizing hormone (LH). FSH and LH are collectively called the gonadotropins and are composed of dimers of the common α-glycoprotein subunit with a distinct β-subunit that confers hormonal specificity. Their release under hypothalamic control is positively mediated by gonadotropin-releasing hormone (GnRH). The gonadotropins act on the gonads to regulate gametogenesis and synthesis of the gonadal sex steroid hormones, which in turn feed back to the hypothalamus and pituitary to modulate FSH and LH secretion by means of complex positive and negative feedback loops. Although the rate of gonadotropin secretion by the pituitary is directly modulated by the hypothalamus via GnRH, the blood level of circulating sex steroids produced by the gonads is the most important physiologic determinant of serum gonadotropin levels.

The gonads (ovary and testis) are composed of both gametogenic and endocrine components. The anatomical and functional units of the ovary are the follicles, corpora lutea, and interstitial-stromal compartment. Follicles are further divided into the theca and granulosa cells that produce steroids (in a temporal and cell-specific manner regulated by the gonadotropins) as well as surround the germ cell (oocyte). Thecal cells possess the full complement of enzymes necessary for estradiol production, whereas granulosa cells are dependent on thecal-derived androgens as substrates for P450 aromatase activity and conversion to estradiol under stimulation by FSH. Follicle rupture and ovulation occur in response to a surge in gonadotropins, at which time the thecal and granulosa cells differentiate into the corpus luteum and there is a shift in steroid synthesis toward progesterone. Units of the testis are the seminiferous tubules where spermatogenesis takes place and the interstitial compartment that includes the steroidogenic Leydig cells. The major regulator of testosterone production is LH, and a major function of testosterone is to act in a paracrine manner on the Sertoli cells of the seminiferous tubule to support spermatogenesis. FSH also acts directly on the Sertoli cell. It should be noted that, in addition to the hormones mentioned, a variety of other locally acting chemical mediators such as growth factors and prostaglandins play an important role in gonadal function by regulating processes of cell proliferation, differentiation, and apoptosis.

## Mutant Phenotypes of the Gonads

From the complex interdependent relationships outlined above, it is apparent that reproductive phenotypes may result from genetic manipulations affecting any one of the cellular or biochemical components of the hypothalamic-pituitary-gonadal axis. A review of the major phenotypes of spontaneous or induced mouse mutations in the literature permits a broad categorization into (1) steroid receptor–deficient mice, (2) mutants with altered pituitary gonadotroph function, (3) mutants with defective steroidogenesis, (4) growth factor mutations, (5) mutations causing germ cell aplasia, (6) mutations affecting gonadal apoptosis, and (7) neoplastic gonadal phenotypes. Major examples in each of these categories are discussed below and listed in Table 22.1.

### SEX STEROID RECEPTOR–DEFICIENT MICE

The proper function of the reproductive system is governed to a large degree by the gonadal sex steroid hormones, acting in concert with the peptide hormones of the anterior pituitary gonadotrophs. The biologic effects of the sex steroid hormones are mediated by receptor proteins that have great specificity and high affinity for their respective steroid ligands. In the reproductive tract, the estrogen receptor (ER), androgen receptor (AR), and progesterone receptor (PR) are all members of the nuclear receptor superfamily that includes the receptors for the sex and adrenal steroids, thyroid hormones, retinoids, vitamin $D_3$, and eicosanoids (Mangelsdorf et al. 1995). These receptors are intracellular proteins acting as nuclear transcription factors (i.e., upon binding with the ligand they will be activated and result in translation/transcription of specific gene products and ultimately a cellular or tissue response). Considerable understanding of the role of hormones and their receptors in homeostasis of the reproductive tract has been derived from studies of mice that are deficient for these receptors.

A naturally occurring mouse mutant with sex steroid receptor deficiency was described in 1970 and referred to as the X-linked testicular feminization (*Tfm*) mutation (Lyon and Hawkes 1970). The *Tfm* mouse has a single point mutation in the AR gene that results in a defective truncated form of the AR protein (Charest et al. 1991). Several phenotypes are observed that are presumably due to lack of testosterone action. The testes of *Tfm* mice are smaller than normal and consistently found in the inguinal region, implying that androgens are critical for testicular migration (Hutson et al. 1994). Spermatogenesis is impaired, Leydig cells are hypertrophied, and testosterone production is reduced due to decreased Leydig cell activity of the 17α-hydroxylase steroidogenic enzyme (Murphy and O'Shaughnessy 1991).

The action of estrogen as mediated by its receptor (ER) is arguably the most well-characterized model of hormone receptor biology today. Decades of study on the role and mechanism of estrogen action preceded the

**TABLE 22.1. Major mutations affecting gonadal structure or function**

| Mutation | Phenotype | Reference |
|---|---|---|
| Spontaneous | | |
| Tfm | Defective androgen receptor; multiple (male) | Lyon and Hawkes 1970; Charest et al. 1991; Hutson et al. 1994; Murphy and O'Shaghnessy 1991 |
| hpg | Defective GnRH; hypogonadism | Cattanach et al. 1977; Mason et al. 1986 |
| | Germ cell aplasia | Witte 1990 |
| Steel (Sl) and dominant spotting (W) | Male germ cell hypoplasia | |
| Jsd | | Beamer et al. 1988 |
| Induced | Multiple (male and femle) | Couse and Korach 1999 |
| ER disruption | Impaired ovulation | Lydon et al. 1995; Chappell et al. 1997 |
| PR disruption | | |
| | Impaired ovarian folliculogenesis | |
| FSH disruption | Impaired ovarian folliculogenesis; subfertile males | Kumar et al. 1997 |
| FSH-R disruption | | Dierich et al. 1998 |
| | Cystic ovaries; granulosa cell tumors | |
| LH overexpression | Multiple (female) | Risma et al. 1995 |
| PRL disruption | Hypogonadism | Bole-Feysot et al. 1998 |
| Glycoprotein α- subunit disruption | Hypogonadism | Kendall et al. 1995 |
| Krox-24 disruption | Female differentiation only due to lack of testosterone; gonadal and adrenal aplasia; absence of ventromedial hypothalamic nucleus | Topilko et al. 1997 |
| SF-1 disruption | | Parker 1998 |
| | Germ cell aplasia | |
| WT1 disruption | Impaired ovulation | Schedl and Hastie 1998 |
| Aromatase disruption | Impaired ovarian folliculogenesis | Fisher et al. 1998 |
| Igf1 disruption | | Baker et al. 1996; Zhou et al. 1997 |
| | Impaired ovarian folliculogenesis | |
| gdf-9 disruption | | Dong et al. 1996; Carabatsos et al. 1998 |
| | Hypogonadism; gonadostromal tumors | |
| α-inhibin disruption | | Matzuk et al. 1992; Matzuk et al. 1996; Nishimori and Matzuk 1996 |
| | Hypogonadism | |
| Activin receptor type II disruption | Impaired ovarian folliculogenesis; seminiferous tubule degeneration | Matzuk et al. 1996; Nishimori and Matzuk 1996 |
| Follistatin overexpression | Impaired ovulation | Guo et al. 1998 |
| Cox-2 disruption | Impaired ovulation | Lim et al. 1997; Davis et al. 1999a |
| C/EBPβ disruption | Impaired ovulation | Sterneck et al. 1997 |
| SOD1 disruption | Enhanced folliculogenesis; increased ovarian teratoma frequency | Matzuk et al. 1998 |
| Bcl-2 overexpression | Decreased ovarian follicular atresia; increased male germ cell apoptosis | Hsu et al. 1996 |
| BAX disruption | Increased male germ cell apoptosis | Perez et al. 1999; Knudson et al. 1995 |
| CREM disruption | Increased male germ cell apoptosis | Nantel et al. 1996; Blendy et al. 1996 |
| Hsp70-2 disruption | Leydig, Sertoli, and ovarian granulosa cell tumors | Dix et al. 1996 |
| Tag overexpression | Testicular teratocarcinomas | Rahman et al. 1998 |
| p53 disruption | Parthenogenesis; ovarian teratomas | Donehower et al. 1995 |
| c-mos disruption | | Colledge et al. 1994; Hashimoto et al. 1994 |
| | Ovarian stromal cell tumors | |
| Lats1 disruption | | St. John et al. 1999 |

development of the first genetically engineered mouse with a targeted disruption of the ERα gene (Lubahn et al. 1993). The discovery of a second type of ER, ERβ, and generation of mice deficient for this protein added further complexity to the field (Krege et al. 1998). The two receptors are not isoforms of one another but instead are distinct proteins encoded by separate genes on different chromosomes and with variable expression patterns. As summarized below (and reviewed in Couse and Korach 1999), studies with ERα-null mice have demonstrated numerous requirements for this protein in estrogenic action, in contrast to studies with ERβ-null mice that have shown no responses mediated solely by ERβ, indicating that ERα is the major biologically active form.

Estrogens are not required for differentiation and initial development of the female reproductive tract (in contrast to testosterone, which is essential to male differentiation); therefore, ERα-deficient female mice have properly developed reproductive tracts. However, the estrogen insensitivity rendered by ERα disruption does result in abnormal morphologic phenotypes in the ovary, uterus, and vagina of adult female ERα-null mice. The characteristic phenotype of the female ERα-null mouse reproductive tract is the presence of an ovary with numerous cystic and hemorrhagic follicles. Growing follicles are present but corpora lutea are notably absent, indicating follicular arrest and anovulation. Thecal cells are hypertrophied, consistent with stimulation by LH, and elevated levels of this hormone are found in these mice. Increased LH is likely due to increased serum estradiol concentrations and loss of normal hypothalamic-pituitary feedback inhibition controls. In aging ERα-null females, there is an approximately 40 percent incidence of ovarian granulosa cell tumors that may be related to the chronic overstimulation of follicle cells by estradiol or gonadotropins.

The estrogen receptor is detectable in all components of the rodent uterus (epithelium, stroma, and myometrium) during early development, through puberty, and into adulthood. However, responses to estrogen, as measured by increases in uterine weight, cannot be seen until after weaning. Therefore, sexual maturation of the uterus is marked not only by the presence of ER but also by the acquisition of the capacity to respond to estrogen-induced signals for proliferation and differentiation. The requirement for a functioning ERα signaling pathway for sexual maturation of this tissue is indicated by the finding of hypoplastic uteri in female ERα-null mice, with reductions in both endometrial and myometrial compartments. Likewise, the requirement for this pathway for mitogenic and stimulatory uterine responses to estrogens is demonstrated in multiple studies in which there is failure to evoke agonist activity in ERα-deficient mice treated with estrogenic compounds.

Similar to the uterus, the vagina is a highly sensitive estrogen target tissue that undergoes cyclic effects in response to the ovarian cycle and estradiol levels. The characteristic changes of vaginal mucosal estrogenization, such as stratification and keratinization, are absent in ERα-deficient females, despite elevated serum levels of estradiol or administration of exogenous estrogens.

Although there is no apparent role for estrogen in the development of the male reproductive tract, there are numerous reports of the effect of estrogen agonists or antagonists on this system, and ER has been detected in the testes and accessory tissues of the male tract. Generation of male mice that lack ERα and exhibit complete infertility has confirmed the requirement for a functional estrogen-signaling system in the adult male (Eddy et al. 1996). Although younger males do produce viable sperm, there is a progressive testicular phenotype characterized by dilatation of the rete testis and atrophy of the seminiferous epithelium with corresponding decreases in sperm counts. Impaired motility of the sperm and abnormal sexual behavior are other characteristics of the adult ERα-deficient male that contribute to its infertility.

Reproductive phenotypes in ERβ-null mice are not readily apparent morphologically. However, continuous mating studies have indicated a deficit in fertility that at present is attributed to ovarian dysfunction. Studies with ERβ-deficient females superovulated by administration of gonadotropins have indicated diminished ovulatory capacity. However, normal physiologic responses to estrogen are maintained in the uterus and vagina of ERβ-deficient females, indicating that ERα is the predominant form responsible for mediating estrogen actions in these tissues. In contrast to ERα-deficient males, male mice with ERβ disruption do not have in any obvious testicular phenotype.

Another receptor-deficient mouse that has contributed new insights into the field of reproductive biology is the progesterone receptor (PR) mutant (Lydon et al. 1995). Viability, sexual differentiation, and male fertility are not affected by the loss of PR. However, homozygous null females are completely infertile. The uteri of PR mutant females develop normally and have normal architecture. However, as expected from the known role of progesterone in preparation of the uterus for pregnancy, the process of induced decidualization is completely abrogated in these mice. Furthermore, an ovarian phenotype develops after superovulation, similar to that of the ERα-deficient ovary, characterized by numerous preovulatory but unruptured follicles, indicating roles for progesterone in ovulation and luteinization that were previously unsuspected. Hormonal characterizations of PR-deficient mice have revealed dysregulation of gonadotropin secretions and resultant inability to effectively recognize ovulatory signals (Chappell et al. 1997).

## MUTATIONS AFFECTING PITUITARY FUNCTION

Normal reproductive function is clearly dependent on the release of pituitary hormones, in particular the gonadotropins, FSH and LH. In addition, although the pituitary hormone prolactin (PRL) is more closely related to growth hormone (GH) than to the gonadotropins, and is primarily considered to be mammotrophic, numerous other functions have been attributed to this multifaceted hormone, including ones involved in gonadal homeostasis (Bole-Feysot et al. 1998). Therefore, abnormal reproductive phenotypes may result from mutations involving the production or action of either the pituitary gonadotropins or PRL. Spontaneous mutations demonstrated this fact prior to genetic engineering experiments. The first spontaneous endocrine mutant described was the autosomal recessive mutation Snell dwarf (dw), the locus of which was subsequently identified as encoding for a nuclear transcription factor termed Pit-1, which activates the transcription of GH, PRL, and thyroid-stimulating hormone (TSH) genes (Camper et al. 1990). Reproductive phenotypes in this mutant are likely associated with PRL deficiency. The hypogonadal (hpg) mutation (Cattanach et al. 1977) is an autosomal recessive mutant allele that proved to code for a partial deletion of the gene for hypothalamic gonadotropin–releasing hormone, GnRH (Mason et al. 1986). The result of homozygosity for the hpg allele is production of a truncated mRNA and translation of an inactive GnRH peptide. Pituitary gonadotrophs are not stimulated to synthesize or release adequate amounts of LH and FSH. Consequently, the hpg/hpg males and females have infantile gonads throughout life and no detectable gonadal sex steroids (Mannan et al. 1988).

A critical structural component of the pituitary glycoprotein hormones is the α-subunit, and disruption of this gene leads to infertility, hypogonadism, and hypothyroidism due to absence of FSH, LH, and TSH (Kendall et al. 1995). Targeted inactivation of the gene for the transcription factor Krox-24 leads to the inability of gonadotropes to synthesize the β-subunit of LH, with resulting infertility of both male and female mutant mice (Topilko et al. 1997). To study the function of FSH alone, mice deficient in this hormone were generated (Kumar et al. 1997), producing infertile females due to a block in folliculogenesis prior to antrum formation. Although FSH was predicted to be essential for spermatogenesis, FSH-defective males are fertile despite having small testes. Similar male and female phenotypes are found in mice lacking the FSH receptors that are localized to testicular Sertoli cells and ovarian granulosa cells (Dierich et al. 1998). Overexpression of LH in transgenic mice leads to a phenotype of multiple hemorrhagic ovarian cysts and granulosa cell tumors (Risma et al. 1995), similar to that described above for ERα-deficient females.

Mice with null mutations of the PRL receptor gene have been generated (Bole-Feysot et al. 1998). In addition to the expected defects in mammary gland development and lactation, PRL-deficient females also exhibit multiple reproductive abnormalities in ovulation and embryo implantation.

## MUTANTS WITH DEFECTIVE STEROIDOGENESIS

Because of their essential roles in reproduction and many other diverse functions, the mechanisms that regulate the biosynthesis of steroids have been the subject of considerable study. One approach has been to study the cytochrome P450 steroid hydroxylases that catalyze most of the reactions in the steroidogenic pathways. Two notable examples of genetically engineered mouse models for this purpose are mice with targeted disruptions of the SF-1 and aromatase genes. SF-1 (steroidogenic factor-1) is a nuclear hormone receptor and transcription factor that regulates the coordinated expression of the steroid hydroxylases within steroidogenic cells (Parker 1998). Consistent with their inability to synthesize steroids, SF-1–deficient mice die shortly after birth, and all exhibit female sexual differentiation due to lack of testicular androgens. More unexpectedly, however, these mice also exhibit absence of the gonads, defects of pituitary gonadotroph function, and failure of the ventromedial hypothalamic nucleus to develop, revealing essential roles of SF-1 in the development of the gonads and at all three levels of the hypothalamic-pituitary-gonadal axis.

Aromatase catalyzes the final step in estrogen biosynthesis, and disruption of this gene is another approach to studying estrogen function by removing the source of the hormone rather than neutralizing its action as is done by receptor-deficient mice (Fisher et al. 1998). Aromatase-null females have an ovarian phenotype of arrested folliculogenesis that has some similarities to that of ER-deficient mice described previously.

## GROWTH FACTOR MUTATIONS

Targeted manipulations of diverse growth factor genes are revealing their roles in reproduction. For example, various growth factors have been implicated as mediators of estrogen action, and this has been supported by studies with mutant mice such as those lacking the epidermal growth factor (EGF) receptor (Hom et al. 1998) and insulinlike growth factor–1 (IGF-1) (Baker et al. 1996), both of which display prominent reproductive phenotypes. The functional relationship between IGF-1 and FSH has been examined in detail (Zhou et al. 1997), revealing that IGF-1 augments the expression of FSH receptors. Growth differentiation factor (GDF) -9 is an oocyte-specific member of the TGFβ superfamily; female mice with targeted deletions of the GDF-9 gene are infertile and exhibit a hypogonadal phenotype with primary follicle arrest (Dong et al. 1996; Carabatsos et al. 1998). Activins, inhibins, and follistatin are structurally related proteins also belonging to the TGFβ family and recognized as peptides that stimulate or inhibit FSH production. Correspondingly, reproductive phenotypes and altered gonadotropin levels have been seen in mice that were generated (1) lacking either inhibin or activin receptors (Matzuk et al. 1996) or (2) overexpressing follistatin (Guo et al. 1998). Another member of the TGFβ family is Müllerian inhibiting substance (MIS), which is secreted by the fetal testis and imposes a male pattern of differentiation. The critical role of this protein in sexual development is confirmed by the altered sexual phenotypes that are found in genetically altered mice either overexpressing or lacking MIS (Behringer et al. 1994).

## MUTANTS WITH GERM CELL APLASIA

Mutants with germ cell aplasia include several spontaneous mutations at the steel (Sl) and dominant spotting (W) loci that may result in absence of germ cells in both sexes (Witte 1990). The Sl locus product has been defined as a growth factor ligand for the c-kit proto-oncogene receptor encoded by the W locus, the interactions of which are critical for stem cell function in multiple cell lineages. Other mutations at the Sl locus result in ovaries with germ cells but with impaired folliculogenesis presumably due to an intrinsic defect in stromal cells (Kuroda et al. 1988). In males, a spontaneous mutation affecting spermatogenesis, juvenile spermatogonial depletion (jsd), is characterized by the presence of only rare spermatogonia and absence of any further stages of spermatogenesis (Beamer et al. 1988). Seminiferous tubules of jsd/jsd mice experience a single wave of spermatogenesis coincident with the peripubertal period that ends at about 7–8 weeks of age. Adults show no further spermatogenesis, perhaps due to defective paracrine mitogenic factors produced within the seminiferous tubules. As described previously, the critical role of testosterone in the development of the male reproductive tract has been demonstrated by the lack of gonadal development in the Tfm mutant (lacking a functional androgen receptor) and in mice homozygous for a disruption of the steroidogenic factor-1 (SF-1) gene. Multiple roles for the Wilms' tumor suppressor gene (WT1) have been identified in genitourinary development, and failure of gonadal and renal development is seen in WT1-null mice (Schedl and Hastie 1998).

## MUTANTS WITH CHANGES IN GERM CELL APOPTOSIS

The fate of most ovarian follicles is atresia, and apoptosis plays a fundamental role in normal follicular atresia. Members of the Bcl-2 family of proteins may act as either positive or negative regulators of apoptotic cell death, and recent studies have shown that one of these proteins, Bax, is central to ovarian cell death (Tilly 1996). A dramatic phenotype in Bax-null females is the presence of threefold more primordial follicles in their reserve than their wild-type sisters at a young age, as well as an extended functional life span of the ovary, as indicated by recovery of fertilization-competent oocytes and absence of age-related ovarian and uterine atrophic changes in later years (Perez et al. 1999). An opposite effect of Bax deficiency is seen in males: there is disorganized spermatogenesis with an accumulation of atypical and apoptotic premeiotic germ cells within the seminiferous tubules (Knudson et al. 1995). Therefore, Bax deficiency may lead to either increases or decreases in the apoptotic cell death pathway, depending on the cell type or lineage and presumably the composition and context of other Bcl-2 family members in that particular tissue. A potential role for the Bcl-2–dependent survival pathway in the ovarian follicle was further elucidated by studies that demonstrated decreased follicle apoptosis and enhanced folliculogenesis in transgenic mice with targeted overexpression of Bcl-2 (Hsu et al. 1996). Interestingly, these mice also display increased germ cell tumorigenesis (see following section, "Phenotypes of Gonadal Neoplasia").

Increased male germ cell apoptosis is seen in several other genetically altered mice. A large number of genes are expressed during spermatogenesis, including CREM (cyclic AMP–responsive element modulator), a transcription activator thought to regulate several germ cell–specific genes involved in the postmeiotic structuring of spermatozoon. Homozygous CREM-deficient mice show reduced seminiferous tubule size with associated absence of developing spermatids and spermatozoa and increased numbers of apoptotic and multinucleated cells (Nantel et al. 1996). The defect in spermiogenesis is not accompanied by changes in the Sertoli or Leydig cells, or by alterations in FSH or testosterone levels, indicating CREM mutant mice may be a model of idiopathic infertility in men in whom there is defective spermatogenesis although gonadotropin and androgen status is normal (Blendy et al. 1996). Some members of the heat shock protein (HSP70) family, such as HSP70-2, are expressed exclusively during the meiotic phase of spermatogenesis; male mice homozygous for mutant Hsp70-2 lack spermatids and mature sperm due to meiotic failure coincident with increased spermatocyte apoptosis (Dix et al. 1996).

## PHENOTYPES OF GONADAL NEOPLASIA

Tumors of the reproductive system are relatively uncommon phenotypes in genetically altered mice (Rahman et al. 1998). Generally a strong oncogenic stimulus is required, such as the large T antigens (Tag) of the SV40 and polyoma viruses. Expression of these oncogenes may be directed to the gonads by the use of promoters for genes endogenous to those tissues, such as the promoters of the mouse inhibin α-subunit gene. The inhibin α-subunit is expressed in ovarian granulosa and theca cells and in testicular Sertoli and Leydig cells and functions as a feedback regulator of FSH synthesis in the pituitary. Utilizing an α-inhibin/Tag construct, transgenic mice were generated that developed gonadal tumors (granulosa and thecal cell tumors in females; Leydig cell tumors in males) at 4–9 months of age with a penetrance of 100 percent (Kananen et al. 1995, 1996). Another transgenic mouse with Tag expression directed to Sertoli cells by Müllerian inhibiting substance regulatory sequence develops Sertoli cell tumors (Peschon et al. 1992). Different testicular tumor phenotypes are observed in two lines of transgenic mice harboring the polyoma virus Tag (PyLT): Sertoli cell tumors form when PyLT is under control of the viral enhancer–promoter region (Paquis-Flucklinger et al. 1993), and Leydig cell adenomas develop with genomic insertion of PyLT linked to the mouse metallothionein-1 promoter (Chalifour et al. 1992). Overexpression of the apoptosis suppression protein Bcl-2, again directed to the ovary by the α-inhibin gene promoter/enhancer, leads to the development of benign ovarian teratomas (Hsu et al. 1996), presumably related to prolonged survival of ovarian cells.

The transformation capacity of Tag is believed to be due to its ability to bind to the cellular tumor suppressor gene, *p53* (Dilworth 1990). Therefore, it is not unexpected that mice with disruptions of the *p53* gene may also be predisposed to gonadal tumors, as is the case. Malignant teratomas occurred with high incidence in *p53*-null mice on the 129/Sv genetic background and with lower incidence in mice with the same genetic disruption on a mixed C57BL/6 × 129/Sv background (Donehower et al. 1995).

As mentioned previously, inhibins, along with activins, are growth factor peptides that are produced and secreted intragonadally and regulate FSH hormone production. Mice with a targeted deletion of the α-inhibin gene develop normally but develop gonadal tumors as early as 4 weeks of age with virtually 100 percent penetrance in both sexes (Matzuk et al. 1992). Histologically the tumors are characterized as mixed or poorly differentiated gonadostromal neoplasms. These studies implicate inhibin as a critical intragonadal negative growth regulator and the first secreted protein to have been identified with tumor suppressor activity.

Prolonged stimulation by gonadotropins is believed to contribute to ovarian cancer, and FSH dysregulation may contribute partly to the ovarian tumor phenotype in the inhibin-deficient mice described above. Further support that hypergonadotropin stimulation plays a role in the development of the ovarian granulosa cell tumor in the mouse is found in the increased incidences of this tumor seen in transgenic mice with overexpression of the LHβ-subunit gene (Risma et al. 1995) and in ERα-null mice (Couse and Korach 1999), both of which have significantly elevated levels of LH.

Recently, another gene with tumor suppressor activity in the gonad has been described. Disruption of the mouse *Lats1* gene resulted in reduced neonatal viability and impaired fertility in both male and female survivors (St. John et al. 1999). By 3 months of age, ovarian stromal tumors developed in all *Lats1*-deficient females examined. Similar to *p53*, *Lats1* is thought to function as a negative cell cycle regulator. The *c-mos* proto-oncogene product is implicated in the control of meiotic maturation events during gametogenesis. An unusual phenotype seen in female mice deficient for *c-mos* was parthogenetic activation of the oocyte, as defined by completion of the second meiotic division, extrusion of the second polar body, and pronucleus formation without fertilization (Colledge et al. 1994). An apparent long-term consequence of this phenotype appearing in older *c-mos*–null females was the development of ovarian teratomas at high frequency (Hashimoto et al. 1994).

Miscellaneous transgenic mouse lines that exhibit gonadal tumorigenesis include male mice expressing the human papilloma virus E6 and E7 genes with a high incidence of Leydig cell tumors (Kondoh et al. 1994) and female mice with an activated v-Ha-*ras* transgene that develop ovarian yolk sac carcinomas (Hansen et al. 1996).

## MISCELLANEOUS MODELS WITH REPRODUCTIVE TRACT PHENOTYPES

Multiple actions of prostaglandins have been implicated in various female reproductive functions, particularly the ovulatory process. The rate-limiting enzyme in prostaglandin biosynthesis is cyclooxygenase (COX), and mice deficient for one isoform of this enzyme, COX-2, have been found to have ovulatory failure as well as abnormal implantation and decidualization reactions (Lim et al. 1998; Davis et al. 1999a). C/EBPβ (CCAAT/enhancer-binding protein β) is a transcription factor that is specifically induced in the granulosa cells of antral follicles following LH receptor signaling. Impaired granulosa cell differentiation and ovulation in response to LH is seen in female mice with a null mutation of the C/EBPβ gene (Sterneck et al. 1997) and is attributed to failure to down-regulate *Cox-2* and P450 aromatase genes. A loss of function mutation in the superoxide dismutase (SOD) 1 gene is associated with reduced gonadotropin levels, lack of ovarian corpora lutea formation, and subfertility (Matzuk et al. 1998). Abnormal ovarian phenotypes are also described in mice deficient for a diverse group of other gene products including cyclin D2 (Sicinski et al. 1996), connexin 37 (Simon et al. 1997), and vitamin D receptor (Yoshizawa et al. 1997) among others (for review, see Elvin and Matzuk 1998).

An unusual phenotype of macroorchidism is seen in male mice with inactivation of the *Fmr1* gene (Slegtenhorst-Eegdeman et al. 1998); testicular enlargement, due to increased perinatal Sertoli cell proliferation, mimics that seen in humans with fragile X syndrome. Additional examples of mutated mice with impaired spermatogenesis may be found in recent reviews by Nishimori and Matzuk (1996) and Simoni (1994).

# REFERENCES

Baker, J., Hardy. M.P., Zhou, J., et al. 1996. Effects of an *Igf1* gene null mutation on mouse reproduction. Mol. Endocrinol. 10:903–918.

Beamer, W.G., Cunliffe-Beamer, T.L., Shultz, K.L., et al. 1988. Juvenile spermatogonial depletion (jsd): a genetic defect of germ cell proliferation of male mice. Biol. Reprod. 38:899–908.

Behringer, R.R., Finegold, M.J., and Cate, R.L. 1994. Müllerian-inhibiting substance function during mammalian sexual development. Cell 79:415–425.

Blendy, J.A., Kaestner, K.H., Weinbauer, G.F., et al. 1996. Severe impairment of spermatogenesis in mice lacking the CREM gene. Nature 380:162–165.

Bole-Feysot, C., Goffin, V., Edery, M., et al. 1998. Prolactin (PRL) and its receptor: actions, signal transduction pathways and phenotypes observed in PRL receptor knockout mice. Endocr. Rev. 19:226–268.

Camper, S.A., Saunders, T.L., Katz, R.W., et al. 1990. The pit-1 transcription factor gene is a candidate for the murine Snell dwarf mutation. Genomics 8:586–590.

Carabatsos, M.J., Elvin, J., Matzuk, M.M. et al. 1998. Characterization of oocyte and follicle development in growth factor differentiation-9-deficient mice. Dev. Biol. 204:373–384.

Cattanach, B.M., Iddon, A., Charlton, H.M., et al. 1977. Gonadotropin releasing hormone deficiency in a mutant mouse with hypogonadism. Nature 269:338–340.

Chalifour, L.E., Mes-Masson, A-M., Gomes, M.L., et al. 1992. Testicular adenoma and seminal vesicle engorgement in polyomavirus large-T antigen transgenic mice. Mol. Carcinog. 5:178–189.

Chappell, P.E., Lydon, J.P., Conneely, O.M., et al. 1997. Endocrine defects in mice carrying a null mutation for the progesterone receptor gene. Endocrinology 138:4147–4152.

Charest, N.J., Zhou, Z., Lubahn, D.B., et al. 1991. A frame shift mutation destabilizes androgen receptor messenger RNA in the Tfm mouse. Mol. Endocrinol. 5:573–581.

Colledge, W.H., Carlton, M.B.L., Udy, G.B., et al. 1994. Disruption of *c-mos* causes parthenogenetic development of unfertilized mouse eggs. Nature 370:65–68.

Couse, J.F. and Korach, K.S. 1998. Exploring the role of sex steroids through studies of receptor-deficient mice. J. Mol. Med. 76:497–511.

Couse, J.F. and Korach, K.S. 1999. Estrogen receptor null mice: what have we learned and where will they take us? Endocr. Rev. 20:358–417.

Davis, B.J., Lennard, D.E., Lee, C.A., et al. 1999a. Anovulation in cyclooxygenase-2-deficient mice is restored by prostaglandin E$_2$ and interleukin-1α. Endocrinology 140:2685–2695.

Davis, B.J., Dixon, D., and Herbert, R.A. 1999b. Ovary, oviduct, uterus, cervix and vagina. In: Maronpot, R.R., Boorman, G.A., and Gaul, B.W. (eds.), Pathology of the Mouse: Reference and Atlas. Vienna, IL: Cache River Press, pp. 409–443.

Dierich, A., Sairam, M.R., Monaco, L., et al. 1998. Impairing follicle stimulating hormone (FSH) signaling *in vivo*: targeted disruption of the FSH receptor leads to aberrant gametogenesis and hormonal imbalance. Proc. Natl. Acad. Sci. USA 95:13612–13617.

Dilworth, S.M. 1990. Cell alterations induced by large T-antigens of SV40 and polyoma virus. Semin. Cancer Biol. 1:407–414.

Dix, D.J., Allen, J.A., Collins, B.W., et al. 1996. Targeted gene disruption of *Hsp70-2* results in failed meiosis, germ cell apoptosis, and male infertility. Proc. Natl. Acad. Sci. USA 93:3264–3268.

Donehower, L.A., Harvey, M., Vogel, H., et al. 1995. Effects of genetic background on tumorigenesis in p53-deficient mice. Mol. Carcinog. 14:16–22.

Dong, J., Albertini, D.F., Nishimori, K., et al. 1996. Growth differentiation factor-9 is required during early ovarian folliculogenesis. Nature 383:531–535.

Eddy, E.M., Washburn, T.F., Bunch, D.O., et al. 1996. Targeted disruption of the estrogen receptor gene in male mice causes alteration of spermatogenesis and infertility. Endocrinology 137:4796–4805.

Elvin, J.A. and Matzuk, M.M. 1998. Mouse models of ovarian failure. Rev. Reprod. 3:183–195.

Fisher, C.R., Graves, K.H., Parlow, A.F., et al. 1998. Characterization of mice deficient in aromatase (ArKO) because of targeted disruption of the *cyp19* gene. Proc. Natl. Acad. Sci. USA 95:6965–6970.

Guo, Q., Kumar, T.R., Woodruff, T., et al. 1998. Overexpression of mouse follistatin causes reproductive defects in transgenic mice. Mol. Endocrinol. 12:96–106.

Hansen, L.A., Trempus, C.S., Mahler, J.F., et al. 1996. Association of tumor development with increased cellular proliferation and transgene overexpression, but not c-Ha-ras mutation, in v-Ha-ras transgenic Tg.AC mice. Carcinogenesis 17:1825–1833.

Hashimoto, N., Watanabe, N., Furuta, Y., et al. 1994. Parthenogenetic activation of oocytes in *c-mos*-deficient mice. Nature 370:68–71.

Hom, Y.K., Young, P., Wiesen, J.F., et al. 1998. Uterine and vaginal growth requires epidermal growth factor receptor signaling from stroma. Endocrinology 139:913–921.

Hsu, S.Y., Lai, R.J-M., Finegold, M., et al. 1996. Targeted overexpression of Bcl-2 in ovaries of transgenic mice leads to decreased follicle apoptosis, enhanced folliculogenesis, and increased germ cell tumorigenesis. Endocrinology 137:4837–4843.

Hutson, J.M., Baker, M., Terada, M., et al. 1994. Hormonal control of testicular descent and the cause of cryptorchidism. Reprod. Fertil. Dev. 6:151–156.

Kananen, K., Markkula, M., Rainio, E., et al. 1995. Gonadal tumorigenesis in transgenic mice bearing the mouse inhibin α-subunit promoter/SV40 T-antigen fusion gene: characterization of ovarian tumors and establishment of gonadotropin-responsive granulosa cell lines. Mol. Endocrinol. 9:616–627.

Kananen, K., Markkula, M., El-Hefnawy, T., et al. 1996. The mouse inhibin α-subunit promoter directs SV40 T-antigen to Leydig cells of transgenic mice. Mol. Cell. Endocrinol. 119:135–146.

Kendall, S.K., Samuelson, L.C., Saunders, T.L., et al. 1995. Targeted disruption of the pituitary glycoprotein hormone alpha-subunit produces hypogonadal and hypothyroid mice. Genes Dev. 9:2007–2019.

Knudson, C.M., Tung, K.S.K., Tourtellotte, W.G., et al. 1995. Bax-deficient mice with lymphoid hyperplasia and male germ cell death. Science 270:96–99.

Kondoh, G., Nishimune, Y., Nishizawa, Y., et al. 1994. Establishment and further characterization of a line of transgenic mice showing testicular tumorigenesis at 100% incidence. J. Urol. 152:2151–2154.

Krege, J.H., Hodgin, J.B., Couse, J.F., et al. 1998. Generation and reproductive phenotypes of mice lacking estrogen receptor-β. Proc. Natl. Acad. Sci. USA 95:15677–15682.

Kumar, T.T., Wang, Y., Lu, N., et al. 1997. Follicle stimulating hormone is required for ovarian follicle maturation but not male fertility. Nat. Genet. 15:201–204.

Kuroda, H., Terada, N., Nakayama, H., et al. 1988. Infertility due to growth arrest of ovarian follicles in Sl/Slᵗ mice. Dev. Biol. 126:71–79.

Lim, H., Paria, B.C., Das, S.K., et al. 1997. Multiple female reproductive failures in cyclooxygenase 2-deficient mice. Cell 91:197–208.

Lubahn, D.B., Moyer, J.S., Golding, T.S., et al. 1993. Alteration of reproductive function but not prenatal sexual development after insertional disruption of the mouse estrogen receptor gene. Proc. Natl. Acad. Sci. USA 90:11162–11166.

Lydon, J.P., DeMayo, F.J., Funk, C.R., et al. 1995. Mice lacking progesterone receptor exhibit pleiotropic reproductive abnormalities. Genes Dev. 9:2266–2278.

Lyon, M.F. and Hawkes, S.G. 1970. X-linked gene for testicular feminization. Nature 227:1217–1219.

Mahler, J.F. and Elwell, M.R. 1999. Pituitary gland. In: Maronpot, R.R., Boorman, G.A., and Gaul, B.W. (eds.), Pathology of the Mouse: Reference and Atlas. Vienna, IL: Cache River Press, pp. 491–507.

Mangelsdorf, D.J., Thummel, C., Beato, M., et al. 1995. The nuclear receptor superfamily: the second decade. Cell 83:835–839.

Mannan, M.A., and O'Shaughnessy, P.J. 1988. Ovarian steroid metabolism during post-natal development in the normal mouse and in the adult hypogonadal (hpg) mouse. J. Reprod. Fertil. 82:727–734.

Mason, A.J., Hayflick, J.S., Zoeller, R.T., et al. 1986. A deletion truncating the gonadotropin-releasing hormone gene is responsible for hypogonadism in the hpg mouse. Science 234:1366–1371.

Matzuk, M.M., Finegold, M.J., Su, J-G.J., et al. 1992. α-inhibin is a tumor-suppressor gene with gonadal specificity in mice. Nature 360:313–319.

Matzuk, M.M., Kumar, T.R., Shou, W., et al. 1996. Transgenic models to study the roles of inhibins and activins in reproduction, oncogenesis, and development. Recent Prog. Horm. Res. 51:123–157.

Matzuk, M.M., Dionne, L., Guo, Q., et al. 1998. Ovarian function in superoxide dismutase 1 and 2 knockout mice. Endocrinology 139:4008–4011.

McEwen, B.S. 1992. Steroid hormones: effect on brain development and function. Horm. Res. 37:1–10.

Murphy, L. and O'Shaughnessy, P.J. 1991. Testicular steroidogenesis in the testicular feminized (Tfm) mouse: loss of 17α-hydroxylase activity. J. Endocrinol. 131:443–449.

Nantel, F., Monaco, L., Foulkes, N.S., et al. 1996. Spermiogenesis deficiency and germ cell apoptosis in CREM-mutant mice. Nature 380:159–162.

Nishimori, K. and Matzuk, M.M. 1996. Transgenic mice in the analysis of reproductive development and function. Rev. Reprod. 1:203–212.

Paquis Flucklinger, V., Michiels, J-F., Vidal, F., et al. 1993. Expression in transgenic mice of the large T antigen of polyomavirus induces Sertoli cell tumors and allows the establishment of differentiated cell lines. Oncogene 8:2087–2094.

Parker, K.L. 1998. The roles of steroidogenic factor 1 in endocrine development and function. Mol. Cell. Endocrinol. 145:15–20.

Perez, G.I., Robles, R., Knudson, C.M., et al. 1999. Prolongation of ovarian lifespan into advanced chronological age by *Bax*-deficiency. Nat. Genet. 21:200–203.

Peschon, J.J., Behringer, R.R., Cate, R.L., et al. 1992. Directed expression of an oncogene to Sertoli cells in transgenic mice using Mullerian inhibiting substance regulatory sequences. Mol. Endocrinol. 6:1403–1411.

Radovsky, A., Mitsumori, K., and Chapin, R.C. 1999. Male reproductive tract. In: Maronpot, R.R., Boorman, G.A., and Gaul, B.W. (eds). Pathology of the Mouse: Reference and Atlas. Vienna, IL: Cache River Press, pp. 381–407.

Rahman, N.A., Rilianawati, K.K., Paukku, T., et al. 1998. Transgenic mouse models for gonadal tumorigenesis. Mol. Cell. Endocrinol. 145:167–174.

Risma, K.A., Clay, C.M., Nett, T.M., et al. 1995. Targeted overexpression of luteinizing hormone in transgenic mice leads to infertility, polycystic ovaries, and ovarian tumors. Proc. Natl. Acad. Sci. USA 92:1322–1326.

Schedl, A. and Hastie, N. 1998. Multiple roles for the Wilms' tumor suppressor gene, WT1, in genitourinary development. Mol. Cell. Endocrinol. 140:65–69.

Sicinski, P., Donaher, J.L., Geng, Y., et al. 1996. Cyclin D2 is an FSH-responsive gene involved in gonadal cell proliferation and oncogenesis. Nature 384:470–474.

Simon, A.M., Goodenough, D.A., Li, E., et al. 1997. Female infertility in mice lacking connexin 37. Nature 385:525–529.

Simoni, M. 1994. Transgenic animals in male reproduction research. Exp. Clin. Endocrinol. 102:419–433.

Slegtenhorst-Eegdeman, K.E., DeRooij, D.G., Verhoef-Post, M., et al. 1998. Macroorchidism in FMR1 knockout mice is caused by increased Sertoli cell proliferation during testicular development. Endocrinology 139:156–162.

Stefaneanu, L. 1997. Pituitary sex steroid receptors: localization and function. Endocr. Pathol. 8:91–108.

Sterneck, E., Tessarollo, L., and Johnson, P.F. 1997. An essential role for C/EBPβ in female reproduction. Genes Dev. 11:2153–2162.

St. John, M.A.R., Tao, W., Fei, X., et al. 1999. Mice deficient of Lats1 develop soft-tissue sarcomas, ovarian tumors, and pituitary dysfunction. Nat. Genet. 21:182–186.

Tilly, J.L. 1996. Apoptosis and ovarian function. Rev. Reprod. 1:162–172.

Topilko, P., Schneider-Maunoury, S., Levi, G., et al. 1997. Multiple pituitary and ovarian defects in Krox-24 (NGFI-A, Egr-1)-targeted mice. Mol. Endocrinol. 12:107–122.

Witte, O.N. 1990. Steel locus defines new multipotent growth factor. Cell 63:5–6.

Yoshizawa, T., Handa, Y., Uematsu, Y., et al. 1997. Mice lacking the vitamin D receptor exhibit impaired bone formation, uterine hypoplasia and growth retardation after weaning. Nat. Genet. 16:391–396.

Zhou, J., Kumar, R., Matzuk, M.M., et al. 1997. Insulin-like growth factor 1 regulates gonadotropin responsiveness in the murine ovary. Mol. Endocrinol. 11:1924–1933.

# 23
# Renal Diseases in Genetically Engineered Mice

Michael A. Eckhaus and Jeffrey B. Kopp

## EMBRYOLOGY

The definitive mammalian kidney is derived from a reciprocal interaction between the ureteric bud and the
metanephric mesenchyme, both of which are derived
from nephrogenic mesoderm (Kaufman 1992). At about
embryonic day (E) 11.5, the ureteric bud enters the
metanephric blastema, composed of undifferentiated mesenchymal cells (Fig. 23.1). Thereafter, the ureteric bud
undergoes sequential bifurcation. The advancing ureteric
bud releases various soluble factors that induce condensation of undifferentiated mesenchyme. These induced mesenchymal cells undergo a conversion to renal epithelium,
and the aggregated epithelial cells form the renal vesicles.
The renal vesicles form comma-shaped bodies that elongate to form S-shaped bodies. The portion of the
S-shaped body closest to the ureteric duct fuses with the
duct to form the distal convoluted tubule. The other end
of the S-shaped body forms the proximal convoluted
tubule, Bowman's capsule, and the glomerulus. At
E12.5–13 the metanephric kidney has a primitive cortical
region, with the medulla composed of undifferentiated
mesenchyme. The cortex expands by E14, with increased
numbers of tubules and renal vesicles present. Primitive
glomeruli are present on E14.5, and the medulla still contains primarily undifferentiated mesenchyme. By
E16.5–17 most glomeruli are concentrated in the peripheral third of the kidney, with less differentiated
metanephric tissue present in the superficial nephrogenic
cap. Increased numbers of proximal and distal convoluted
tubules are present by E17.5, with little undifferentiated
mesenchyme remaining in the medulla. The kidney continues to grow and mature during the first several weeks

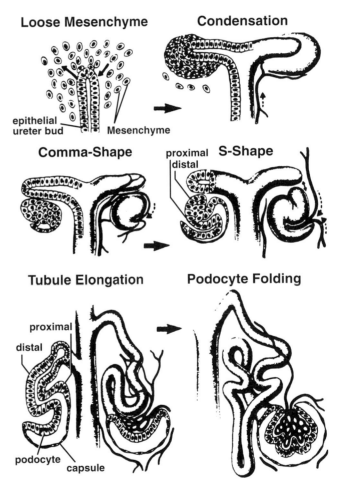

**FIGURE 23.1** Development of the metanephric
kidney. Reciprocal interaction between the ureteric
epithelium and metanephric mesenchyme leads to an
ordered progression of steps resulting in formation of
the nephron. (Reproduced with permission, Mugrauer
et al. 1988)

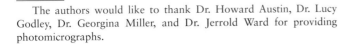

The authors would like to thank Dr. Howard Austin, Dr. Lucy
Godley, Dr. Georgina Miller, and Dr. Jerrold Ward for providing
photomicrographs.

347

postpartum, attaining adult glomerular and tubular morphology by approximately 3 weeks of age in the mouse.

## ANATOMIC FEATURES

The kidneys in mice and rats are unilobular with a single pyramidal-shaped renal papilla (Fig. 23.2A). This contrasts with the human kidney, in which the medulla is organized into multiple pyramids separated by cortical columns. The right kidney is located cranial to the left kidney and tends to be slightly heavier. Average kidney weight in 12-week-old mice ranges from 0.5 to 0.8 percent body weight. An excellent review of mouse kidney anatomy and histology is available (Liebelt 1986).

Mouse kidneys manifest sexual dimorphism, which becomes apparent between days 20 and 30 of life. The kidneys in male mice are larger than in female. N-acetylglucosaminidase, an enzyme present in abundance in lysosomes of the proximal tubular epithelial cell, is present in urine at concentrations eightfold higher in male mice compared with female mice (Funakawa et al. 1984). In most strains, the glomerular parietal epithelial cells lining Bowman's capsule are cuboidal in male mice and more flattened in female mice (Figs. 23.2C–D) (Liebelt 1986).

The normal mouse kidney contains approximately 4000–7000 glomeruli, depending upon the strain and upon environmental conditions, including humidity. Glomerular number reaches a peak value at 10 weeks of age and undergoes a slight but significant decline by 50 weeks of age (Sato et al. 1975). Glomerular numbers can be readily evaluated by digestion of the kidney with hydrochloric acid, with direct counting of the free glomeruli under phase microscopy (MacKay et al. 1987).

## TISSUE PROCESSING

For routine examination of the kidney, fixation with 10 percent neutral buffered formalin (or 4 percent paraformaldehyde, which provides the same amount of formaldehyde) is quite adequate. Fixation with a zinc-based fixative may enhance the ability to perform immunohistochemical studies on the kidney. Immunostaining may be enhanced by using a non–cross-linking fixative, in which an alcohol serves as a denaturing agent. Types of this fixative include 70 percent ethanol, Carnoy's solution, and methanol Carnoy's solution (methacarn, composed of 60 percent methanol, 30 percent chloroform, 10 percent glacial acetic acid). The Carnoy solutions should be stored in glass, and tissues should not be left longer than 48 hours before being changed to 70 percent ethanol, since otherwise substantial dehydration will occur.

Fixed tissue may be embedded in paraffin. While multitissue blocks provide the opportunity to survey many tissues economically, the best histology may be obtained by embedding the kidney in a single block and sectioning to produce a coronal view through the precise center of the kidney (also known as a bivalve section). This allows the inspection of cortex, outer medulla, and inner medulla, including the renal papilla (Fig. 23.2A). Paraffin kidney sections are best cut as thinly as possible, ideally 4 µm. The mouse glomerulus has a high volume fraction of cells, appearing hypercellular when compared with the rat or human kidney, and thin sections are essential for evaluating proliferative glomerulonephritis. Alternatively, fixed tissue may be embedded in plastic (such as glycol methacrylate), which permits sectioning at 2 µm. These sections may be stained with conventional stains (although the reduced amount of tissue will cause the staining to appear fainter than with 4 µm sections) and will facilitate detailed examination of renal structure.

Tissue for transmission electron microscopy should be fixed in fresh 2.5 percent glutaraldehyde in either phosphate-buffered saline or cacodylate buffer. Glutaraldehyde is an excellent fixative, acting very quickly, but it is a larger molecule than formaldehyde and penetrates tissue more slowly. As a consequence, tissue specimens for electron microscopy must be small, ideally with no dimension larger than 1 mm. Tissue is then embedded in glycol methacrylate. Thick sections (2 µm) can be stained with toluidine blue or trichrome stain, suitable for high-power light microscopy and particularly suitable for detailed examination of the glomeruli. Thin sections (0.5 µm) are stained, typically with uranyl acetate, for transmission electron microscopy.

Routine histologic analysis of the kidney can be made using routine hematoxylin and eosin (H&E) stains. A variety of additional histochemical stains are extremely useful for evaluation of glomeruli and tubules. The periodic acid-Schiff stain (PAS) is particularly helpful in staining glomerular and tubular basement membranes, as well as proteinaceous tubular fluid. Some investigators working on kidneys rely largely on the PAS stain and omit the H&E stain. The PAS stain combined with methenamine silver (PAMS) is also particularly useful in staining basement membranes. Masson trichrome is valuable for staining interstitial or intraglomerular matrix. Congo red differentially stains amyloid deposits in the glomeruli, blood vessels, and interstitium. Sections stained with Congo red should be prepared at a thickness of 10 µm. Special procedures including apoptosis assays and in situ hybridization may be valuable in some instances.

Evaluation of renal histology should include detailed consideration of the following four compartments: (1) glomeruli—glomerular number, glomerular size,

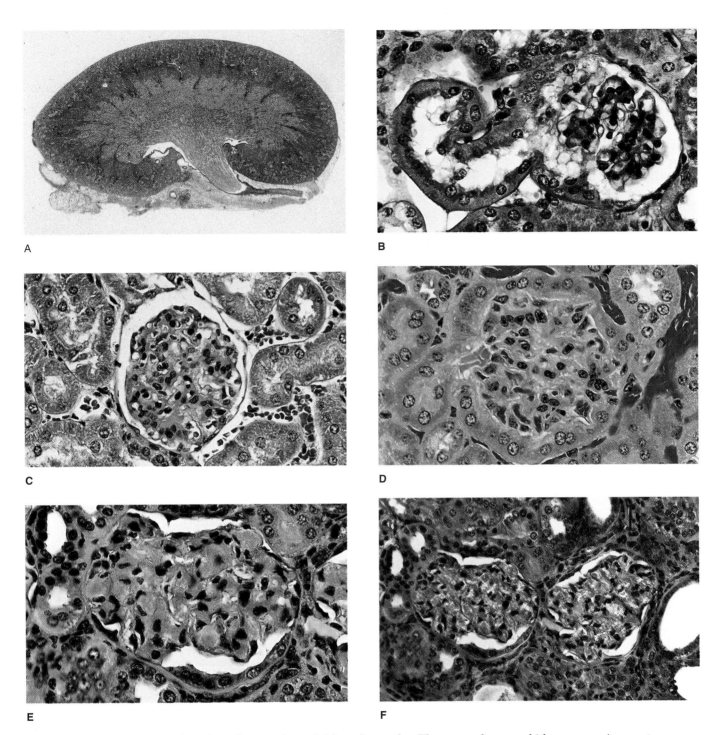

**FIGURE 23.2**  Normal kidney histology and amyloid nephropathy. The normal mouse kidney comprises cortex, outer medulla, and inner medulla. The inner medulla terminates in a single renal pyramid, or papilla (**A,** PAS). In FVB/N mice, Bowman's capsule is lined by parietal epithelial cells that are flat at the vascular pole and cuboidal at the tubular pole (**B,** PAS). A C57BL/6 mouse exhibits sexual dimorphism in the morphology of the glomerular parietal epithelial cells, with flat cells in female mice (**C,** H&E) and cuboidal cells in male mice (**D,** H&E). Secondary amyloid in a 129 × C57BL mouse with chronic dermatitis appears as orange-red extracellular matrix material within the glomeruli on Congo red stain (**E**), which exhibits apple green birefringence when viewed under polarizing light (**F**).

glomerular cellularity, mesangial matrix expansion, patency of capillary loops, and crescents within Bowman's space; (2) tubules—epithelial cell integrity, tubular atrophy, and tubular casts; (3) interstitium—fibrosis and cellular infiltrates; (4) vessels—hypertrophy, intimal proliferation, medial proliferation and cellular infiltrates.

Renal structure is well suited to quantitative assessment of pathology. There are several available approaches using light microscopy. First, glomerulosclerosis, tubular dilatation/atrophy, and interstitial fibrosis may be assessed using a semiquantitative scale (Okada et al. 1995; Raij et al. 1984). Second, the number of glomerular cell nuclei may be counted. Third, using the light microscope and a point-counting method, one can quantitate the volume of renal cortex occupied by glomeruli, tubules, interstitium, and fluid space (Möller and Skriver 1985). Fourth, light microscopic images may be digitized and the area of glomeruli or the extent of glomerulosclerosis, defined as stained matrix exceeding a particular optical density threshold, may be measured. Fifth, ultrastructural photographs may be subjected to direct measurement or point counting to determine glomerular basement membrane thickness or the volume density of glomerular components (Jensen et al. 1979; Pagtalunan et al. 1997).

Immunologic renal disease is typically associated with the deposition of one or more immunoglobulins, sometimes in association with complement (Kopp et al. 1994a). These molecules can be identified using immunofluorescence of frozen sections or immunoperoxidase technique on paraffin-embedded tissue (alkaline phosphatase is best avoided in the kidney, where the tubular cells express high levels of alkaline phosphatase). The detecting antibodies must be specific for mouse or rat protein. While immunofluorescence requires a microscope equipped for epifluorescence, the staining protocols for using this approach are easier to use and may involve lower background staining as compared with immunoperoxidase techniques. To detect IgG, IgA, and IgM, specific antibody directed against the appropriate heavy chain (δ, α, and μ, respectively) are used. Immunoglobulin light chain is detected with antibodies specific for κ or λ light chain. Since the classical and alternate complement activation cascades unite with the activation and deposition of C3, it is common to screen for complement deposition using an antibody that identifies C3. The presence of blood-derived fibrinogen, particularly within Bowman's space, indicates severe disruption of capillary integrity, such as seen with florid glomerulonephritis associated with crescents. Finally, when albumin is detected throughout the glomerulus, this indicates nonspecific capillary leakage and thus provides a control for the specificity of the deposition of other proteins within the glomerulus.

# RENAL FUNCTION

Routine screening for renal function should be carried out on mice, even if they lack histologic abnormalities (Ragan 1989). The initial assessment should include urinalysis. Urine can be simply obtained by gently lifting the mouse from its cage and placing it on a square of Parafilm (American Can, Greenwich, CT). Mice often void spontaneously when placed on the Parafilm or may void when abdominal pressure is applied gently, in a sweeping motion beginning in the midabdomen and extending down over the bladder (a procedure know as a Crede maneuver). A microscopic examination can be conducted on freshly voided urine, preferably following centrifugation to concentrate the sample as much as feasible (e.g., from 100 μl to 25 μl). This exam can be used to identify formed elements in the urine, such as white blood cells, red blood cells, and cellular casts.

A urine dipstick (Boehringer Mannheim, Indianapolis, IN) can be used to measure multiple parameters in a semiquantitative fashion. The most useful of these include urine protein, urine blood, and urine glucose (a reflection of both serum glucose and tubular function). Each test will require approximately 10 μl of urine. Proteinuria can be quantitatively measured by use of a metabolic cage; since the mouse urine volume is typically 1–2 ml/day, obtaining an adequate collection may be difficult. Protein concentration can be measured in a random collection, but since urine concentration may vary in a given animal and between animals, protein concentration is not a sensitive measure of renal disease. It is worth noting that with renal injury, one of the first tubular functions to be lost is the ability to concentrate urine; therefore urine volumes are frequently large early in the course of chronic renal disease. An alternative is to measure urine protein and urine creatinine in a random urine specimen. The daily urine excretion of creatinine is constant, assuming the presence of stable renal function (not necessarily normal function) and the absence of ongoing muscle injury. The urine protein/urine creatinine ratio is a dimensionless number that provides an index of proteinuria independent of urine concentration (Abitbol et al. 1990).

Large proteins (particularly >40–60 kDa) and anionic proteins experience restricted passage across the glomerular filtration barrier. Glomerular filtrate therefore contains mostly small molecular weight proteins, although detectable amounts of albumin (67 kDa) are also present. Normal tubules reabsorb most of this protein. Tubular injury manifests as an increase in low–molecular weight proteins, of which β2-microglobulin (12 kDa) is a commonly measured example. By contrast, glomerular proteinuria is characterized by the appearance in urine of the full range of serum proteins, including both large proteins (intact immunoglobulin, 150 kDa, and albumin) and small proteins. The distinction between glomerular and tubular proteinuria may therefore be made with either SDS-PAGE or nondenaturing gel electrophoresis.

Other urinary tests are available to assess tubular cell injury. Several proximal tubular cell enzymes, including N-acetylglucosaminidase and lysozyme, enter urine with tubular cell injury (Suzuki et al. 1995). As with total protein, values should be normalized to urine creatinine concentration to correct for differences in urine concentration. N–acetylglucosaminidase is also present in serum; therefore glomerular injury will also be associated with the presence of N–acetylglucosaminidase in urine.

Blood may be obtained by retro-orbital puncture or tail vein incision (following tail warming) as a survival procedure or cardiac puncture at the time of sacrifice. Useful and commonly available serologic tests include blood urea nitrogen (BUN), creatinine, and albumin. BUN is a more sensitive measure of renal function in mice than is creatinine but may also be elevated with saline losses. The most definitive test for glomerular filtration rate is inulin clearance, for which detailed protocols exist (Kiberd 1991; Konikowski et al. 1970).

Hypertension may be a feature of early renal disease, particularly glomerulonephritis, and is a common feature of advanced or end-stage renal disease of all etiologies. Typically, hypertension due to renal disease is a result of impaired sodium excretion and/or increased production of renin. Direct intra-arterial assessment (for example of the carotid artery) in unanesthetized, unrestrained animals is generally considered the optimal method of determining blood pressure (Schlager 1966). Limitations of this approach include technical difficulty, the invasiveness of the procedure, and the difficulty of obtaining long-term observations from a single animal. An alternative is tail cuff measurement, which when coupled with the appropriate computer algorithm, can be a reliable approach (Krege et al. 1995).

## RENAL DISEASE SYNDROMES

Glomerular disease is conventionally classified as nephritis (nephritic syndrome) or nephrosis (nephrotic syndrome). Glomerulonephritis in its most full-blown manifestation is characterized by systemic hypertension, impaired glomerular filtration (elevated BUN and serum creatinine), hematuria, proteinuria, and the presence of red blood cell casts in urine (Fig. 23.3A-D). In certain immunologic forms of glomerulonephritis, serum levels of complement proteins are reduced, and complement deposits are present in the kidney. Nephrosis is characterized by low serum albumin, elevated serum cholesterol, edema (manifested in the mouse as total body

swelling, including ascites within the peritoneal cavity but with the edema sparing the limbs), and proteinuria. In both glomerulonephritis and nephrotic syndrome, the progression of glomerular disease is associated with progressive glomerulosclerosis, characterized by accumulation of extracellular matrix material that typically includes collagen I and III, fibronectin, and small leucine-rich proteoglycans, biglycan and decorin.

Another form of renal disease is interstitial nephritis, in which the glomeruli are spared, at least in the early forms. Manifestations include dilated tubules, sometimes with proteinaceous casts, and interstitial inflammatory cell infiltrates, usually composed predominantly of mononuclear cells (lymphocytes and macrophages). Ultimately, interstitial fibrosis develops, in which the tubules, initially located back-to-back, are separated by matrix material rich in collagen.

With progressive glomerular disease, tubular injury and interstitial nephritis also develop. With progressive interstitial nephritis, tubular injury is associated with glomerular atrophy and sclerosis. Therefore, the late stages of many diverse renal diseases appear remarkably similar, with widespread glomerular, tubular, and interstitial changes. An important corollary of this observation is that the specific pathways of renal injury in a given model are best elucidated by studying the earliest phases of renal injury. Clues to which ages and which specific animals to sacrifice to study these early phases may be derived from serum and urine tests outlined above, or it may be necessary to sacrifice animals from a range of ages.

## SPONTANEOUS RENAL DISEASE

A number of spontaneous conditions may affect the kidney in a variety of inbred and outbred murine strains (Table 23.1). Many of these conditions manifest morphologic characteristics similar to the phenotypes observed in transgenic and knockout models. Familiarity with these conditions will avoid possible confusion with phenotypes observed in genetically engineered murine models.

Hydronephrosis is a condition in which there is dilatation of the renal pelvis and calyces containing urinary filtrate. With long-term hydronephrosis, of at least a few weeks duration, pressure atrophy results in thinning of the renal cortex, which may transform the kidney into a fluid-filled sac. Hydronephrosis may occur secondary to obstruction of the urinary outflow tract due to urethral calculi or, in male mice, seminal plugs. Hereditary hydronephrosis has been described in STR/N, NZC, C3H, and C57BL mice. It is associated with the presence of mutant genes for luxate (lx),

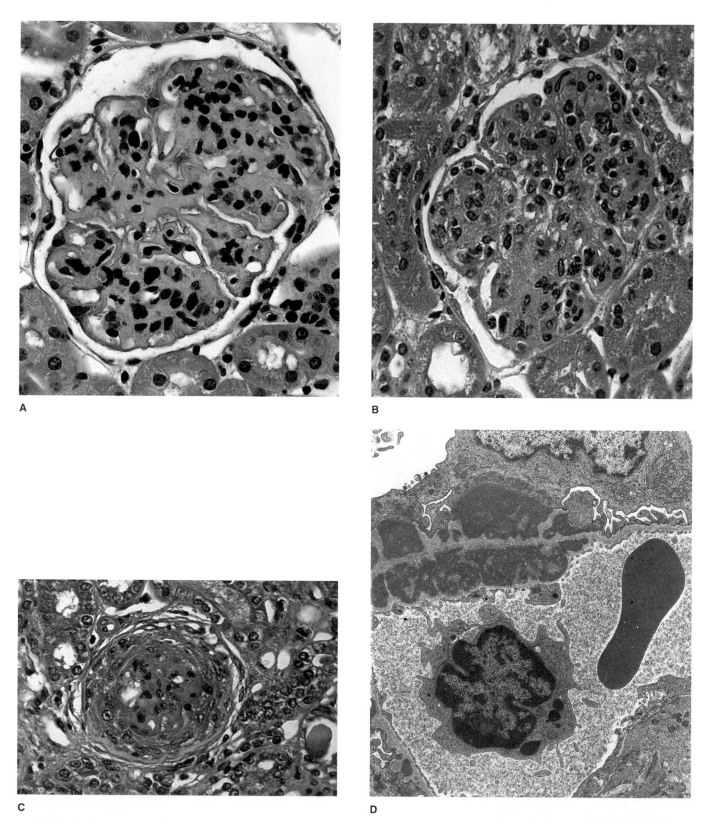

**FIGURE 23.3** Proliferative glomerulonephritis. Spontaneous proliferative glomerulonephritis develops in 129 × C57BL/6 mice with aging (**A**, H&E). *lpr/lpr* mice also manifest proliferative glomerulonephritis (**B**, H&E), which in some cases manifests as fibrocellular epithelial crescents within Bowman's space (**C**, H&E). Ultrastructrural study of the *lpr/lpr* mouse reveals subendothelial and subepithelial deposits within peripheral glomerular capillary loops; an erythrocyte and a lymphoid cell are visible in the vessel lumen (**D**).

**TABLE 23.1. Spontaneous renal disease**

| | |
|---|---|
| Hydronephrosis | STR/N, NZC, C3H, C57BL *lx, my, os, se, ur* |
| Nephronophthisis | CBA/CaH |
| Amyloidosis | AB/J, A/J, CD-1 |
| Chronic progressive nephropathy | B6C3F1 |
| Glomerulonephritis | AKR, BALB/c, HI, NZB, NZB × NZW, C57BL/6, 129 |

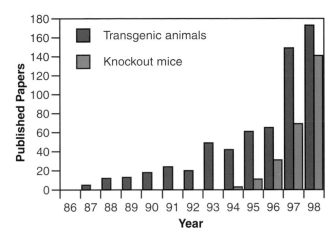

**FIGURE 23.4** Transgenic mouse and knockout mouse publications concerning the kidney. Since the development of the first transgenic mouse in 1974 and the first knockout mouse in 1985, there has been a progressive increase in the numbers of transgenic and knockout papers that have relevance for kidney anatomy, physiology, or pathology, as indicated by Medline references.

myelencephalic blebs (*my*), oligosyndactyly (*os*), short ear (*se*), and urogenital recessive (*ur*) (Hsu 1986).

Nephronophthisis is a progressive nephropathy that has been described in CBA/CaH mice (Lyon and Hulse 1971). The disease is due to the expression of an autosomal recessive gene located on chromosome 10. Tubular atrophy of convoluted tubules, with protein-filled tubules and glomerulosclerosis, are the principal morphologic changes. Affected mice generally die of renal failure by 5 to 7 months of age.

Amyloidosis is a disease process that occurs secondary to an underlying disease condition or associated with senescence. Amyloid is an extracellular eosinophilic homogenous hyaline material, composed of fibrils arranged in β pleated sheets. Deposition may lead to dysfunction due to pressure atrophy of adjacent cellular elements. Secondary amyloidosis in mice is associated with increased deposition of amyloid-associated (AA) protein within glomeruli and within the subintimal region of small renal blood vessels. In age-associated amyloidosis, the amyloid tends to be deposited in the interstitium of the renal cortex and at the corticomedullary junction (Wolf and Hard 1996). Amyloid can be demonstrated in tissue sections using the Congo red stain in thick sections (10 μm), where it stains orange-red and exhibits a typical apple-green birefringence when viewed with polarized light (Figs. 23.2E-F).

Chronic progressive nephropathy has been noted in aging B6C3F1 mice, and the disease process is morphologically similar to the spontaneous nephropathy of aging rats (Wolf and Hard 1996). Renal tubular degeneration and regeneration are prominent along with dilated proteinaceous fluid–filled tubules and variable glomerulosclerosis.

Spontaneous glomerulonephritis develops in a variety of inbred mouse strains with an increased incidence noted in AKR, BALB/c, HI, NZB × NZW, and C57BL/6 mice (Sass 1986). In addition to light microscopy, these lesions are best characterized by utilizing transmission electron microscopy to identify immune deposits adjacent to or in the glomerular basement membrane. Additionally, immunohistochemistry can document the presence of immunoglobulins and complement within the immune

deposits. The incidence of glomerulonephritis in C57BL/6 mice is notable, since this strain is frequently used in gene-targeting models. Recent analyses of aging 129/SvTer mice have identified a similar glomerulonephritis (Fig. 23.3A; J.M. Ward, personal communication).

The recently available technology for creating genetically engineered murine models has allowed substantial strides to be made in the areas of renal development, disease, and physiology. The number of published manuscripts utilizing either transgenic or gene-targeting technology has significantly increased in recent years (Fig. 23.4). These models include investigations in developmental biology, with emphasis on specific transcription factors and oncogenes. Other studies have concentrated on examining the basic roles of hormones, cytokines, matrix proteins, and inflammatory mediators on renal disease and physiology. Models examining the role of specific viral genes have increased the understanding of the pathogenesis of viral-mediated renal disease. Excellent reviews of these models have been published (Grandaliano et al. 1995; Kone 1998; Kopp 1997; Kopp and Klotman 1995a, 1995b; Matsuka and Ichikawa 1997; Ryffel 1996; Saito et al. 1997; Schieren et al. 1996; Striker et al. 1995).

A variety of promoters are used to increase the specificity and activity of gene constructs within renal tissues. Tables 23.2 and 23.3 list the principle viral and mammalian promoters that have been used in transgenic investigations and that might be used in conditional gene-targeting investigations.

**TABLE 23.2. Expression of gene constructs using viral promoters**

|  | Renal expression | Extrarenal expression |
|---|---|---|
| CMV | Glomerulus, tubule | Widespread |
| SV40 | Glomerulus, DT | Thymus, choroid plexus |
| BK | Epithelium | Thymus |
| MMTV | DT, CT | Mammary, lung, prostate, salivary |
| HIV-1 | GEC, PT | Lymphoid, intestine, skin, muscle |

Note: DT = distal convoluted tubule; CT = collecting tubule; GEC = glomerular epithelial cell; PT proximal tubule.

**TABLE 23.3. Expression of gene constructs using mammalian promoters**

|  | Renal expression | Extrarenal expression |
|---|---|---|
| Vimentin | Glomerulus, tubules | Heart, brain |
| ICAM-2 | Endothelial cells | Endothelial, monocytes, neutrophils |
| von Willebrand factor | Endothelial cells | Endothelial cells |
| pre-proET-1 | Endothelial, mesangial | Endothelial cells |
| $\gamma$-GT type II | PT | None |
| Angiotensinogen | PT | Liver, heart, adrenal, ovary |
| PEPCK | PT | Liver, fat, muscle, intestine, mammary |
| Kidney Androgenic protein | PT | None |
| Cadherin | CT | None |
| Insulin II | PT | Pancreas |
| Erythropoietin | PT, interstitial cell | Liver |
| DARPP-32 | MTAL | Brain |
| Bumetanide-sensitive Na-K-Cl cotransporter | MTAL | None |
| Tamm-Horsfall glycoprotein | MTAL | None |
| Epidermal growth factor | MTAL, DT | Salivary gland |
| Keratin 18 | DT, CT | Lung, liver, intestine |
| Metallothionein I | Tubules | Testes, lymphoid, mammary |
| NaCl-coupled betaine transporter | Medulla | None |
| Renin | JGA | None |
| PTH receptor | Kidney | Liver |

Note: ICAM-2 = intracellular adhesion molecule–2; ET-1 = endothelin 1; $\gamma$-GT = $\gamma$ glutamyl transpeptidase; PEPCK = phosphoenolpyruvate carboxykinase; DARPP-32 = dopamine and camp-regulation phosphoprotein–32; PTH parathyroid hormone; PT = proximal tubule; MTAL = medullary thick ascending limb; DT = distal tubule; CT = collecting tubule; JGA = juxtaglomerular apparatus.

# DEVELOPMENTAL ABNORMALITIES

Renal development requires a well-ordered reciprocal interaction between the ureteric bud and the metanephric mesenchyme. A number of transgenic and gene-targeted deletion models have been described that further define the role of these regulatory genes (Table 23.4).

The expression of *WT-1* and *Wnt-4* are necessary for mesenchymal condensation in the developing metanephric kidney. Null mutation of these genes leads to renal agenesis (Kreidberg et al. 1993; Stark et al. 1994). Following initial induction by the ureteric bud, the metanephric mesenchyme expresses *WT-1* mRNA, leading to mesenchymal condensation and the formation of renal vesicles. Targeted deletion of *WT-1* results in absence of the ureteric bud, indicating the crucial role of communication between the mesenchyme and the ureteric bud to promote ureteric bud differentiation, and consequent failure of mesenchymal differentiation. *Wnt-4* is expressed in mesenchymal condensates and comma-shaped body; targeted deletion of this gene also interferes with nephronogenesis.

Glial-cell-line–derived neurotropic factor (GDNF) is a dopaminergic neurotropic factor expressed in the developing metanephric mesenchyme, as well as in the mesenchymal layer of the gastrointestinal tract. In the developing kidney, GDNF plays an important role in the induction of the ureteric epithelium to stimulate branching of the ureteric bud. Mice homozygous for a

**TABLE 23.4. Developmental renal abnormalities in transgenic and knockout mice**

| Gene | Renal phenotype | Reference |
|---|---|---|
| *WT-1* (KO) | Agenesis | Kreidberg et al. 1993 |
| *Wnt-4* (KO) | Agenesis | Stark et al. 1994 |
| *GDNF* (KO) | Agenesis, dysgenesis | Pichel et al. 1996 |
| *c-ret* (KO) | Agenesis, hypoplasia | Schuchardt et al. 1994 |
| *p53* (T) | Small kidneys, decreased number glomeruli, glomerulosclerosis | Godley et al. 1996 |
| *Pax2b* (T) | Glomerular and tubular disease | Dressler et al. 1993 |
| *Pax2b* (KO) | Agenesis, hypoplasia, cysts | Keller et al. 1994 |
| *ld* locus (KO) | Agenesis | Messing et al. 1990 |
| *inv* locus (KO) | Glomerular and tubular disease | Yokoyama et al. 1993 |
| *PDGFB* chain (KO) | Glomerular tuft does not form | Levéen et al. 1994 |
| Cyclooxygenase II (KO) | Immature glomeruli, dysplastic tubules | Dinchuk et al. 1995 |

targeted deletion of the GDNF gene have significant renal abnormalities, including bilateral agenesis and dysgenesis, with mice dying shortly after birth (Pichel et al. 1996). Gastrointestinal lesions include an absence of myenteric neurons, resulting in defective peristalsis.

The oncogene *c-ret* encodes a receptor tyrosine kinase that transduces signals for cell growth and differentiation and is required for renal differentiation. *c-ret* is normally expressed in the wolffian duct and ureteric bud epithelium, as well as in the developing central and peripheral nervous system. Targeted deletion of *c-ret* leads to renal aplasia and dysplasia. Mice with a null mutation develop to term but die shortly after birth (Schuchardt et al. 1994).

Transgenic mice with overexpression of wild-type *p53* manifest small kidneys with reduced numbers of nephrons, and subsequently these mice develop glomerulosclerosis (Fig. 23.5; Godley et al. 1996). Expression of *c-ret*, *Dolichos biflorus (DB)* lectin, and aquaporin-2, normally expressed in ureteric bud derivatives, was abnormal in *p53* transgenic mice. Increased apoptosis of mesenchymal cells in the nephrogenic cap was noted. This increase in apoptosis resulted in a decrease in functional nephrons that was not directly due to *p53* expression, as expression of *p53* was restricted to the ureteric bud. Asynchrony of ureteric bud induction of the metanephric mesenchyme was likely responsible for the decreased numbers of functional nephrons. Subsequent hyperfiltration injury of existing nephrons was the probable cause of secondary glomerular injury and glomerulosclerosis.

*Pax2* encodes a transcription factor expressed in the embryonic development of the kidney, as well as the optic cup, optic stalk, otic vesicle, and neural tube. *Pax2* is normally expressed in the induced metanephric mesenchyme, the ureteric bud epithelium, and the renal epithelial structures that derive from the induced mesenchyme. The spontaneous null mutation *(krd/krd)* of *Pax2* leads to a combination of renal defects including agenesis, hypoplasia, and cyst formation (Keller et al. 1994). Ocular manifestations include hypoplasia of the inner cell layer and ganglion cell layers of the retina. Transgenic mice overexpressing *Pax2* develop neonatal microcystic tubular dilatation associated with atrophic glomeruli (Dressler et al. 1993). Ultrastructural analysis reveals effacement of podocytes and poorly developed endothelial fenestrations.

Renal aplasia has also been documented in *ld* (limb deformity) knockout mice (Messing et al. 1990). Approximately one-third of the null mutation mice develop unilateral renal aplasia along with a variety of lesions affecting the appendicular skeleton.

There are *inv* locus knockout mice that have been reported to develop situs inversus. Mice with a null mutation have renal lesions including glomerulonephropathy and microcystic tubular dilatation and die during the first week of postnatal life (Yokoyama et al. 1993).

Targeted deletion of the gene encoding PDGF-B causes significant abnormalities in glomerular morphology (Levéen et al. 1994). Mice with the null mutation have renal vesicles containing Bowman's capsule and loss of the glomerular tuft. No abnormalities are detected in embryonic comma- or S-shaped bodies, and normal numbers of glomeruli are present. Mice typically die between E17 and 18.5 or at birth. During formation of the glomerular tuft, expression of PDGF-B shifts from the epithelium to the mesangial cells. Ultrastructural analyses reveal Bowman's capsule to contain one to several capillary aneurysmal-like structures, with normal basement membrane, podocytes, and endothelial cells but an absence of mesangial cells.

Cyclooxygenase (COX)-2 knockout mice develop renal dysplasia (Dinchuk et al. 1995). Neonatal mice with the null mutation have underdeveloped kidneys with immature glomeruli, tubular cysts at the corticomedullary junction, and medullary hypoplasia. COX-2 may play a role in the normal induction of the metanephric mesenchyme between E15 and 18.

# CYSTIC RENAL DISEASE

Multiple murine models of cystic and polycystic renal disease have been described (Table 23.5). Several models involve transgenic mice expressing oncogenes, in which expression is associated with hyperplasia of renal tubular epithelium. These include the oncogenes *c-erb B*, *c-myc*, H-*ras*, and *v-src* (Boulter et al. 1992; Schaffner et al. 1993; Stöcklin et al. 1993; Trudel et al. 1991) Increased proliferation of tubular epithelium is associated with the development of tubular epithelial cysts and sometimes tubular epithelial adenomas. SV40 T antigen transgenic mice exhibit similar phenotypes due to hyperplasia of renal tubular epithelium (Kelley et al. 1991).

Other murine models of cystic renal disease involve targeted deletions of genes involved in the regulation of apoptosis. Knockout models of *bcl-2* and AP-2β transcription factor are associated with an inhibition of apoptosis, leading to cystic tubular disease (Moser et al. 1997; Nakayama et al. 1994). Inhibition of apoptosis during the critical stages of nephrogenic development is the underlying mechanism leading to cyst development.

Gene-targeted deletion of the tensin gene in mice also leads to renal tubular cyst formation (Lo et al. 1997). Deficiency of tensin in the renal tubules causes a

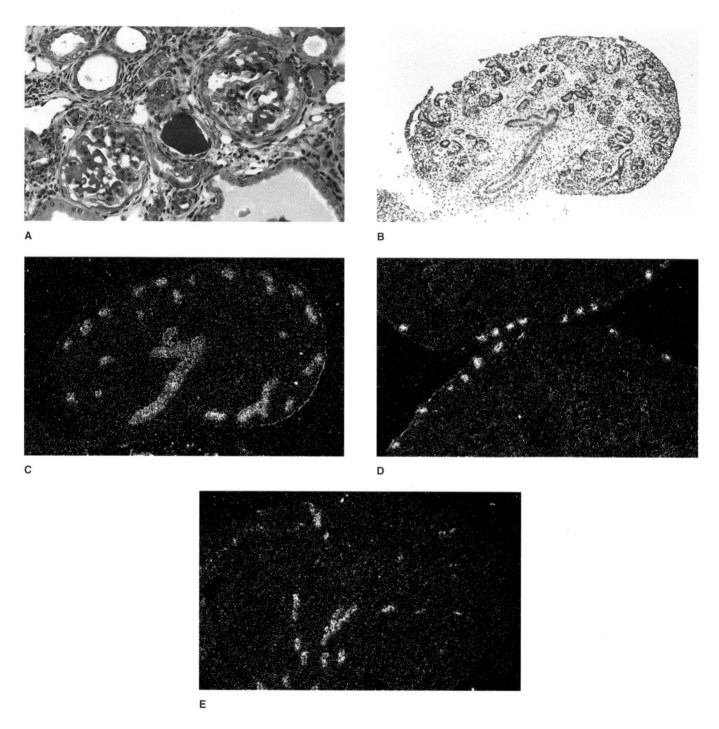

**FIGURE 23.5** *p53* transgenic mice: reduced glomerular numbers. MMTV-*p53* mice were found to have small kidneys and reduced glomerular numbers. With age, these mice develop secondary focal segmental glomerulosclerosis as a consequence of reduced nephron numbers (**A**, PAS). In situ hybridization for transgene RNA at E14.5 indicates expression in the ureteric bud derivatives, both within the central portion of the kidney and in the nephrogenic zone of the peripheral cortex (**B**, H&E, bright-field; **C**, dark-field). In situ hybridization for c-*ret* mRNA, the receptor for glial-derived growth factor, shows normal expression in the tips of the ureteric bud in wild-type mice at E18.5 (**D**). c-*ret* MRNA expression in MMTV-*p53* mice at E18.5 is confined to the more proximal portions of the ureteric bud derivatives, with minimal expression in the nephrogenic zone of the outer cortex (**E**). These findings suggest that overexpression of wild-type *p53* alters the differentiation program of the ureteric bud and impairs its ability to induce metanephric mesenchyme. (Figures reproduced with permission, Godley et al. 1996)

**TABLE 23.5. Cystic renal disease in transgenic and knockout mice**

| Gene | Affected tubule | Reference |
|------|-----------------|-----------|
| SV40 T Ag (T) | DT, CT | Kelley et al. 1991 |
| HIV-1 (T) | NS | Kopp et al. 1992 |
| *Pax-2b* (T) | NS | Dressler et al. 1993 |
| *c-erb B-2* (T) | NS | Stöcklin et al. 1993 |
| *c-myc* (T) | CT | Trudel et al. 1991 |
| H-*ras* (T) | PT | Schaffner et al. 1993 |
| *bcl-2* (KO) | NS | Nakayama et al. 1994 |
| SR2-3 (KO) | NS | Boulter et al. 1992 |
| 737 Rpw (KO) | PT, CT | Moyer et al. 1994 |
| tensin (KO) | PT | Lo et al. 1997 |
| *Pkd2* (KO) | DT, CT | Wu et al. 1998 |
| AP-2β transcript factor (KO) | DT, CT | Moser et al. 1997 |

Note: DT = distal convoluted tubule; CT = collecting tubule; NS = not specified; PT = proximal convoluted tubule.

disruption and weakening of cell-matrix junctions and lack of tubular epithelial polarity, which subsequently lead to cyst formation. *Pkd2* is a gene implicated in autosomal dominant polycystic kidney disease in humans. Targeted deletion of the *Pkd2* locus in mice causes polycystic kidney disease similar to the human disease (Wu et al. 1998).

# RENAL PHYSIOLOGY

Genetic engineering has enabled the creation of multiple murine models focusing on parameters of renal physiologic function. Transgenic and knockout models have been created that allow in-depth investigation of the hemodynamic mediators of hypertension and hypotension (Table 23.6).

# GLOMERULAR AND TUBULAR DISEASE

Genetically engineered models of renal glomerulonephropathy are varied and involve overexpression or inactivation of genes encoding transcription factors, cytokines, growth factors, inflammatory mediators, and viral genes (Table 23.7).

The role of a variety of growth factors associated with the development of glomerulonephropathy has been investigated utilizing primarily transgenic mice. Doi and colleagues have evaluated mice transgenic for growth hormone (GH), growth hormone releasing factor (GHRF), and insulinlike growth factor-1 (IGF-1) (Doi et al. 1988, 1990, 1991). Transgenic mice in all three models developed phenotypic glomerular

**TABLE 23.6. Alterations in renal physiology in transgenic and knockout mice**

| Gene | Phenotype | Reference |
|------|-----------|-----------|
| Bradykinin B2 receptor (T) | Hypotension | Wang et al. 1997 |
| Bradykinin B2 receptor (KO) | Hypertension | Alfie et al. 1996 |
| Kallikrein-binding protein (T) | Hypotension | Chen et al. 1996 |
| Atrial natriuretic peptide (T) | Hypotension | Veress et al. 1995 |
| Pro-ANP (KO) | Hypertension | John et al. 1995 |
| Angiotensinogen (T) | Hypertension | Kimura et al. 1992 |
| Angiotensinogen (KO) | Hypotension | Nagata et al. 1996 |
| Renin (T) | Hypertension | Springate et al. 1997 |
| Guanylyl cyclase-A receptor (KO) | Hypertension | Lopez et al. 1995 |

**TABLE 23.7. Glomerular and tubular disease in transgenic and knockout mice**

| Gene | Renal phenotype | Reference |
|------|-----------------|-----------|
| IGF-1 (T) | Increased glomerular size | Doi et al. 1990 |
| GH (T) | GEC hyperplasia | Doi et al. 1991 |
| GHRF (T) | Mesangial sclerosis | Doi et al. 1988 |
| HGR/SF (T) | Progressive GN, cysts | Takayama et al. 1997 |
| TGF-α (T) | Mesangial proliferation, renal cysts | Lowden et al. 1994 |
| TGF-β1 (T) | Increased mesangial matrix | Böttinger and Kopp 1998 |
| *bcl-2*-Ig (T) | Immune complex GN | Strasser et al. 1991 |
| *Fli-1* (T) | Immune complex GN | Zhang et al. 1995 |
| Interleukin-4 (T) | Immune complex GN | Erb et al. 1997 |
| Interleukin-6 (T) | Membranous GN | Fattori et al. 1994 |
| endothelin-1 (T) | Glomerulonephritis | Hocher et al. 1997 |
| endothelin-2 (T) | Glomerulonephritis | Hocher et al. 1996 |
| prorenin (T) | Renovascular lesions | Veniant et al. 1996 |
| hemoglobin SAD (T) | Renovascular lesions | De Paepe and Trudel 1994 |
| ACE (KO) | Renovascular lesions | Hilgers et al. 1997 |
| uteroglobin (KO) | Fibronectin deposit GN | Zhang et al. 1997 |
| *COL4A3* (KO) | Glomerulonephritis | Cosgrove et al. 1996 |
| SV40 T/t Ag (T) | FSGS | MacKay et al. 1987 |
| HIV-1 (T) | FSGS | Dickie et al. 1991 |

Note: GEC = glomerular epithelial cell; GN = glomerulonephritis; FSGS = focal and segmental glomerulosclerosis; ACE = angiotensin II converting enzyme.

abnormalities. GH and GHRF transgenic mice developed progressive glomerulosclerosis. Mesangial proliferation was detected in GH transgenic mice as early as 4 weeks of age. Increased amounts of extracellular matrix were noted with increased production of types I and IV collagen, laminin, and basement membrane heparan sulfate proteoglycan in the mesangium. Advanced glomerulosclerosis and mesangial cell proliferation were present in GHRF transgenic mice by 14 weeks of age. Secondary tubulointerstitial lesions were present in both GH and GHRF transgenic mice. Albuminuria was present and became more severe with advanced glomerulosclerosis. The pathogenesis of glomerulosclerosis is likely due to the dysregulation of glomerular cell function resulting in increased extracellular matrix proteins.

Mice transgenic for hepatocyte growth factor/scatter factor (HGF/SF) develop progressive glomerulosclerosis along with cystic tubular disease (Takayama et al. 1997). HGF/SF is a pleiotrophic cytokine that regulates cell growth and regeneration. HGF/SF and its tyrosine kinase receptor *c-met* are expressed in the developing kidney at E11. HGF/SF is expressed in the mesenchyme and *c-met* in the developing tubular epithelium. HGF/SF is not required for normal embryonic renal development because mice with null mutations for HGF/SF or *c-met* have no evidence of renal abnormalities (Schmidt et al. 1995). Transgenic mice developed cystic tubular lesions as early as 2 weeks of age. Tubular cyst formation was likely due to failure of autocrine regulation leading to tubular epithelial cell hyperplasia.

TGF-α transgenic mice develop renal cysts and glomerular enlargement with mesangial cell proliferation (Lowden et al. 1994). TGF-α is produced in the developing kidney within tubular segments and glomeruli. Tubular cyst formation is secondary to the effect of TGF-α on epithelial growth and hyperplasia. While there is an increase in number of mesangial cells and cell processes, no increase in extracellular matrix was noted by Lowden et al.

Transgenic mice that overexpress porcine TGF-β1 develop progressive glomerulosclerosis and interstitial fibrosis (Kopp et al. 1996; Sanderson et al. 1995). TGF-β1 is expressed in the liver, and transgenic mice develop hepatic fibrosis with increased collagen deposition around hepatocytes and in the space of Disse. Increased plasma levels of TGF-β1 correlate with transgene expression in the liver and lead to renal phenotypic abnormalities. TGF-β1 transgenic mice exhibit glomerular lesions as early as 3 weeks with increased mesangial matrix and deposition of collagen I and III (Fig. 23.6). Uremia develops by 5–20 weeks of age with a significant number of mice having a nephrotic syndrome.

Several transgenic murine models of immune-mediated glomerulonephritis have been described, including *bcl*-2-Ig (Strasser et al. 1991), *Fli*–1 (Zhang et al. 1995), *IL-4* (Erb et al. 1997), and *IL-6* (Fattori et al. 1994). Progressive glomerular disease with deposition of IgM, IgG, and C3 is evident in each of these models.

Transgenic mice and rats that overexpress either endothelin-1 or -2 have been developed that exhibit progressive glomerulosclerosis, renal cysts, and interstitial fibrosis (Hocher et al. 1996, 1997). ET-1 transgenic mice develop glomerulosclerosis by 14 months of age. ET-1 stimulates mesangial cell proliferation and extracellular matrix synthesis.

Several genetically engineered murine models have been developed that exhibit variably severe renovascular lesions. Transgenic mice that produce a modified sickle cell hemoglobin (Hb-SAD) serve as a model of sickle cell anemia (DePaepe and Trudel 1994). The transgenic mice develop microvascular occlusions and vascular thrombi, resulting in cortical infarcts and papillary necrosis. In addition, they develop glomerular hypertrophy and progressive glomerulosclerosis. Ultrastructural analysis reveals electron-dense mesangial deposits. Immunocytochemistry is positive for IgG and C3 deposition within the mesangium. The glomerulosclerosis is similar to that seen in a percentage of individuals with sickle cell disease.

Prorenin transgenic rats have been developed that express renin in the liver, lack hypertension, and develop glomerulosclerosis and renal arteriolar disease (Veniant et al. 1996). The vascular lesions are characterized by medial hypertrophy and fibrinoid degeneration. Renovascular lesions have also been seen in mice with targeted deletion of the angiotensin-converting enzyme gene (Hilgers et al. 1997). These mice develop tubular atrophy and dilatation. Arterioles are thickened and hypercellular, and there is an abnormal distribution of renin immunopositive cells.

Murine models involving targeted deletions of the uteroglobin gene and the *COL4A3* gene have been established that exhibit glomerulosclerosis. Uteroglobin knockout mice develop increased glomerular deposition of fibronectin and also have multifocal interstitial fibrosis and renal tubular hyperplasia (Zhang et al. 1997). Uteroglobin binds fibronectin to form fibronectin-uteroglobin heteromers preventing fibronectin aggregation and deposition. *COL4A3*-deficient mice are a model for Alport's disease (Cosgrove et al. 1996). These mice develop progressive glomerulosclerosis and have end-stage renal disease by 14 weeks of age. Glomerular basement membranes are thickened, and there is increased deposition of fibronectin, heparan sulfate proteoglycan, laminin-1, and entactin.

Several transgenic murine models have been developed using viral transgenes that develop focal and seg-

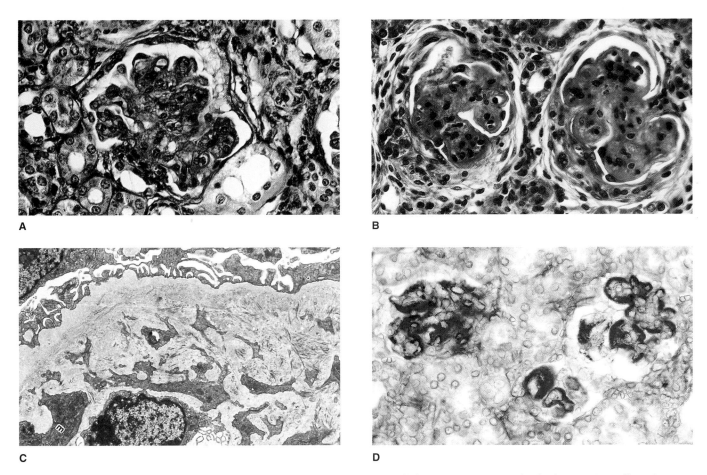

A  B  C  D

**FIGURE 23.6** TGF-β transgenic mice: global glomerulosclerosis. Alb/TGF-β1 mice, in which the murine albumin promoter and enhancer drive expression of TGF-β1, develop diffuse global glomerulosclerosis, as shown by PAS stain (**A**) and Masson trichrome stain (**B**). Extracellular matrix protein stains red with PAS stain and blue with Masson trichrome stain. Electron microscopy reveals subendothelial accumulation of flocculent extracellular matrix material, including collagen fibrils (**C**, ×10500). Immunostaining for collagen I, normally present in kidney only in trace amounts, shows abundant deposits, particularly within the glomeruli (**D**). (Figures reproduced with permission, Kopp et al. 1994a and Mozes et al. 1999)

mental glomerulosclerosis. Mice transgenic for the SV40 T antigen develop progressive focal and segmental glomerulosclerosis. Models have been created utilizing the large T, small T, and both large and small T antigens. Renal disease manifestations are similar in all three models (MacKay et al. 1987). The SV40 T antigen is expressed in glomeruli, mesangium, endothelial cells, and epithelial cells of the kidney. Tubular lesions in these mice include epithelial cell proliferation, tubular dilatation, and tubular atrophy. Ultrastructural analysis of the glomeruli reveals diffuse thickening of the mesangium with increased mesangial matrix, with no evidence of electron-dense deposits.

HIV-1 transgenic mice have been produced that lack *gag* and *pol* (Dickie et al. 1991; Kopp et al. 1992, 1994). These mice develop focal and segmental glomerulosclerosis, microcystic tubular dilatation, and interstitial fibrosis (Fig. 23.7). Proteinuria develops by day 18–25, and a high percentage of mice develop a

nephrotic syndrome. Mesangial deposition of IgM and lesser amounts of IgA and C3, in a pattern typical of mesangial trapping. Transmission electron microscopy reveals increased mesangial matrix, basement membrane thickening, and no evidence of electron-dense deposits. Immunostaining of the mesangium shows increased accumulation of laminin, collagen type IV, perlecan, and fibronectin. The morphology of the renal disease is similar to HIV-1–associated nephropathy, with the exception that tubulo-reticular inclusions are not present in the transgenic mice. The transgenic mice do not bear the complete HIV-1 genome, and no viral particles or viral replication are present in these mice. Also, g*ag-pol-nef*–deleted transgenic lines have been established with disease manifestations being similar to the *gag-pol*–deleted transgenic mice (Kajiyama et al. 2000). gp120 viral envelope protein and viral RNA were detected in glomerular and tubular epithelial cells.

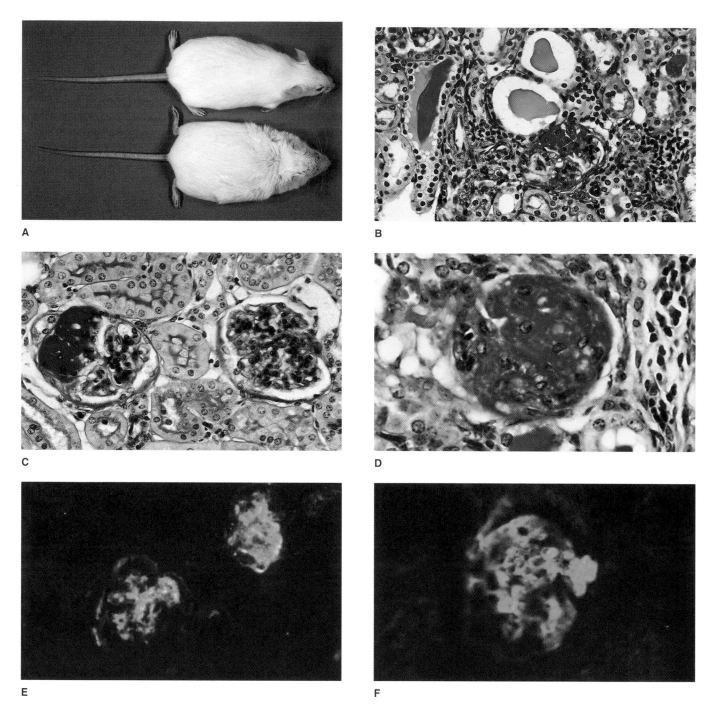

**FIGURE 23.7** HIV-1 transgenic mice: focal segmental glomerulosclerosis. Transgenic mice bearing a *gag-pol*–deleted HIV-1 genome develop nephrotic syndrome, characterized by edema (**A:** lower mouse, transgenic with edema; upper mouse, wild-type control), hypercholesterolemia, hypoalbuminemia, and proteinuria. Renal histology reveals focal segmental glomerulosclerosis, tubular atrophy and dilatation, and mononuclear cell infiltration (**B-D,** PAS). The sclerotic glomeruli have increased deposition of IgM (**E**) but not other immunoglobulins, and the HIV-1 protein Rev is also present in sclerotic glomeruli (F). (Figures reproduced with permission, Kopp et al. 1992)

The genetically engineered murine models of renal disease share many similarities of morphologic lesions, particularly at the light microscopic level. The cytokines, growth factors, viral genes, transcription factors, and inflammatory mediators that are associated with renal disease may tend to act through similar mechanisms affecting renal glomerular epithelial, mesangial, and endothelial cells, as well as tubular epithelial cells, to lead to the varied manifestations of renal disease.

# CONCLUSIONS

The development of transgenic and knockout methodology has greatly expanded the experimental tool kit available to investigators interested in renal development, physiology, and pathology. A plethora of new models is available, and the universe of models is likely to expand rapidly in the near future. New technologies and refinement of existing technologies, such as induced transgene expression and conditional knockout systems, will be exploited in the renal field as they have been in other areas.

A frequent problem is uncovering a latent phenotype in a genetically engineered mouse. A major challenge at the moment is to develop and refine useful and widely applicable methods to challenge various cellular and molecular pathways in the kidney in order to detect subtle evidence of dysregulation. Handling of water, sodium, and potassium may be assessed by dietary restriction, administration of diuretics, or other specific antagonists of tubular transport. As discussed above, blood pressure can be measured. Acute renal failure may be modeled in the mouse with ischemia-perfusion injury (Kelly et al. 1996) and with nephrotoxins such as folic acid (Cowley et al. 1989; Mullin et al. 1976) and mercury (Tanaka-Kagawa et al. 1998; Nielsen et al. 1991). Interstitial nephritis may be induced by ureteral obstruction (Maxwell et al. 1997; Ophascharoensuck et al. 1998).

A variety of approaches have been used to induce glomerulonephritis in mice (Furness and Harris 1994). The most commonly used model of glomerulonephritis in mice has been nephrotoxic serum nephritis, characterized by Masugi in the 1930s and often referred to as Masugi nephritis. This may be induced by immunization of the mouse with basement membrane components to induce autologous antibody or by the administration of heterologous antibodies directed against glomerular matrix components (Masuda et al. 1989; Assmann et al. 1985). Further, heterologous nephritis with an accelerated autologous phase may be induced, in which mice are preimmunized with antibody from another species (e.g., sheep) and subsequently the mice

are given antibody of the species with antiglomerular specificity (e.g., sheep antiglomerular basement membrane antibody) (Neugarten et al. 1995). Another approach has been to induce circulating immune complexes that deposit in the kidney, producing a model of serum sickness (Chen et al. 1995; Gesualdo et al. 1990; Iskandar et al. 1988). Recently, we have developed a model of acute glomerulonephritis in the mouse involving the administration of antiserum directed against murine mesangial cells; the model resembles anti-Thy1 nephritis in the rat (X.-J. Yao and J.B. Kopp, unpublished data). This list of maneuvers to induce glomerulonephritis is still limited, and it is likely that more precisely targeted interventions and approaches will become available in the future.

# REFERENCES

Abitbol, C., Zilleruelo, G., Freundlich, M., et al. 1990. Quantitation of proteinuria with urinary protein/creatinine ratios and random testing with dipsticks in nephrotic children. J Pediatr 116:243–247.

Alfie, M.E., Yang, X.P., Hess, F., et al. 1996. Salt-sensitive hypertension in bradykinin B2 receptor knockout mice. Biochem Biophys Res Commun 224:625–630.

Assmann, K.J., Tangelder, M.M., Lange W.P., et al. 1985. Anti-GBM nephritis in the mouse: severe proteinuria in the heterologous phase. Virchows Arch A Pathol Anat Histopathol 406:285–299.

Böttinger, E.P., and Kopp, J.B. 1998. Lessons from TGF-α transgenic mice. Mineral Electrolyte Metab 24:154–160.

Boulter, C.A., Aguzzi A., Evans, M.J., et al. 1992. A chimaeric mouse model for autosomal-dominant polycystic kidney disease. In M.H. Breuning, M. Devoto, and G. Romeo (eds.), Contributions to Nephrology (pp. 60–70). Basel, Switzerland: Karger.

Chen, A., Wei, C.H., Sheu, L.F., et al. 1995. Induction of proteinuria by adriamycin or bovine serum albumin in the mouse. Nephron 69:293–300.

Chen, L.M., Ma, J., Liang, Y.M., et al. 1996. Tissue kallikrein binding protein reduces blood pressure in transgenic mice. J Biol Chem 271:27590–27594.

Cosgrove, D., Meehan, D.T., Grunkemeyer, J.A., et al. 1996. Collagen COL4A3 knockout: a mouse model for autosomal Alport syndrome. Genes Dev 10:2981–2992.

Cowley, B.D., Jr., Chadwick,, L.J., Grantham, J.J., et al. 1989. Sequential protooncogene expression in regenerating kidney following acute renal injury. J Biol Chem 264:8389–8393.

De Paepe, M.E., and Trudel, M. 1994. The transgenic SAD mouse: a model of human sickle cell glomerulopathy. Kidney Int 46:1337–1345.

Dickie, P., Felser, J., Eckhaus, M., et al. 1991. HIV-associated nephropathy in transgenic mice expressing HIV-1 genes. Virology 185:109–119.

Dinchuk, J.E., Car, B.D., Focht, R.J., et al. 1995. Renal abnormalities and an altered inflammatory response in mice lacking cyclooxygenase II. Nature 378:406–409.

Doi, T., Striker, L.J., Quaife, C., et al. 1988. Progressive glomerulosclerosis develops in transgenic mice chronically expressing growth hormone and growth hormone releasing factor but not in those expressing insulinlike growth factor-1. Am J Pathol 131:398–403.

Doi, T., Striker, L.J., Gibson, C.C., et al. 1990. Glomerular lesions in mice transgenic for growth hormone and insulinlike growth factor-I. I. Relationship between increased glomerular size and mesangial sclerosis. Am J Pathol 137:541–552.

Doi, T., Striker, L.J., Kimata, K., et al. 1991. Glomerulosclerosis in mice transgenic for growth hormone. Increased mesangial extracellular matrix is correlated with kidney mRNA levels. J Exp Med 173:1287–1290.

Dressler, G.R., Wilkinson, J.E., Rothenpieler, U.W., et al. 1993. Deregulation of Pax-2 expression in transgenic mice generates severe kidney abnormalities. Nature 362:65–67.

Erb, K.J., Ruger, B., von Brevern, M., et al. 1997. Constitutive expression of interleukin (IL)-4 in vivo causes autoimmune-type disorders in mice. J Exp Med 185:329–339.

Fattori, E., Della, R.C., Costa, P., et al. 1994. Development of progressive kidney damage and myeloma kidney in interleukin-6 transgenic mice. Blood 83:2570–2579.

Funakawa, S., Itoh, T., Miyata, K., et al. 1984. Sex difference of N-Acetyl-beta-D-glucosaminidase activity in the kidney, urine, and plasma of mice. Ren Physiol 7:124–128.

Furness, P.N., and Harris, K. 1994. An evaluation of experimental models of glomerulonephritis. Int J Exp Pathol 75:9–22.

Gesualdo, L., Ricanati, S., Hassan, M.O., et al. 1990. Enzymolysis of glomerular immune deposits in vivo with dextranase/protease ameliorates proteinuria, hematuria, and mesangial proliferation in murine experimental IgA nephropathy. J Clin Invest 86:715–722.

Godley, L.A., Kopp, J.B., Eckhaus, M., et al. 1996. Wild-type p53 transgenic mice exhibit altered differentiation of the ureteric bud and possess small kidneys. Genes Dev 10:836–850.

Grandaliano, G., Choudhury, G.G., and Abboud, H.E. 1995. Transgenic animal models as a tool in the diagnosis of kidney diseases. Semin Nephrol 15:43–49.

Hilgers, K.F., Reddi, V., Krege, J.H., et al. 1997. Aberrant renal vascular morphology and renin expression in mutant mice lacking angiotensin-converting enzyme. Hypertension 29:216–221.

Hocher, B., Liefeldt, L., Thone-Reineke, C., et al. 1996. Characterization of the renal phenotype of transgenic rats expressing the human endothelin-2 gene. Hypertension 28:196–201.

Hocher B., Thone-Reineke, C., Rohmeiss, P., et al. 1997. Endothelin-1 transgenic mice develop glomerulosclerosis, interstitial fibrosis, and renal cysts but not hypertension. J Clin Invest 99:1380–1389.

Hsu, H.H. 1986. Hereditary hydronephrosis, mouse. In T.C. Jones, U. Mohr, and R.D. Hunt (eds.), Monographs on Pathology of Laboratory Animals—Urinary System (pp. 273–275). New York: Springer-Verlag.

Iskandar, S.S., Gifford, D.R., and Emancipator, S.N. 1988. Immune complex acute necrotizing glomerulonephritis with progression to diffuse glomerulosclerosis. A murine model. Lab Invest 59:772–779.

Jensen, E.B., Gundersen, H.J., and Osterby, R. 1979. Determination of membrane thickness distribution from orthogonal intercepts. J Microsc 115:19–33.

John, S.W., Krege, J.H., Oliver, P.M., et al. 1995. Genetic decreases in atrial natriuretic peptide and salt-sensitive hypertension. Science 267:679–681.

Kajiyama, W., Kopp, J.B., Marinos, N.J., et al. 2000. Glomerulosclerosis and viral gene expression in HIV-transgenic mice. Kidney Int. In press.

Kaufman, M.H. 1992. The Atlas of Mouse Development. London: Academic Press.

Keller, S.A., Jones, J.M., Boyle, A., et al. 1994. Kidney and retinal defects (Krd), a transgene-induced mutation with a deletion of mouse chromosome 19 that includes the Pax2 locus. Genomics 23:309–320.

Kelley, K.A., Agarwal, N., Reeders, S., et al. 1991. Renal cyst formation and multifocal neoplasia in transgenic mice carrying the simian virus 40 early region. J Am Soc Nephrol 2:84–97.

Kelly, K.J., Williams, W.W., Jr., Colvin, R.B., et al. 1996. Intercellular adhesion molecule-1-deficient mice are protected against ischemic renal injury. J Clin Invest 97:1056–1063.

Kiberd, B.A. 1991. Murine lupus nephritis. A structure-function study. Lab Invest 65:51–60.

Kimura, S., Mullins, J.J., Bunnemann, B., et al. 1992. High blood pressure in transgenic mice carrying angiotensinogen gene. Embo. J. 11:821–827.

Kone, B. 1998. Molecular approaches to renal physiology and therapeutics. Semin Nephrol 18:102–121.

Konikowski, T., Haynie, T.P., and Farr, L.E. 1970. Inulin clearance in mice as a standard for radiopharmaceutical bioassay. Proc Soc Exp Biol Med 135:320–324.

Kopp, J.B. 1997. Gene expression in kidney using transgenic approaches. Exp Nephrol 5:157–167.

Kopp, J.B., and Klotman, P.E. 1995a. Animal models of lentivirus-associated renal disease. In J. Berns and P. Kimmel (eds.), Renal and Urologic Aspects of HIV Infection (pp. 389–404). New York: Churchill Livingstone.

Kopp, J.B., and Klotman, P.E. 1995b. Transgenic animal models of renal development and pathogenesis. Am J Physiol 269:F601–620.

Kopp, J.B., Klotman, M.E., Adler, S.H., et al. 1992. Progressive glomerulosclerosis and enhanced renal accumulation of basement membrane components in mice transgenic for human immunodeficiency virus type 1 genes. Proc Natl Acad Sci USA 89:1577–1581.

Kopp, J.B., Ray, P.E., Adler, S.H., et al. 1994. Nephropathy in HIV-transgenic mice. In H. Koide and T. Hayashi (eds.), Contributions to Nephrology (pp. 194–204). Basel, Switzerland: Karger.

Kopp, J.B., Factor, V.M., Mozes, M., et al. 2000. Transgenic mice with increased plasma levels of TGF-beta 1 develop progressive renal disease. Lab Invest 74:991–1003.

Krege, J.H., Hodgin, J.B., Hagaman, J.R., et al. 1995. A noninvasive computerized tail-cuff system for measuring blood pressure in mice. Hypertension 25:1111–1115.

Kreidberg, J.A., Sariola, H., Loring, J.M., et al. 1993. WT-1 is required for early kidney development. Cell 74:679–691.

Levéen, P., Pekney, M., Gebre-Medhin, S., et al. 1994. Mice deficient for PDGF B show renal, cardiovascular, and hematological abnormalities. Genes Dev 8:1875–1887.

Liebelt, A.G. 1986. Unique features of anatomy, histology, and ultrastructure, kidney, mouse. In T.C. Jones, U. Mohr, and R.D. Hunt (eds.), Monographs on Pathology of Laboratory Animals—Urinary System (pp. 24–44). New York: Springer-Verlag.

Lo, S.H., Yu, Q.C., Degenstein, L., et al. 1997. Progressive kidney degeneration in mice lacking tensin. J Cell Biol 136:1349–1361.

Lopez, M.J., Wong, S.K., Kishimoto, I., et al. 1995. Salt-resistant hypertension in mice lacking the guanylyl cyclase A receptor for atrial natriuretic peptide. Nature 378:65–68.

Lowden, D.A., Lindemann, G.W., Merlino, G., et al. 1994. Renal cysts in transgenic mice expressing transforming growth factor-alpha [see comments]. J Lab Clin Med 124:386–394.

Lyon, M., and Hulse E. 1971. An inherited disease of mice resembling human nephronophthisis. J Med Genet 8:41–48.

MacKay, K., Striker, L.J., Pinkert, C.A. et al. 1987. Glomerulosclerosis and renal cysts in mice transgenic for the early region of SV40. Kidney Int 32:827–837.

Masuda, Y., Ishizaki, M., Yamanaka, N., et al. 1989. Evidence of delayed mesangial transport of human IgA in glomeruli of ddY mice pretreated with sheep anti-type IV collagen serum. Acta Pathol Japan 39:289–295.

Matsuka, T., and Ichikawa, I. 1997. Gene targeting in nephrology. Exp Nephrol 5:168–173.

Maxwell, P.H., Ferguson, D.J., Nicholls, L.G., et al. 1997. The interstitial response to renal injury: fibroblast-like cells show phenotypic changes and have reduced potential for erythropoietin gene expression. Kidney Int 52:715–724.

Messing, A., Behringer, R.R., Slapak, J.R., et al. 1990. Insertional mutation at the ld locus (again!) in a line of transgenic mice. Mouse Genome 87:107.

Möller, J.C., and Skriver, E. 1985. Quantitative ultrastructure of human proximal tubules and cortical interstitium in chronic renal disease (hydronephrosis). Virchows Arch A Pathol Anat Histopathol 406:389–406.

Moser, M., Pscherer, A., Roth, C., et al. 1997. Enhanced apoptotic cell death of renal epithelial cells in mice lacking transcription factor AP-2β. Genes Dev 11:1938–1948.

Moyer, J.H., Lee-Tischler, M.J., Kwon, H.-Y., et al. 1994. Candidate gene associated with a mutation causing recessive polycystic kidney disease in mice. Science 264:1329–1333.

Mozes, M., Böttinger, E., Jacot, T., et al. 1999. Increased renal expression of TGF-β and fibrotic matrix proteins in TGF-β transgenic mice. J Am Soc Nephrol 10: 271–280.

Mugrauer, G., Alt, F.W., and Ekblom, P. 1988. N-myc proto-oncogene expression during organogenesis in the developing mouse as revealed by in situ hybridization. J Cell Biol 107:1325–1335.

Mullin, E.M., Bonar, R.A., and Paulson, D.F. 1976. Acute tubular necrosis. An experimental model detailing the biochemical events accompanying renal injury and recovery. Invest Urol 13:289–294.

Nagata, M., Tanimoto, K., Fukamizu, A., et al. 1996. Nephrogenesis and renovascular development in angiotensinogen-deficient mice. Lab Invest 75:745–753.

Nakayama, K., Nakayama, K.-I., Negishi, I., et al. 1994. Targeted disruption of Bcl-2 alpha beta in mice: occurrence of gray hair, polycystic kidney disease, and lymphocytopenia. Proc Natl Acad Sci USA 91:3700–3704.

Neugarten, J., Feith, G.W., Assmann, K.J., et al. 1995. Role of macrophages and colony-stimulating factor-1 in murine antiglomerular basement membrane glomerulonephritis. J Am Soc Nephrol 5:1903–1909.

Nielsen, J.B., Andersen, H.R., Andersen, O., et al. 1991. Mercuric chloride-induced kidney damage in mice: time course and effect of dose. J Toxicol Environ Health 34:469–483.

Okada, H., Suzuki, H., Kanno, Y., et al. 1995. Renal responses to angiotensin receptor antagonist and angiotensin-converting enzyme inhibitor in partially nephrectomized spontaneously hypertensive rats. J Cardiovasc Pharmacol 26:564–569.

Ophascharoensuk, V., Fero, M.L., Hughes, J., et al. 1998. The cyclin-dependent kinase inhibitor p27Kip1 safeguards against inflammatory injury. Nat Med 4:575–580.

Pagtalunan, M.E., Miller, P.L., Jumping-Eagle, S., et al. 1997. Podocyte loss and progressive glomerular injury in type II diabetes. J Clin Invest 99:342–348.

Pichel, J.G., Shen, L., Sheng, H.Z., et al. 1996. Defects in enteric innervation and kidney development in mice lacking GDNF. Nature 382:73–76.

Ragan, H.A. 1989. Markers of renal function and injury. In W.F. Loeb and F.W. Quimby (eds.), The Clinical Chemistry of Laboratory Animals (pp. 321–343). New York: Pergamon.

Raij, L., Azar, S., and Keane, W. 1984. Mesangial immune injury, hypertension, and progressive glomerular damage in Dahl rats. Kidney Int 26:137–143.

Ryffel, B. 1996. Gene knockout mice as investigative tools in pathophysiology. Int J Exp Pathol 77:125–141.

Saito, A., Yamazaki, H., Nakagawa, Y., et al. 1997. Molecular genetics of renal diseases. Intern Med 36:81–86.

Sanderson, N., Factor, V., Nagy, P., et al. 1995. Hepatic expression of mature transforming growth factor beta 1 in transgenic mice results in multiple tissue lesions. Proc Natl Acad Sci USA 92:2572–2576.

Sass, B. 1986. Glomerulonephritis, Mouse. In T.C. Jones, U. Mohr, and R.D. Hunt (eds.), Monographs on Pathology of Laboratory Animals—Urinary System (pp. 273–275). New York: Springer-Verlag.

Sato, F., Tsuchihahsi, S., and Kawashima, N. 1975. Age changes in number and size of the murine renal glomeruli. Exp Gerontol 10:325–331.

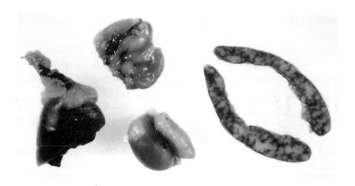

**FIGURE 24.1** Enlarged cervical mediastinal and renal nodes. Enlarged spleen with cut surface showing nodular architecture in follicular lymphoma. (Courtesy of J.M. Ward)

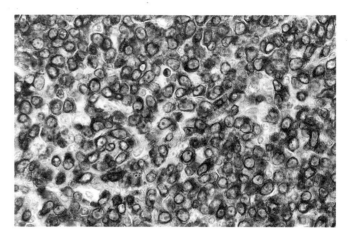

**FIGURE 24.2** CD3 immunohistochemistry, thymus. Uniformly positive T cell lymphoblastic lymphoma. (Courtesy of J.M. Ward)

in a fixative such as Bouin's or 10 percent neutral buffered formalin. Other fixatives, such as methacarn and paraformaldehyde, can be used to preserve immunoreactivity in paraffin-embedded tissues. Cut sections of tissues, placed in mounting medium and snap frozen, can be used for immunohistochemistry. Tissue samples can also be frozen for molecular analysis, solid blocks for preparation of DNA, and material frozen in commercially available solutions containing phenol and quanidine hydrochloride for analysis of RNA. Single-cell suspensions prepared from affected tissue can be used to make cytospins, which are stained for morphology and further evaluated using cytochemistry and immunofluorescence. In addition, the cell suspensions can be stained with antibodies specific for any large number of cell surface antigens and examined by flow cytometry. These suspensions can also be further transplanted into normal or immunocompromised mice to propagate the tumors.

## SPECIAL TECHNIQUES

Although morphologic evaluation remains the preeminent diagnostic modality, hematopoietic neoplasms are best evaluated utilizing the full range of diagnostic methods available (Pattengale and Taylor 1983). Immunohistochemical studies have proven to be quite useful in analysis of murine lymphomas (Ward and Rehm 1990). Staining sections from frozen or paraffin-embedded tissues with antibodies specific for T cells (e.g., anti-CD3; Fig. 24.2) and B cells (e.g., CD45R; Fig. 24.3) establishes the phenotype of neoplastic cells. Flow cytometry, while lacking simultaneous morphologic evaluation, has advantages over immunohistochemistry in being 10- to 100-fold more sensitive than immunohistochemistry and in allowing analysis of a

large number of cells using mouse monoclonal antibodies to surface molecules characteristic for each hematopoietic lineage (Fredrickson et al. 1985). Using flow cytometry, neoplastic T cells may be found to express markers characteristic of normal mature cells such as CD4 or CD8 (Fig. 24.4). Other T cell lymphomas simultaneously express both subset markers on single cells, appearing as double-positive cells (Fig. 24.4), or lack such expression and appear as double-negative cells (Fig. 24.4). CD4+CD8+ and CD4−CD8− phenotypic patterns are abnormal for peripheral T cells. Similarly, B cell lineage lymphomas can exhibit the surface Ig− phenotype of normal precursor B cells (Fig. 24.5) or resemble mature B cells expressing surface IgM (Fig. 24.5) or other Ig isotypes. Anomalous expression of lineage markers allows the detection of a neoplastic clone even in small numbers, as exemplified by the CD5+ B cell lymphoma in Fig. 24.5 (Davidson et al. 1984). CD5+ B cells make up less than 2 percent of normal mouse spleen (Hardy et al. 1994). Nonlymphoid neoplasms of granulocytic or histiocytic origin can also be detected using cell surface markers such as Gr-1 and CD11b (Mac-1), respectively (Fig. 24.5).

The tools of molecular biology offer powerful means for evaluating lineage as well as clonality of hematopoietic neoplasms in humans and mice (Fredrickson et al. 1993). Southern blot hybridization analyses of immunoglobulin heavy chain and T cell receptor (TCRβ) gene organization using J$_H$ and TCRβ probes show nongermline bands ranging from multiple and faint bands in hyperplastic lesions, indicative of early oligoclonal selection, to distinct monoclonal bands in more advanced lymphomas (Fig. 24.6A and B). Cytogenetic studies, used in screening human neoplasms for chromosomal abnormalities, are difficult to perform in mice. Recently, however, the technique of spectral karyotyping,

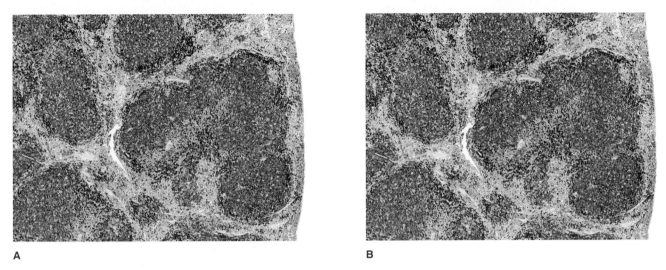

**FIGURE 24.3** CD45R immunohistochemistry, spleen. Diffuse staining and obliteration of periarteriolar lymphoid sheath (PALS) T cell zone in follicular lymphoma (**A**). Normal C57BL/6 mouse (**B**). (Courtesy of J.M. Ward)

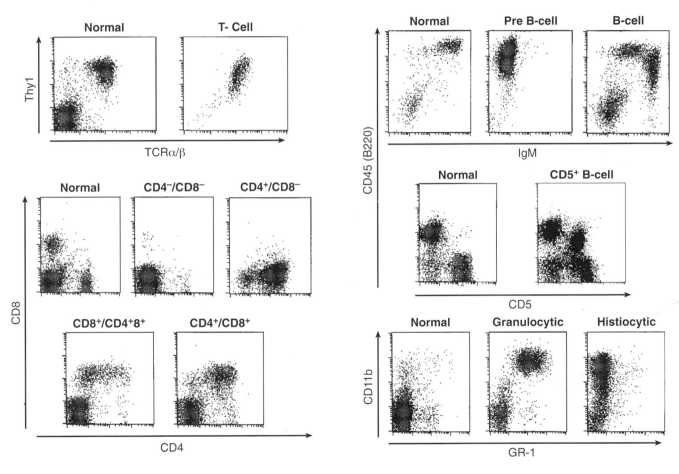

**FIGURE 24.4** Flow cytometric analyses of mouse spleen double stained with antiThy1 and TCRα/β. Normal C57BL/6 mouse (upper left). Homogenous population of T cells and loss of B cells in lymphoblastic lymphoma (upper right). AntiCD4 and CD8 double staining shows the normal distribution (middle left) and neoplastic T cell with immature (middle center and right, lower right) and/or mature (lower left) surface marker phenotypes.

**FIGURE 24.5** Flow cytometric analyses of mouse spleen double stained with CD45 and IgM showing the various B cell lymphoma phenotypes. Surface IgM⁻ precursor B-lymphoblastic lymphoma (upper middle) and surface IgM bright mature B cell lymphoma (upper right). AntiCD45R and CD5 double staining shows the CD5 dull B cell lymphoma (middle right). GR-1 and CD11b⁺ granulocytic leukemia (lower middle) and CD11b⁺ histiocytic sarcoma (lower right).

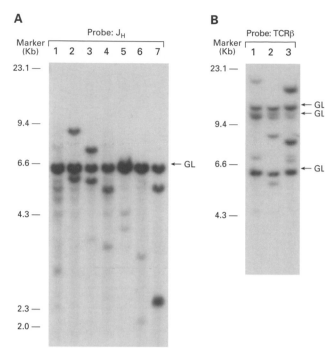

**A**

Probe: J_H

Marker (Kb)    1  2  3  4  5  6  7

23.1 —

9.4 —

6.6 —                                          ← GL

4.3 —

2.3 —
2.0 —

**B**

Probe: TCRβ

Marker (Kb)    1  2  3

23.1 —

                                               ← GL
                                               ← GL
9.4 —

6.6 —                                          ← GL

4.3 —

**FIGURE 24.6** Southern blot analysis for IgH and TCRβ gene rearrangement in spleen of *p53*⁻/⁻ mice showing a range from oligo to monoclonal bands in a variety of B cell (**A**) and T cell (**B**) lymphomas.

**FIGURE 24.7** Normal spleen, C57BL/6 mouse. Note thin marginal zones.

known as SKY, which combines fluorescence in situ hybridization (FISH) with spectral imaging, has proven useful in detecting and identifying chromosomal abnormalities in mice (Liyanage et al. 1996). Reverse transcription (RT) and DNA-PCR, as well as studies of single-strand conformational polymorphisms (SSCP), may also be helpful in some settings.

# CORRELATION OF LYMPHOMA AND NORMAL HISTOLOGY

A thorough familiarization with normal histology, as well as nonneoplastic proliferative lesions of the hematopoietic organs, is necessary for the proper evaluation of lymphomas, since proliferative lesions may be difficult to distinguish from neoplastic processes (Frith et al. 1996). In the mouse spleen, unlike the human, megakaryocytes are normally found in the red pulp along with erythroid and granulocytic cells and their precursors at different stages of maturation (Fig. 24.7). Reactive hyperplasias of the red pulp with marked erythropoiesis, granulopoiesis, and megakaryocytosis may lead to marked enlargement of the spleen (Frith et al. 1996).

The splenic white pulp in the mouse is composed of the follicle, separated into functionally and anatomi-

cally distinct T and B cell zones. The T cell zone surrounds the central arteriole and is called the periarteriolar lymphoid sheath (PALS) (Fig. 24.3). The B cell area surrounds the PALS and comprises naive B cells in the mantle zone, surrounded by a thin outer layer of pale-staining marginal zone cells. Although there is some strain variation, the marginal zone in mice forms a thin halo around the splenic follicle, one to three cell layers in thickness (Fig. 24.7). Germinal centers are found in the secondary follicle of activated spleens (Fig. 24.8A). Marked splenic follicular hyperplasia may be difficult to distinguish from follicular lymphomas. The morphologic differentiation is based on cell distribution and architecture (Frith et al. 1996). The presence of a heterogeneous population of small lymphocytes, plasma cells, and tingible body macrophages among cleaved (centrocytes) and noncleaved (centroblasts) cells, with preservation of the normal T and B cell architecture, favors the diagnosis of reactive follicular hyperplasia (Fig. 24.8B). In follicular lymphoma, the majority of cells are composed of centrocytes and/or centroblasts, with a paucity of small lymphocytes and macrophages. In addition, there is loss of normal architecture with obliteration of the T cell region (Fig. 24.3) and sometimes light chain restriction, as evidenced by immunohistochemical staining (Ward 1990a). It must be recognized that over 95 percent of normal B cells in the mouse express κ light chains, so only lymphomas expressing λ light chains could be diagnosed as clonal by immunohistochemistry. In cases where morphologic distinction between hyperplastic and neoplastic lesions is equivocal, genetic analysis of immunoglobulin and TCR gene organization can be a valuable aid in discriminating between diagnoses; hyperplastic lesions are polyclonal, whereas neoplastic lymphoid lesions are clonal.

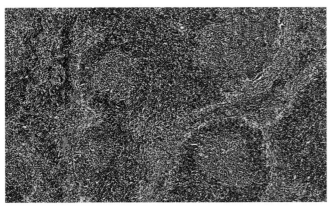

A

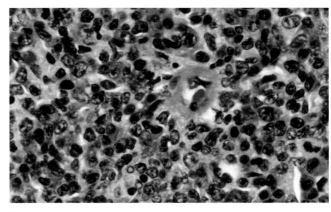

B

**FIGURE 24.8**   Follicular hyperplasia of spleen with numerous germinal centers (pale zones) (**A**). It comprises a mixed population of small lymphocytes, plasma cells, centrocytes, and centroblasts (**B**).

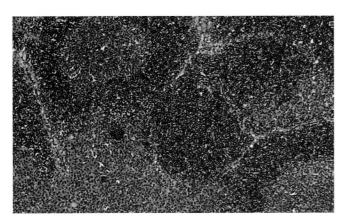

**FIGURE 24.9**   Reactive hyperplasia of lymph node with germinal centers in the cortex and reactive plasmacytosis in medulla (pale zones).

In lymph nodes, B cells are mostly found in the primary and secondary follicles of outer cortex and the medullary sinuses, while T cells occupy the paracortical regions. The spectrum of reactive lesions of lymph nodes includes follicular hyperplasia and marked medullary plasmacytosis (Fig. 24.9), as well as sinus histiocytosis (Ward 1990b). Lymphomas cause a partial or complete effacement of the normal nodal architecture. In the thymus, neoplastic processes obliterate the normal distinction between the cortex and medulla. Reactive cortical or medullary hyperplasias can be seen in mice, while age-related involution results in thymic atrophy.

To accurately classify the lymphomas, it is necessary to evaluate neoplastic lesions with respect to origin, pattern, and cytology. In cases where the lymphoma is confined to one organ or has minimally involved others, the origin as well as growth pattern—diffuse versus nodular and splenic white pulp versus red pulp—may provide important diagnostic information. In addition, a detailed cytologic assessment should be undertaken that includes size, shape, and uniformity of the cell and the nucleus; amount and color of cytoplasm; chromatin pattern; prominence and number of nucleoli; and mitotic activity. Furthermore, cytologic evaluation of metastatic lesions and pattern of involvement in various tissues, especially liver and lungs, supplements information obtained from the primary tumor.

Every attempt should be made to correlate the neoplastic cells with their normal cellular counterparts using morphologic, immunophenotypic, and genetic data (Pattengale 1994). This has an important bearing on understanding the biologic behavior of the various types of lymphomas that arise from lymphoid cells at different stages of maturation. Thus, lymphomas that express surface antigens characteristic of B cell lineage and are positive for cytoplasmic immunoglobulin but lack surface immunoglobulin resemble normal pre-B cells from the bone marrow, while others express a mature B cell phenotype with surface IgM. These various B cell lymphomas mirror the various stages of B cell differentiation morphologically, phenotypically, and in anatomic location (Fig. 24.10). Similarly, T cell lymphomas mirror the various stages of T cell differentiation (Fig. 24.11). For the most part, neoplastic cells retain the morphologic characteristics of their normal counterparts, enabling recognition and classification, while some may show variation in size, nuclear characteristics, and proliferative fraction, indicating transformation to a higher grade. Evaluation of grade in the mouse is based mainly on morphologic assessment of invasiveness and proliferative index (number of mitoses, apoptosis, etc.).

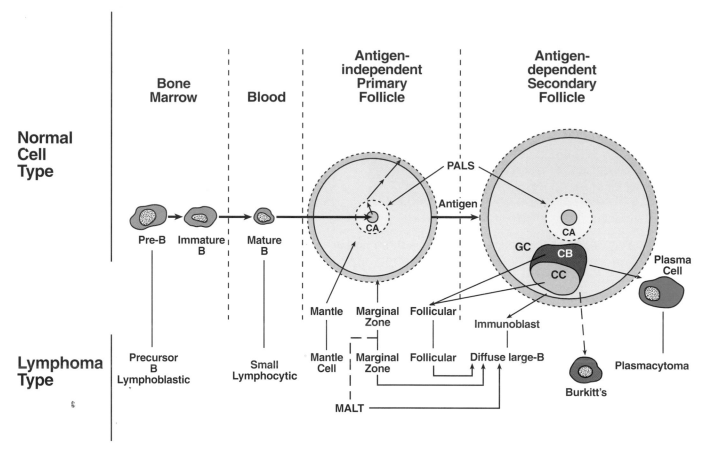

**FIGURE 24.10**  Schematic representation of B cell development and differentiation and corresponding B cell lineage lymphomas. CB = centroblast; CC = centrocyte; CA = central arteriole; GC = germinal center.

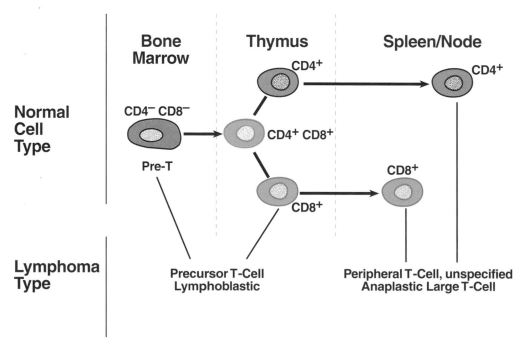

**FIGURE 24.11**  Schematic representation of T cell development and differentiation with corresponding T cell lineage lymphomas.

# CLASSIFICATION OF LYMPHOMAS

Both human and mouse lymphoma classification systems have undergone numerous changes over the years. In some cases, different terminologies used for the same lesions make interpretation and exchange of information difficult. In the mouse, many classification systems have been proposed beginning with Dunn (1954). Development of a classification system for mice is important for (1) relating neoplastic diseases of the mouse hematopoietic system to neoplasms seen in humans (identification of true parallels potentially establishes a model system in the mouse for dissecting the pathogenesis of the human disorder) and (2) enhancing diagnostic accuracy and reproducibility for mouse disorders. In proposing a system for classification of mouse neoplasms, there are several lessons to be learned from the efforts to develop classification systems for human hematopoietic tumors. First, schemes that rely mainly on morphology fail to distinguish neoplasms derived from separate cell lineages (precursor T cell versus precursor B cell lymphoblastic lymphomas) or stages of differentiation within the same lineage (lymphoblastic lymphomas of precursor B cells versus sIg+ B cells) (Figs. 24.12-24.17). Second, it is difficult to distinguish between certain phenotypically similar lymphomas on a morphological basis. These and other problems are largely addressed in the proposed

World Health Organization (WHO) classification of human hematopoietic and lymphoid neoplasms developed by consensus of over 50 international experts (Jaffe et al. 1999). This system, modeled after the Revised European American Classification of Lymphoid neoplasms (REAL) (Harris et al. 1994), recognizes that individual disease entities are best defined by taking into account morphology, immunophenotype, and genetic and clinical features and indicates that, when possible, the malignancies should be classified in relation to the normal counterpart of the neoplastic cell.

Not all of the modalities for diagnosis that exist for human neoplasms are routinely available for studies in mice. Nonetheless, it is clear that there are mouse counterparts for lymphomas in the WHO classification of human lymphomas. These include splenic marginal zone B cell lymphoma (MZL) (Fredrickson et al. 1999), MZL of mucosa-associated lymphoid tissue (Enno et al. 1995), and Burkitt's lymphoma (unpublished observations). It is therefore important to revise the classification of mouse lymphomas to include these newly described entities, to allow addition of lymphomas that parallel human disorders as they are discerned, and to provide a uniform nomenclature system. Consistency in the classification of hematopoietic neoplasms is absolutely essential for comparative analysis and meaningful interpretation and application of various studies

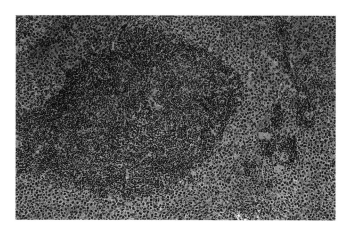

**FIGURE 24.13** Marginal zone lymphoma in spleen of a *p53*[-/-] mouse.

Size: medium, uniform
Cytoplasm: abundant, grayish
Nuclei: round; chromatin: stippled to vesicular
Nucleoli: variable
Mitosis: low
Pattern: diffuse, red pulp
Phenotype: mature B cell, (CD45R+, sIg+)
Molecular: IgH gene rearrangement
Characteristic: uniform, grayish cytoplasm, early
    marginal zone hyperplasia, infiltrate red pulp, low
    grade with progression to high grade (centroblastic)

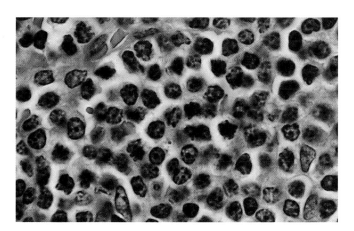

**FIGURE 24.12** Small lymphocytic lymphoma.

Size: small, uniform size and shape
Cytoplasm: scant, basophilic
Nuclei: round; chromatin: clumped
Nucleoli: inconspicuous
Mitosis: low
Pattern: diffuse
Phenotype: mature B (CD45R+, sIg+) or T cells (CD3+)
Molecular: IgH/TCR gene rearrangement
Characteristic: low grade, resembles small mature
    lymphocyte

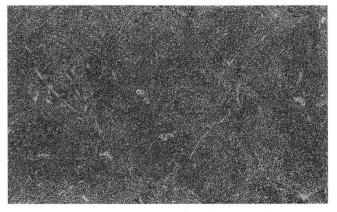

A

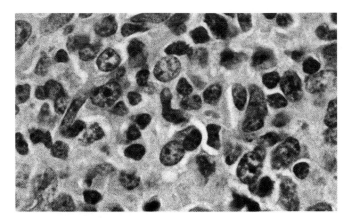

B

C

**FIGURE 24.14** Follicular lymphoma in spleen of an aged B6,129 mouse showing a nodular pattern (**A**). Grade 1 is composed predominantly of small cleaved cells (centrocytes) (**B**). The larger noncleaved vesicular cells (centroblasts) predominate in grade III (**C**).

Size: small, large, and mixed
Cytoplasm: scant, large cells basophilic
Nuclei: cleaved/round; chromatin: clumped/vesicular
Nucleoli: inconspicuous/prominent
Mitosis: variable
Pattern: nodular/diffuse

Phenotype: mature B cell (CD45R⁺, sIg⁺)
Molecular: IgH gene rearrangement
Synonym: Centroblastic-centrocytic/centroblastic
Characteristic: low grade to high grade, mixed cell
    population resembling those of germinal center

(Frith et al. 1999). Thus, in Table 24.1 we list with the proposed WHO classification for human lymphomas/leukemias a parallel system for the mouse and relate this proposed National Institute of Allergy and Infectious Diseases/National Cancer Institute (NIAID/NCI) classification to those of (1) Frith et al. (1996), based on the Lukes-Collins classification (1992) of human tumors, and (2) Fredrickson et al. (1995), which is based on the Kiel system for classification of human lymphoma (Lennert and Feller 1992). Both of these mouse nomenclature systems have used immunophenotypic data in addition to morphology to classify the neoplasms; however, this is limited to distinguishing between T and B lymphomas and not precursor versus mature types.

Follicular lymphomas are nodular lesions. Three grades of this neoplasm are recognized in the WHO classification based on the predominant cell population: small (centrocytic), large (centroblastic), and mixed. Diffuse follicular lymphomas, composed of large cells (centroblastic), are morphologically difficult to distinguish from B-immunoblastic lymphomas (Fig. 24.16); therefore they are classified together as diffuse large B cell lymphomas (DLCL) in the proposed WHO and NIAID/NCI classification. Follicular lymphoma and/or MZL sometimes coexist with DLCL, reflecting progression of the neoplasm from a low to a higher grade. T-immunoblastic lymphomas have been reported in mice (Fredrickson et al. 1985; Pals et al. 1986). These are

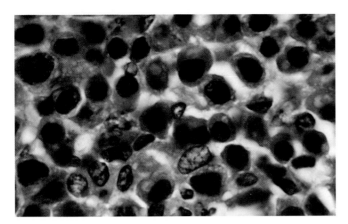

**FIGURE 24.15** Plasmacytoma in lymph node of a pristane-induced *p16⁻/⁻* mouse. Note a mixture of plasma cells and plasmablasts.

Size: small to large
Cytoplasm: abundant, amphophilic
Nuclei: eccentric, round; chromatin; marginated
Nucleoli: variable
Mitosis: variable
Pattern: diffuse
Phenotype: mature B cell (cIg⁺)
Molecular: IgH gene rearrangement
Characteristic: mixture of plasma cells and plasmablasts

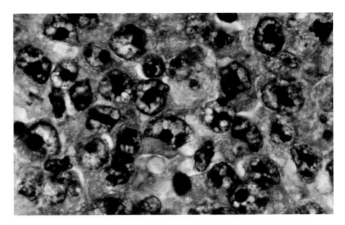

**FIGURE 24.16** Immunoblastic lymphoma large cells with abundant amphophilic cytoplasm and prominent nucleoli.

Size: large
Cytoplasm: abundant, amphophilic
Nuclei: round; chromatin: vesicular
Nucleoli: prominent
Mitosis: high, apoptosis
Pattern: diffuse
Phenotype: mature B (CD45R⁺, sIg⁺) or T cell (CD3⁺)
Molecular: IgH/TCR gene rearrangement
Characteristic: High grade, large noncohesive cells, prominent, eosinophilic central nucleolus

included in the peripheral T-unspecified category of the proposed WHO and NIAID/NCI classification. The lymphoblastic lymphoma (LL) morphologic category in mice comprises three distinct lymphoma groups that can be recognized by immunophenotype: precursor T, precursor B, and mature B. We therefore suggest that the term "lymphoblastic lymphoma" should be used as a morphologic description and not a diagnostic term unless qualified. Whether all T-LLs in mice are precursor T neoplasms, which have an immature TdT⁺ phenotype as in humans, remains to be determined. Lymphomas that originate from the thymus and/or exhibit markers of immature CD4/CD8 double-negative or double-positive cells are clearly precursor T-LLs. In cases where LLs arise in the spleen or lymph nodes without apparent thymic involvement, it is unclear whether these neoplasms represent precursor T or peripheral T cell lymphomas. Since LLs in the WHO classification are considered precursor neoplasms, LLs of sIg⁺ mature B cells in mice need to be better defined, especially since some of these tumors now appear to be homologues of Burkitt's and possibly atypical Burkitt's lymphoma in humans (Pattengale and Taylor 1983). The diagnosis of murine Burkitt's lymphoma and its relation to human disease is supported by morphologic, immunophenotypic, and genetic similarities including deregulated expression of *c-Myc* in certain strains of mice.

# LYMPHOMAS IN GENETICALLY ENGINEERED MICE

Several examples of lymphomas arising in transgenic and gene knockout mice have been reported. A summary of some of these mice and their lymphomas is presented in Table 24.2. Lymphomas in genetically engineered mice appear to be mostly LLs of T, B, or pre-B cell phenotype. Some strains of mice have a high frequency of spontaneous LLs: precursor T-LL in AKR, B-LL in NFS.V⁺ (Fredrickson et al. 1995), and pre–B-LL in SL/KH (Shimada et al. 1993). These neoplasms may originate in the thymus, spleen, or lymph nodes and are high-grade tumors with a propensity to diffusely metastasize, often presenting as leukemias (Fig. 24.17).

Other lymphomas, however, have also been reported in genetically engineered mice. These include a high incidence of splenic MZL in retired breeder *p53*-deficient mice (Ward et al. 1999). MZLs were first described in NZB mice (Yumoto et al. 1980). Fredrickson et al. reported these tumors in NFS.V⁺ mice (1995) and subsequently showed that MZLs were the most common B cell lymphomas in these mice, accounting for 36 percent of hematopoietic neoplasms (1999). MZLs are low-grade lesions that remain confined to the spleen with late

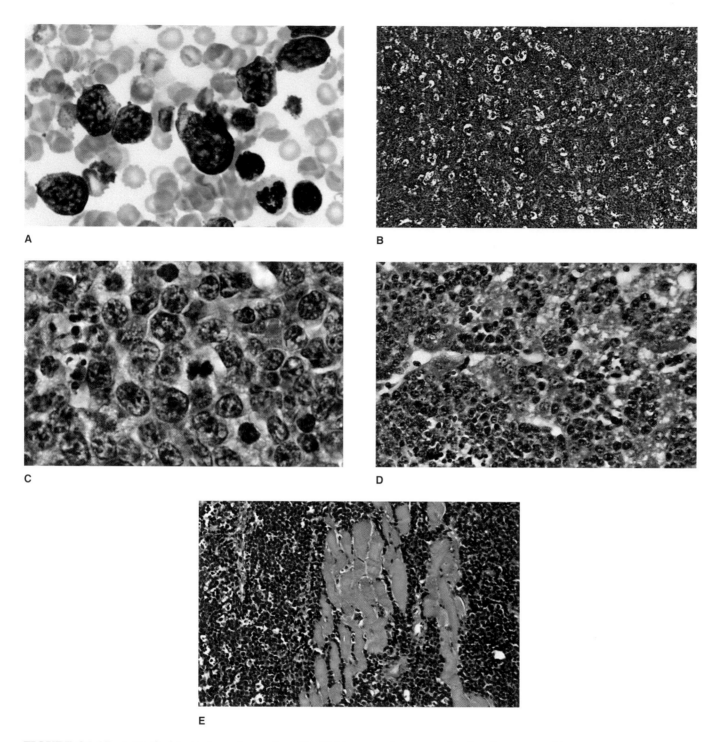

**FIGURE 24.17** Lymphoblastic lymphoma in a *Bcr/Abl* transgenic mouse. Leukemic smear with numerous lymphoblasts (**A**). Spleen with starry sky pattern (**B**). Round, uniform lymphoblasts with prominent nucleoli (**C**). Diffuse infiltration of liver (**D**) and muscle (**E**).

Size: medium/large, uniform
Cytoplasm: scant
Smear: leukemic, lymphoblasts
Nuclei: round; chromatin: fine
Nucleoli: multiple, small/prominent
Mitosis: high
Pattern: diffuse, starry sky

Phenotype: precursor B (CD45R⁺, cIg⁺, sIg), mature B
    (CD45⁺, sIg⁺), or T cell (CD3⁺)
Molecular: IgH/TCR gene rearrangement
Characteristic: High grade, starry sky, sheets of
    hyperchromatic tumor lymphocytes; diffuse
    infiltration, lung, liver, soft tissue

**TABLE 24.1.  Classifications for neoplastic diseases of the lymphoid tissues**

| | Proposed WHO human | Mouse | | |
| --- | --- | --- | --- | --- |
| | | Proposed NIAID/NCI | Frith et al. 1996 | Fredrickson et al. 1995 |
| B cell neoplasms of Precursor cells (preB) | Precursor B cell lymphoblastic leukemia/lymphoma | Precursor B cell lymphoblastic leukemia/lymphoma | Lymphoblastic leukemia/ lymphoma | Lymphoblastic leukemia/ lymphoma |
| Mature B cells | B cell chronic lymphocytic leukemia/small lymphocytic lymphoma | Small lymphocytic leukemia/lymphoma | Small lymphocytic leukemia/ lymphoma | Lymphocytic leukemia/ lymphoma |
| | B cell prolymphocytic leukemia | Not defined | Not defined | Not defined |
| | Lymphoplasmacytic lymphoma | Lymphoplasmacytic lymphoma | Not defined | Not defined |
| | Mantle cell lymphoma | Mantle cell lymphoma | Not defined | Not defined |
| | Follicular lymphoma | Follicular lymphoma | Follicular center cell lymphoma –Mixed cell –Pleiomorphic | Centroblastic-centro- cytic lymphoma Centroblastic, follicular |
| | Marginal zone B cell lymphoma of MALT type | Marginal zone B cell lymphoma, MALT type | Not defined | Not defined |
| | Nodal marginal zone lymphoma ± monocytoid B cells | Not defined | Not defined | Not defined |
| | Splenic marginal zone B cell lymphoma | Splenic marginal zone B cell lymphoma | Not defined | Splenic marginal zone B cell lymphoma |
| | Hairy cell leukemia | Not defined | Not defined | Not defined |
| | Diffuse large B cell lymphoma | Diffuse large B cell lymphoma | Immunoblastic | Immunoblastic, Centroblastic-diffuse, marginal zone |
| | Burkitt's lymphoma | Burkitt's lymphoma | Lymphoblastic | Lymphoblastic |
| | Plasmacytoma | Plasmacytoma | Plasma cell | Plasmacytoma/anaplastic plasmacytoma |
| | Plasma cell myeloma | Not defined | Not defined | Not defined |
| T cell neoplasms of Precursor cells (preT) | Precursor T cell lymphoblastic leukemia/lymphoma | Precursor T cell lymphoblastic leukemia/lymphoma | Lymphoblastic T cell lymphoma | Lymphoblastic T cell lymphoma |
| Mature T cells | T cell prolymphocytic leukemia | Not defined | Not defined | Not defined |
| | T cell large granular lymphocytic leukemia | Not defined | Not defined | Not defined |
| | Mycosis fungoides | Not defined | Not defined | Not defined |
| | Sézary syndrome | Not defined | Not defined | Not defined |
| | Angioimmunoblastic T cell lymphoma | Not defined | Not defined | Not defined |
| | Peripheral T cell lymphoma (unspecified) | Peripheral T cell lymphoma (unspecified) | Not defined | Lymphoblastic T cell lymphoma Immunoblastic T cell lymphoma Lymphocytic T cell lymphoma |
| | Systemic anaplastic large T cell lymphoma | Systemic anaplastic large T cell lymphoma | Not defined | Large anaplastic T cell lymphoma |
| | Primary cutaneous anaplastic large cell lymphoma | Not defined | Not defined | Not defined |
| | Subcutaneous panniculitis-like T cell lymphoma | Not defined | Not defined | Not defined |
| | Enteropathy-type intestinal T cell lymphoma | Not defined | Not defined | Not defined |
| | Hepatosplenic γ/δ T cell lymphoma | Not defined | Not defined | Not defined |
| Hodgkin's lymphoma | Nodular lymphocyte–predominant Hodgkin's lymphoma | Not defined | Not defined | Not defined |
| | Classic Hodgkin's lymphoma | Not defined | Not defined | Not defined |

Note: MALT = mucosa-associated lymphoid tissue.

TABLE 24.2.  **Transgenic and knockout mice with lymphoma/leukemia**

|  | Knockout | | | | Transgenic | |
|---|---|---|---|---|---|---|
| T-lymphoblastic lymphoma | E2A, Atm | p53, Pten | Brca2, MMR | Ku70, Ikaros | Pim-1 | Eμ-Nras |
| B-lymphoblastic lymphoma | Aiolos | Ink4a | p53 | | | |
| Pre-B–lymphoblastic lymphoma | c-Myc, IL-7 | n-Myc | Blk | Bcr/Abl | | |
| Marginal zone lymphoma | p53 | | | | Hox11 | |
| Plasmacytoma | p16 | | | | IL-6 | |
| Burkitt's lymphoma | | | | | Eλ-Myc | |
| Granulocytic leukemia | Icsbp | NF 1 | | | PML-RAR | |
| Erythroleukemia | | | | | Tg.AC | |
| Histiocytic sarcoma | | | | | Eμ-Nras | |

Sources: Adams et al. 1985; Bain et al. 1997; Donehower et al. 1992; Fisher et al. 1995; Friedman et al. 1998; Grisolano et al. 1997; Hough et al. 1998; Li et al. 1998; Malek et al. 1998; Prolla et al. 1998; Serrano et al. 1996; Sheppard et al. 1998; Suzuki et al. 1998; van Lohuizen et al. 1989; Voncken et al. 1992; Wang et al. 1998; Winandy et al. 1995; Xu et al. 1996.

metastasis limited to the abdominal nodes. The growth pattern, initially limited to the perifollicular area, is characterized by an outward expansion of proliferating cells, leading to coalescence of adjacent marginal zones and eventual obliteration of the red pulp (Fig. 24.13). Fredrickson et al. described progression of MZL through distinct grades, including the early, prelymphomatous expansion of the marginal zone to a high-grade lesion marked by cytologic changes, with centroblastlike morphology and increased mitotic activity (1999). Progression of lymphomas from low to high grade had not been previously well established in mice (Frith et al. 1996).

Follicular lymphomas appear to be uncommon in genetically engineered mice but occur frequently in aged mice, usually involving the spleen, mesenteric node, and Peyer's patches (Fig. 24.14; Pattengale 1994). Spontaneous plasmacytomas are rare in mice but can be readily induced in BALB/c or NZB mice by pristane (Anderson and Potter 1969) and have been observed in IL-6 transgenic (Suematsu et al. 1989) and pristane-treated p16 knockout mice (unpublished observations). These neoplasms vary in composition from mature plasma cells to immature plasmablasts and should be differentiated from plasma cell hyperplasia, which is a common finding in cervical lymph nodes of older mice (Fig. 24.15). The pristane-induced plasmacytomas are characterized by chromosomal translocation involving c-Myc (Shen-Ong et al. 1982).

Leukemias and histiocytic sarcomas can involve the spleen and lymph nodes. The nonlymphoid leukemias include, among others, granulocytic and erythroleukemia (Frith et al. 1996). In general, these neoplasms occur only rarely in untreated conventional mice; however, murine models of chronic granulocytic leukemias have been established in Icsbp (Holtschke et al. 1996) and Nf1 knockout mice (Jacks et al. 1994). In the

spleen, neoplastic proliferation of granulocytes occurs in the red pulp and, in cases where the cells appear mature, they must be distinguished from a reactive granulopoiesis (Long et al. 1986). Widespread obliteration of the red pulp with follicular atrophy, leukemic presentation with numerous myeloid cells and their precursors (Fig. 24.18), and multiorgan involvement, particularly periportal infiltration of the liver, aid in distinguishing the neoplastic nature of the proliferation. Granulocytic cells are immunoreactive for lysozyme (Ward and Reynolds 1990).

Erythroleukemias have been reported in Tg.AC transgenic mice (Trempus et al. 1998). This type of neoplasm involves the splenic red pulp and leads to marked splenic enlargement (Fredrickson 1990). The infiltrating erythroblasts obliterate the splenic cords and lead to atrophy of the white pulp. Although erythroleukemias rarely involve lymph nodes, they often infiltrate the sinusoids of the liver, leading to marked hepatomegaly (Fig. 24.19; Fredrickson 1990).

Histiocytic sarcoma is the most common nonlymphoid neoplasm in mice (Frith and Ward 1988). In some cases, it may resemble or occur together with follicular lymphoma in the same tissue, making morphologic distinction difficult (Frith et al. 1999). The histiocytic cells, however, have abundant eosinophilic cytoplasm with elongated nuclei having nuclear grooves or folds, and many cases have characteristic multinucleated giant cells (Fig. 24.20). The tumors express antigens of the mononuclear phagocytic system (Ward and Sheldon 1993) and have been reported in the Eμ-Nras transgenic mice (Harris et al. 1988).

Use of the term "composite lymphoma" in humans denotes the presence of two different morphologic types of non-Hodgkin's lymphoma in the same tissue (Kim et al. 1977). Most of these are composite B cell lymphomas and are thought to represent different phases of clonal evolu-

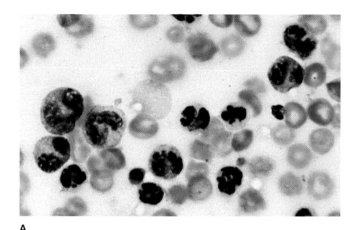

A

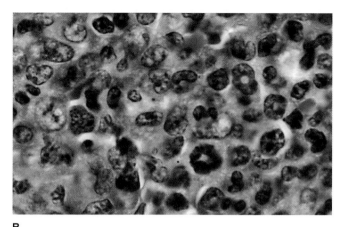

B

C

**FIGURE 24.18**   Myelogenous leukemia. Granulocytic leukemia in a *Icsbp*-/-mouse. Leukemic smear with numerous myeloid cells at different stages of differentiation (**A**). Infiltration of splenic red pulp (**B**) and liver (**C**) by mature and immature granulocytic cells.

Size: small to large
Smear: leukemic, myeloid cells
Cytoplasm: moderate
Nuclei: segmented/round
Nucleoli: prominent in blasts

Mitosis: variable
Pattern: diffuse, red pulp
Phenotype: Gr-1+; cytochemistry: lysozyme
Characteristic: mixed granulocytes and myeloblasts, multiple organ infiltration

tion of the same tumor rather than simultaneous occurrence of unrelated tumors. The histogenesis is unclear for composite lymphomas composed of B and T cells (Kim 1993). Della Porta et al. (1979) first suggested the term "composite lymphoma" in mice to include ill-defined tumors and possible association of different neoplastic elements in the same tumor. Composite lymphomas occur spontaneously in wild-type mice and in genetically engineered mice. They comprise composite B or T cells, are made up of a combination of T and B cells (Fig. 24.21), or may occur in conjunction with nonlymphoid neoplasms. In NFS.V+ mice, most cases of composite lymphomas observed had MZL as one component (Fredrickson and Harris in press). In humans, two different lymphomas can

be seen in different anatomic sites; most are considered to represent histologic conversion from a lower to a higher grade within the same lymphoma (Kim 1993). This also applies to some composite lymphomas in mice, but histogenetically unrelated lymphomas may occur at different anatomic sites. For these, the term "parallel lymphomas" was recommended (Fredrickson and Harris in press). These lymphomas may be useful in understanding lymphoma pathogenesis, and their presence should be noted.

The cytologic and histopathologic characteristics of hematopoietic neoplasms, with special emphasis on distinct morphologic, immunophenotypic features, and correlation with normal cellular counterparts, are outlined in each figure legend.

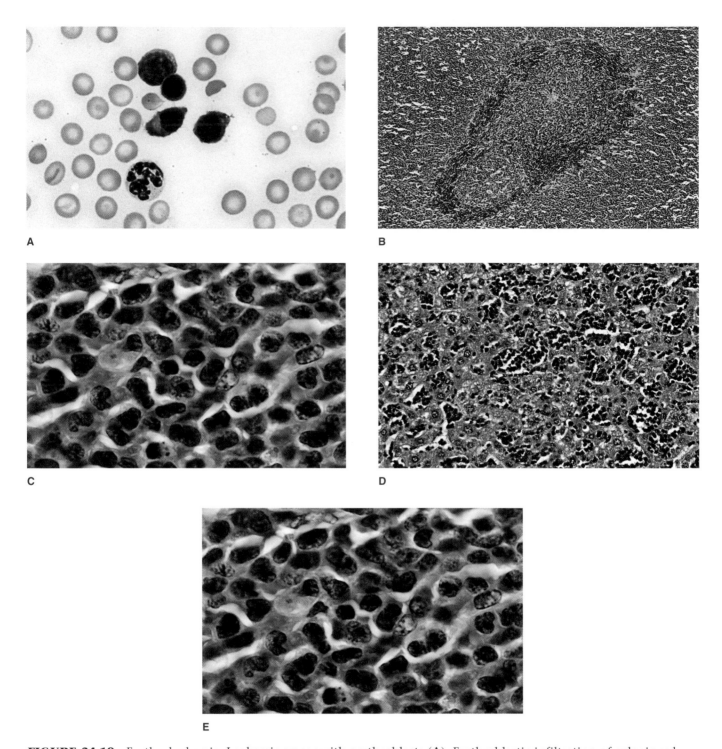

**FIGURE 24.19** Erythroleukemia. Leukemic smear with erythroblasts (**A**). Erythroblastic infiltration of splenic red pulp with follicular atrophy (**B** and **C**) and diffuse infiltration of liver (**D**) showing numerous erythroblasts within the sinusoids (**E**).

Size: medium
Smear: leukemic, erythroblast
Cytoplasm: dense basophilic
Nuclei: round, dark basophilic; chromatin: coarsely
  clumped

Nucleoli: prominent in blasts
Mitosis: low
Pattern: diffuse, red pulp
Characteristic: liver: sinusoidal infiltration, marked
  hepatomegaly

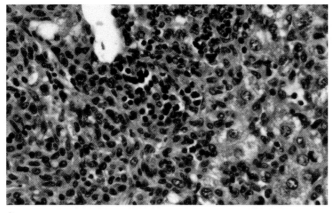

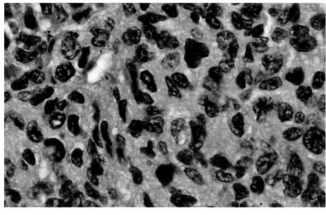

**FIGURE 24.20** Histiocytic sarcoma. Periportal infiltration of liver (**A**) and spleen (**B**) by histiocytes with spindle-shaped nuclei and numerous giant cells.

Size: medium/large, monomorphic
Cytoplasm: abundant, eosinophilic
Nuclei: spindle-shaped/grooved/round
Nucleoli: variable
Mitosis: variable
Pattern: diffuse/nodular
Phenotype: CD11b+ (Mac-1), Mac-2, lysozyme
Characteristic: spindle-shaped or grooved nuclei, giant cells

# REFERENCES

Adams, J.M., Harris, A.W., Pinkert, C.A., et al. 1985. The c-myc oncogene driven by immunoglobulin enhancers induces lymphoid malignancy in transgenic mice. Nature 318:533–538.

Anderson, P.N. and Potter, M. 1969. Induction of plasma cell tumors in BALB/c mice with 2,6,10,14-tetramethylpentadecane (pristane). Nature 222:994–995.

Bain, G., Engel, I., Maandag, E.C.R., et al. 1997. E2A deficiency leads to abnormalities in αβ T-cell development

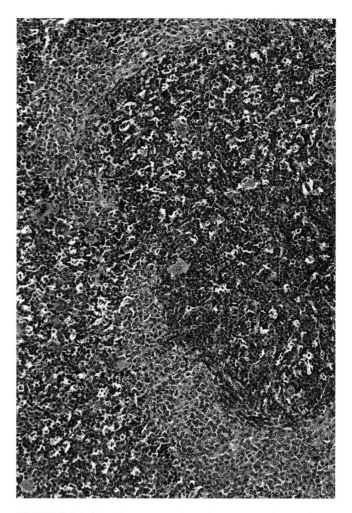

**FIGURE 24.21** Composite lymphoma in spleen of p53$^{-/-}$ mouse composed of lymphoblastic lymphoma ("starry sky" pattern on right side and lower left side of figure) and marginal zone lymphoma (pale wide marginal zone).

and to rapid development of T-cell lymphomas. Mol. Cell. Biol. 17:4782–4791.

Davidson, W.F., Fredrickson, T.N., Rudikoff, E.K., et al. 1984. A unique series of lymphomas related to the Ly-1+ lineage of B lymphocyte differentiation. J. Immunol. 133:744–753.

Della Porta, G., Chieco-Biachi, L., and Pennselli, N. 1979. Tumors of the hematopoietic system. In Pathology of Tumors in Laboratory Animals, vol. II—Tumors of the mouse, ed. V.S. Tursov, pp. 527–576. Lyon: International Agency for Research on Cancer.

Donehower, L.A., Harvey, M., Slagle, B.L., et al. 1992. Mice deficient for p53 are developmentally normal but susceptible to spontaneous tumors. Nature 356:215–221.

Dunn, T.B. 1954. Normal and pathologic anatomy of reticular tissue in laboratory mice. Natl. Cancer Inst. Monogr. 14:1281–1433.

Enno, A., O'Rourke, J.L., Howlett, C.R., et al. 1995. MAL-Toma-like lesions in the murine gastric mucosa after long-term infection with *Helicobacter felis*. A mouse model of *Helicobacter pylori*-induced gastric lymphoma. Am. J. Pathol. 147:217–222.

Erickson, R.P. 1996. Mouse models of human genetic disease: which mouse is more like a man? Bioessays 18:993–998.

Fisher, A.G., Burdet, C., Bunce, C., et al. 1995. Lymphoproliferative disorders in IL-7 transgenic mice: expansion of immature B cells which retain macrophage potential. Int. Immunol. 7:415–423.

Fredrickson, T.N. 1990. Erythroleukemia, Mouse. In Hematopoietic System. Monographs on Pathology of Laboratory Animals, ed. T.C. Jones et al., pp. 205–211. Berlin: Springer-Verlag.

Fredrickson, T.N. and Harris, A.W. In press. Atlas of mouse hematology.

Fredrickson, T.N., Morse, H.C. III., Yetter, R.A., et al. 1985. Multiparameter analyses of spontaneous non-thymic lymphomas occurring in NFS/N mice congenic for ecotropic murine leukemia viruses. Am. J. Pathol. 121:349–360.

Fredrickson, T.N., Hartley, J.W., and Morse, H.C. III. 1993. Early divergence of erythroid lineage suggested by gene rearrangements in mouse hematopoietic neoplasms. Exp. Hematol. 21:354–357.

Fredrickson, T.N., Hartley, J.W., Morse, H.C. III., et al. 1995. Classification of mouse lymphomas. Curr. Top. Microbiol. Immunol. 194:109–116.

Fredrickson, T.N., Lennert, K., Chattopadhyay, S.K., et al. 1999. Splenic marginal zone lymphomas of mice. Am. J. Pathol. 154:805–812.

Friedman, L.S., Thistlethwaite, F.C., Patel, K.J., et al. 1998. Thymic lymphomas in mice with a truncating mutation in Brca2. Cancer Res. 58:1338–1343.

Frith, C.H. and Ward, J.M. 1988. Color Atlas of Neoplastic and Non-neoplastic Lesions in Aging Mice. Amsterdam: Elsevier, pp. 77–86.

Frith, C.H., Ward, J.M., Fredrickson, T.N., et al. 1996. Neoplastic lesions of the hematopoietic system. In Pathobiology of the Aging Mouse, eds. U. Mohr et al., pp. 219–235. Washington, DC: ILSI.

Frith, C.H., Ward, J.M., Harleman, J.H., et al. 1999. Proliferative and nonproliferative lesions of the hematopoietic system in mice. In Guides for Toxicologic Pathology. Washington, DC: STP/ARP.

Grisolano, J.L., Wesselschmidt, R.L., Pelicci, P.G., et al. 1997. Altered myeloid development and acute leukemia in transgenic mice expressing PML-RARα under control of cathepoin G regulatory sequences. Blood 89:376–387.

Hardy, R.R., Carmack, C.E., Li, Y.S., et al. 1994. Distinctive developmental origins and specificities of murine CD5⁺ B cells. Immunol. Rev. 137:91–118.

Harris, A.W., Langdon, W.Y., Alexander, W.S., et al. 1988. Transgenic mouse models for hematopoietic tumorigenesis. Curr. Top. Microbiol. Immunol. 141:82–93.

Harris, N.L., Jaffe, E.S., Stein, H., et al. 1994. A revised European-American classification of lymphoid neoplasms: a proposal from the International Lymphoma Study-Group. Blood 84:1361–1392.

Holtschke, T., Lohler, J., Kanno, Y., et al. 1996. Immunodeficiency and chronic myelogenous leukemia-like syndrome in mice with a targeted mutation of the ICSBP gene. Cell 87:307–317.

Hough, M.R., Reis, M.D., Singaraja, R., et al. 1998. A model for spontaneous B-lineage lymphomas in IgH mu-HOX11 transgenic mice. Proc. Natl. Acad. Sci. USA 95:13853–13858.

Jacks, T., Shih, T.S., Schmitt, E.M., et al. 1994. Tumour predisposition in mice heterozygous for a targeted mutation in Nf1. Nat. Genet. 7:353–361.

Jaffe, E.S., Harris, N.L., Diebold, J., et al. 1999. World Health Organization classification of neoplastic diseases of the hematopoietic and lymphoid tissues. A progress report. Am. J. Clin. Pathol. 111:S8–S12.

Kim, H. 1993. Composite lymphoma and related disorders. Am. J. Clin. Pathol. 99:445–451.

Kim, H., Hendrickson, R., and Dorfman, R.F. 1977. Composite lymphoma. Cancer 40:959–976.

Lennert, K. and Feller, A.C. 1992. Histopathology of Non-Hodgkin's Lymphomas (Based on the Updated Kiel Classification). Berlin: Springer-Verlag.

Li, G.C., Ouyang, H., Li, X., et al. 1998. Ku70: a candidate tumor suppressor gene for murine T-cell lymphoma. Mol. Cell. 2:1–8.

Liyanage, M., Coleman, A., duManoir, S., et al. 1996. Multicolour spectral karyotyping of mouse chromosomes. Nat. Genet. 14:312–315.

Long, R.E., Knutsen, G., and Robinson, M. 1986. Myeloid hyperplasia in the SENCAR mouse: differentiation from granulocytic leukemia. Environ. Health Perspect. 68:117–123.

Lukes, R.J. and Collins, R.D. 1992. Tumors of the hematopoietic system. In Atlas of Tumor Pathology. Bethesda, MD: Universities Associated for Research and Education in Pathology, p. 409.

Malek, S.N., Dordai, D.I., Reim, J., et al. 1998. Malignant transformation of early lymphoid progenitors in mice expressing an activated Blk tyrosine kinase. Proc. Natl. Acad. Sci. USA 95:7351–7356.

Pals, S.T., Zijlstra, M., Radaszkiewicz, T., et al. 1986. Immunologic induction of malignant lymphoma: graft versus host reaction-induced B cell lymphomas contain integration of predominantly ecotropic murine leukemia proviruses. J. Immunol. 136:331–339.

Pattengale, P.K. 1994. Tumors of the lymphohematopoietic system. In Pathology of Tumors in Laboratory Animals, vol. II, Tumors of the Mouse, 2nd ed., eds. V. Tursov and U. Mohr, pp. 651–670. Lyon: International Agency for Research on Cancer.

Pattengale, P.K. and Taylor, C.R. 1983. Experimental models of lymphoproliferative disease. The mouse as a model for human non-Hodgkin's lymphomas and related leukemias. Am. J. Pathol. 113:237–265.

Prolla, T.A., Baker, S.M., Harris, A.C., et al. 1998. Tumour susceptibility and spontaneous mutation in mice deficient in Mlh1, Pms1 and Pms2 DNA mismatch repair. Nat. Genet. 18:276–279.

Serrano, M., Lee, H.W., Chin, L., et al. 1996. Role of the INK4a locus in tumor suppression and cell mortality. Cell 85:27–37.

Shen-Ong, G.L., Keath, E.J., Piccoli, S.P., et al. 1982. Novel myc oncogene RNA from abortive immunoglobulin-gene recombination in mouse plasmacytomas. Cell 31:443–452.

Sheppard, R.D., Samant, S.A., Rosenberg, M., et al. 1998. Transgenic N-myc mouse model for indolent B-cell lymphoma: tumor characterization and analysis of genetic alterations in spontaneous and retrovirally accelerated tumors. Oncogene 17:2073–2085.

Shimada, M.O., Yamada, Y., Nakakuki, Y., et al. 1993. SI/KH strain of mice: a model of spontaneous pre-B-lymphomas. Leuk. Res. 17:573–578.

Suematsu, S., Matusda, T., Aozasa, K., et al. 1989. IgG1 plasmacytosis in interleukin 6 transgenic mice. Proc. Natl. Acad. Sci. USA 86:7547–7551.

Suzuki, A., de la Pompa, J.L., Stambolic, V., et al. 1998. High cancer susceptibility and embryonic lethality associated with mutation of the PTEN tumor suppressor gene in mice. Curr. Biol. 8:1169–1178.

Trempus, C.S., Ward, S., Farris, G., et al. 1998. Association of v-Ha-ras transgene expression with development of erythroleukemia in Tg.AC transgenic mice. Am. J. Pathol. 153:247–254.

van Lohuizen, M., Verbeek, S., Krimpenfort, P., et al. 1989. Predisposition to lymphomagenesis in pim-1 transgenic mice: cooperation with c-myc and n-myc in murine leukemia-virus induced-tumors. Cell 56:673–682.

Voncken, J.W., Griffiths, S., Greaves, M.F., et al. 1992. Restricted oncogenicity of BCR/ABL p190 in transgenic mice. Cancer Res. 52:4534–4539.

Wang, J.H., Avitahl, N., Cariappa, A. et al. 1998. Aiolos regulates B cell activation and maturation to effector state. Immunity 9:543–553.

Ward, J.M. 1990a. Early follicular center cell lymphoma, mouse. In Hematopoietic System. Monographs on Pathology of Laboratory Animals, eds. T.C. Jones et al., pp. 212–216. Berlin: Springer-Verlag.

Ward, J.M. 1990b. Classification of reactive lesions of lymph nodes. In Hematopoietic System. Monographs on Pathology of Laboratory Animals, eds. T.C. Jones et al., pp. 155–161. Berlin: Springer-Verlag.

Ward, J.M. and Rehm, S. 1990. Applications of immunohistochemistry in rodent tumor pathology. Exp. Pathol. 40:301–312.

Ward, J.M. and Reynolds, C.W. 1990. Sources of antibodies and immunological reagents used for immunocytochemistry. In Hematopoietic System. Monographs on Pathology of Laboratory Animals, eds. T.C. Jones et al., pp. 126–128. Berlin: Springer-Verlag.

Ward, J.M. and Sheldon, W. 1993. Expression of mononuclear phagocyte antigens in histiocytic sarcoma of mice. Vet. Pathol. 30:560–565.

Ward, J.M., Taddesse-Heath, L., Perkins, S.N., et al. III. 1999. Splenic marginal zone B-cell and thymic T-cell lymphomas in p53-deficient mice. Lab. Invest. 79:3–14.

Winandy, S., Wu, P., and Georgopoulos, K. 1995. A dominant mutation in the Ikaros gene leads to rapid development of leukemia and lymphoma. Cell 83:289–299.

Xu, Y., Ashley, T., Brainerd, E.E., et al. 1996. Targeted disruption of ATM leads to growth retardation, chromosomal fragmentation during meiosis, immune defects and thymic lymphoma. Genes Dev. 10:2411–2422.

Yumoto, T., Yoshida, Y., Yoshida, H., et al. 1980. Prelymphomatous and lymphomatous changes in splenomegaly of New Zealand Black mice. Acta. Pathol. Jap. 30:171–186.

# General References

## MOUSE INFORMATION WEB SITES

Trans-NIH Mouse Initiative
http://www.nih.gov/science/mouse/

The Jackson Laboratory Mouse Genome Informatics
http://www.informatics.jax.org/

TBASE
http://tbase.jax.org/

NetVet Rodents
http://netvet.wustl.edu/rodents.htm

NCI Veterinary Pathology
http://www.ncifcrf.gov/vetpath/

BioMedNet (Knockout mouse database)
http://www.biomednet.com/

The Whole Mouse Catalog
http://www.rodentia.com/wmc/

The Virtual Mouse Necropsy
www.ncifcrf.gov/vetpath/necropsy.html

## GENERAL MOUSE PATHOLOGY AND BIOLOGY REFERENCES

Faccini, J.M., Abbott, D.P., and Paulus, G.J.J. 1990. Mouse Histopathology: A Glossary for Use in Toxicity and Carcinogenicity Studies. Amsterdam: Elsevier.

Feldman, D.B. and Seely, J.C. 1988. Necropsy of Rodents and the Rabbit. Boca Raton, FL: CRC Press.

Frith, C.H. and Ward, J.M. 1988. Color Atlas of Neoplastic and Non-neoplastic Lesions in Aging Mice. Amsterdam: Elsevier, 109 pp.

Green, E.L. (ed.). 1966. Biology of the Laboratory Mouse. New York: Dover, 706 pp.

Jones, T.C. (ed.). 1983–98. Monographs on Pathology of Laboratory Animals. Series Volumes. Washington, DC: ILSI Press and Springer Verlag. http://www.ilsi.org/animal.html.

Lyon, M.F., Rastan S., and Brown, S.D.M., 1996. Genetic Variants and Strains of the Laboratory Mouse. Third edition, volumes 1 and 2. Oxford: Oxford University Press.

Maronpot, R.R. (ed.). 1999. Pathology of the Mouse: Reference and Atlas. Vienna, IL: Cache River Press, 699 pp.

Mohr, U., Dungworth, D.L., Ward, J.M., et al. (eds.). 1996. Pathobiology of the Aging Mouse. Volumes 1 and 2. Washington, DC: ILSI Press. http://www.ilsi.org/animal.html

Percy, D.H. and Barthold, S.W. 1993. Pathology of Laboratory Rodents and Rabbits. Ames: Iowa State University Press.

Rugh, R. 1968. The Mouse: Its Reproduction and Development. Minneapolis, MN: Burgess.

Silver, L.M. 1995. Mouse Genetics. New York: Oxford, 362 pp.

Sundberg, J.P. and Boggess, B. (eds.). 1999. Systematic Approach to Evaluation of Mouse Mutations. Boca Raton, FL: CRC Press, 199 pp.

Turusov, V. and Mohr, U. (eds.). 1994. Pathology of Tumours in Laboratory Animals. Volume 2, Tumours of the Mouse. Lyon: IARC Scientific Publications.

# Index

ISBN 0-8138-2521-0